Essential Endodontology
Prevention and Treatment of Apical Periodontitis

牙髓病学基础
根尖周炎的预防和治疗

原著第 3 版

主　编　[挪] 达格·奥斯塔维克（Dag Ørstavik）
主　审　余　擎
主　译　程小刚　王可境
副主译　肖　敏　张芯华　王志华

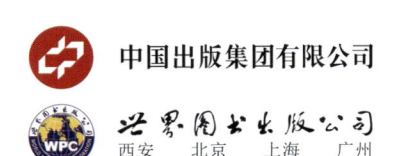

中国出版集团有限公司

世界图书出版公司
西安　北京　上海　广州

图书在版编目（CIP）数据

牙髓病学基础：根尖周炎的预防和治疗：原著第3版 /（挪）达格·奥斯塔维克（Dag Ørstavik）主编；程小刚，王可境主译 . -- 西安：世界图书出版西安有限公司，2025.5. -- ISBN 978-7-5232-2078-8

Ⅰ . R781.3

中国国家版本馆 CIP 数据核字第 20255ME292 号

Essential Endodontology: Prevention and Treatment of Apical Periodontitis by Dag Ørstavik
ISBN: 9781119271956
This edition first published 2020
© 2020 John Wiley & Sons Ltd
Edition History
Blackwell Munksgaard Ltd (2e, 2008), Blackwell Science Ltd (1e 1998)
All Rights Reserved. Authorised translation from the English language edition published by John Wiley & Sons Limited. Responsibility for the accuracy of the translation rests solely with World Publishing Xi'an Corporation Limited and is not the responsibility of John Wiley & Sons Limited. No part of this book may be reproduced in any form without the written permission of the original copyright holder, John Wiley & Sons Limited.

本书简体中文版专有翻译出版权由 John Wiley & Sons Limited. 公司授予世界图书出版西安有限公司。翻译的准确性由世界图书出版西安有限公司负责，John Wiley & Sons Limited 对此不负责。未经许可，不得以任何手段和形式复制或抄袭本书内容。

书　　名	牙髓病学基础：根尖周炎的预防和治疗（原著第3版） YASUIBINGXUE JICHU: GENJIANZHOUYAN DE YUFANG HE ZHILIAO
主　　编	[挪] 达格·奥斯塔维克（Dag Ørstavik）
主　　译	程小刚　王可境
责任编辑	马元怡　杨菲
装帧设计	新纪元文化传播
出版发行	世界图书出版西安有限公司
地　　址	西安市雁塔区曲江新区汇新路 355 号
邮　　编	710061
电　　话	029-87214941　029-87233647（市场营销部） 029-87234767（总编室）
网　　址	http://www.wpcxa.com
邮　　箱	xast@wpcxa.com
经　　销	新华书店
印　　刷	西安市久盛印务有限责任公司
开　　本	889mm×1194mm　1/16
印　　张	18.25
字　　数	530 千字
版次印次	2025 年 5 月第 1 版　2025 年 5 月第 1 次印刷
版权登记	25-2025-061
国际书号	ISBN 978-7-5232-2078-8
定　　价	278.00 元

医学投稿　xastyx@163.com　‖　029-87279745　029-87285296

☆如有印装错误，请寄回本公司更换☆

译者名单

主　审　余　擎

主　译　程小刚　王可境

副主译　肖　敏　张芯华　王志华

译　者（按姓氏笔画排序）

王可境　王志华　王罗千慧　白　玉　白庆霞
李　桐　李菲菲　肖　敏　吴昊泽　余　擎
况金鑫　张　劢　张　晓　张芯华　林欣芳
徐　宁　梅笑寒　程　庚　程小刚

郑重声明

本书的内容旨在促进科学研究，并不为特定患者推荐或推广特定的诊断、治疗方法。出版商、作者、译者没有就本书内容的精确性和完整性做任何保证，并且明确否认任何负责任的保证，例如针对特定的健康和疗效的保证。针对正在进行的研究、设备升级、仪器更新换代、政府法规的变化、设备和用药等信息的不断完善，有读者要求审查和评估其包含的详尽信息，例如每种药物、设备和装置的各种信息，并希望对部分问题提供详细的指示、警告和预防措施，对于这种情况读者应适当咨询专家。任何组织或网站在本书中被引用时，并不意味着作者或出版商认可该组织或网站提供或建议的任何信息。读者还应意识到，本书所列的互联网网站在著书和阅读时可能发生变化甚至消失，本作品的任何推广声明，不为其提供任何担保。无论是出版商还是作者，都不对由此产生的任何损害负责。

原著主编

Dag Ørstavik cand. odont. & dr. odont.

Professor Emeritus
Department of Endodontics
Institute of Clinical Dentistry
University of Oslo
Oslo, Norway

原著作者

Lars Bjørndal, DDS, PhD
Associate Professor
Department of Odontology – School of Dentistry
University of Copenhagen
Copenhagen, Denmark

Conor Durack BDS NUI, MFDS RCSI, MClinDent (Endo), MEndo RCS Edin.
Specialist Endodontist and Practice Partner
Riverpoint Specialist Dental Clinic
Limerick, Ireland

Ashraf F. Fouad, DDS, MS
Freedland Distinguished Professor and Chair of Endodontics
Adams School of Dentistry, University of North Carolina
Chapel Hill, NC, USA

Kerstin M. Galler, Prof. Dr. med. dent., Ph.D.
Associate Professor
Department of Conservative Dentistry and Periodontology
University Hospital Regensburg
Regensburg, Germany

Bekir Karabucak, DMD, MS
Associate Professor and Chair
Department of Endodontics
Penn Dental Medicine
The Robert Schattner Center
University of Pennsylvania
School of Dental Medicine
Philadelphia, PA, USA

Asma A. Khan, BDS, PhD
Associate Professor
Department of Endodontics
Dental School
UT Health San Antonio
San Antonio, TX, USA

Lise-Lotte Kirkevang cand. odont., ph. d., dr. odont.
Associate Professor
Department of Dentistry and Oral Health
Aarhus University
Aarhus, Denmark

Dag Ørstavik cand. odont. & dr. odont.
Professor Emeritus
Department of Endodontics
Institute of Clinical Dentistry
University of Oslo
Oslo, Norway

Susanna Paju, DDS, PhD, Dipl. Perio.
Specialist in Periodontology
Adjunct Professor
Department of Oral and Maxillofacial Diseases
Clinicum, Faculty of Medicine
University of Helsinki
Helsinki, Finland

Shanon Patel, BDS, MSc, MClinDent, MRD, FDS, FHEA, PhD
Consultant/Senior Lecturer
Postgraduate Endodontic Unit
King's College London Dental Institute
London, UK

Isabela N. Rôças, DDS, MSc, PhD
Professor
Department of Endodontics
School of Dentistry
Iguaçu University
Nova Iguaçu, RJ, Brazil

Frank C. Setzer, DMD, PhD, MS
Assistant Professor
Department of Endodontics
School of Dental Medicine
University of Pennsylvania
Philadelphia, PA, USA

José F. Siqueira Jr, DDS, MSc, PhD
Professor
Department of Endodontics
School of Dentistry
Iguaçu University
Nova Iguaçu, RJ, Brazil

Asgeir Sigurdsson
Presley Elmer Ellsworth Professor and Chair
Endodontics
New York University College of Dentistry,
New York City, NY, USA

Leo Tjäderhane, DDS, PhD; Spec. Cariology and Endodontology
Professor, Chief Endodontist
Department of Oral and Maxillofacial Diseases
Faculty of Medicine; Helsinki University Hospital HUS
University of Helsinki
Helsinki, Finland

Michael Vaeth
Faculty Member, Public Health
Aarhus University
Aarhus, Denmark

John Whitworth
Professor of Endodontology
School of Dental Sciences, Newcastle University
Newcastle upon Tyne, UK

序

根尖周炎是发生于根尖周组织的炎症性疾病，是临床中最常见的口腔疾病之一，其病因及病理机制较为复杂，目前尚未形成成熟完整的理论。此外，致病因素、患牙解剖因素的复杂性为根尖周炎的临床诊疗带来了较大的困难。近年来，随着理论、技术、材料、器械的不断发展，根尖周炎的研究取得了丰硕的成果。

《牙髓病学基础：根尖周炎的预防和治疗》第 3 版由 Dag Ørstavik 教授主编，该系列专著被牙髓病学业内人士称作关于根尖周炎的"科学论文"。本书以科学研究为基础，将根尖周炎的解剖学、组织学、微生物学、流行病学相关知识与诊断治疗实践相结合，侧重于牙髓病学的生物学和临床特征，探索了牙髓病学的科学基础，对现有的临床和实验室证据进行了系统分析，使这一复杂的问题更容易理解，以帮助医生预防、诊断和治疗该病。本书配有大量全彩插图，使复杂概念实现可视化，有助于读者更直观地理解。每个章节都包含明确的学习目标，使学生和牙髓病学从业者能够明确重点，从而获得良好的阅读学习效果。在第 3 版中引入的全新内容——牙髓再生，这部分内容系统介绍了该领域的研究进展和新兴的治疗方法，扩展了书籍内容的广度。

我在牙体牙髓领域深耕多年，深知知识的传承与交流对于学科发展的重要意义。很荣幸我能作为本书的主审并全程参与翻译工作。本书的翻译工作由空军军医大学第三附属医院牙体牙髓病科的优秀团队承担。他们凭借扎实的专业功底和对学术的敬畏之心，反复研讨专业术语，逐句斟酌语句表达，力求译文既要确保专业内容的准确传达，又要符合中文读者的阅读习惯。此次翻译工作的每一个环节都凝聚着团队的心血，在此，衷心感谢他们的辛勤付出。

我们希望本书能够为根尖周炎的诊断、预防和治疗提供宝贵的理论支持，成为牙髓病学学生和专业人士不可或缺的学习资料。同时，我们也深知，尽管团队全力以赴，但由于时间有限和语言差异，书中或许仍存在不足之处，敬请广大专家、同行批评指正。

2025 年 4 月

前 言

有两种感染会影响牙齿的生存：牙龈/牙周的感染和牙髓/根尖周组织的感染。这两种疾病引起的疼痛和功能丧失也可能严重损害感染者的生活质量。牙髓和根尖周组织的感染属于牙髓病学的范畴。虽然其他条件和疾病构成了这个学科的重要组成部分，但目前根管充填或根尖外科手术仍是牙髓炎或根尖周炎最重要的治疗手段。

《牙髓病学基础：根尖周炎的预防和治疗》尝试将根尖周炎的基础、生物学和微生物学知识与诊断治疗实践相结合。本书侧重于牙髓病学中最重要疾病的生物学和临床特征，以促进医生不断改进该病的预防、诊断和治疗。

有人可能会问是否还需要编写这类图书。任何学生或从业者都可以在社交媒体上或从公共数据库中直接获得最先进、最新颖的技术和方法。然而，有人可能会说，如今对更先进的纸质图书的需求甚至比以前更大。图1中显示了近年来与牙髓病学相关的出版物数量激增。在2008年第2版之前的10年间，新的牙髓病学出版物的数量比10年前增加了38%；而在接下来的10年里，增幅为125%，共计14 685篇。

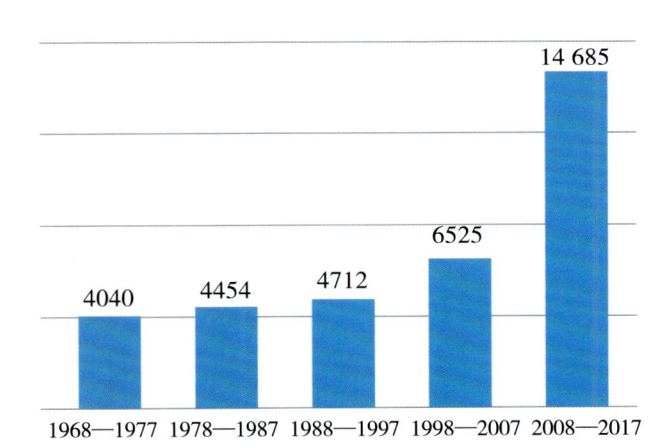

图1 在PubMed中搜索到的有关牙髓病学出版物的数量

显然，现有的该学科的科学贡献总量远远超过了任何研究人员、科学家或临床医生能够阅读或吸收的内容。对于该领域的新手来说，也难以在一个信息质量参差不齐的领域探索。因此，作为进一步研究的起点，由各领域专家提供的精炼的知识基础是必不可少的，它提供了知识和见解的骨架。本书的目标读者仍然是研究生、教师，以及专注于牙髓病学的研究人员。本书也可作为牙髓病学本科生的补充读物。

2008年，本书第2版出版不满1年，前两版的共同编辑Thomas R. Pitt Ford就去世了。他对前两版的贡献是完成这两版书的必要条件，在编写第 3 版时，我们非常怀念他的专业能力和素养。我希望读者会发现前两版的精神在本版中得到了体现，并认识到对质量和深度的关注是 Thomas R. Pitt Ford 的特点。

Dag Ørstavik

目 录

第1章	根尖周炎微生物感染和宿主的反应	1
第2章	牙髓-牙本质复合体与牙周组织的解剖生理学	8
第3章	牙髓病与根尖周病的病因及发病机制	45
第4章	根尖周炎的微生物学	69
第5章	根尖周炎的流行病学、疗效和风险因素	106
第6章	根尖周炎的影像学检查	133
第7章	临床表现和诊断	156
第8章	牙髓修复和再生的生物学基础	174
第9章	牙髓-牙本质复合体暴露的预防和治疗	185
第10章	牙髓摘除术	201
第11章	根尖周炎的根管治疗	228
第12章	根管外科	250

第 1 章 根尖周炎微生物感染和宿主的反应

Dag Ørstavik

1.1 概述

牙髓病学包括牙髓及根尖周的生物学和病理学。牙髓病学作为一门临床学科，主要涉及根管治疗和根管充填，以及牙髓外科手术治疗。与治疗相关的技术过程主要集中在根管系统的无菌和消毒的问题上。保存活髓是牙体牙髓科的共同责任，其中包括牙科创伤学的特定治疗技术。最近的研究表明，无菌和消毒对于治疗因龋病或创伤而意外露髓的患牙十分重要，其将经典的根管治疗原则扩展到深龋的治疗（详见第9章）。

对于需要部分或全部切除牙髓的活髓牙，初始诊断和治疗难点可能与牙髓的状态相关，但治疗的目的不再是保存牙髓，而是预防和消除根管系统中的感染。这个治疗的最终生物学目的是预防根尖周炎的发生。对于有感染或坏死牙髓或者确有根尖疾病的患牙，治疗的生物学目标是治愈根尖周炎。因此，在牙髓疾病中，根尖周炎是比较重要的，因为它是根管治疗的主要指征，也是迄今为止根管治疗不完善或失败时最常见的后遗症（图1.1）。保护牙髓活力所采取的措施，也是从根本上预防根管感染和根尖周炎发生。

微生物在根尖周炎的发生、发展和持续存在中的作用已经被充分证明（详见第4章）。本书重点聚焦根尖周炎感染的病因学以及治疗中应用的杀菌方法和无菌原则。此外，新的研究结果对牙髓病学的诊断、治疗、预后和预后评估等方面都有影响。因此，对医生而言，利用所获得的知识有逻辑地建立治疗原则，并将其应用于临床实践是十分重要的。

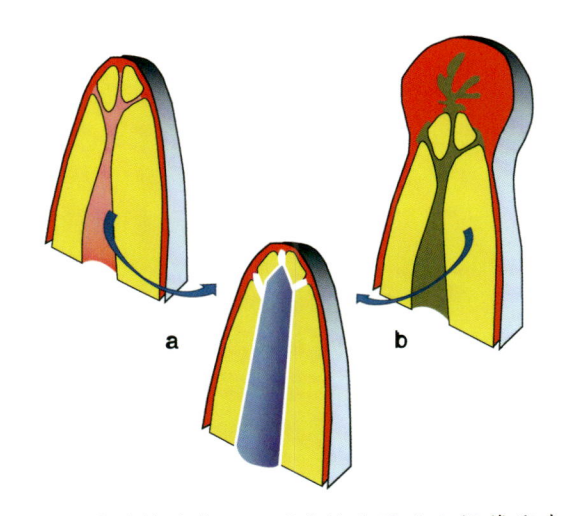

图 1.1 牙髓摘除术。a. 预防根尖周炎和根管消毒。b. 治疗根尖周炎。两者都需要根管的严密充填

1.2 术语

牙髓和牙髓－牙周病都受到许多可变术语的分类系统的影响。由牙髓系统感染引起的牙周炎被称为根尖周炎（apical periodontitis）、根尖周肉芽肿/囊肿、根尖周骨炎（periapical osteitis）和根尖周炎（periradicular periodontitis）。亚分类为急性/慢性、加重/由慢性根尖周肉芽肿发展而来的急性根尖周脓肿，有症状/无症状等[18]。两种最被认可的分类方案见表1.1。这两个方案非常相似，但对国际疾病分类标准（ICD）分类中有急性根尖周炎的牙齿而言，根据美国牙体牙髓学会（AAE）

表 1.1　根尖周炎的分类 [18]

AAE	ICD-10
有症状的根尖周炎（SAP）[1]	K04.4 牙髓源性急性根尖周炎 [2]
无症状的根尖周炎（AAP）	K04.5 慢性根尖周炎
慢性根尖周脓肿	K04.6 有窦道的根尖周脓肿 [3]
急性根尖周脓肿	K04.7 无窦道的根尖周脓肿
致密性骨炎 [4]	
根尖周囊肿	K04.8 根尖周囊肿

1. 表现出广泛的症状
2. 表现为强烈的疼痛
3. 根据表面窦道的位置进一步细分
4. 可能被视为 AAP 或慢性根尖周炎的一种变体

分类有症状的牙齿可能包括更多的病例。ICD 是指有主观需要立即治疗的病例，而有症状的牙齿可能包括仅对患者有轻微影响的患牙和通过椅旁测试诊断的患牙（详见第 7 章）。术语"慢性"一词对于预后和随访研究很有用：无论是否有症状，它都意味着影像学低密度透射影像病变的存在，而这种低密度影像是否存在是预测治疗能否成功的主要因素 [24]。术语"有症状的"是有客观体征证实的诊断。

根尖周炎包括根尖周脓肿、肉芽肿和囊肿，为同一基本疾病的不同表现。毒性和感染程度与身体反应之间的平衡，决定了该疾病是有症状/急性，还是无症状/慢性。曾经强调的囊肿与肉芽肿的鉴别诊断的观念已被舍弃。原因如下：①不管是 X 线片，还是 CBCT，在鉴别囊肿和肉芽肿方面均不敏感 [6]；②它们具有相同的病因和基本的疾病进程（详见第 3、第 4 章）；②两者治疗和预后也很相似（详见第 11、第 12 章）。然而，从根管感染中分离出来的所谓真性囊肿可能显示愈合不良 [27]，需要手术切除，但如果不对摘除物进行仔细的组织学活检，就没有办法诊断这类病例 [32]。

术语不应成为作者或临床医生的限制。因此，在本书和其他文献中，术语的变化和对其他诊断方案的描述是不可避免的，甚至是可取的。但是，鉴于保险公司和其他第三方报销的代码或条款规定，法律规定要求将明确的基本诊断作为治疗的

基础，因此选择和使用公认的分类方案是必须的。

1.3　牙髓感染及根尖周炎症

口腔是皮肤/黏膜屏障向外部环境的延伸。在消化道中，口腔可能被视为机体维持体内平衡并防止体内脆弱部位感染的第一战场。当致病性或机会性微生物浸润或穿透身体表面时，就会发生感染。对于口腔/牙齿，其表面或是黏膜，或是牙釉质/牙本质覆盖底层软组织。牙髓治疗旨在重建从冠方到根尖严密封闭的黏膜−牙髓屏障，而修复过程中的空隙或渗漏可能为细菌的定植并最终进入身体内部创造机会。冠方和根尖区细菌及其产物影响的重要性是确定这一原则的原因之一。

牙列中具有多种功能的恒牙的进化是动物进化中不可或缺的一部分 [40]，灵长类动物和人类更是如此。然而，这些牙齿如果发生断裂，微生物可能会进入牙齿内部，并在暴露的牙本质和牙髓组织中建立一个据点。除非牙齿保护机制形成，否则这些感染将威胁年轻恒牙，甚至导致牙齿拔除 [40]。根尖周炎利用并调整炎症的一般作用机制，对抗和控制受损牙髓感染。这些感染会通过牙髓分支和牙本质小管扩散（图 1.2）。因此，在定义疾病时，根尖周炎的表述对我们有利；真正值得关注的是其潜在的感染。

组织反应的保护作用是有代价的。炎症导致

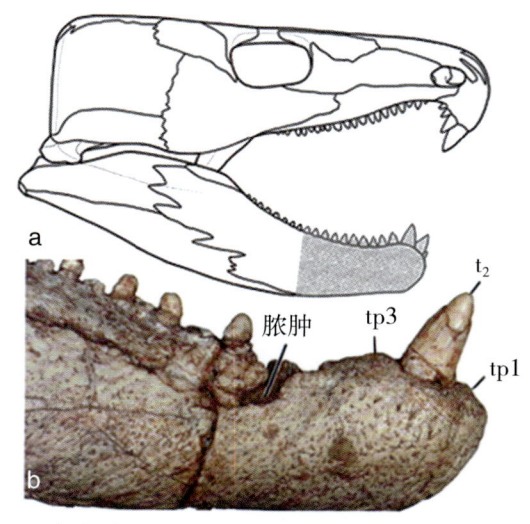

图 1.2　来自俄克拉荷马州下二叠纪的基底爬行动物拉比达龙的牙齿和下颌骨病理证据。a. 右侧视颅骨重建。b. 右侧下颌骨侧视图（经许可转载 [40]）

的临床症状可能会使患者感到疼痛，而肉芽肿或囊肿并不能总是有效地控制入侵的微生物。牙髓和根尖周组织的炎症性有时会导致剧烈疼痛，这也证明了感染的潜在危险。这种疼痛也是人类试图对抗牙科疾病的出发点。因此，急性牙髓炎和根尖周炎是牙科首先关注的问题之一。

牙齿、口腔前庭、舌隐窝、扁桃体不规则区、龈沟和其他解剖结构是口腔微生物的安全聚集处。不同毒性的微生物可能从这些区域迁移并引起感染，如扁桃体炎、牙龈炎、冠周炎、边缘性牙周炎、龋齿、牙髓炎和根尖周炎。虽然生理性的和机械的清洁活动倾向于降低口腔中的微生物的水平，但环境因素有时有利于感染，而不是预防感染。目前对口腔微生物群落的研究强调生物膜的形成和发展的概念，还有由生物膜内条件决定的微生物特定的生理、遗传和致病性质（详见第4章）。

几十年来，龋齿一直是牙齿主要的感染类疾病，而牙髓和根尖周组织的感染和炎症往往是龋齿发展的结果。作为龋齿调查研究的一部分，研究人员研究了根尖周炎的发生和流行病学。根尖周炎具有感染性，其潜在的扩散风险与并发症表明，有必要针对牙髓疾病的公共卫生影响开展独立的系统性调查，并以此为基础制定更全面的防治策略。

1.4 根尖周炎的生物学及临床意义

1.4.1 根尖周炎——感染

在考古研究的头骨中经常发现感染根管和根尖周炎（图1.3）。在没有抗生素的时代，牙髓和根尖周组织的感染可能是严重的，并且需要密切观察。在抗生素使用的早期，人们发现青霉素对大多数这类感染均有作用，因此可以通过抗生素来控制感染的扩散。今天，人们认识到牙髓感染可能是由具有不同毒性的微生物引起的（详见第4章），而且难以有效地控制。

幸运的是，口腔菌群中的致病菌相对较少，通常毒力较低，且大多数是机会致病菌，只在混合感染或伴有其他疾病的宿主中引起疾病。然而，口腔内通常不致病的微生物如果进入牙髓或根尖周组织，可能表现出毒力特征。对感染牙髓的研究表明，感染牙髓中存在定植于口腔内的通常不

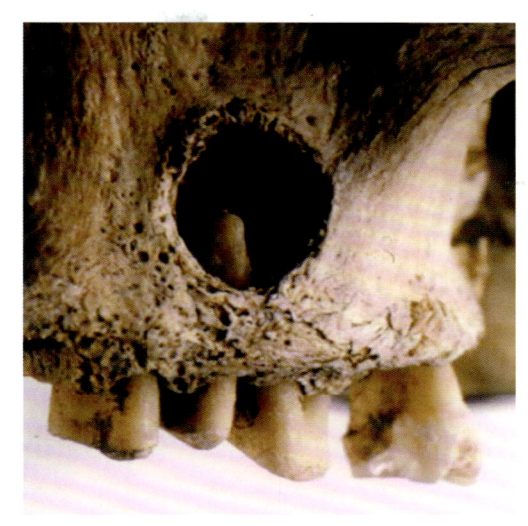

图1.3 在冰岛发现的一名女性头骨上颌前磨牙患有根尖周炎，其可追溯到12世纪。创伤或磨损导致牙髓暴露，感染和病变发展

致病的细菌。根尖周炎对牙髓感染的反应，可以被看作是一种控制和应对感染生物体毒力表达的方式。因此，在疾病发展的早期阶段，大多数疼痛通常会因组织反应而消退。此外，根尖周炎病变初期扩展后，很快就会出现一段静止期，甚至可能消退或至少病变相对稳定。这一动态过程随着来自根管内菌群再次进入根尖区的变化而变化。

一些类型的根尖周炎与根管内特定优势菌群有关。然而，来自分子分析的证据表明，根管的感染可能更多的是机会性感染，而不是特异性感染，并且涉及的菌种数量远超既往认知（详见第4章）。为了提高诊断的准确性和治疗的成功率，研究根尖周炎的微生物学原因和相互作用是必要的，尤其是所谓的"治疗耐受"的根尖周炎病例，即根管治疗完善但是感染仍然持续存在，以及再治疗的病例。现代微生物学技术[19, 53]已经证明了根管内感染的复杂性和可变性是无穷无尽的，这为研究和增强医生对该疾病的理解开辟了新的途径。

1.4.2 感染控制

根管治疗的效果取决于使用无菌技术和消毒措施来预防和（或）消除感染，但感染控制的关键性通常得不到重视。肝炎病毒的传播是一个长期存在的问题，人们担心病毒通过受污染的器械

传播。污染的牙科器械的灭菌有局限性，因此一次性器械的使用有明显增加的趋势。大多数现代仪器操作的器械是为单次使用而设计的，这种做法有利于局部治疗和防止交叉感染。

1.4.3　微生物的特异性和对宿主的防御

宿主对根管感染的反应一直是许多研究的目标。边缘性牙周炎和根尖周炎（marginal and apical periodontitis）的致病过程非常相似，牙周研究中的许多发现与根尖周炎直接相关。医生对参与根尖周炎发展的免疫学过程的理解正在增加（详见第 3 章）。感染根管中微生物的变异和毒力因素已被证实，菌群可能随着所涉及牙齿的临床情况（持续感染、耐药感染）而发生变化（详见第 4 章、第 11 章）。因此，采取不同的抗菌措施是可能的，甚至是可取的，这取决于特定病例的微生物学诊断。

关于根尖周炎伴有特异侵袭性微生物感染的相关报道非常罕见。有报道表明，根管感染细菌引起的坏死性筋膜炎是非常严重的，甚至危及生命[48]，对普通抗生素耐药的细菌可能会造成严重问题，免疫系统受损的患者更是如此[5]。重要的是，不完全和不充分的根管治疗导致的感染可能需要住院治疗和进一步的医治[17]。

1.4.4　牙髓感染及一般健康状况

病灶感染理论对于牙科治疗和研究而言一直是挫折和灵感的来源。几十年来，不相关的、有时是不正确的论点和概念都被用来决定一些健康个体中不必要的拔牙。关于这一课题的未经证实的观点长期限制了牙髓病学领域的临床发展。然而，这一争议也引发了重要的新发现，即使在今天，病灶感染理论也是根管微生物学和宿主防御机制研究参考框架中的重要组成部分。

1.4.4.1　一般健康状况对根尖周炎的影响

根尖周炎与其他疾病过程可能相互影响。根管对感染的反应由宿主的状况决定，并依赖遗传和体质因素，包括系统性疾病。这种可变的组织反应可能会限制或导致根尖病变的扩大，并可能促进或损害在感染治疗期间和治疗后的愈合反应。

糖尿病会减少患者对感染的防御能力，患者可能有更严重的病变[41, 45]。

抽烟对感染防御普遍有不良影响，并对边缘性牙周炎和伤口愈合有负面影响；也可能影响根尖周炎的发生率和愈合率[25, 36]，但影响力可能较弱或存疑，混淆因素（年龄、边缘性牙周炎）对其影响的结论尚不明确[25]。

有研究推测，水痘带状疱疹病毒感染可能与牙根吸收和根尖周炎[35, 47]的发展有因果关系，但证据非常有限且不确定[22]。同样，其他病毒感染也与其他细菌引发的根尖周炎的发病机制有关[20-21, 26, 29]。

镰状细胞性贫血可引起牙髓坏死，多发生于下颌骨，无明显微生物感染[12]。继发的感染会导致典型的根尖周炎。这种易感性增加的机制尚不清楚，但患者多表达高水平的炎症细胞因子[13]。

影响患者免疫和宿主反应状态的全身药物也将影响与根尖周炎相关的生物学过程[9]。此外，随着研究设计和研究方法变得更加复杂，研究发现牙科疾病与其他部位的疾病有关。炎症性肠病患者根尖周炎的患病率较高，病变较大[37]，就像血糖控制不良的糖尿病患者一样。一般来说，免疫抑制药物或其他使用免疫抑制剂药物的疾病，可能不会显著影响根管治疗的愈后[2, 33]。其他药物可能有利于愈合，一项研究发现使用他汀类药物可改善根管治疗的愈合率[1]。

边缘性牙周炎与先兆子痫和早产之间有显著相关性[34]，这在传统上与炎症性血液标志物水平的升高有关[10, 50]。同样，先兆子痫更常发生于有根尖周炎的患者中[23]。

抗生素和止痛药物在治疗根尖周炎中有作用。然而，当应用于其他适应证时，这些药物可能掩盖症状[38]，同时可能损害身体防御能力[52]，微生物种群有可能对抗生素产生耐药性。

接受免疫抑制剂治疗的患者或其他免疫系统受损的患者需要特别关注。许多血液功能障碍（特别是白血病）与根尖周炎的潜在严重后遗症有关：感染很容易传播，可能需要广谱的抗菌药物治疗。放疗患者是一种特殊的患者群体：为了避免口腔手术后放射性骨坏死[8]的发生，需要高要求的、有效的、保守的根管治疗。同样，接受静脉注射双膦酸盐治疗的患者在牙髓外科治疗后可能有组织坏死的风险[31]。抵抗力较低的患者根管治疗并发症的病例报告指出：细致和完善的根管治疗对这类患者具有重要作用[5, 46]。

1.4.4.4.2 根尖周炎对其他组织和器官的影响

根尖周炎的远隔效应和全身性影响是另一个重要方面。

鼻窦炎可由上颌磨牙的根管感染引起，或在极少数情况下由第二前磨牙根管感染引起[49]。下颌炎症可能导致下颌神经或颏神经感觉异常。这些并发症通常在患牙成功治疗后消退[51]。

一般来说，任何菌血症造成的其他危险疾病在牙髓病学中都是值得关注的，特别是有感染性心内膜炎、先天性心脏病、风湿性心脏病或存在人工心脏瓣膜或其他易受感染的血管植入物病史的患者，在根管治疗时可能需要使用抗生素。由牙源性菌血症引起心血管并发症的风险很低，需要控制轻微和慢性口腔感染，包括根尖周炎[39]的观点可能会受到的质疑[11]。内科医生和牙医共同制定抗生素预防需求的指南，以确保有风险患者的安全，从而更容易制定治疗决策[28]。

动脉粥样硬化是心血管疾病（CVD）发展的关键因素[14]。动脉斑块可能是短暂菌血症期间微生物循环的定植点，因此口腔感染可能是CVD的一个危险因素[44]。具体来说，根尖周炎与心血管疾病的发病率增加相关[3-4, 15-16, 43]。由于缺乏严格的评估根尖周感染性质的标准，使这种关联的研究变得复杂；影像学检查只给出拍摄时的状态，不能区分正在进行的感染和正在愈合的病变。根管填充的牙齿，有或没有病变，可能代表有牙髓炎或根尖周炎的病史。在个体中将所有已行根管充填的牙齿与未经治疗的根尖周炎牙齿混合，已被用作衡量"牙髓病学的负担"；这与CVD独立相关[16]。然而，从其他因素来看，已完成的根管充填与心血管疾病发病率降低有关[30]。在这个阶段，根尖周炎可能在CVD发展中发挥作用纯粹只是推测。然而，根尖周炎患者血液中与CVD相关的几种细胞因子和其他化合物水平升高[3]。

1.4.5 牙齿脱落和更换

未经治疗的根尖周炎是一种口腔组织的慢性感染，发病部位靠近许多重要的组织。虽然这些感染可能保持静止几十年，但它们也可能发展和扩散，并造成严重后果。面对这种慢性感染的风险，拔除患牙和使用种植体替代患牙作为一种可行的替代牙髓治疗方案已经被提出和讨论。根据严格的标准（详见第5章），根尖周炎治疗的不同成功率有时被用作支持种植治疗的一个论点。但很少有证据表明牙髓治疗后的牙齿存活率较低[7]，保存牙齿相对于替代牙齿的优势使其应该作为一种生物学优先原则。对于牙髓病学，其他治疗方案应该作为一个驱动力，以产生更科学可靠的证据，以治愈和预防的方式对待医生感兴趣的疾病——根尖周炎。

1.5 结论

牙髓和根尖周炎症引起的相关疼痛和根管感染的后果仍然是当今口腔医生需要考虑的重要方面。新的理论和见解为患者提供了更好的治疗机会，并引导学者们实施进一步的研究。根尖周炎的预防和控制具有坚实的科学基础，但其临床表现差异较大，仍存在有待解决的技术和生物学问题。治疗技术的进步使得以前被认为无法治疗的牙齿的有效治疗成为可能，微生物学、宿主生物学和成像技术的发展肯定会在不久的将来改善牙髓病学的科学基础。

参考文献

[1] Alghofaily M, et al. Healing of apical periodontitis after nonsurgical root canal treatment: the role of statin intake. J Endod, 2018, 44: 135–136.

[2] Azim A A, Griggs J A, Huang G T. The Tennessee study: factors affecting treatment outcome and healing time following nonsurgical root canal treatment. Int Endod J, 2016, 49: 6–16.

[3] Berlin-Broner Y, Febbraio M, Levin L. Apical periodontitis and atherosclerosis: Is there a link? Review of the literature and potential mechanism of linkage. Quintessence Int, 2017, 48: 527–534.

[4] Berlin-Broner Y, Febbraio M, Levin L. Association between apical periodontitis and cardiovascular diseases: a systematic review of the literature. Int Endod J, 2017, 50: 847–859.

[5] Blount C A, Leser C. Multisystem complications following endodontic therapy. J Oral Maxillofac Surg, 2012, 70: 527–530.

[6] Chanani A, Adhikari H D. Reliability of cone beam computed tomography as a biopsy-independent tool in differential diagnosis

of periapical cysts and granulomas: an in vivo study. J Conserv Dent, 2017, 20: 326–331.

[7] Chercoles-Ruiz A, Sanchez-Torres A, Gay-Escoda C. Endodontics, endodontic retreatment, and apical surgery versus tooth extraction and implant placement: a systematic review. J Endod, 2017, 43: 679–686.

[8] Chronopoulos A, et al. Osteoradionecrosis of the jaws: definition, epidemiology, staging and clinical and radiological findings. A concise review. Int Dent J, 2018, 68: 22–30.

[9] Cotti E, et al. An overview on biologic medications and their possible role in apical periodontitis. J Endod, 2014, 40: 1902–1911.

[10] da Silva H E C, et al. Effect of intra-pregnancy nonsurgical periodontal therapy on inflammatory biomarkers and adverse pregnancy outcomes: a systematic review with meta-analysis. Syst Rev, 2017, 6: 197.

[11] Dayer M, Thornhill M. Is antibiotic prophylaxis to prevent infective endocarditis worthwhile? J Infect Chemother, 2018, 24: 18–24.

[12] Demirbas Kaya A, Aktener B O, Unsal C. Pulpal necrosis with sickle cell anaemia. Int Endod J, 2004, 37: 602–606.

[13] Ferreira S B, et al. Periapical cytokine expression in sickle cell disease. J Endod, 2015, 41: 358–362.

[14] Frostegard J. Immunity, atherosclerosis and cardiovascular disease. BMC Med, 2013, 11: 117.

[15] Garg P, Chaman C. Apical periodontitis-is it accountable for cardiovascular diseases? J Clin Diagn Res, 2016, 10: Ze08–12.

[16] Gomes M S, et al. Apical periodontitis and incident cardiovascular events in the Baltimore Longitudinal Study of Ageing. Int Endod J, 2016, 49: 334–342.

[17] Gronholm L, et al. The role of unfinished root canal treatment in odontogenic maxillofacial infections requiring hospital care. Clin Oral Investig, 2013, 17: 113–121.

[18] Gutmann J L, et al. Identify and define all diagnostic terms for periapical/periradicular health and disease states. J Endod, 2009, 35: 1658–1674.

[19] Iriboz E, et al. Detection of the unknown components of the oral microflora of teeth with periapical radiolucencies in a Turkish population using next-generation sequencing techniques. Int Endod J, 2018, 5（12）: 1349–1357

[20] Jakovljevic A, Andric M. Human cytomegalovirus and Epstein-Barr virus in etiopathogenesis of apical periodontitis: a systematic review. J Endod, 2014, 40: 6–15.

[21] Jakovljevic A, et al. Epstein-Barr virus infection induces bone resorption in apical periodontitis via increased production of reactive oxygen species. Med Hypotheses, 2016, 94: 40–42.

[22] Jakovljevic A, et al. The role of varicella zoster virus in the development of periapical pathoses and root resorption: a systematic review. J Endod, 2017, 43: 1230–1236.

[23] Khalighinejad N, et al. Apical periodontitis, a predictor variable for preeclampsia: a case-control study. J Endod, 2017, 43: 1611–1614.

[24] Kirkevang L-L, et al. Prognostic value of the full-scale Periapical Index. Int Endod J, 2015, 48（11）: 1051–1058

[25] Kirkevang L-L, et al. Risk factors fordeveloping apical periodontitis in a general population. Int Endod J, 2007, 40（4）: 290–299.

[26] Lee M Y, et al. A case of bacteremia caused by Dialister pneumosintes and Slackia exigua in a patient with periapical abscess. Anaerobe, 2016, 38: 36–38.

[27] Lin L M, et al. Nonsurgical root canal therapy of large cyst-like inflammatory periapical lesions and inflammatory apical cysts. J Endod, 2009, 35: 607–615.

[28] Lockhart P B, et al. Acceptance among and impact on dental practitioners and patients of American Heart Association recommendations for antibiotic prophylaxis. J Am Dent Assoc, 2013, 144: 1030–1035.

[29] Makino K, et al. Epstein-Barr virus infection in chronically inflamed periapical granulomas. PLoS One, 2015, 10: e0121548.

[30] Meurman J H, et al. Lower risk for cardiovascular mortality for patients with root filled teeth in a Finnish population. Int Endod J, 2017, 50: 1158–1168.

[31] Moinzadeh A T, et al. Bisphosphonates and their clinical implications in endodontic therapy. Int Endod J, 2013, 46: 391–398.

[32] Nair P N. New perspectives on radicular cysts: do they heal? Int Endod J,1998,31: 155–160.

[33] Ng Y L, Mann V, Gulabivala K. A prospective study of the factors affecting outcomes of nonsurgical root canal treatment: part 1: periapical health. International Endodontic Journal, 2011, 44: 583–609.

[34] Parihar A S, et al. Periodontal Disease: A Possible Risk-Factor for Adverse Pregnancy Outcome. J Int Oral Health, 2015, 7:137–142.

[35] Patel K, et al. Multiple apical radiolucencies and external cervical resorption associated with varicella zoster virus: a case report. J Endod, 2016, 42: 978–983.

[36] Persic Bukmir R, et al. Influence of tobacco smoking on dental periapical condition in a sample of Croatian adults. Wien Klin Wochenschr, 2016, 128: 260–265.

[37] Piras V, et al. Prevalence of apical periodontitis in patients with inflammatorybowel diseases: a retrospective clinical study. J Endod, 2017, 43: 389–394.

[38] Read J K, et al. Effect of ibuprofen on masking endodontic diagnosis. J Endod, 2014, 40: 1058–1062.

[39] Reis L C, et al. Bacteremia after endodontic procedures in patients with heart disease: culture and molecular analyses. J

[40] Reisz R R, et al. Osteomyelitis in a Paleozoic reptile: ancient evidence for bacterial infection and its evolutionary significance. Naturwissenschaften, 2011, 98: 551–555.

[41] Segura-Egea J J, et al. Association between diabetes and the prevalence of radiolucent periapical lesions in root-filled teeth: systematic review and meta-analysis. Clin Oral Investig, 2016, 20: 1133–1141.

[42] Segura-Egea J J, Martin-Gonzalez J, Castellanos-Cosano L. Endodontic medicine: connections between apical periodontitis and systemic diseases. Int Endod J, 2015, 48: 933–951.

[43] Singhal R K, Rai B. sTNF-R Levels: apical periodontitis linked to coronary heart disease. Open Access Maced J Med Sci, 2017, 5: 68–71.

[44] Slocum C, Kramer C, Genco C A. Immune dysregulation mediated by the oral microbiome: potential link to chronic inflammation and atherosclerosis. J Intern Med, 2016, 280: 114–128.

[45] Smadi L. Apical periodontitis and endodontic treatment in patients with type II diabetes mellitus: comparative cross-sectional survey. J Contemp Dent Pract, 2017, 18: 358–362.

[46] Stalfors J, et al. Deep neck space infections remain a surgical challenge. A study of 72 patients. Acta Otolaryngol, 2004, 124: 1191–1196.

[47] Talebzadeh B, et al. Varicella zoster virus and internal root resorption: a case report. J Endod, 2015, 41: 1375–1381.

[48] Treasure T, Hughes W, Bennett J. Cervical necrotizing fasciitis originating with a periapical infection. J Am Dent Assoc, 2010, 141: 861–866.

[49] Vidal F, et al. Odontogenic sinusitis:a comprehensive review. Acta Odontol Scand, 2017, 75: 623–633.

[50] Vivares-Builes A M, et al. Gaps in knowledge about the association between maternal periodontitis and adverse obstetric outcomes: an umbrella review. J Evid Based Dent Pract, 2018, 18: 1–27.

[51] von Ohle C, ElAyouti A. Neurosensory impairment of the mental nerve as a sequel of periapical periodontitis: case report and review. Oral Surg Oral Med Oral Pathol Oral Radiol Endod, 2010, 110: e84–99.

[52] Yang J H, et al. Antibiotic-induced changes to the host metabolic environment inhibit drug efficacy and alter immune function. Cell Host Microbe, 2017, 22: 757–765.

[53] Zandi H, et al. Antibacterial effectiveness of 2 root canal irrigants in root-filled teeth with infection: a randomized clinical trial. J Endod, 2016, 42: 1307–1313.

第 2 章 牙髓－牙本质复合体与牙周组织的解剖生理学

Leo Tjäderhane, Susanna Paju

2.1 概念

虽然牙本质和牙髓在本质上不同，牙本质是一种矿化组织，而牙髓是一种软组织，但它们在发育上相互依赖，并且在整个牙齿生命周期中，在解剖学和功能上也保持紧密的关联。因此，这两种组织通常被称为牙髓－牙本质复合体。

在牙齿发育的钟状期，牙本质和牙髓由颅神经嵴的胚胎结缔组织的外胚间充质细胞发育而来（图2.1）。"钟状"内层的牙上皮包裹着致密的间充质。上皮－外胚叶间充质的相互作用在牙乳头周围启动了第一个成牙本质细胞的分化，其余的间充质将形成未来的牙髓。分化的成牙本质细胞开始分泌牙本质蛋白，并激发成釉细胞启动釉质基质的分泌[138]。

当牙冠形态发生后牙根开始形成时，赫特维希上皮根鞘（HERS）由成釉器颈部的上皮发育而来。当HERS向根尖方向生长时，相邻的牙乳头细胞分化为成牙本质细胞，形成根部牙本质。HERS对牙根牙本质的形成至关重要：如果HERS被破坏，牙乳头细胞就无法分化；同时，分化中的成牙本质细胞与HERS之间的相互作用对于根部形成也是必需的。HERS的断裂使牙囊细胞与牙根牙本质表面接触，分化为成牙骨质细胞形成牙骨质。此外，部分HERS细胞也可能经历转变，直接分化成为成纤维细胞。牙囊细胞分泌的胶原纤维嵌入牙骨质基质，形成牙周膜。HERS的部分残余细胞留在牙髓和牙周结缔组织中（图2.2），称为马拉瑟（Malassez）上皮剩余[88, 112, 221]。同时，侧支根管以及根尖区域副根管系统形成，而非单一的根尖孔，这可能是生物个体的正常变异，也可能与HERS的异常有关。

牙髓的软组织通过根尖孔与牙周膜（PDL）直接相连。有时，根尖区域由一个三角形的副根管系统组成，该系统包含多个牙髓与PDL之间的

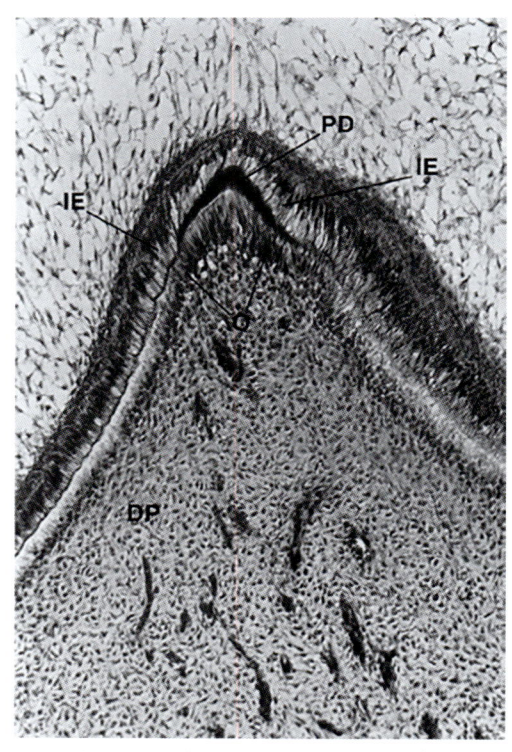

图2.1 牙本质发生在牙齿发育的钟状期。DP: 牙乳头。O: 成牙本质细胞。PD: 前期牙本质。IE: 内牙上皮

连通点。除此之外，PDL 的其余部分与牙髓 – 牙本质复合体被一层牙骨质隔开。嵌入牙骨质和牙槽骨的穿通纤维称作夏普（Sharpey）纤维，具有将牙齿固定在牙槽骨上的作用（图 2.3）。

2.2 牙本质

牙本质是人类牙齿最主要的组成部分，为牙釉质提供支持，防止牙釉质在承担咬合负荷时断裂；它还保护牙髓免受潜在的有害刺激，并参与硬组织和软组织（通常称为牙髓 – 牙本质复合体）的整体保护。牙齿不同部位的牙本质在性质上可能会有所不同，这种差异性确保了牙本质能够满足特定位置的具体需求。

牙本质是一种矿化的结缔组织，纳米晶相的胶原生物复合物，这种独特有特征使牙本质在承受较大的咬合力时能为牙齿提供机械强度。牙本质的大致组成为：约 70% 的质量百分比（55% 的体积百分比）为矿物质，约 20% 的质量百分比（30% 的体积百分比）为有机成分，其余为水。由于牙本质在牙齿内部的结构会随位置而变化，因此这些值仅为平均值[208]。约 90% 的牙本质有机基质是高度交联的 I 型胶原蛋白，其余为非胶原蛋白，如蛋白多糖、其他蛋白质、生长因子、酶以及少量脂质。该矿化物主要成分是羟基磷灰石 $[Ca_{10}(PO_4)_6(OH)_2]$，还含有杂质（CO_3、Mg、Na、K、Cl）和氟化物，因此应称为生物磷灰石[208]。

构成牙本质的主要部分是管间牙本质，由牙本质 – 牙髓交界处的成牙本质细胞形成。几乎整个牙本质的有机成分都位于管间牙本质。在形成牙本质的过程中，成牙本质细胞会留下牙本质小管，在小管周围形成牙本质。

管周牙本质形成会导致小管缓慢闭塞。由于管周牙本质高度矿化，矿物 – 有机基质比例从牙本质 – 牙髓边缘向牙本质 – 牙釉质交界处增加，并且随年龄增长而增长[208–209]。

2.2.1 牙本质的形成

2.2.1.1 成牙本质细胞、前期牙本质与矿化前沿

成牙本质细胞是牙髓最外层的细胞，由乏细胞层（Weil 层）将其与其余牙髓组织（固有牙髓）分隔开。在分化过程中和分化完成后，成牙本质细胞会排列成一个独特的成牙本质细胞层，有机基质的矿化则完成了罩牙本质的形成（图 2.4）。在牙冠部分，胶原合成细胞的形态特征和细胞膜极化是独一无二的[39, 205]。成牙本质细胞是有丝分裂后的终末分化细胞，这意味着它们已经退出细胞周期，不能被细胞分裂所更新取代[39, 209]。冠方成牙本质细胞在形态学上和细胞膜极性上都高度极化，并形成假复层栅状结构，而在根部形成单细胞层。细胞体位于牙本质的髓壁上，成牙本质细胞突起伸入牙本质小管（图 2.5）。细胞体高 20~40μm，这取决于成牙本质的活性，在细胞的基部包含一个大的细胞核、高尔基体、粗面内质网、几个线粒体和其他细胞内结构[39]。

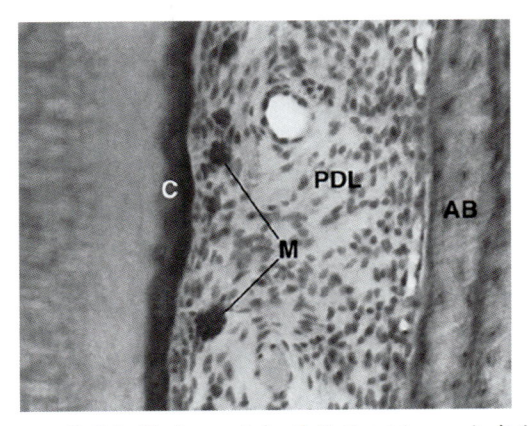

图 2.2 牙周韧带（PDL）切面显示 Malassez 上皮剩余（M）、邻近牙骨质（C）。AB：牙槽骨

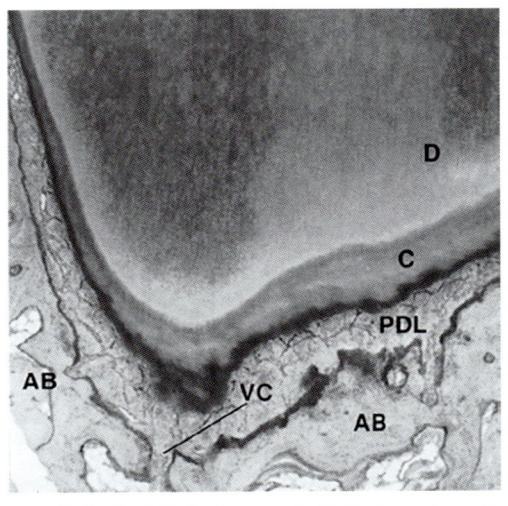

图 2.3 牙齿的顶端部分显示牙槽骨（AB），牙周韧带（PDL）、牙骨质（C）、牙本质（D）、福尔克曼管（VC）

相邻的成牙本质细胞通过广泛的紧密连接相连，在细胞体之间形成一个稳定的屏障，但在受到创伤或龋坏时[23, 40, 209]，这个屏障可能被破坏。成牙本质细胞突起伸入矿化的牙本质小管。主干直径为0.5~1μm，还有较细的侧支，通过这些侧支，突起可以相互连接[27, 39, 209]（图2.6）。成牙本质细胞突起作为一个受体区域，被认为可以用来检测该区域的完整性。任何刺激都会传递到细胞体，引发一系列反应以维持牙齿的整体健康。同时这些突起收缩会留下空管，在横截面上这种现象表现为所谓的"死区"[127]。关于成牙本质细胞进入牙本质小管的程度仍然是一个有争议的问题，因为不同的研究方法和可能的物种差异所获得的结

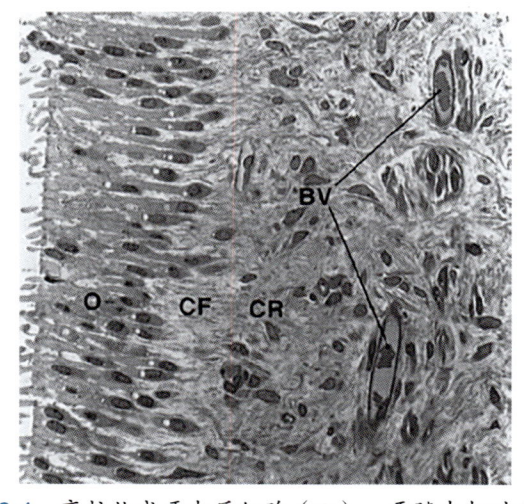

图 2.4 高柱状成牙本质细胞（O），牙髓中相对无细胞区（CF）和相对富细胞区（CR）。BV：血管

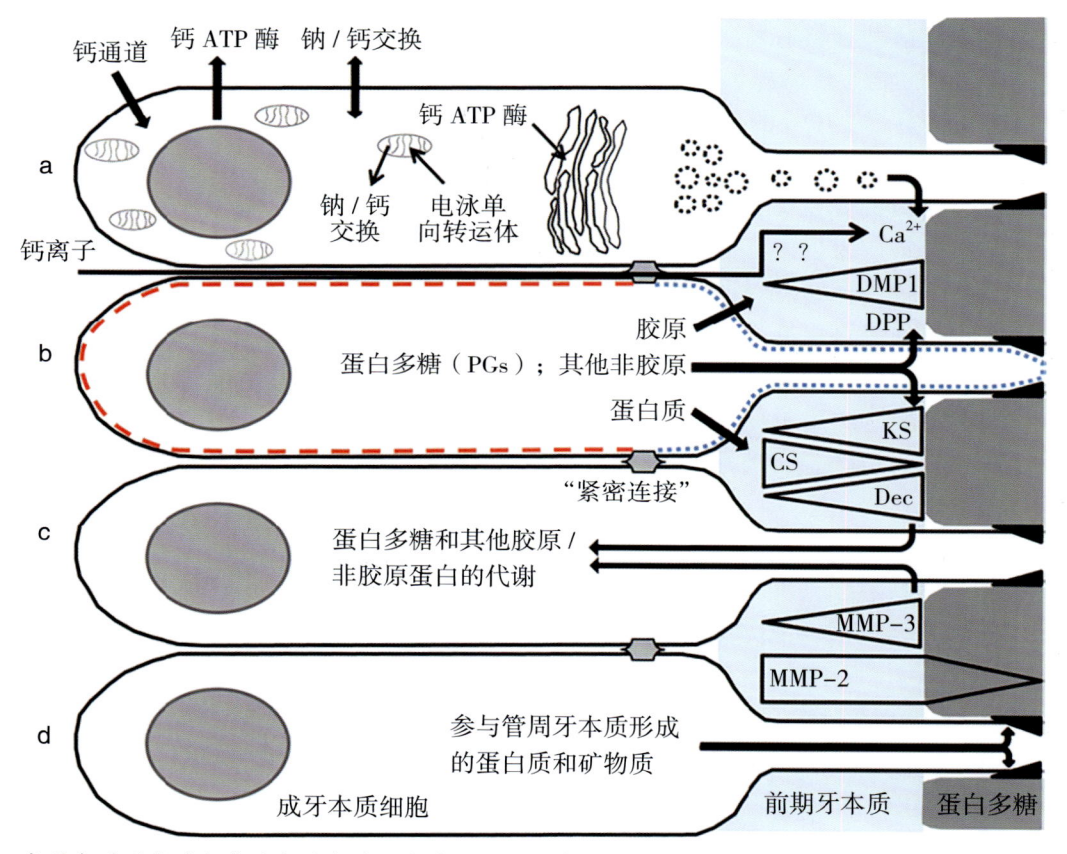

图 2.5 成牙本质形成过程中的成牙本质功能涉及牙本质基质形成、成熟和矿化的因素。a. 成牙本质细胞内 Ca^{2+} 的运输和调控，以提供钙矿化所需的钙和维持胞质 Ca^{2+} 浓度。囊泡内依赖于钙 ATP 酶的 Ca^{2+} 积累是矿化前沿受控运输所必需的。尽管存在紧密连接，一些钙也可能通过细胞间途径进入，至少在成牙本质细胞层完整性被破坏的情况下（带问号箭头所示）会进入。b. 牙本质有机基质成分被成牙本质细胞加工，并在准确的位置分泌到前期牙本质，如牙本质磷蛋白（DPP）直接或接近矿化前沿。牙本质基质蛋白-1（DMP1）、蛋白多糖[PGs，如 decorin（Dec）]或其侧链 [硫酸角蛋白（KS）、硫酸软骨素（CS）] 的差异表明，前期牙本质中蛋白质的酶修饰可控制矿化。基质金属蛋白酶（如 MMP-2 和 MMP-3）等酶参与前期牙本质成熟过程中的蛋白质加工。细胞膜高度极化为基底外侧突（蓝色虚线）和顶端细胞体膜（红色虚线），由紧密连接分隔[205]。c. 成牙本质细胞也有一个运输系统，可以排除前期牙本质不需要的蛋白质和降解产物。d. 成牙本质细胞也负责管周牙本质的形成（修改自文献209）

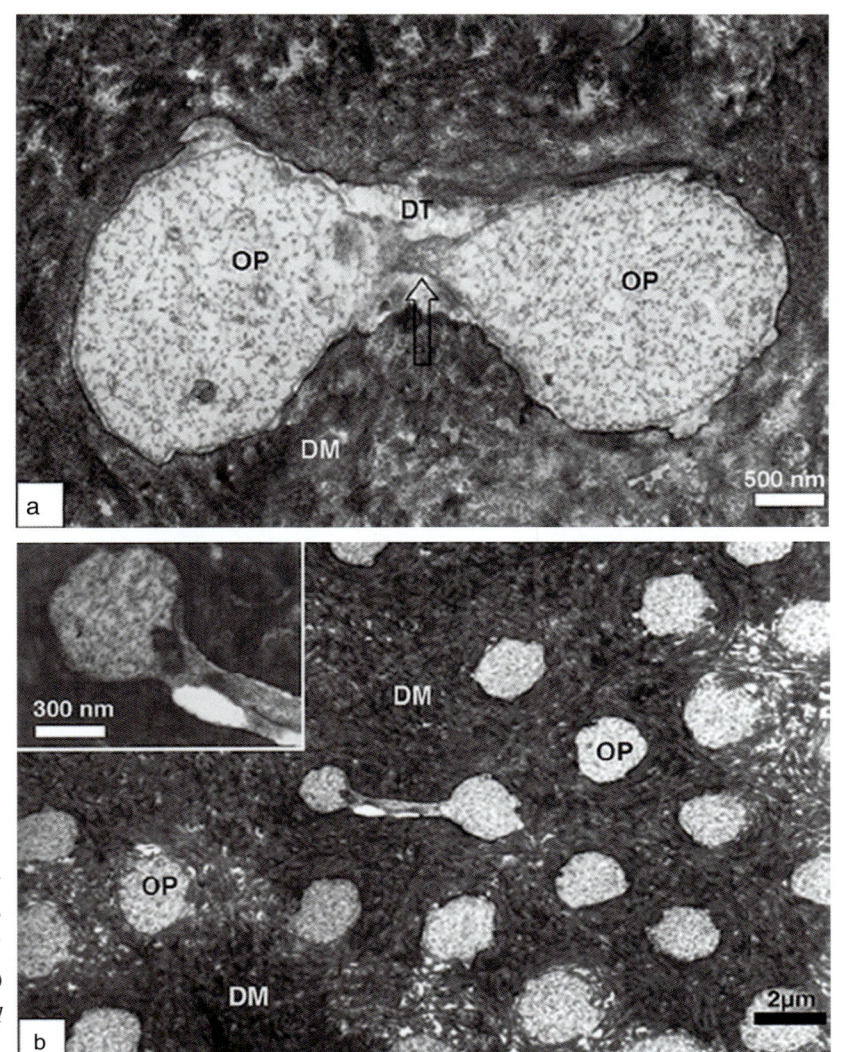

牙髓 – 牙本质复合体与牙周组织的解剖生理学 | 第 2 章

图 2.6 成牙本质细胞突起（OP）存在细胞间连接（空箭头），这些突起填充在被管间牙本质基质（DM）包围的牙本质小管（OT）中。a.10 000 倍。b.2500 倍；插图 20 000 倍（经 Tissue and Cell 许可引用）[27]

果存在争议。在大鼠的磨牙中，成牙本质细胞的突起一直延伸到釉质牙本质界[127]。在人类牙齿中，大多数研究表明，成牙本质细胞突起不会从牙本质 – 牙髓边界（200~700μm）延伸太远[27, 209]。

在成牙本质细胞和矿化牙本质之间，存在一层 10~30μm 的未矿化的前期牙本质（图 2.5）。在这里，牙本质有机基质得以组织排列[14]，随后在矿化前沿进行可控的矿化过程，从而形成管间牙本质[14]。有机基质的主要成分是Ⅰ型胶原蛋白，而非胶原蛋白质（糖蛋白、蛋白聚糖和酶），它控制基质的成熟和矿化（图 2.5）。牙本质胶原的矿化是通过胶原间隙区的蛋白 – 聚糖 – 胶原相互作用发生的（纤维内矿化）[43, 209]。有趣的是，导致未成熟骨和钙化软骨矿化的基质囊泡参与了

罩牙本质和修复性牙本质的矿化，但囊泡不参与原发性或继发性牙本质的矿化[193]。矿化前沿通常被认为是线性的，但实际上球形矿化突起更为常见，称为钙化球粒[209, 213]。

2.2.2 牙本质的结构

牙本质也可以根据形成时间分为：釉质牙本质界（DEJ）、牙本质基质（前期牙本质）、原发性牙本质、继发性牙本质，以及第三期牙本质。根据结构和负责形成的牙本质可进一步分为反应性牙本质和修复性牙本质。

2.2.2.1 釉质牙本质界与牙本质基质

在人体中，釉质牙本质界（DEJ）是一个 7~15μm 宽的波状扇形结构[59, 131, 169, 213]，与牙釉质和牙本质[59]都不同。扇形界面被认为可以增强

11

牙釉质与牙本质之间的机械附着。罩牙本质是牙本质最外部的一层，厚度在5~30μm。罩牙本质形成于成牙本质细胞终末分化期间及之后，是含有牙乳头的有机残余，其矿化机制与矿化前沿的不同[193, 209]。罩牙本质中没有大的小管，每个小管都有小分支（图2.7）。与其他牙本质不同，罩牙本质包含Ⅲ型胶原（von Korff 纤维）。自罩牙本质至牙髓，牙本质矿化率逐渐变化[197]，这可能会产生高达500μm的"弹性带"，以防止在较大咬合力作用下牙齿发生折裂[197, 208, 231-232]。

2.2.2.2 原发性牙本质及继发性牙本质

原发性牙本质形成（原发性牙本质发生）发生在大部分冠和根的形成和生长过程中，构成牙本质的主要部分。之后，牙本质以大约1/10的速率继续形成继发性牙本质[208]。原发性牙本质形成"结束"的确切时间尚不清楚，实际上原发性牙本质的形成是逐渐减慢的[100]。即使在组织学或电子显微镜图像中，也很难区分原发性和继发性牙本质，并且没有临床相关性。继发性牙本质的形成持续终生，导致牙髓腔和根管逐渐消失[208]。

2.2.2.3 牙本质小管及管周牙本质

牙本质的管状特性对其机械性能[11-13, 129]和牙本质粘接[202]有利。通常，小管从DEJ以直角延伸并以S形平滑地延伸向牙髓–牙本质边界，但在牙釉质下方时方向可能不同[232]。牙本质小管的方向在上下颌牙弓中也有所不同[232]，这可能会影响咬合时牙齿对负荷的机械反应[208, 232]。小管的密度根据牙齿的位置而变化，但在牙髓–牙本质边界中是最高的，并且向DEJ逐渐降低[142]（图2.8）。小管的数量向根尖缓慢减少，并且在根部牙本质中，特别是在根尖区域存在广泛分支[77, 129, 142-143]。在冠部，牙本质小管最多，且在牙尖下方的方向更直，成牙本质细胞突[212, 229]和密集的支配神经[23]在此处也更深地穿透牙本质

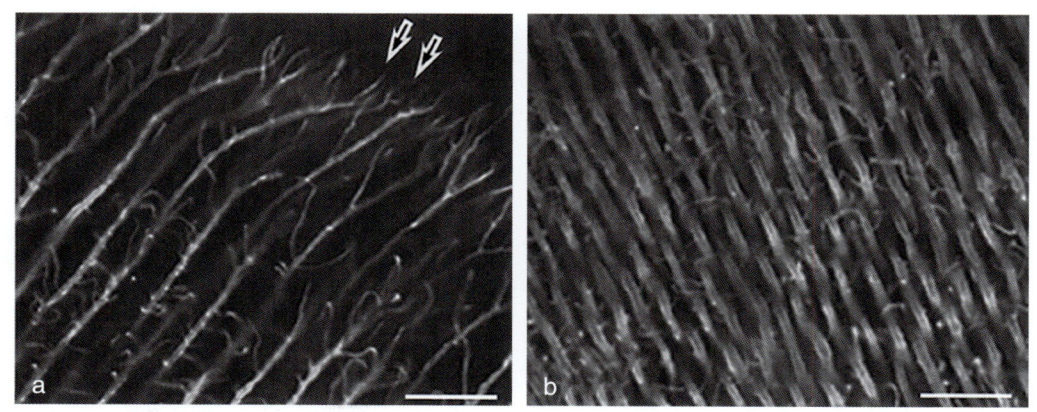

图2.7 a. 靠近DEJ的人牙本质小管分支密集（箭头）。b. 牙本质中部牙本质小管分支密集（比例尺：20μm）（经 *Tissue and Cell* 许可引用[101]）

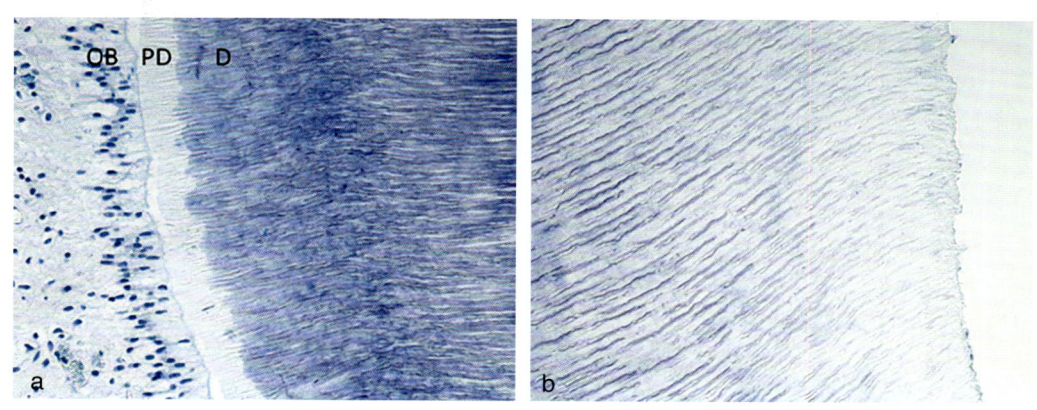

图2.8 靠近牙本质–牙髓边界的致密牙本质小管（a）和靠近DEJ的稀疏牙本质小管（b）。一名年轻患者的第三颗磨牙的甲苯胺蓝染色。OB：牙本质细胞。PD：前期牙本质。D：牙本质

小管。这可能与感知外部刺激有关，并有助于调节牙髓-牙本质复合体的防御反应。

管周（管内）牙本质以规则的圆形方式在牙本质小管的壁上形成（图2.9）。这种高度矿化的结构导致管腔直径增龄性减小，甚至完全闭塞，称为牙本质硬化。在磨损严重或龋齿的情况下，再沉积或来自牙本质液的矿物离子可能导致牙本质小管被矿物晶体阻塞。通常，这种现象也称为牙本质硬化，但称为"反应性（牙本质）硬化"会更合适[208]。管周牙本质通常是不均匀的，并且被小管分支和一些小穿孔[70]贯穿，牙本质液及其组分可通过上述结构穿过管周牙本质。

2.2.2.4 第三期牙本质

第三期牙本质是牙本质对外部刺激应答反应所形成的，包括生理性和病理性的磨损和侵蚀，如创伤、龋齿（病变的大小及活动性都会影响[16]）、龋坏窝洞的制备以及化学刺激。生长因子及其他生物活性分子存在于矿化牙本质中，并在龋齿或磨损期间释放出来，这些分子被认为启动了第三期牙本质的形成和并控制其结构[187]。第三期牙本质增加了口腔微生物和其他刺激物与牙髓组织之间的矿化屏障厚度，目的是保持牙髓组织的活力，维持牙髓未感染的状态。牙本质的形态和规律取决于刺激的强度和持续时间。三期牙本质有两种：由原始成牙本质细胞形成的反应性牙本质和由新分化的替代成牙本质细胞形成的修复性牙本质[16,138,171,173,209]（图2.10）。反应性牙本质是管状的，在结构上与继发性牙本质相似；修复性牙本质也称为纤维牙本质或钙化瘢痕组织[16,138,171,209]，通常无管状结构，或小管化程度较低，也可能呈现多种不同的形态（图2.11）。修复性牙本质被认为是相对不可渗透的，在管状牙本质和牙髓组织之间形成屏障。

2.2.2.5 根部牙本质

根部牙本质与冠部牙本质有一些明显的区别，紧挨着牙骨质下，Tomes颗粒层类似于冠部前期牙本质，伴薄层管状及融合不良的球状结构。这些颗粒含有未钙化或钙化不良的胶原纤维束，并被认为具有类似于罩牙本质的"弹性区"[102]。如上所述，根部牙本质的管状密度低于冠部牙本质，特别是最靠近根尖的部分[77,129,142-143]（图2.12）。年龄相关的根管硬化症从根尖区域开始并向冠部方向发展[149,216]，影响根部牙本质渗透性[164,198]。其他区域牙本质也有差异，如根管颊侧和舌侧牙本质有开放的小管，而近中和远中牙本质可以完全闭塞[164,198]（图2.13）。这些小管的开放或闭塞可能与咬合负荷下的应力分布相对应[208]，并且会影响细菌的渗透和消毒[164,198]。

根尖部分也有相对大量的副根管、根尖分支（根尖delta区）以及根尖管壁的牙骨质样内衬[208]（图2.14）。根尖delta区的发生百分比在5.7%（上颌前牙）到16.5%（下颌磨牙），平均拥有4个

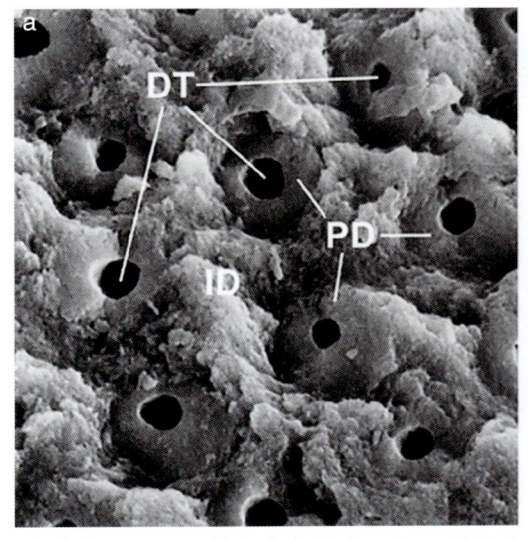

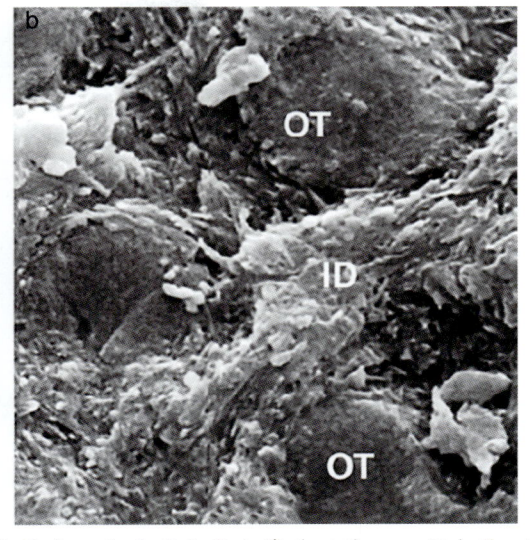

图2.9 牙本质断面，显示管间牙本质（ID）、管周牙本质（PD）和牙本质小管（DT）。a.新出牙。b.老年人牙齿中牙本质小管闭塞（OT）

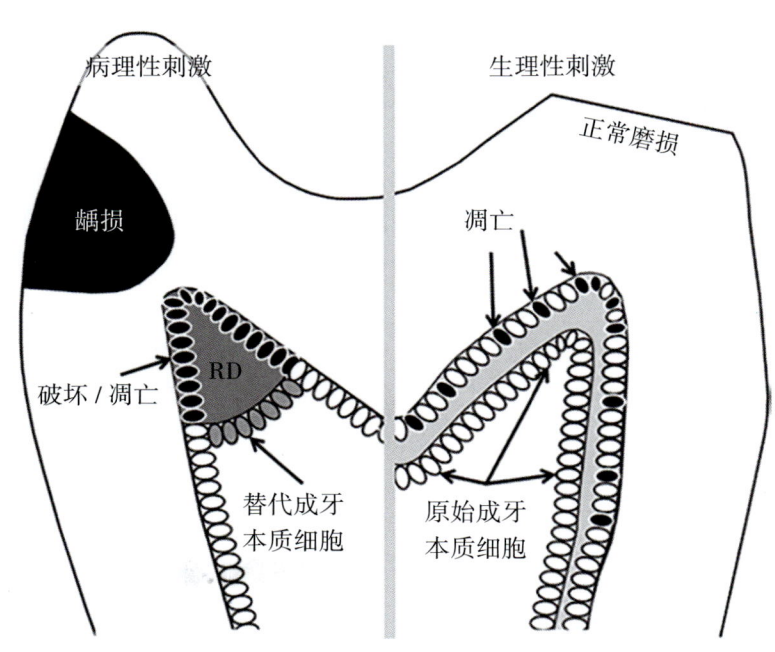

牙髓病学基础：根尖周炎的预防和治疗

图 2.10 强烈的刺激（如深部龋病）诱导局部成牙本质细胞的破坏、凋亡和分化形成修复牙本质（RD）。正常磨损或其他轻度刺激可诱导原发性牙本质形成。成牙本质细胞的聚集会导致特定的细胞（黑色细胞）凋亡（修改自文献 209）

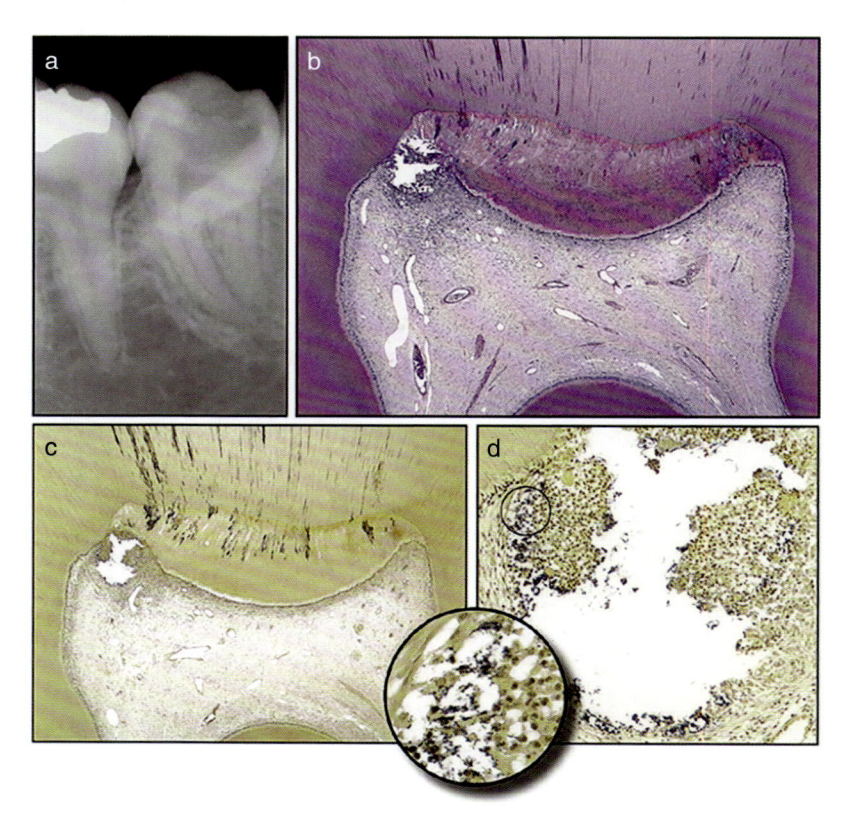

图 2.11　a. 下磨牙深龋的 X 线片。b. 三期牙本质，包括反应性和修复性两种。近中髓角局部坏死（苏木精－伊红，放大倍数 16 倍）。c. 与图 b 相近的切片（Taylor 改良的革兰氏深色，放大 16 倍）。d. 局部微脓肿详细图。右侧细菌被炎症性中性粒细胞包围，左侧是成纤维细胞（原图放大 100 倍；插图 400 倍）（经 Journal of Endodontics 许可引用[172]）

14

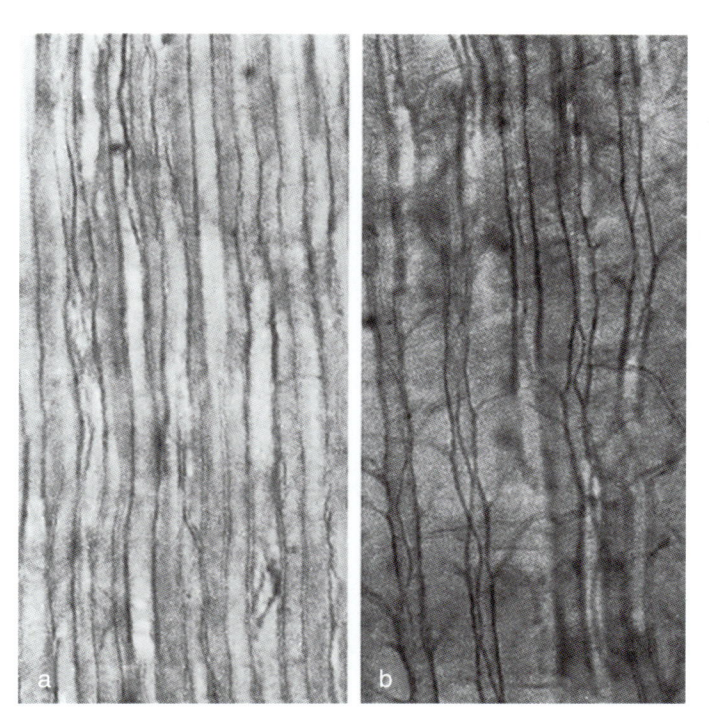

图 2.12 牙本质小管纵切面。a. 冠内。b. 根中的小管比冠中的小管间距更大，根中有许多细小的分支

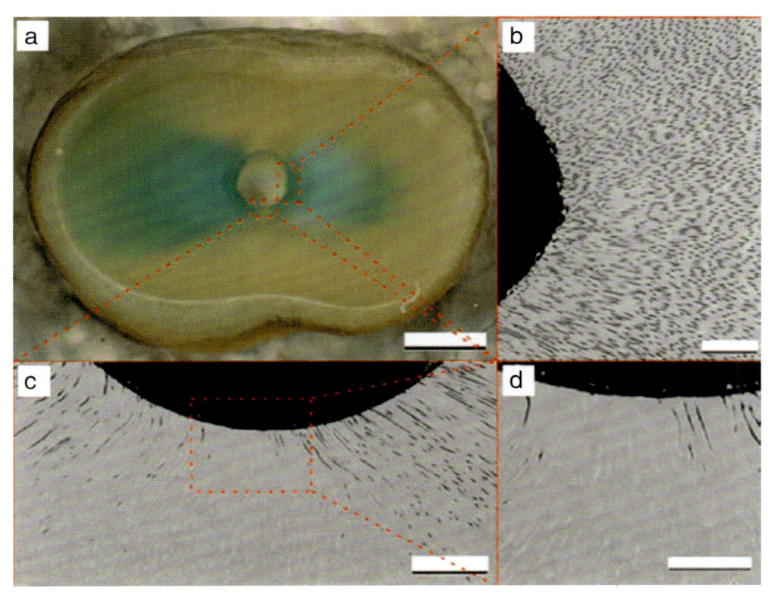

图 2.13 a. 典型舌颊染料渗透的牙齿横切面。b~d. 有染料渗透区域（b）和没有染料渗透区域（c、d）的背散射电子显微图。染色透入区牙本质小管通畅，未染色区可见明显的小管硬化（c、d）。放大倍数：16 倍（a），1000 倍（b、c），3000 倍（d）（经 *Journal of Endodontics* 许可引用[164]）

根管（范围 3~18），大约 87% 的根管垂直延伸长度不超过 3mm[60]。最近的显微 CT 研究对传统认为的单一的根尖缩窄的形式提出了质疑，该研究发现长度大于 1 mm 的平行形式是最常见的，同时在所有类型的牙齿中，没有明显缩窄的锥形形式也相对常见[179]（图 2.15）。

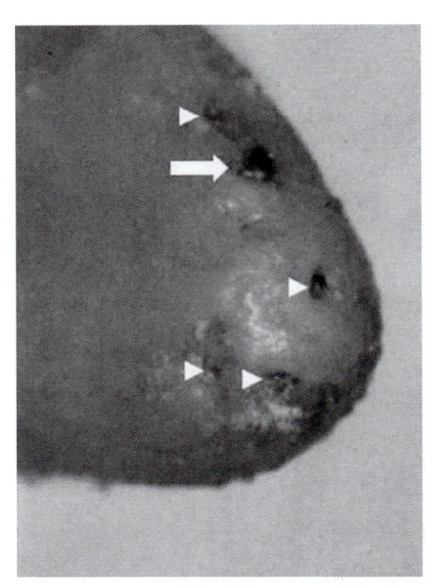

牙髓病学基础：根尖周炎的预防和治疗

受到成牙本质细胞的严格控制[209]（图 2.5）。牙本质还含有多种人血白蛋白，已知的有白蛋白、IgG、转铁蛋白、胎球蛋白 A 和超氧化物歧化酶 3（SOD3）[135]，这些蛋白主要存在于牙本质小管中。除转铁蛋白[160]外，其他蛋白质并不是由成牙本质细胞表达的。因此，在完整的牙齿中，人血白蛋白也可以进入牙本质液。与血清[200]相比，牙本质中存在 SOD3[165]，甚至胎球蛋白 A 的浓度是血清的 100~200 倍，这些都说明成牙本质细胞具有活跃的转运系统[209]。

有证据表明，牙本质液的生理流动可能受内分泌系统的控制。一种被称为腮腺激素的因子被认为能够影响牙本质液流速。这种激素在下丘脑控制下分泌，已从牛、大鼠和猪腮腺中分离出来，并存在于血浆中[175, 209]。合成的腮腺激素与相应的腮腺纯化激素具有同等的生物活性，可增强腺体内液体运动[233]。

牙本质液对整体牙本质内的应力-应变分布具有明显的调节作用，能增加弹性（加载时弹性吸收能量的能力）和韧性（抵抗断裂的能力）[109]。在龋齿中，牙本质液不仅被认为是通过封闭牙本质小管（特别是在缓慢进展的慢性病变中）起到

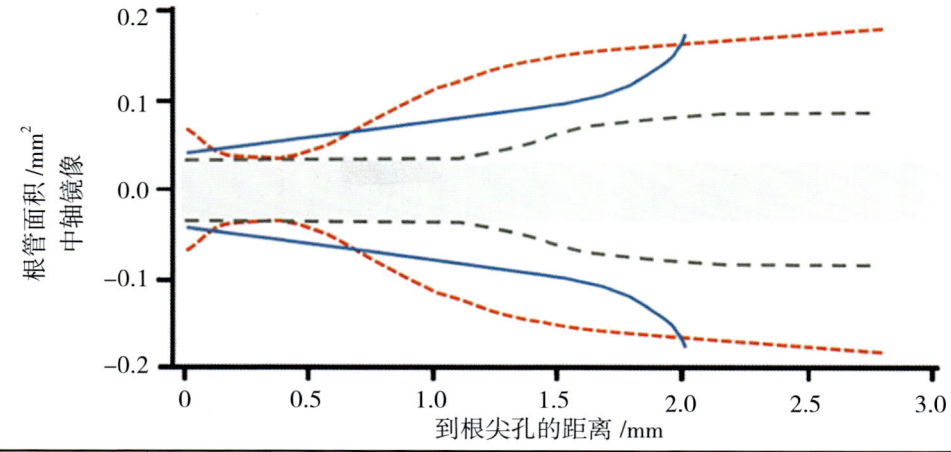

图 2.14 人类尖牙根尖的主根尖孔（箭头）和四个副孔（白色三角）大到足以轻松通过 10#K 锉

2.2.3 牙本质液

成牙本质细胞突和小管壁之间的空间充满了牙本质液。成牙本质细胞层形成功能屏障，主要功能是抑制液体、离子和其他分子沿着细胞外途径通过。在没有组织损伤（如龋齿、窝洞制备、磨损）的牙齿中，一般认为牙本质液的含量

标记	形态	前牙		前磨牙		磨牙	
		横截面积 /mm²	95%CI	横截面积 /mm²	95%CI	横截面积 /mm²	95%CI
-----	常规样	20	7~46	6	1~24	14	6~30
——	锥状	12	3~37	8	2~28	12	5~28
- - -	平行样	68	43~86	86	65~95	74	57~86

图 2.15 不同根尖缩窄形式的根尖根管横截面面积及其在不同牙中的分布（95% 可信区间）。每个点代表一条根管的横截面。X 轴：到根尖孔的距离（mm）。Y 轴：管面积（mm²），反映在零轴上（修改自文献 179）

保护作用[141]，而且通过在小管内沉积的免疫球蛋白[73]成为牙本质-牙髓复合体先天免疫反应的一部分。即使在未感染的小管中，免疫球蛋白的质量和数量似乎也根据龋病的深度和强度而改变[73]。重要的是要认识到：向内流动的液体持续存在，直至牙髓[23, 117]，甚至穿过釉质，至少年轻牙齿是这样[23]。对不同大小的微球研究发现：微球的渗透性与尺寸相关，较大的微球（0.2~1 μm，接近小微生物的大小）能渗透到牙本质内部的三分之一，最小的微球（0.02~0.04 μm）甚至能到达牙髓[117]。因此，向外流动的液体不能"洗掉"小管中的有害刺激。牙本质液也影响粘接修复的成功率。由于牙本质小管的大小的增加和液体流动，牙本质的湿度增加，使得在深窝洞（靠近牙髓）粘接比在浅层牙本质更加困难[166]。牙本质液不仅可能导致亲水性粘接剂降解，也会增加混合层中胶原蛋白降解率，导致粘接剂强度和耐久性降低[202]。

2.3 牙髓组织及其稳态

牙髓组织（有时称为固有牙髓）是松散的结缔组织，含有Ⅰ型和Ⅲ型胶原蛋白。细胞和结构嵌在凝胶状基质中，主要含有硫酸软骨素、透明质酸盐、蛋白多糖和间质液。细胞依赖间质液体作为营养和氧气运输的媒介，并清除代谢废物（图2.16）。神经和血管通过根尖孔或其他开孔进入牙髓（图2.17）。它们紧密地排列在一起，直到在冠部牙髓中发出主要分支，最后在成牙本质细胞/成牙本质细胞下层形成丰富而密集的分支（图2.18）。

2.3.1 牙髓细胞

牙髓组织的主要细胞群是成纤维细胞。在成牙本质层的正下方是乏细胞层（Weil），富含腱生蛋白和纤维连接蛋白，但Ⅲ型胶原蛋白含量较低[134]。在此层之下是多细胞层，其中含有大量成纤维细胞（图2.4）。成纤维细胞在牙髓其余部分的分布较稀疏且相对均匀。牙髓中还含有类似间充质干细胞的牙源性干细胞，具有自我更新能力和多向分化潜能[18]。周细胞是围绕血管的星状细胞，与毛细血管周围的内皮细胞紧密接触，形成不连续的细胞层，而在微血管周围形成连续的细胞层[176]。它们被认为是血管生成和血压的调节因子。目前，周细胞（或其前体）被认为具有间充质干细胞的特征，包括多向分化潜能。它们可以特异性地分化为脂肪细胞、形成硬组织的细胞（成骨细胞和软骨细胞）[95, 176]，在牙髓中也是如此[162, 230]，而且可能与其他非周细胞来源的间充质干细胞[55]一起发生这种分化。

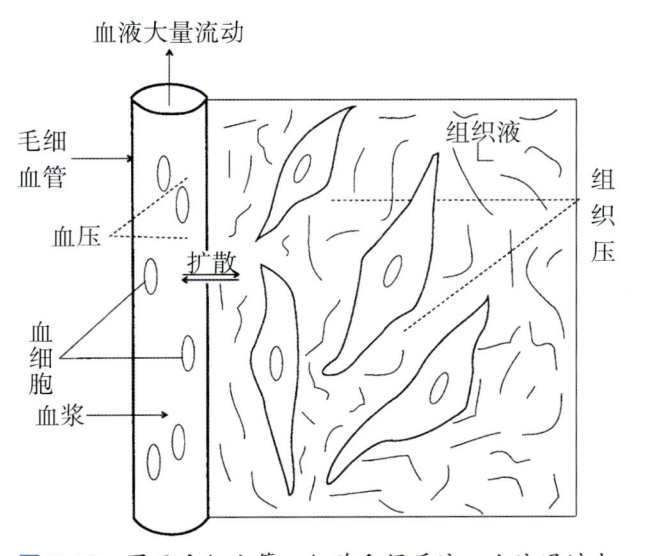

图2.16 图示毛细血管、细胞和间质液。血液通过大量流动进入毛细血管，扩散作用连接血浆和间质液。细胞被间质液包围，间质液作为血浆的延伸发挥作用

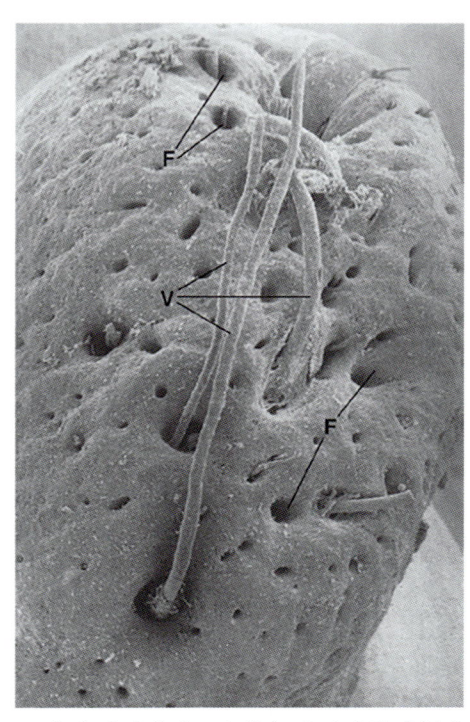

图2.17 在狗的牙齿中，血管（V）通过许多根尖孔（F）进入/离开牙髓。人类牙齿根尖孔的数量并不具有代表性（经 Journal of Endodontics 许可引用[192]）

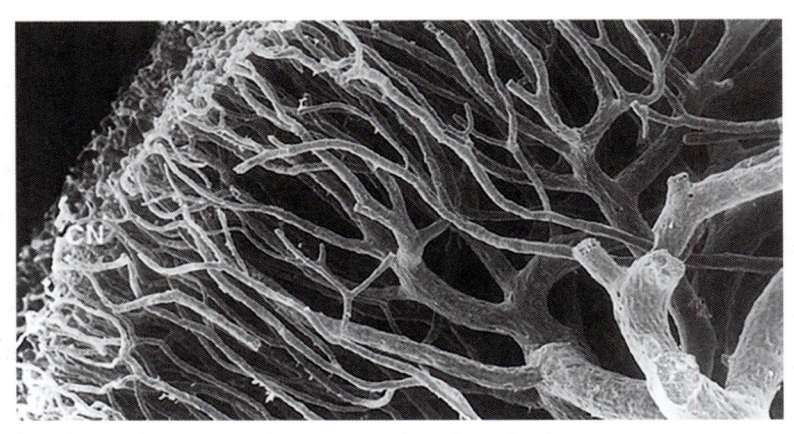

图 2.18 牙髓里有血管。前期牙本质下可见末端毛细血管网（CN）（经 *Journal of Endodontics* 许可引用[192]）

2.3.2 血管和淋巴管

就像在其他组织中一样，牙髓需要血液流动来为细胞提供氧气和营养，并清除二氧化碳和代谢废物。牙髓的血液由上颌动脉供应，上颌动脉分支形成牙动脉和进一步的小动脉，这些小动脉通过根尖孔和侧支根管进入牙齿内。小动脉位于中央，其中一些直接进入冠髓，而另一些则供应根部牙髓。血液流入微静脉，微静脉大体上遵循与小动脉相同的路线，在中央牙髓中经常发现小动脉、微静脉和神经的三联结构（图 2.19）。牙冠和牙根的脉管系统不同。在牙根中，血管穿透牙髓的根尖区域并形成细小的分支。在牙冠区，毛细血管形成一个由连续的肾小球样结构组成的成牙本质细胞下层丛状结构，每个肾小球样结构为 100~150μm 的成牙本质细胞下层区域和成牙本质细胞区供血[90]。在牙本质发育迅速的年轻牙齿中，毛细血管进入成牙本质细胞层以确保其营养供给。牙髓毛细血管壁相对较薄，可能是不连续的，且有窗孔结构[28, 52, 90]。周细胞嵌入毛细血管基底膜内，在那里它们可能迁移并转变为成纤维细胞表型[28]，调节炎症反应（如血浆蛋白泄漏），并可能与血管钙化有关[186]，从而与髓石的形成有关。牙髓的血管由感觉神经和交感神经纤维支配（图 2.20）[23, 81]。

牙髓组织间质液的胶体渗透压低于血浆，有利于毛细血管吸收。这有助于保持较低的组织压力，对包裹着的牙本质在低顺应性环境中的血管内完成正常功能至关重要。不过令人惊讶的是，牙髓中是否存在淋巴管仍然存在争议，尤其是在

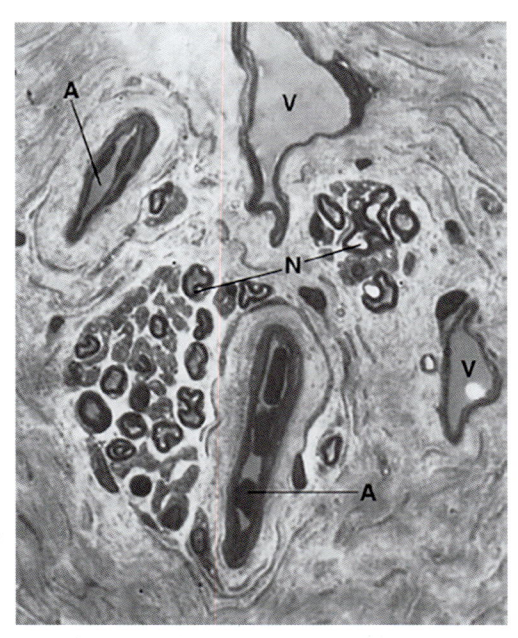

图 2.19 来自牙髓中央部分，显示三联小动脉（A）、静脉（V）和神经（N）

早期使用特定淋巴标记物研究牙髓内淋巴毛细血管的研究最近受到了争议[64, 119, 133, 218]后。

2.3.3 神经

牙髓中存在有髓神经和无髓神经（图 2.21），其中大多数是感觉神经。牙髓的感觉神经支配非常有效，主要终止于成牙本质层、前期牙本质和 0.1mm 矿化的冠部牙本质的内部，在那里神经与成牙本质突非常接近[27, 41]（图 2.22）。至少有 6 种牙齿感觉神经纤维类型，它们的分布有特定的区域，集中在血管、冠部牙髓和牙本质的特定区域（表 2.1）。感觉纤维在牙髓角尖端附近特别

密集，此处的敏感度也最高，然后逐渐向釉牙本质交界处（DEJ）减少。只有少数神经末梢存在于根髓和牙本质-牙髓边界[23]。牙髓的神经支配与微血管密切相关[90]。血管由感觉纤维和交感神经纤维支配，并且在颈部牙髓中也有一些其他的交感神经纤维[23, 90]。痛觉神经纤维可以感知损伤，并引起反射性收缩，限制了初始损伤的程度；它们还通过增强炎症、免疫和愈合机制促进修复。牙髓周围神经纤维分泌各种神经肽，激活靶细胞质膜上的受体，影响组织稳态、

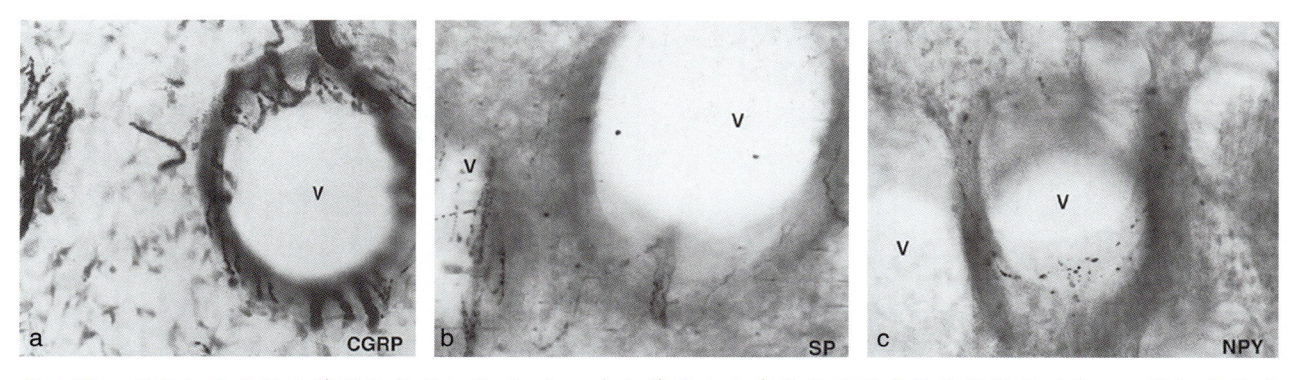

图 2.20 猫的尖牙牙髓血管的连续横切面（V）。在血管壁中含有神经肽的感觉神经纤维网络。a. 降钙素基因相关肽。b. P 物质（SP）。c. 神经肽 Y（NPY）（经 Acta Odontologica Scandinavica 许可引用[81]）

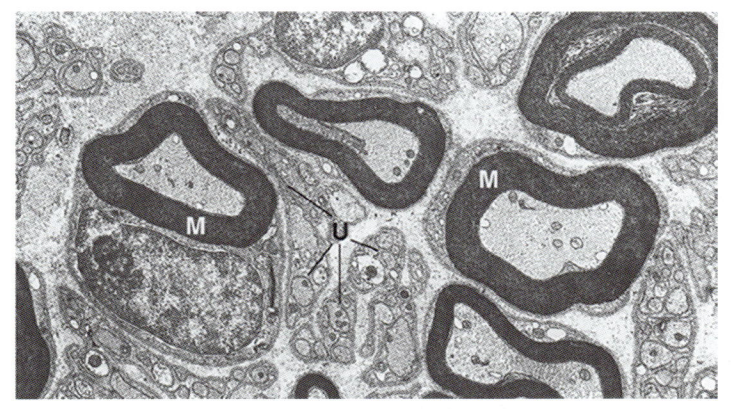

图 2.21 电子显微图显示了髓鞘中央部分的神经纤维，有髓鞘（M）和无髓鞘（U）神经纤维（经 Acta Odontologica Scandinavica 许可引用[41]）

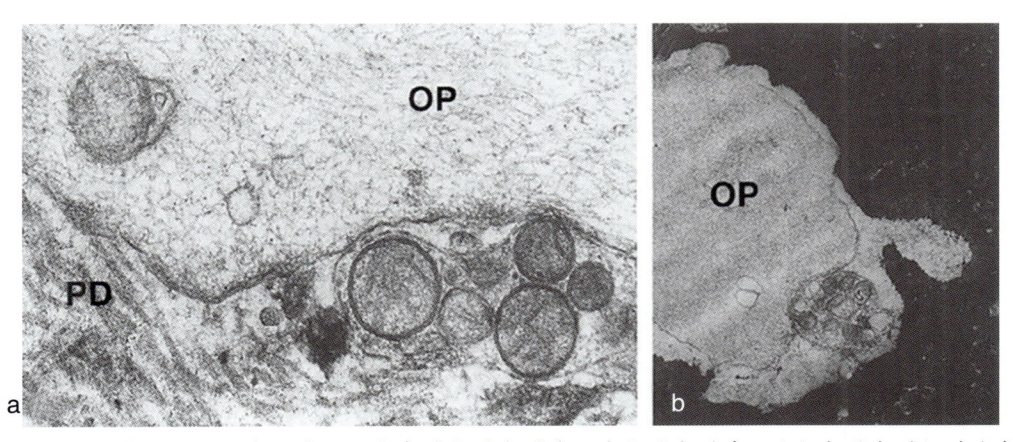

图 2.22 成牙本质细胞突周间隙中的神经纤维在前期牙本质（PD）和牙本质中，毗邻成牙本质细胞突起（OP）（经 Acta Odontologica Scandinavica 许可引用[41]）

血流、免疫细胞功能、炎症和愈合。这种现象被称为神经源性炎症，它发生在没有直接的化学、热或微生物刺激的情况下[19, 23, 30]。一方面，神经纤维能调整其自身的功能、细胞化学成分和结构以适应组织条件[23, 65]。另一方面，肾上腺素能激动剂（具有血管收缩作用）可能直接抑制牙齿伤害感受器传入神经纤维[31, 76]，环境条件（如pH）可以调节伤害感受器传入神经活动，并可能对牙痛的临床发展和缓解具有重要意义[69]。这些例子证明了组织-神经的双向相互作用和神经可塑性，尤其突出表现在痛觉感觉纤维上，这是牙齿神经支配的主要组成部分（图2.20）[23]。

2.3.4 髓石

髓石是不连续的或弥漫的牙髓钙化。一颗牙齿可能含有一个或多个髓石，分布在冠部或根部牙髓中，大小不一。牙髓钙化的具体原因在很大程度上仍然是个谜。外部刺激（龋齿、磨损）可能诱发牙髓钙化，但髓石也会出现在没有明显原因的牙齿上（如阻生的第三磨牙）。随着年龄的增长，其发生率似乎会增加，特别是在外部刺激的累积作用下[67]。与年龄有关的牙髓钙化已发现与血管和神经纤维有关。从结构上看，有"真性"髓石，其内有成牙本质细胞（或类成牙本质细胞），并含有牙本质小管；还有"假性"髓石，有或多或少的管状钙化，也被称为萎缩性钙化[171]。区分"真"和"假"牙髓结石可能是人为的，因为单个髓石中可以同时存在有小管和无小管的牙本质（图2.23）。髓室中大的髓石可能会堵塞根管口或根管，这可能会使器械进入根尖的过程变得复杂[67, 208]。除了给根管治疗带来困难外，髓石似乎没有任何其他意义[67]。

2.4 牙髓炎症

牙髓被包裹在牙本质和牙釉质中，形成了一个低顺应性环境，这在人体炎症组织反应方面是独一无二的。无论牙髓性质如何（化学、机械或热），外部刺激都会引起牙髓的局部炎症反应，

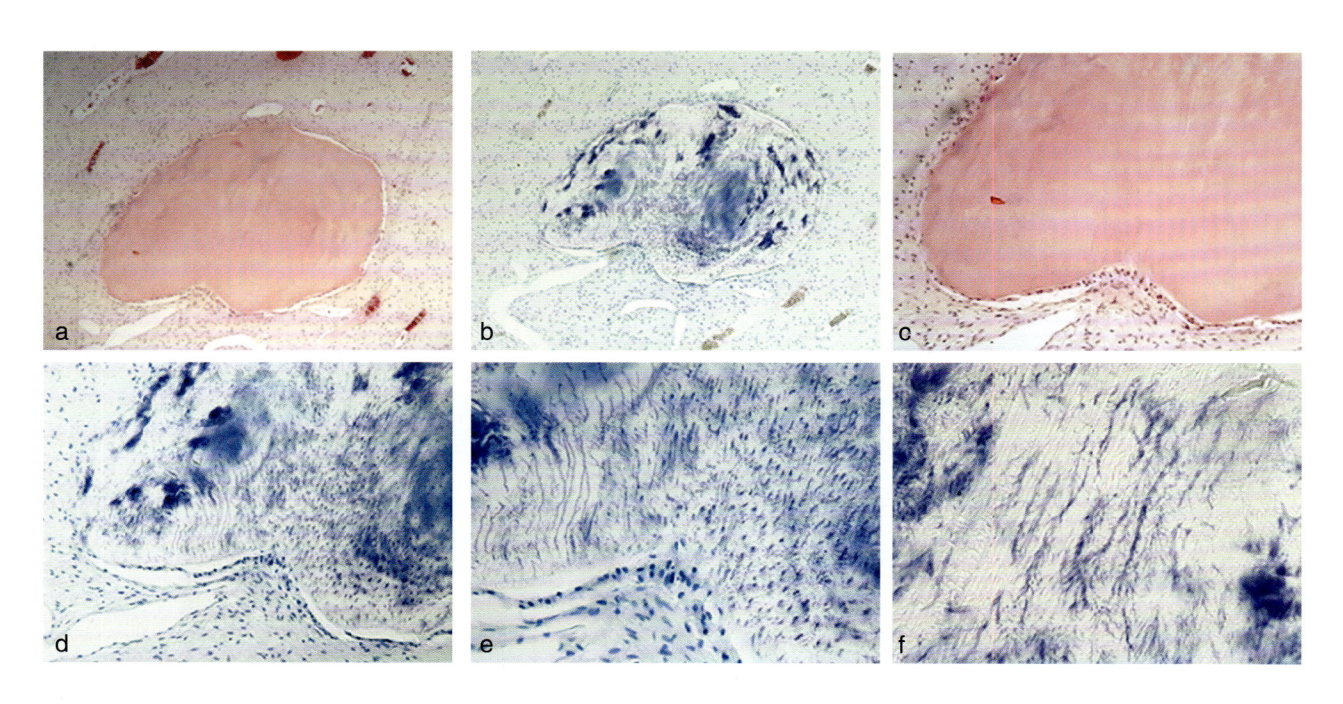

图2.23 约3mm髓石，用苏木精-伊红（HE）染色（a、c）和甲苯胺蓝（b、d~f）染色。a、b.甲苯胺蓝呈异质结构，而HE染色呈固体状。c.a图的左下角放大。成牙本质细胞样细胞排列在牙髓结石的下缘，左侧无细胞。d.甲苯胺蓝染色的相同区域显示成牙本质细胞样细胞处的管状结构，而没有细胞的区域则没有小管。e.d图放大。左侧为纵向切开形成良好的小管，右侧为沿小管方向切开的组织较松散的小管。f.在髓石的另一部分，小管稀疏，有许多细支和微支（经 Endodontic Topics 许可引用[208]）

其特征是血管扩张和血流阻力降低（图 2.24）。血管扩张和免疫细胞的早期募集主要由感觉神经通过释放血管活性神经肽来调节（表 2.1）（图 2.25）[30]。感觉神经的相关作用在研究中得到了证实，其中去神经支配导致免疫潜能细胞显著减少[57]，并在牙髓暴露后急剧加速牙髓坏死[24]。血管扩张和阻力降低导致血管内压和毛细血管血流增加，进而引起白细胞渗出，血清蛋白和液体渗入组织，这主要发生在成牙本质细胞层下区域[201]。血管通透性的增加和蛋白质的积累可能发生得很快，在窝洞制备 4 h 后就可以明显观察到[201]。血管反应的目的是提供炎症细胞和消除该区域的微生物毒素和代谢废物。然而，如果外部刺激超过了一定的阈值水平（如来自龋齿病变的持续和加剧的微生物刺激），牙髓反应就有可能不限于限定的区域。蛋白质和液体的渗入以及细胞含量的增加导致组织水肿，组织压力随之升高。在几乎所有的其他组织中，这将导致肿胀。但在牙髓的低顺应性环境中组织压力可能增加到超过了静脉压力，导致静脉被压迫（图 2.24）。随后，由于静脉回流受阻，流动阻力增加，血流量也随之减少。缓慢的血流导致红细胞和其他血细胞的聚集和局部血液黏度的升高，这进一步减少了血流。随之而来的局部缺氧、代谢废物和二氧化碳的增加以及 pH 的降低会导致邻近血管结构的血管扩张，从而导致炎症的扩散（图 2.24）。局部炎症反应有时会导致局部坏死（局部牙髓脓肿），有时被称为渐进性坏死，即部分牙髓坏死和感染，其余部分则出现不可逆的炎症[2, 115]（图 2.11）。基质金属蛋白酶（MMP）是降解胶原和其他细胞外基质蛋白的酶，由成牙本质细胞[206-207, 211]，尤其是由炎症细胞（PMN，即白细胞、巨噬细胞和浆细胞）产生，旨在限制感染的扩散。无论是化学因素[204]还是遗传因素[136, 220]，MMP 功能的损伤都会引起根尖病变的发生。然而，不受控制的酶活性也可能导致组织破坏的增加[4, 72, 183, 211, 219]。如果这种恶性循环继续下去，它将慢慢扩散并最终导致牙髓的完全坏死（图 2.24）。

表 2.1　牙髓神经纤维

纤维类型	感觉	激活	终端位点
感觉神经			
Aβ	前期疼痛 锐痛	机械：振动、牙本质液流动 电流（低压） 化学物质：芥子油、血清素	原发：前期牙本质、成牙本质细胞 继发：牙本质、牙髓
Aδ（快速）	前期疼痛 锐痛	极低温度 机械：振动、牙本质液流动 电流（中压） 化学物质：芥子油、血清素	原发：牙本质、前期牙本质、成牙本质细胞 继发：牙髓
Aδ（慢速）	疼痛	极低温度 电流（高压） 牙髓损伤（ATP） 化学物质：辣椒素	原发：牙髓 继发：血管
多模态 C 纤维	疼痛	极高温度 电流（高压） 牙髓损伤（ATP）	原发：牙髓 继发：血管
沉寂型 C 纤维	疼痛	化学成分：辣椒素、组胺、缓激肽	原发：牙髓 继发：血管
C 纤维类	疼痛	电流（高压）、组织损伤（？）	原发：成牙本质细胞、牙髓、血管
交感神经			
C 纤维		交感神经激活、炎症介质	原发：血管、牙髓

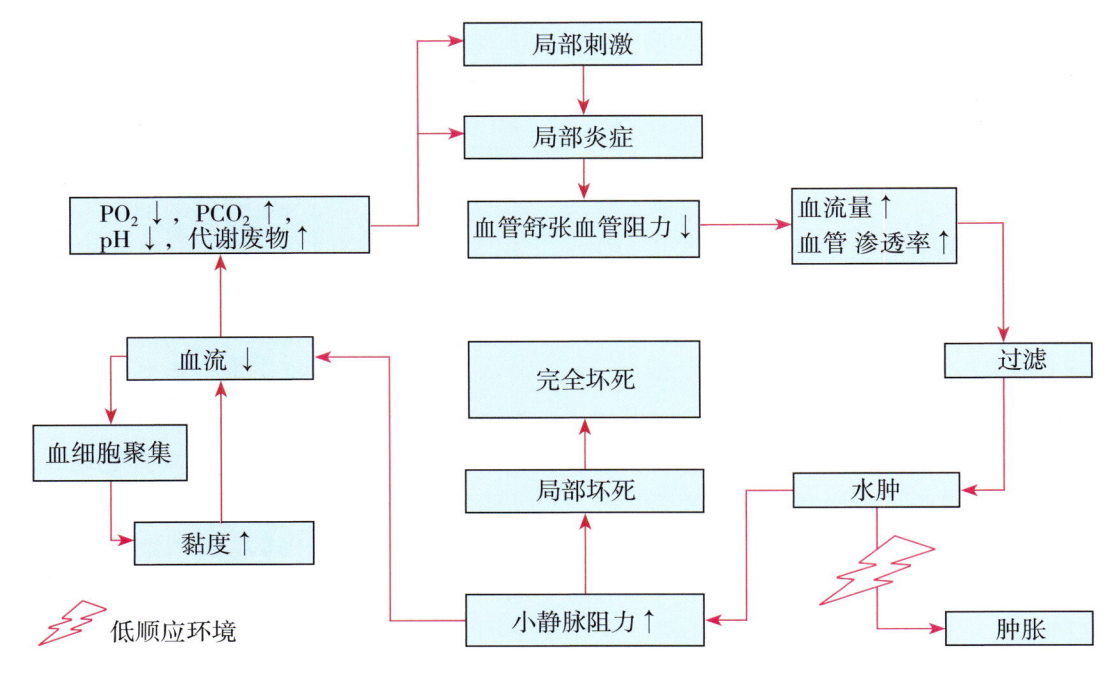

图 2.24　龋病导致的牙髓组织局限性炎症反应，其邻近组织完整性未受破坏。在炎症部位，炎症因子会导致血管大小和血液流速改变。如果炎症反应持续存在，炎症因子不断释放，如此恶性循环将先导致牙髓局部坏死，直至牙髓全部坏死（改变自文献 201）

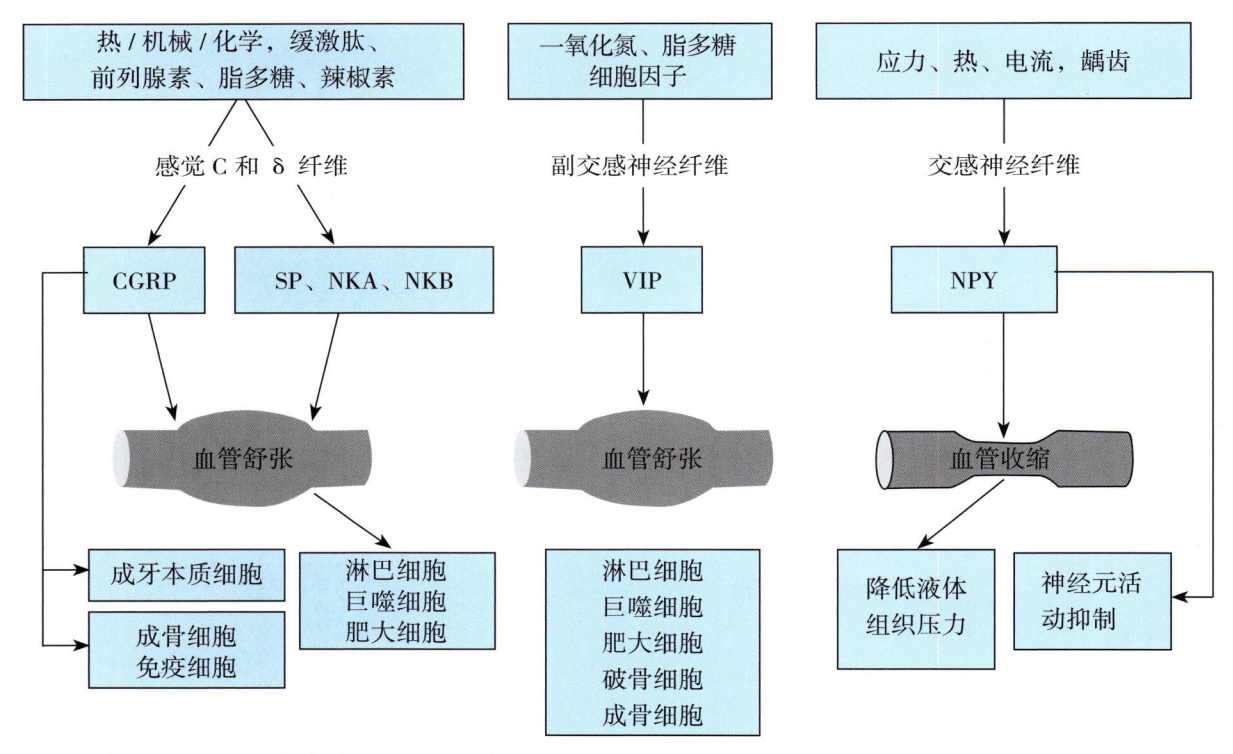

图 2.25　神经肽的释放及其在神经源性炎症中的作用。不同的刺激和炎症介质，如缓激肽（BK）和前列腺素（PG）、脂多糖（LPS）和辣椒素可导致 C 纤维和 Aδ 感觉纤维释放降钙素基因相关肽（CGRP）和速激肽 P 物质（SP）、神经激肽 A（NKA）和神经激肽 B（NKB）。除了血管舒张，它们还能激活免疫细胞和成牙本质细胞。血管活性肠多肽（vascular active intestinal polypeptide，VIP）是由一氧化氮（NO）、脂多糖（LPS）和细胞因子刺激的副交感神经纤维释放出来，可舒张血管，并对不同的免疫细胞发挥免疫调节作用。交感神经纤维释放神经肽 Y（NPY），导致血管收缩和减少液体组织压力。在正常情况下，NPY 也会抑制神经元活动（改编自文献 30）

牙髓血管具有控制炎症反应和坏死扩散的功能。动脉 U 形回路和动静脉吻合（AVA）可使部分动脉血流偏离炎症区（图 2.26）。此外，动脉分支点处存在狭窄或括约肌，可以调控流向炎症区域的微动脉的血流量。控制血流可以调节组织压力的水平，从而使炎症区及其周围的血管能够发挥充分的功能[201]。交感神经纤维释放的神经肽 Y 也会引起血管收缩，这也会导致液体组织压力降低[30]。牙髓的愈合和再生过程需要血管生成。从牙本质或牙髓细胞中释放的促血管生成因子和抗血管生成因子、神经肽和缺氧状态共同调控牙髓血管化的过程[3, 10, 71, 174, 218]，而炎症导致毛细血管生成。

2.4.1 牙髓中的免疫细胞

人类牙髓中含有常驻的免疫活性细胞。这些细胞参与维持组织稳态，并能够对即将发生的感染产生先天适应性免疫应答[73-74]。引发这些反应的炎症介质从龋坏牙本质或牙髓常驻细胞中释放出来[38, 187, 189]。炎性趋化因子、调节免疫和炎症反应的细胞因子构成的复杂网络进一步调控了初始炎症的消退或进展[73-74, 82]。它们或由成牙本质细胞[73-74, 85, 116, 159]、牙髓细胞[38, 73-74]产生，或由被吸引到炎症部位的免疫细胞产生（主要方式）。介质的作用具有时间依赖性：如果炎症消退，低水平的促炎介质可能会促进组织修复，而在慢性炎症中，修复机制则会受到抑制[38]。

未成熟的树突状细胞（DCs）和 T 细胞作为机体对龋齿先天性免疫反应的一部分，在免疫监测中有重要作用。Ⅱ类主要组织相容性复合体（MHC）阳性的未成熟树突状细胞主要位于成牙本质细胞层下，也位于成牙本质细胞-前期牙本质区[40, 52, 153]，其中一些树突状细胞将其细胞质突起延伸至牙本质小管中[153-154]。它们检测微生物抗原，启动成熟过程，然后转移到区域淋巴结，将抗原呈递给初始 T 细胞。在体外，变形链球菌可以在 24h 内将单核细胞迅速转化为成熟的 DCs[75]，这可能有助于炎症牙髓内 DCs 的局部成熟。作为对龋病的反应，位于牙本质下层的 DCs 浸润成牙本质细胞层，并侵入反应性牙本质，这一过程受到从牙本质中释放或由成牙本质细胞[54]分泌的 TGF-β 的吸引[40]。在成熟过程中，DCs 产生促炎细胞因子和趋化因子，将循环中未成熟的 DCs、DC 前体细胞和 T 细胞招募到炎症组织中[114]。

健康牙髓中主要的 T 细胞类型是记忆性 CD8+T 细胞[54, 61, 94]，它们比 CD4+T 细胞具有更强的跨内皮细胞迁移能力。CD8+T 细胞在正常牙髓中的功能尚不清楚，但通常认为 CD8+T 细胞具有免疫监测作用[110]。自然杀伤（NK）细胞存在于血液中，可通过外渗进入炎症部位影响炎症趋化因子。在健康的牙髓中可能存在非常少量的 NK 细胞，它们也可能参与免疫监测[61]。在健康人牙髓中，调节性 T 细胞（T-reg）[20]不存在或仅以非常低的数量存在[61]。

中性粒细胞和巨噬细胞是先天性免疫反应中的专职吞噬细胞。组织巨噬细胞一般来源于循环中的单核细胞[73]，异质性高，且受其微环境的影响。在完整牙齿的牙髓中，可能存在少量巨噬细胞[93]，甚至更少的中性粒细胞[61]。当龋病局限于 DEJ 或外层牙本质时，巨噬细胞的数量在龋病损害早期会显著增加[93-94]。巨噬细胞可能在牙髓炎早期被激活，通过增加血管通透性来保护牙髓，并通过蛋白酶来清除外来抗原和受损组织[73, 94]。活化的巨噬细胞在先天性和适应性免疫反应中都能有效地消除病原体，同时通过清除衰老细胞而

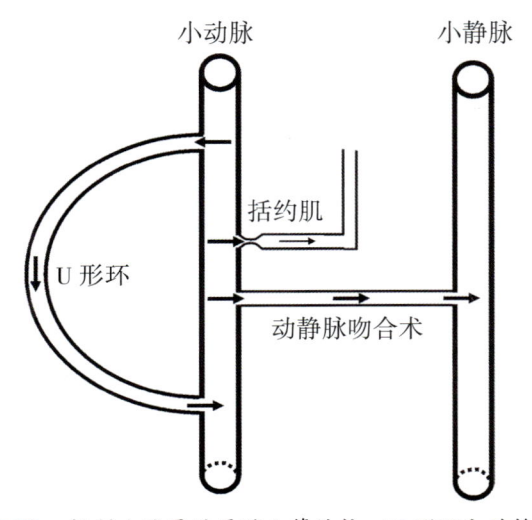

图 2.26 控制血流量的牙髓血管结构。U 形环和动静脉吻合术（AVA）可以被打开，使血流从炎症区重新流出，从而降低间质组织压力。小动脉分支的平滑肌收缩可以限制或阻塞小动脉的血流（修改自文献 201）

在组织稳态中发挥重要作用，并在炎症后组织的重塑和修复中发挥重要作用。中性粒细胞在早期和可复性牙髓炎中可能并不重要，因为浅龋的牙髓组织中的中性粒细胞很少，但当龋损接近牙髓时，中性粒细胞的数量显著增加[94]。

2.4.2 成牙本质细胞作为免疫细胞

在牙髓-牙本质复合体中，成牙本质细胞是抵御外部刺激的第一道细胞防线，它们通过多种方式参与牙髓-牙本质复合体炎症和（或）免疫反应的启动和发展[53, 68, 116, 217]。成牙本质细胞表达Toll样受体（TLR），这是一组跨膜糖蛋白，可识别微生物和病毒颗粒、真菌蛋白、病毒和细菌的RNA和DNA[194]。TLR启动先天性免疫反应的早期激活，如炎症细胞的募集、抗菌肽的产生和DCS[53]的成熟，并可能参与反应性牙本质的形成[33]。在人类中已确定的10种TLR中，*TLR1~TLR9*基因在成熟的人成牙本质细胞或体外培养的成牙本质细胞样细胞中表达[48, 53, 158]，其中对分别识别革兰氏阳性细菌的脂磷壁酸（LTA）、革兰氏阴性细菌的脂多糖（LPS）和病毒RNA的*TLR2*、*TLR4*和*TLR8*的研究最为广泛[53, 98, 147, 158, 217]（图2.27）。原则上，成牙本质细胞表达的TLR能够识别几乎所有重要的微生物成分。

防御素是一组小分子（3k~5 kDa）多肽，具有广谱抗菌、免疫细胞趋化和灭活细菌毒素活性[97]。在人类中发现了两个亚家族的17种防御素，即α-防御素和β-防御素[97]。人β-防御素-1（hBD-1）和hBD-2在体内和体外均由成牙本质细胞表达[46-47]，并被认为参与了人牙髓[46]的先天宿主防御。hBD-2是TLR4[15]的宿主衍生配体，抑制TLR信号传导的核心通路[80]，可阻断变异链球菌诱导的体外成牙本质细胞样细胞[45]中IL-6和IL-8基因表达的增加。因此，成牙本质细胞衍生的hBD也可能参与成牙本质细胞免疫防御的自分泌或内分泌调节。

蛋白酶激活受体（PAR）是一类G蛋白偶联受体，可通过蛋白酶进行不可逆的蛋白水解激活。它们参与调控多种生物过程，如炎症、止血、血栓形成和胚胎发育[156]，以及骨骼生长和骨修复[62]。PAR-2存在于牙髓成纤维细胞样细胞中[121, 145]，PAR-1和PAR-12存在于人成牙本质细胞[9]中。在龋病刺激下，成牙本质细胞和牙髓组织中的PAR的表达水平显著增加[121, 145]，表明PAR在修复性牙本质形成和（或）牙髓炎症中发挥调节作用。

尽管成牙本质细胞似乎在调节牙髓-牙本质复合体炎症反应的启动和进展方面具有独特的作用，但在任何临床治疗方法得到证实之前，还需要进行更多的研究。例如，最具潜力的修复性牙本质生成诱导因子[转化生长因子β（TGF-β）]会

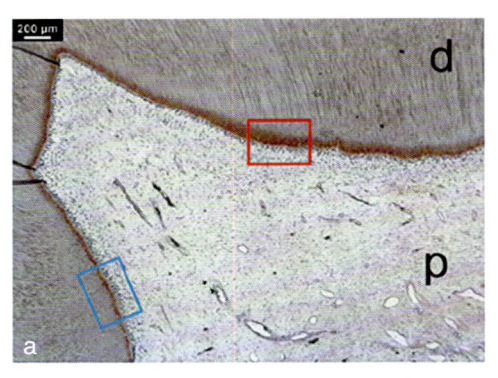

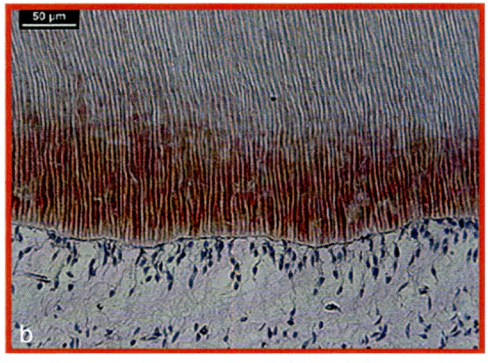

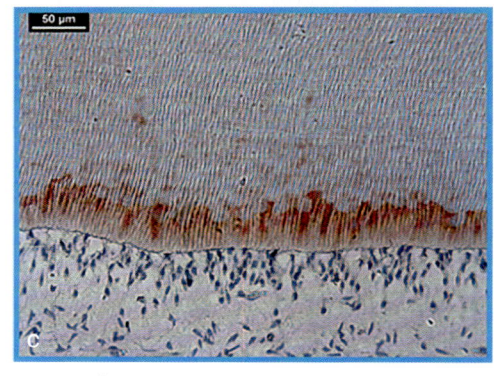

图2.27 人第三磨牙TLR8免疫组化染色。a. 牙齿所有部位的牙本质-牙髓边缘都有强烈的染色，不同部位的染色模式不同。b. 咬合面的牙本质-牙髓边界（图a中红色方框标记区放大）。c. 近髓腔壁（图a中蓝色方框标记区放大）（经*International Endodontic Journal*许可引用[158]）

影响成熟人成牙本质细胞的炎性白细胞介素生成[159]，抑制 TLR2 和 TLR4 的表达，并降低体外成牙本质样细胞对龋病病原体的反应[86]。目前大部分数据来自体外研究，这与临床实际情况存在较大差异。牙髓-牙本质复合体的复杂性要求进行详细的体内或原位研究，并尽可能采用接近临床实际的研究方法。

2.5　牙髓痛觉和过敏

对人类的心理学研究表明，牙齿只能感知三种主要感觉。首先是基于 A_β 和 A_δ 纤维快速传导的，最初定义不明确的低刺激"预疼痛"感觉。这种感觉会在更高的刺激强度下转变为剧烈的疼痛。此外，还有与 C 纤维和可能的慢速 A_δ 信号有关的钝痛感觉。牙齿的伤害感受神经元可能具有与其他组织不同的特性[36]。牙神经的一个不寻常的特征是所有类型的神经纤维对牙齿的强烈冷刺激都极为敏感[23]。牙齿疼痛与其他组织的疼痛有几个显著区别。特别是在牙髓炎时，轻微的热或空气刺激，在其他部位可能仅被感知为冷、热或是轻柔的"微风"，却在牙齿上容易引发疼痛。牙髓的低顺应性环境、神经末梢的增生以及牙齿传入神经元的神经肽表达变化可能导致痛觉灵敏度的增加[181]。因此，任何类型的刺激作用于牙齿都会导致疼痛感，这与身体其他组织的情况不同[23, 36]。

在完全健康的牙髓中，感觉神经也会传递疼痛感，但炎症会加剧这些感觉。痛觉感受器增生被认为是牙本质损伤的早期神经反应，与反应性牙本质形成有关，但与修复性牙本质形成无关[23, 40]。对动物单神经纤维的分析显示，在这些条件下，A 类纤维激活的牙本质感受区扩大[150]，中枢神经系统可塑性增强[181]。

牙本质过敏是由支配牙髓的三叉神经节痛觉神经元（牙本质的主要传入神经）被激活而引起的。这种激活的确切机制尚不完全清楚。流体动力学机制（牙本质小管内的液体运动被靠近牙本质-牙髓边界的神经末梢检测到）已被广泛接受，并成为牙齿痛觉感觉的主导理论。然而，越来越多的关于其他潜在机制的证据导致了其他可能的理论：①神经理论，牙本质小管中的神经末梢直接对外界刺激作出反应；②成牙本质传感器理论，成牙本质细胞本身可以作为疼痛传感器[36, 126]（图 2.28）。

在流体动力学理论中，牙本质小管中伤害感受性传入神经的机械感受器提供了一种潜在的疼痛传导机制（图 2.28），而不仅仅是简单的机械拉伸。即使正常的咀嚼力也可以产生足够的流体流动，以激发假定的机械感受器[163]，尤其是在水平负荷的情况下[191]。瞬时受体电位 TRPV1、TRPV2，瞬时受体电位锚蛋白 1（TRPA1）和瞬时受体电位（TRPM8）在牙齿传入神经中的表达[36, 105-106]，使其成为这一机制的理想候选者。在疼痛性的不可逆牙髓炎中，TRPA1 阳性轴突的显著增加[106]和 TRPA1 在冷感知中的作用[103]进一步表明该受体在牙齿过敏中的重要性。

电压门控 Ca^{2+}、Na^+ 和 K^+ 通道，Ca^{2+} 激活的 K^+ 通道，钙库操纵性钙离子通道和 Na^+/Ca^{2+} 交换器[7-8, 26, 89, 120, 125-126, 182, 222]的表达表明成牙本质细胞具有兴奋性。实际上，体外电刺激可以在成牙本质细胞中诱发动作电位[8, 91, 126]。人成牙本质细胞还具有电耦合特性，允许信息在大量相邻细胞间传输，使得在电刺激后，对外界刺激的感受野可能远大于刺激区域[91]。人成牙本质细胞至少表达 TRPV1、TRPV4、TRPA1、TRPM8，机械敏感的 TWIK 相关的 K^+ 通道（TREK-1），pH 敏感的上皮 Na^+（EnaC）通道和大麻素受体（CB1）[35, 49-50, 106, 125, 168, 188, 195]。由于成牙本质细胞和神经传入纤维之间不存在突触结构，ATP[37, 49, 118, 182]和谷氨酸[35, 107, 152]被认为是成牙本质细胞和神经传入物之间的信号介质。嘌呤能受体（P2X）[6, 99, 105]和谷氨酸受体（mGluR5）[107, 152]均存在于牙髓神经纤维、Raschkow 的成牙本质细胞下丛、成牙本质细胞层甚至牙本质小管中。

成牙本质细胞感觉功能的另一种可能机制是初级纤毛（primary cilia）。初级纤毛是几乎存在于所有脊椎动物细胞上的单个非运动鞭毛细胞器，具有多种信号传导功能[63]。初级纤毛在成骨细胞、骨细胞和软骨细胞中也起着血流传感器的作用[128, 223]。在骨细胞中，纤毛负责细胞活动的变化[128]，提示其在骨重塑中发挥作用。成牙本质细胞表达初级纤毛[39, 123, 199]，它们可能参与成牙本质细胞的极化和终末分化，以及影响细胞向牙髓

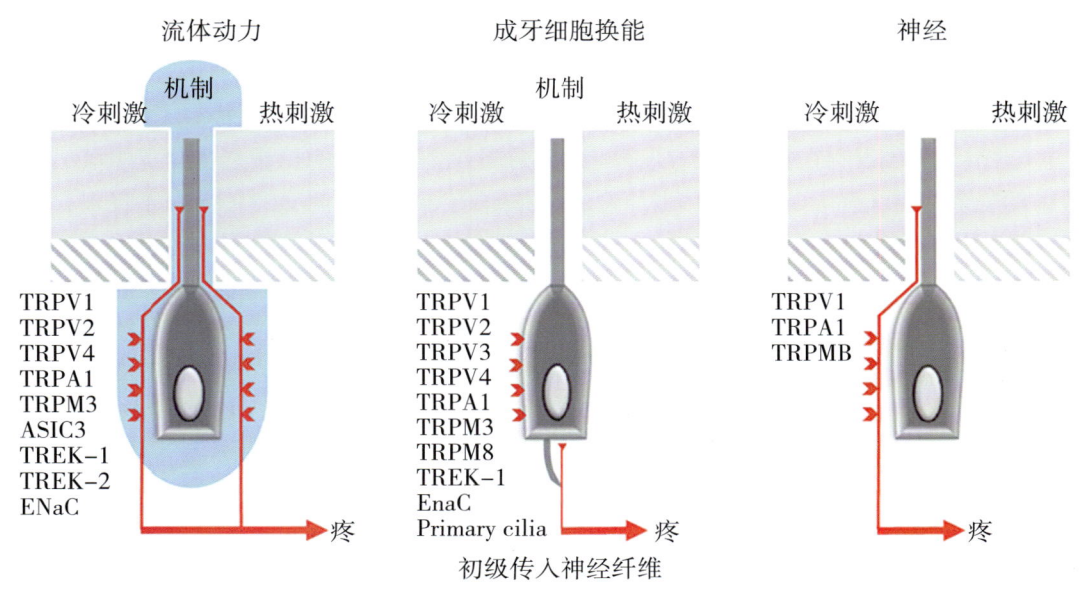

图2.28 流体动力学机制、成牙细胞换能器和牙痛觉神经理论。不同的外部刺激引起的流体运动最终激活口腔初级传入的机械感受器。在神经理论中，牙本质小管的神经传入受外界刺激的直接激活。列出了机械敏感分子和热敏分子的候选分子（改编自文献36）

移动的信号[39, 63, 123]。纤毛可能对牙本质液流动的机械刺激[124]或来自牙本质或牙髓细胞外环境或两者的其他信号作出反应。在成牙本质细胞中，初级纤毛位于体内细胞的顶端[39,199]，这与骨细胞的情况相似[128]。这种假定的传感器功能、成牙本质初级纤毛和神经纤维之间的密切关系（图2.29）以及产生动作电位的能力表明，成牙本质细胞的初级纤毛可能在牙齿疼痛传递中发挥作用[199]。

神经理论基于牙齿传入神经元表达的受体，这些受体参与了将特定刺激转化为电脉冲[36]。在冠部牙本质中，特别是在牙髓角区，传入神经纤维可深入牙本质小管约100μm[23, 27]。牙齿传入神经元中存在伤害感受和热敏性TRP受体，有助于直接感知疼痛，而不需要流体力学或成牙本质细胞传导刺激（图2.28）。

2.6 牙髓－牙本质复合体增龄性变化

尽管成牙本质细胞形成牙本质的能力终身存在，但也会表现出衰老的迹象。最初的迹象出现在原发性牙本质形成的过渡阶段，此时成牙本质表型[39]发生显著变化（图2.30），这与转录活性的差异[185]和因拥挤导致的成牙本质细胞凋亡增加有关[56, 137]。人类成熟的成牙本质细胞还会形成与年龄相关的自噬溶酶体系统，其中具有自噬泡以促进细胞成分[39]的更新和降解。自噬是一个具有"抗衰老"功能的调节过程，在大多数寿命长的细胞中活跃，该功能由溶酶体介导的自我消化途径维持细胞稳态。在成牙本质细胞中，自噬活性被认为是一种重要的生存机制。自噬也可以构成细胞死亡的另一种机制，称为"自噬Ⅱ型程序性细胞死亡"（Type Ⅱ型PCD）[39]。

随着牙髓的衰老和修复性牙本质的逐渐积累，牙髓组织趋于纤维化，与冠部牙髓相比，根部牙髓中成牙本质细胞和成纤维细胞的数量减少[42, 87, 146]。成牙本质细胞和成纤维细胞的减少更为明显[42, 146]。毛细血管内皮细胞形态和细胞骨架发生改变，包括跨内皮运输[52]增加、神经支配减弱并改变其细胞化学特性[23]。一项对年轻人和老年人牙齿的基因表达的全面比较研究表明，衰老牙齿中与细胞和组织发育、细胞生长和增殖、血液和免疫系统发育和功能有关的功能基因组表达降低；而凋亡相关基因表达增加[210]。总体而言，这些变化可能反映了组织破坏时再生和修复能力的下降。

2.6.1 牙本质的增龄性变化

在临床牙髓病学中，牙髓－牙本质复合体最重要的年龄相关变化是即使在完整的牙齿中，牙髓腔和根管也会逐渐闭塞[5, 130, 146, 167]，这是因为继发性牙本质缓慢形成（图2.31）。与冠部相比，根部牙本质厚度的相对增加得更为显著[146]。外部刺激（如龋齿、修复治疗等）可能会显著加速这一过程。在切牙、尖牙和前磨牙中，闭塞始于冠部方向；但在磨牙中，牙髓腔底部牙本质也经常向顶部生长。这种闭塞可能会使根管的定位变得困难[170]，并导致初始根管准备和顺滑通路的建立也更加困难。

增龄变化对牙本质机械性能的影响一直存在争议，但最近的研究强烈表明，增龄变化会导致矿化牙本质的强度和弹性变化。牙本质的抗拉强度可能会随着小管闭塞而增加[129]，但这是以降低弯曲强度为代价的[184]。最重要的是，在老化的牙本质中，由于牙本质小管的管周牙本质闭塞，导致矿物质与胶原比增加[11, 144, 184]，从而增加了硬度，特别是外层牙本质[144]。因此，与年轻牙本质相比，老化牙本质的疲劳裂纹扩展指数降低了40%左右[13]，持久强度降低了48%左右[12]，疲劳裂纹扩展速度加快了100倍以上[13]。牙本质弯曲强度降低约20 MPa/10年，并且与小管闭塞密切相关[11, 184]（图2.32）。根部牙本质中的小管同样会闭塞[198]（图2.33）。

人类根部牙本质的弯曲强度可能高于冠部牙本质[51, 184]，但同样会随着年龄的增长而降低[184, 228]，矿物质含量和硬度也会增加[226]。

有机成分的增龄变化似乎也对牙本质的机械性能有影响[12, 184, 228]。老化牙本质的交联程度更高[228]，并具有高水平的戊糖苷交联胶原[184]。这种非酶促晚期糖基化终末产物（AGE）在单

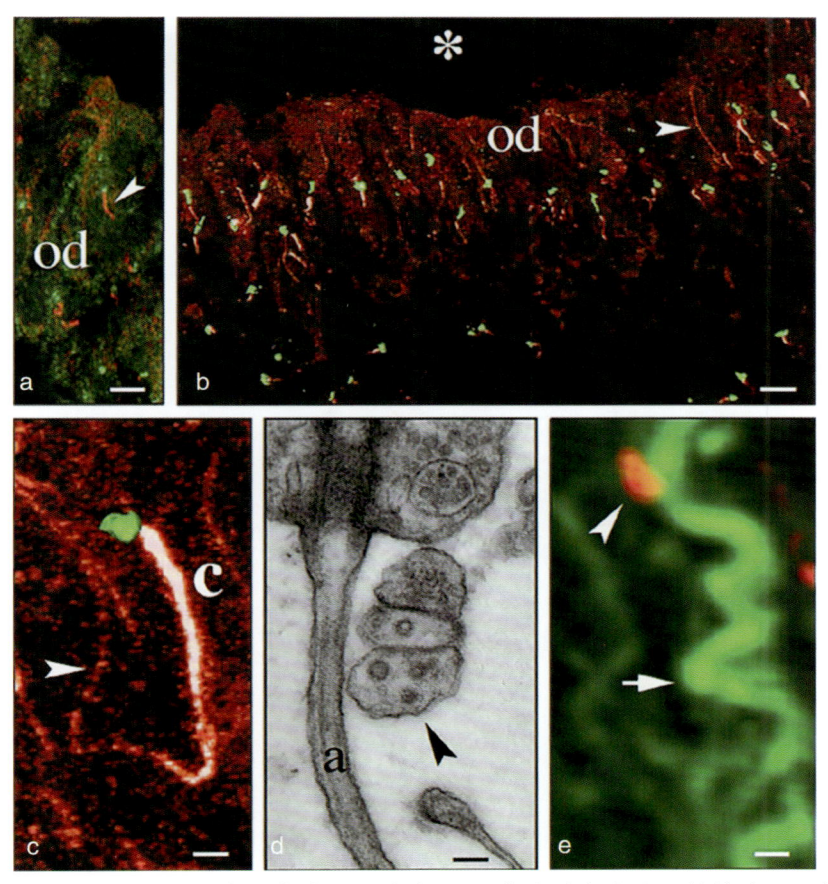

图2.29 人成牙细胞的原生纤毛，激光共聚焦显微镜（a~c、e）和透射电子显微镜（TEM）分析（d）。a. 箭头表示成牙本质细胞（od）原生纤毛轴突（比例尺：10 μm）。b. 绿色代表基部纤毛中的小根，红色代表纤毛；箭头为神经纤维。*：牙本质（比例尺：10 μm）。c. 初级纤毛轴突（尾巴）（c）与神经纤维（箭头）的密切关系；绿色表示成牙本质细胞细胞膜上纤毛基底体（比例尺：1.25μm）。d. 成牙细胞通过基底体产生的初生纤毛的TEM图像，与类似神经的结构密切接触（箭头）（比例尺：0.20μm）。e. 纤毛结构之间的密切接触（红色；箭头）和神经纤维（绿色；箭头）（比例尺：0.65μm）（经 *Journal of Dental Research* 许可用[199]）

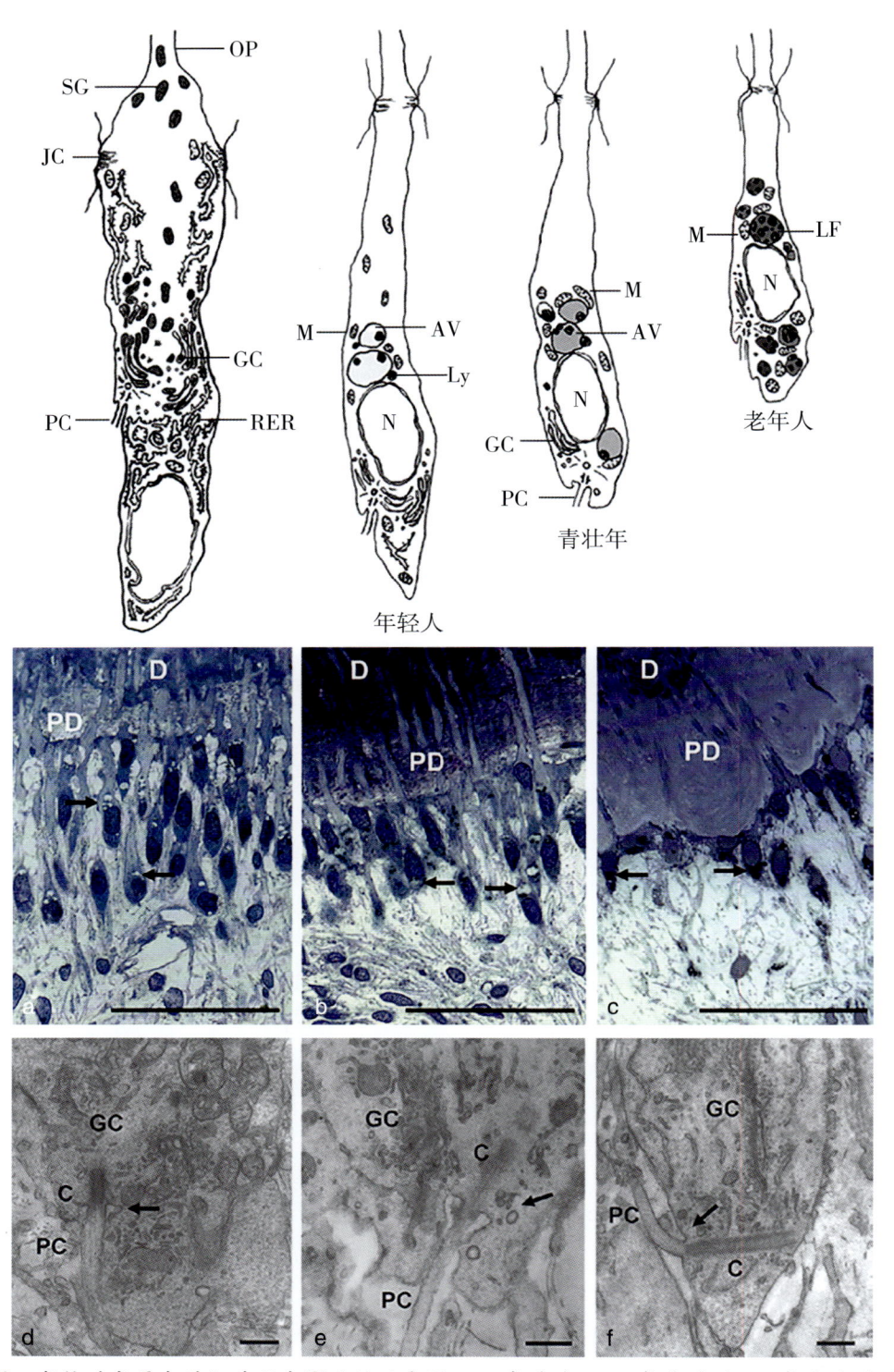

图 2.30 上图：年龄对成牙本质细胞形态影响的示意图。15 岁（a）、25 岁（b）和 75 岁（c）患者牙齿冠状面成牙细胞层的光学显微镜图像。在年轻和青壮年个体中，成牙本质细胞是柱状细胞，具有大的自噬空泡（图 a、图 b 中的箭头），而在老年患者的牙齿中，成牙本质细胞变得更短、更扁平，并在自噬空泡中积累致密的沉积物（图 c 中箭头）。d~f. 不同年龄的初生纤毛（PC）的透射电镜图像，显示 PC 在成牙本质细胞中是一个持久的结构。C：中心体。D：牙本质。GC：高尔基体。PD：前期牙本质。SG：分泌颗粒。JC：连接复合体。RER：粗面内质网。N：细胞核。Ly：溶酶体。比例尺：50μm（a~c）和 0.5μm（d~f）（经 *Journal of Dental Research* 许可引用[39]）

个胶原分子之间的交联使胶原基质变硬，且更加脆弱，并参与了骨质疏松患者的骨强度降低改变[177, 215]。同样，在人牙本质中，高水平的 AGE 显著降低了牙本质的弯曲强度，并在体外实验[139]和体内研究中都导致了老化牙本质的的机械强度降低[184]。

随着年龄的增长，牙本质有机基质也可能发生其他变化：基质降解酶的减少和丧失已经得到证实[132, 151, 196]，这可能也意味着其底物，即胶原蛋白和非胶原蛋白的变化。

2.6.2 龋病对牙本质的影响

龋病对牙的损害随着年龄的增长而发展和加重，对牙齿的修复具有极大的临床影响。牙科微创修复的目的是避免不必要地去除牙齿结构，龋齿窝洞制备仅限于去除受龋损感染的牙本质，将修复体与未受龋损影响的牙本质粘接。受龋损影响的牙本质的矿物质含量较低，牙本质有机成分的结构和组成发生了改变，包括胶原蛋白。这些变化降低了牙本质的硬度、刚度、拉伸强度、弹性模量和干燥时的收缩率[203]。因此，由于聚合应力和咬合力，复合体-牙本质界面及其下方的牙本质更容易发生内聚性破坏[202]。牙本质短时间暴露于乳酸[34]（乳酸是致龋菌产生的最重要的酸）也会导致牙本质疲劳强度显著降低，裂纹扩增速

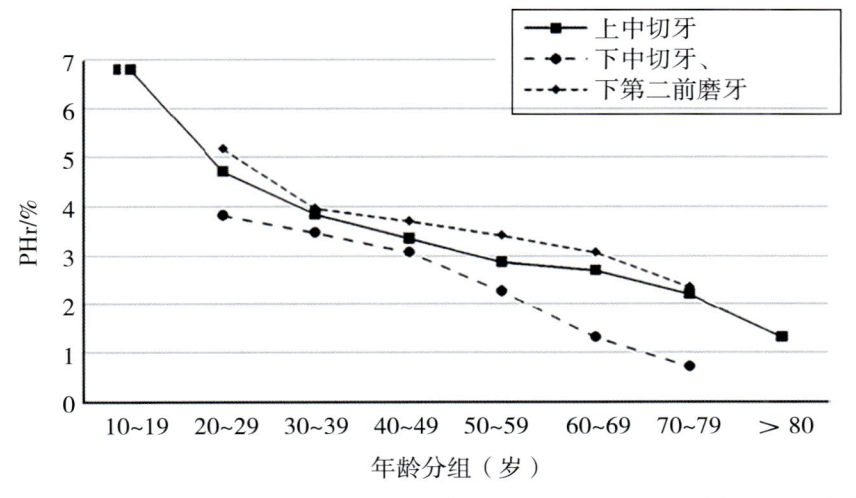

图 2.31 随着年龄的增长，髓腔缩小。PHr：牙髓体积占总硬组织体积的百分比（数据改编自文献 5 和 167）

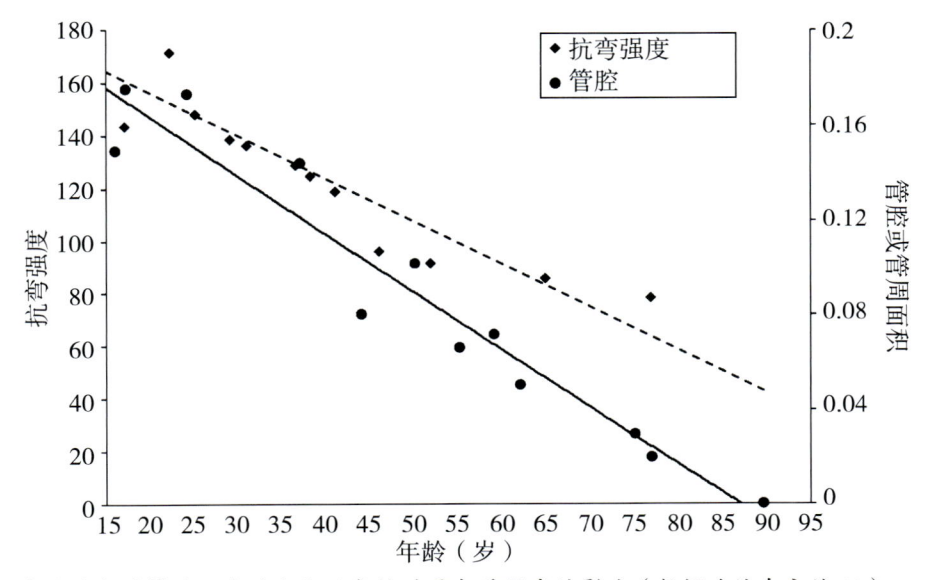

图 2.32 人第三磨牙牙本质管腔尺寸的变化及年龄对牙本质强度的影响（数据改编自文献 11）

率加快，疲劳裂纹扩展阻力降低[44, 155]。由于疲劳裂纹是不稳定断裂的前兆，乳酸暴露增加了在低咬合力下修复后牙齿折裂的可能性[155]。特别是牙髓治疗后的牙齿更容易折裂，这不仅是由于组织损失导致结构较弱，还因为与表层牙本质相比，深层牙本质中裂纹扩增所需的循环应力较低[92]。为了避免灾难性且不可修复的牙齿折裂，应以保护和保存剩余牙齿结构的方式进行修复治疗，特别是在牙髓治疗后。

2.7 牙周组织

牙周组织包括牙龈、牙周韧带（PDL）、牙槽骨和牙骨质（图2.34）。牙周组织的主要功能是辅助牙齿附着到牙槽骨。牙周组织实际上是一种嵌合型的纤维关节，其中锥形结构（牙根）通过纤维韧带插入牙槽窝。在人体中，牙周组织是唯一的嵌合型的关节，允许牙齿的位置进行微小的调整。牙组织是一种有弹性的悬吊装置，为咀嚼功能提供最佳条件。根尖周组织包括PDL、牙骨质和牙槽骨，对牙髓病学至关重要，下文将详细介绍这部分的牙周组织。

2.8 牙周韧带

PDL是致密的结缔组织，在致密的胶原纤维束之间散布着疏松的、岛状的间质结缔组织（图2.2，图2.34）。PDL的主要纤维从牙骨质延伸到牙槽骨。然而，每一根纤维并不完全跨越牙骨质和牙槽骨之间的全部距离，它们构成了一个复杂的分支和重新连接的纤维模式。它们以夏普（Sharpey）纤维（穿通纤维）的形式深深嵌入两个矿化组织中（图2.34，图2.35）。插入牙骨质的纤维比进入牙槽骨的纤维更细小，数量更多。

PDL中有四组主要纤维。牙槽嵴纤维从牙颈部的牙骨质向下延伸至牙槽嵴；水平纤维占据颈部三分之一的PDL；斜向纤维从牙槽骨向根尖方向延伸到牙骨质；根尖纤维从牙骨质向牙槽骨呈放射状延伸。

PDL的主要纤维具有功能性排列，不同组纤维对抗不同类型的力，包括抵抗牙齿旋转的力。虽然胶原蛋白是无弹性的，但由于纤维的波浪形走向，牙齿仍能进行轻微移动，使纤维在受力时拉伸。PDL血流和血压的变化可引起牙齿轻微的移动。血液和组织液也起到流体动力系统的作用，吸收咬合力。

2.8.1 牙周膜中的细胞

成纤维细胞是PDL中的主要细胞，位于主纤维之间的成纤维细胞呈细长形，而位于间质组织中的细胞则呈不规则或星形。成纤维细胞的功能是在正常更新和修复过程中维持胶原纤维，以及构成基质的糖胺聚糖和糖蛋白。巨噬细胞和肥大细胞，包括相关的细胞因子，也存在于正常的PDL中，并且在炎症期间显著增加。成牙骨质细胞位于牙骨质侧，成骨细胞位于牙槽骨侧。破骨细胞和破牙骨质细胞可以吸收骨质和牙齿。它们

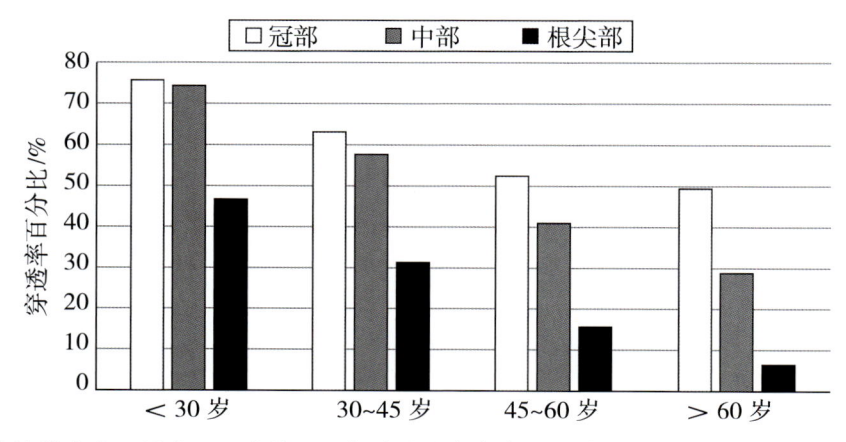

图2.33 在预备的根管内广泛孵育亚甲基蓝后，相对平均染色穿透率（占牙本质完整面积的百分比）（数据改编自文献198）

在 PDL 的更新、牙周（包括根尖）疾病和牙齿正畸移动期间发挥重要作用，在根尖周炎的发展中也起着重要的作用。破牙骨质细胞和破骨细胞在乳牙脱落和恒牙萌出过程中也发挥着重要作用。

交感神经切除可增加破骨细胞介导的骨吸收[113]和根部牙本质吸收[78]，这表明交感神经对破骨细胞和破牙骨质细胞有抑制作用。实验性牙齿移动研究证实，PDL 中的交感神经对粒细胞的募集也很重要[78]。在实验性诱导的根尖周病变中，交感神经对病变的大小、病变边缘破骨细胞的数量和病变内 IL-1α（白细胞介素-1α）的含量具有抑制作用[79]。

2.8.2 上皮细胞剩余

无论是发育中的牙齿还是成熟的牙齿，都被源自赫特维希上皮根鞘的一层连续的、呈网状分布的上皮细胞包围。这些所谓的 Malassez 上皮剩余（图 2.2）位于根部牙骨质附近，并在牙齿的整个生命周期内持续存在于牙周膜中[225]。Malassez 上皮剩余在 PDL 中持续存在的原因尚不清楚，但有观点认为这些细胞对防止牙齿固连和阻止骨向内生长具有重要作用[225]。刺激这些上皮细胞可诱导细胞增殖[66]，从而在病变周围形成囊肿内壁。这些上皮细胞会发生凋亡，并伴随增殖，这可能在牙周组织中 Malassez 上皮剩余的减少和（或）更新中发挥作用[32]。

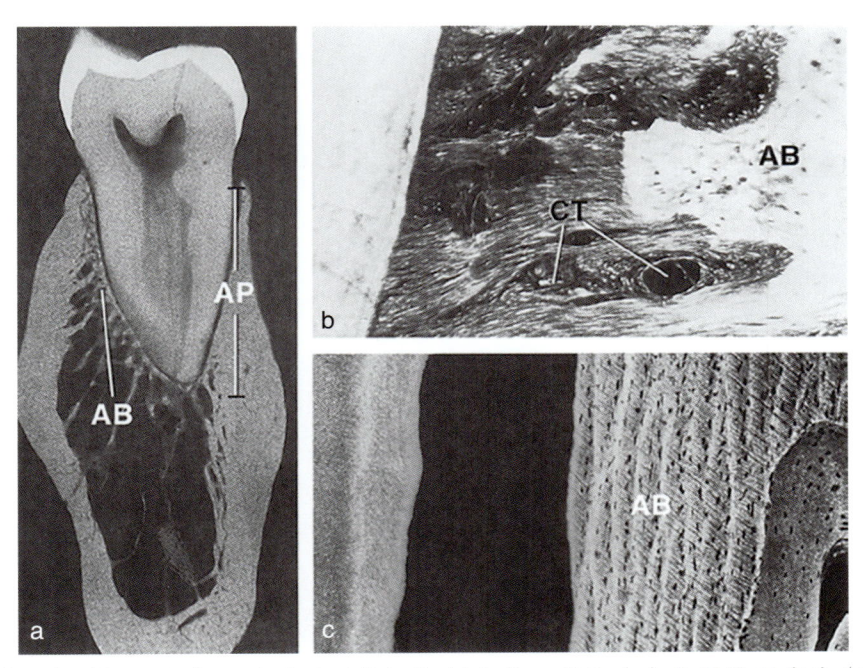

图 2.34 牙槽骨（AB）矿化不足（a、c）和去矿化切片（b）的 X 线片（a）和显微 X 线片（b、c）。注意附着在牙槽骨上的牙周韧带纤维和透光夏普纤维之间的血管岛和疏松结缔组织（CT）。AP：下颌骨牙槽突

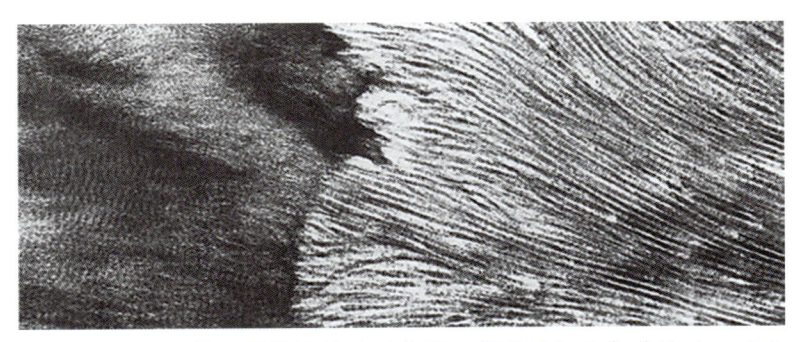

图 2.35 电子显微照片显示细胶原纤维以夏普纤维的形式插入牙骨质细胞中（经 *Acta Odontologica Scandinavica* 许可引用[58]）

Malassez 细胞可能是牙周神经发育的靶点。Ruffini 样受体和游离神经末梢与这些细胞密切相关（图 2.36）[81]。此外，免疫组化研究表明 Malassez 细胞含有神经肽（如 CGRP 和 SP），因此可能具有功能性内分泌作用[81]。Malassez 上皮剩余也可能通过矿化作用在牙骨质小体的形成中发挥作用。它们可能是附着的或游离的状态，并且可能包含类似于在牙齿根尖区域发现的髓石样的细胞残余（图 2.37）。

2.8.3 转换

值得注意的是，骨是比牙骨质更具活力的组织。骨的正常更替也影响牙槽突的形态。一方面，牙骨质通常被一层薄的未矿化的前牙骨质覆盖，缓慢的牙骨质形成可补偿牙齿的磨损。另一方面，骨组织仅在骨形成期间被类骨质覆盖。未矿化的基质往往能抵抗破牙骨质细胞的活动[190]。因此，在 PDL 中，破骨细胞的活动似乎比破牙骨质细胞

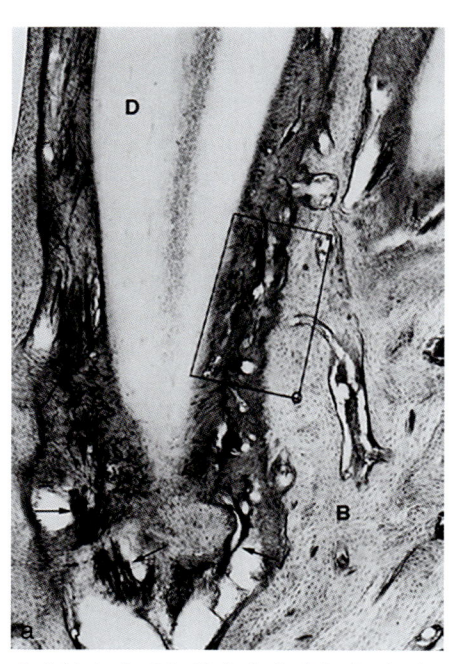

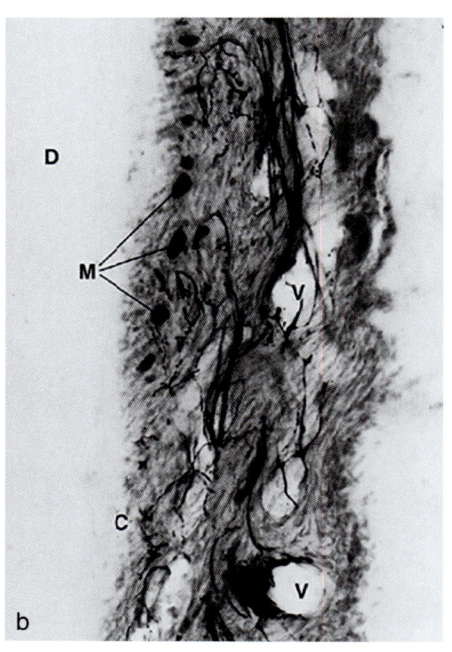

图 2.36 a. 猫切牙的根尖牙周韧带富含来自根尖（B）的蛋白基因产物（PGP）免疫反应神经（箭头）。b. 框区扩大图，显示神经纤维供应血管（V）和神经向根牙骨质（C）和 Malassez 上皮细胞（M）的广泛分支。D：牙本质（经 *Acta Odontologica Scandinavica* 许可引用[81]）

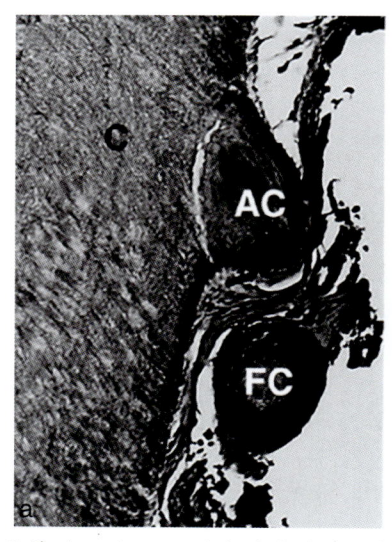

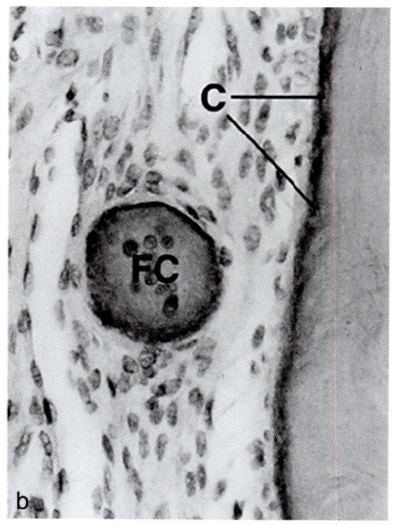

图 2.37 a. 牙周韧带附着（AC）。b. 游离牙骨质（FC）。C：牙骨质

或破牙细胞的活动更为显著，并且在骨缺损中，豪希普腔隙比牙齿吸收更常见。上述两种吸收过程可以同时发生。细胞性牙骨质可通过修复性牙骨质的形成填充骨吸收的缺陷。

PDL中骨和牙骨质吸收活性的差异是正畸牙齿移动的基础。对牙齿施加适度的力会导致压力侧的骨吸收而张力侧的骨形成，且不会引起牙骨质吸收。这样，牙齿就会沿着施加力的方向移动。然而，过大的力也可导致牙骨质吸收，甚至达到出现临床症状的程度。

2.8.4　PDL 的血液循环

PDL的血液供应系统很复杂。虽然PDL是腱性组织，但PDL呈现高度血管化。据计算，PDL总血管容积约占组织的20%，而大多数其他组织仅为3%~4%。PDL的血液供给来自牙槽骨、骨膜、牙龈和牙髓的血管。主要的血管供应自骨内动脉。由于动脉供应来自不同来源，并且静脉和小静脉同时引流骨髓和牙龈，因此PDL的血管床不应被视为孤立的功能单元。这意味着周围邻近组织中的血流，组织液压或血压的炎症和病理变化也会影响牙周循环。牙槽骨或牙龈中平行耦合血管的炎性血管扩张可能导致PDL中的血流减少，这是因为供给PDL的小动脉的压力下降。

PDL的主要血管位于纤维之间的疏松结缔组织隔室中，沿牙齿长轴方向走行。小动脉分支形成毛细血管，毛细血管排列成围绕牙根表面的扁平网状网络。毛细血管网更靠近牙槽骨，而非牙骨质，根尖区三分之一处穿通牙槽壁的血管最为丰富。PDL中的血流似乎主要由引起血管收缩的交感神经纤维和引起血管舒张的感觉纤维控制[104]。然而，由于缺乏合适的方法来测量这样体积微小且位于骨和牙齿之间的组织的血流，因此目前缺乏可靠的PDL血流量的定量测量数据。

PDL血流的定性测量显示交感神经血管收缩纤维参与了PDL血流的调节。α肾上腺素能受体拮抗剂可以显著减弱这种收缩效应，但无法完全消除，这表明支配PDL的一些交感神经纤维含有神经肽Y（NPY），这已通过免疫组织化学研究得到证实[81,157]（图2.36）。此外，在PDL中也发现了β受体的激活引起交感神经性血管舒张，这些β受体可能位于毛细血管后阻力血管中[1]。

PDL血流的变化会影响牙齿位置，而施加在牙冠上的外力可能会极大地影响PDL的血流[29,161]。正常情况下的这种变化可能与PDL组织液压的变化有关[111]。与大多数其他组织相比，PDL的组织液压力的记录值相对较高[111,161]，据称其会影响牙齿的位置、血液流动、牙齿的萌出力，以及可能与疼痛感觉有关。与牙髓一样，PDL也被封闭在牙槽骨和牙齿之间的刚性低顺应性环境中。因此，静脉淤滞或心脏骤停引起的血容量变化会迅速传递到PDL的组织液压力中[111]。

与牙髓主要感受疼痛不同，PDL还能识别牙齿的触觉、压力、移动和位置。在PDL中发现了多种类似Ruffini的机械感受器结构[22]，其中一些完全包裹的机械感受器结构位于血管旁的间质疏松结缔组织中。因此，PDL血流增加导致组织压力增加很可能引起机械感受器的兴奋。PDL中血容量增加会升高组织压力并导致牙齿伸长，而血容量减少会导致牙齿压低并降低组织压力[1,111]。PDL中低顺应性的表现有组织压力的变化可能会影响疼痛感知，即组织液体压力增加导致感觉Aδ和C纤维的活动增加，这与牙髓中的情况大致相同。

2.8.5　PDL 中的神经支配

尽管PDL的神经支配不如牙髓丰富，但PDL仍富含从根尖和侧面牙槽骨进入的神经（图2.36，图2.38）。PDL的根尖部分神经支配最密集，大部分似乎是感觉神经来源，而携带NPY的交感神经纤维则较为少见。然而，下颌管中的一些较大的血管壁上密集分布着NPY纤维[81]。在牙髓暴露后，发炎的PDL中可能观察到含有NPY的交感神经纤维增生[79]。这种增生的意义尚不清楚，但可能会影响血流和免疫调节。由于外周内源性交感神经递质是血管生长因子的重要调节因子[30]，这可能表明交感神经在炎性的PDL的修复和愈合过程中对血运重建起到一定的作用。

牙周韧带包含有髓鞘神经纤维和无髓鞘神经纤维。在PDL的各个层次中，降钙素基因相关肽比SP纤维更为常见[81]。PDL中的大多数神经集中于根尖三分之一，与血管密切相关。它们经常

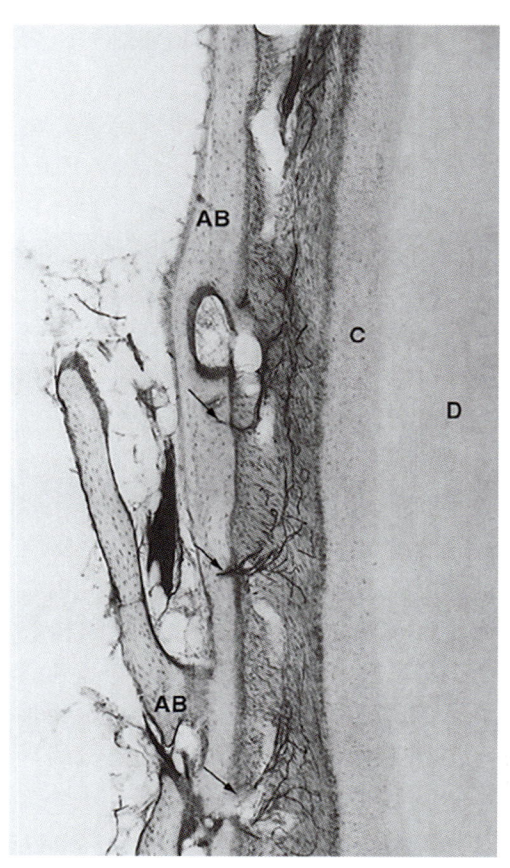

图 2.38 猫尖牙根尖三分之一处的牙周韧带切面，可见许多神经纤维（箭头）从牙槽骨（AB）向韧带靠近。D：牙本质。C：牙骨质（经 *Acta Odontologica Scandinavica* 许可引用[81]）

出现在 PDL 和细胞性牙骨质的交界处，其中一些形成圆形卷曲状、神经样末端。其他与 Malassez 上皮剩余密切相关（图 2.36）[81, 122]。在猫的 PDL 的根尖部分，形成网状结构的免疫反应细胞规律地分布在 Malassez 上皮剩余中，周围环绕着大量神经纤维。位于 Malassez 上皮剩余中的一些细胞含有 CGRP 和 SP。与来自其他部位的特化上皮细胞一样[148]，Malassez 上皮细胞可能包含一些由于其神经肽含量而可归类为内分泌细胞的细胞。根尖周炎症和正畸牙齿移动会诱导感觉轴突在根尖周区域的短暂增生[25,108,214]。较大的轴突通常形成专门的末端，主要在根尖区域，称为 Ruffini 样末端。较细的轴突通常以游离神经末梢的形式终止。电生理和组织学数据均表明，Ruffini 样末端以及游离神经末梢均可能起着机械感受器的作用[122]。牙骨质似乎没有神经支配[81]，但是根尖细胞性牙骨质附近常发现感觉神经的广泛分支，该区域血管较少（图 2.36）。

2.9 牙骨质

牙骨质是覆盖在牙根表面的无血管矿化结缔组织。牙骨质的主要功能是将 PDL 的主纤维附着到牙齿上。通常，牙骨质的牙冠部分是无细胞的，而根尖部分是有细胞的，并且牙骨质细胞嵌入其基质中。无细胞牙骨质薄[227]，厚度为 50~200μm。有细胞牙骨质较厚，通常为多层结构，单层厚度为 10~100μm[227]。无细胞牙骨质对牙齿的支持功能起重要作用，而有细胞牙骨质对牙齿萌出后位置的调节起重要作用。

牙骨质 – 牙本质交界（CDJ）处是牙骨质与牙本质连接的区域，是一个 100~200 μm 厚的间隙，其中包含 10~50 μm 富含亲水性的蛋白多糖的层[83, 227]。CDJ 处牙骨质与牙本质的紧密附着是由连续的胶原纤维桥介导的[83, 208]（图 2.39）。亲水性的 CDJ 也被认为是一种嵌合关节，即牙骨质和牙根牙本质之间的纤维连接，能够以类似牙骨质和牙槽骨之间的方式适应功能负荷[83-84]。

随着年龄的增长，牙骨质的物理化学性质会发生变化，表明其具有适应性[96]。牙骨质硬度随年龄增长而增加，但从牙骨质 – 牙釉质交界处到根尖 CDJ 的宽度减小[96]。细胞牙骨质厚度随年龄增长而增加。代偿性牙骨质沉积发生在根尖区，以抵消咬合磨耗。有时牙骨质的形成可能超过这一生理限度，导致牙骨质增生，这可能影响单个牙齿或所有牙齿。局部牙骨质的异常增厚可能与慢性根尖周炎相关。更广泛的牙骨质增生可能与某些全身性疾病有关，还有曾被描述过的牙骨质瘤，即产生牙骨质的肿瘤。如果发生牙根折，牙骨质可能在牙根碎片之间和折断的周围部位形成。如果发生牙根吸收，则可通过细胞牙骨质形成修复缺损。

牙骨质小体是矿化结构，可以自由存在于 PDL 中或附着于牙根表面（图 2.37）。它们可能由退化的上皮剩余或形成血栓的血管矿化形成。牙骨质小体含有骨涎蛋白（BSP）和骨桥蛋白，这两种非胶原基质蛋白通常存在于骨和牙骨质中[17]。当牙骨质小体存在时，通常可见于大多数牙齿上。

牙髓-牙本质复合体与牙周组织的解剖生理学 | 第 2 章

移动期间，将发生牙周纤维的重新附着，并且牙骨质中的纤维以不同的角度向表面排列。在细胞牙骨质中，细胞固有纤维牙骨质层形成横向和纵向排列的两种类型的交替板层结构，这种排列可以由成牙骨质细胞控制[227]。

牙骨质的细胞成分包括成牙骨质细胞和牙骨质细胞。排列在牙根表面的成牙骨质细胞具有能够合成胶原蛋白和蛋白质-多糖复合物的细胞超微结构特征。在牙根的根尖部分形成细胞牙骨质期间，一些成牙骨质细胞转变为成牙骨质细胞。牙骨质细胞位于牙骨质基质中的陷窝中。牙骨质细胞的功能尚不清楚，但最近它们被用来与骨细胞进行了比较；牙骨质细胞和骨细胞在转化、通讯和特异性标记物方面具有许多共同点，提示牙骨质细胞可能具有与骨细胞相似的动态功能[234]。

牙骨质的纤维间基质中含有蛋白多糖和糖蛋白，与其他牙周组织相似。其中两种主要成分是骨唾液酸蛋白（BSP）和骨桥蛋白。在牙骨质中，胶原纤维的特征比其他成分更为明确，但在细胞外基质的组成方面不断有新的研究进展。最近的小鼠实验揭示了一种新的结构成分——纤维蛋白4在牙骨质中表达[180]。小鼠牙骨质的蛋白质组学分析确定了一个蛋白质-蛋白质相互作用网络，其中包括代谢功能指标，这可能反映了牙骨质细胞的活性[178]。

前期牙骨质是覆盖在牙骨质上一层薄的未矿化层，在一定程度上能够防止牙根吸收。如果前期牙骨质矿化，可能会发生牙根吸收。

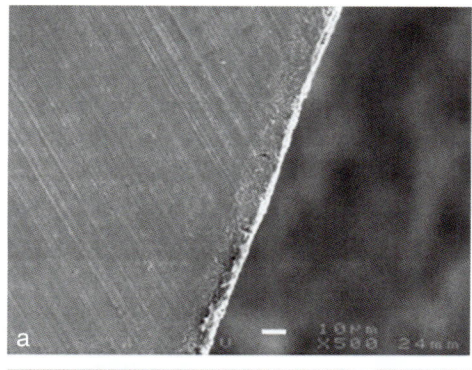

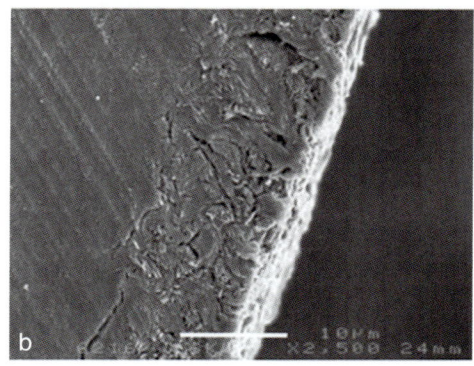

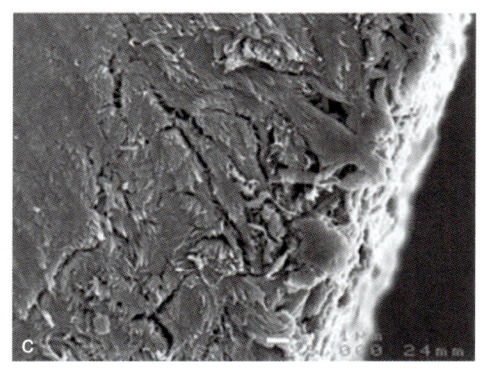

图 2.39 人牙骨质-牙本质连接的场发射扫描电子显微镜（FE-SEM）图像。a. 与牙本质密切接触的牙骨质厚度为 10~15μm。放大倍数：500 倍。比例尺：10μm。b、c. 高倍镜显示矿化胶原纤维从牙骨质到底层牙本质的连续性。放大率：2500 倍（b）和 5000 倍（c）。比例尺：10μm（b）和 1μm（c）（经 *Endodontic Topics* 许可引用[208]）

2.9.1 牙骨质的结构和组成

胶原纤维是牙骨质的主要有机成分。牙骨质中存在两种类型的胶原纤维，Sharpey 纤维和基质纤维。细小的 Sharpey 纤维（外在纤维）代表 PDL 主纤维的末端并穿透牙骨质（图 2.35）。基质纤维沿根面平行排列，并与 Sharpey 纤维交织在一起。Sharpey 纤维由 PDL 中的成纤维细胞形成，而基质纤维由成牙骨质细胞形成。当牙齿的位置改变时，例如在牙齿萌出期间或在正畸牙齿

2.10 牙槽骨

牙槽骨是上下颌窝排列骨牙槽突的一部分，围绕牙齿的牙槽窝排列（图 2.40）。它具有皮质骨的所有特征，但还具有来自牙周韧带的 Sharpey 纤维的独特属性。牙槽骨具有许多从松质骨延伸到 PDL 的供血管和淋巴管（福尔克曼管）通过的通道，因此通常被称为筛状板。尽管有许多通道通过，但它在临床 X 线片上显示为一条阻射线（图 2.41a），因此得名为硬骨板。硬骨板是一个重要的诊断标志。X 线片上硬骨板连续性的破坏可能是吸收的迹象，通常与牙

35

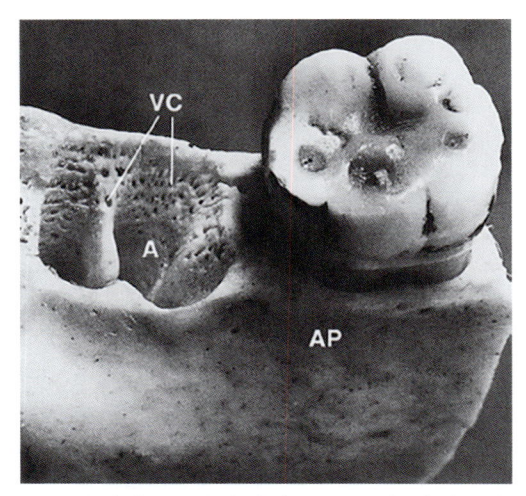

图 2.40 牙槽骨与福尔克曼（Volkmann）管（VC）穿过牙槽骨。AP：下颌牙槽突。A：牙槽窝（经 Munksgaard 许可引用）[140]

2.10.1 牙槽骨的结构

牙槽骨具有骨组织的基本特征，包括成骨细胞、骨细胞和破骨细胞（图 2.43）。它的发育与牙齿的存在密切相关。如果牙齿脱落，牙槽骨就会发生吸收。如果牙齿未萌出，牙槽骨也不会发育。

成骨细胞是产生基质的细胞，具有发达的高尔基体、颗粒内质网和线粒体。嵌入骨基质的成骨细胞称为骨细胞。它们失去了许多细胞器，但仍与邻近的骨细胞保持细胞质接触。骨细胞在控制对机械力的反应中具有重要的作用，因此可能在牙齿萌出、生理性和病理性牙齿移动和正畸治疗中发挥重要作用[21]。胶原形成可能发生在骨细胞和骨陷窝壁之间的骨细胞周围间隙中。陷窝可能发生矿化，形成"堵塞的陷窝"。骨陷窝也可能发生骨溶解，这是骨组织矿物质代谢的一部分[224]。然而，与骨重塑相关的主要过程涉及破骨细胞活动（图 2.43）和成骨细胞形成新骨。

牙槽骨的正常更新率导致牙槽突中的骨组织因年龄不同而呈现多样性，在任何时候，牙槽骨都存在不同矿化程度的骨。骨板是骨组织的增量生长线，是可辨别的。类骨质存在于骨形成发生的任何地方，但它不会完全覆盖已形成的骨。相对较厚的 Sharpey 纤维插入牙槽骨时，其未矿化的核心在显微 X 线片中呈现条纹状外观（图 2.34c）。

髓感染或牙周病有关。然而，在牙槽突中，牙槽骨的矿化程度与其他部分皮质骨没有区别（图 2.41b）。牙槽骨在 X 线片上的切线重叠赋予了硬骨板特有的放射密度。

上下颌牙槽突的颊侧和舌侧骨板厚度会因在口腔内位置的不同而不同。颊侧（唇侧）骨板通常比舌侧（腭侧）骨板薄；但在下颌磨牙区，舌侧骨板较薄。这种关系在拔牙时以及从根尖区域引流脓肿时非常重要，因为脓液倾向于沿着阻力最小的路径扩散。牙槽窝和上颌窦之间的密切关系（图 2.42a）在外科拔牙、种植体植入和根管治疗过程中也很重要（图 2.42 b）。

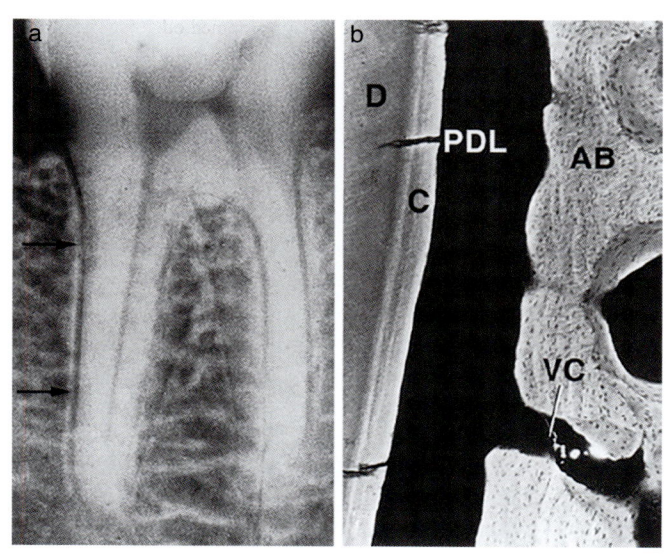

图 2.41 a. 磨牙的 X 线片显示放射密集的牙槽骨（箭头），由此得名骨硬板。b. 牙本质（D）、牙骨质（C）、牙周韧带间隙（PDL）和牙槽骨（AB）。VC：福尔克曼管

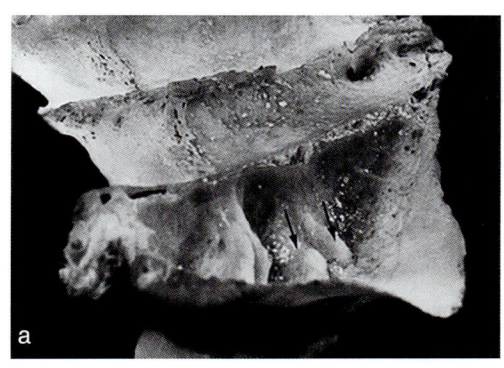

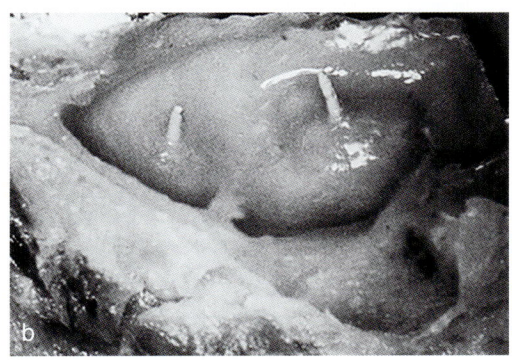

图 2.42 a.硬腭水平截开的上颌骨，显示第一恒磨牙（箭头）的根尖伸入上颌窦（经 Munksgaard 许可引用[140]）。b.在猴子身上进行的一系列牙髓治疗实验的解剖标本显示牙胶尖穿孔进入上颌窦（D. Ørstavik 博士及 I.A. Mjör 博士提供）

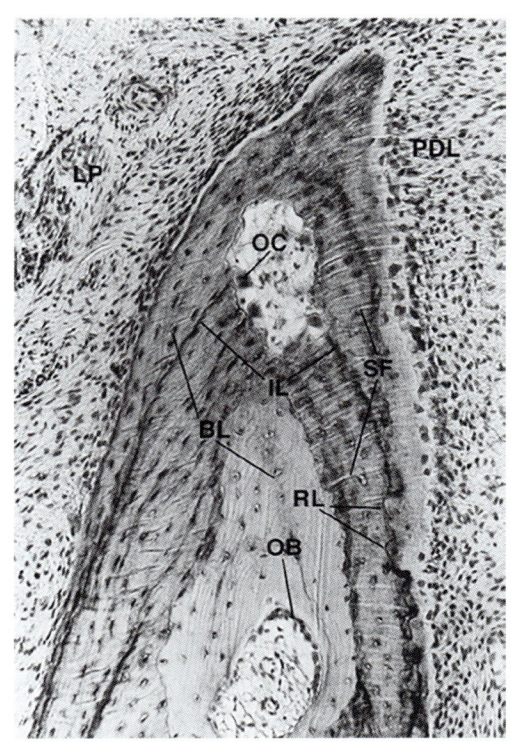

图 2.43 脱矿切片显示人牙槽嵴及邻近组织。PDL：牙周韧带。OB：成骨细胞。SF：Sharpey 纤维。LP：附着龈固有层。BL：有骨细胞的骨陷窝。OC：破骨细胞。IL：增量线。RL：反转线（K. Reitan 博士提供）

参考文献

[1] Aars H. The influence of vascular beta-adrenoceptors on the position and mobility of the rabbit incisor tooth. Acta Physiol Scand, 1982, 116: 423–428.

[2] Abbott P V, Yu C. A clinical classification of the status of the pulp and the root canal system. Aust Dent J, 2007, 52: S17–31.

[3] About I. Dentin regeneration in vitro: the pivotal role of supportive cells. Adv Dent Res, 2011, 23: 320–324.

[4] Accorsi-Mendonca T, et al. Evaluation of gelatinases, tissue inhibitor of matrix metalloproteinase-2, and myeloperoxidase protein in healthy and inflamed human dental pulp tissue. J Endod, 2013, 39: 879–882.

[5] Agematsu H, et al. Three dimensional observation of decrease in pulp cavity volume using micro-CT: age-related change. Bull Tokyo Dent Coll, 2010, 51: 1–6.

[6] Alavi AM, Dubyak GR, Burnstock G. Immunohistochemical evidence for ATP receptors in human dental pulp. J Dent Res, 2001, 80: 476–483.

[7] Allard B, et al. Characterization and gene expression of high conductance calcium-activated potassium channels displaying mechanosensitivity in human odontoblasts. J Biol Chem, 2000, 275: 25556–25561.

[8] Allard B, et al. Voltage-gated sodium channels confer excitability to human odontoblasts: possible role in tooth pain transmission. J Biol Chem, 2006, 281: 29002–29010.

[9] Alvarez M M, et al. PAR-1 and PAR-2 expression is enhanced in inflamed odontoblast cells. Journal of Dental Research, 2017, 96: 1518–1525

[10] Aranha A M, et al. Hypoxia enhances the angiogenic potential of human dental pulp cells. J Endod, 2010, 36: 1633–1637.

[11] Arola D, et al. Microstructure and mechanical behavior of radicular and coronal dentin. Endodontic Topics, 2009, 20: 30–51.

[12] Arola D, Reprogel R K. Effects of aging on the mechanical behavior of human dentin. Biomaterials, 2005, 26: 4051–4061.

[13] Bajaj D, et al. Age, dehydration and fatigue crack growth in dentin. Biomaterials, 2006, 27: 2507–2517.

[14] Beniash E, et al. A transmission electron microscope study using vitrified ice sections of predentin: structural changes in the dentin collagenous matrix prior to mineralization. J Struct Biol, 2000, 132: 212–225.

[15] Biragyn A, et al. Toll-like receptor 4-dependent activation of dendritic cells by beta-defensin 2. Science, 2002, 298:

1025–1029.

[16] Bjørndal L. The caries process and its effect on the pulp: the science is changing and so is our understanding. J Endod, 2008, 34:S2–5.

[17] Bosshardt D D, Nanci A. Immunocytochemical characterization of ectopic enamel deposits and cementicles in human teeth. Eur J Oral Sci, 2003, 111: 51–59.

[18] Botelho J, et al. Dental stem cells: recent progresses in tissue engineering and regenerative medicine. Ann Med, 2017: 1–8.

[19] Bowles W R, et al. Beta 2-adrenoceptor regulation of CGRP release from capsaicin-sensitive neurons. J Dent Res-2003-82: 308–311.

[20] Bruno K F, et al. Characterization of inflammatory cell infiltrate in human dental pulpitis. Int Endod J, 2010, 43: 1013–1021.

[21] Bumann E E, Frazier-Bowers S A. A new cyte in orthodontics: osteocytes in tooth movement. Orthod Craniofac Res, 2017, 20 Suppl 1: 125–128.

[22] Byers M R, Dong W K. Comparison of trigeminal receptor location and structure in the periodontal ligament of different types of teeth from the rat, cat, and monkey. J Comp Neurol, 1989, 279: 117–127.

[23] Byers M R, Suzuki H, Maeda T. Dental neuroplasticity, neuro-pulpal interactions, and nerve regeneration. Microsc Res Tech, 2003, 60: 503–515.

[24] Byers M R, Taylor P E. Effect of sensory denervation on the response of rat molar to exposure injury. J Dent Res, 1993, 72: 613–618.

[25] Byers M R, et al. Effects of injury and inflammation on pulpal and periapical nerves. J Endod, 1990, 16: 78–84.

[26] Byers M R, Westenbroek R E. Odontoblasts in developing, mature and ageing rat teeth have multiple phenotypes that variably express all nine voltage-gated sodium channels. Arch Oral Biol, 2011, 56: 1199–1220.

[27] Carda C, Peydro A. Ultrastructural patterns of human dentinal tubules, odontoblasts processes and nerve fibres. Tissue Cell, 2006, 38: 141–150.

[28] Carlile M J, et al. The presence of pericytes and transitional cells in the vasculature of the human dental pulp: an ultrastructural study. Histochem J, 2000, 32:239–245.

[29] Caviedes-Bucheli J, et al. Angiogenic mechanisms of human dental pulp and their relationship with substance P expression in response to occlusal trauma. Int Endod J, 2017, 50: 339–351.

[30] Caviedes-Bucheli J, et al. Neuropeptides in dental pulp: the silent protagonists. J Endod, 2008, 34: 773–788.

[31] Caviedes-Bucheli J, et al. The effect of different vasoconstrictors and local anesthetic solutions on substance P expression in human dental pulp. J Endod, 2009, 35: 631–633.

[32] Cerri P S, Katchburian E. Apoptosis in the epithelial cells of the rests of Malassez of the periodontium of rat molars. J Periodontal Res, 2005, 40: 365–372.

[33] Charadram N, et al. Regulation of reactionary dentin formation by odontoblasts in response to polymicrobial invasion of dentin matrix. Bone, 2012, 50: 265–275.

[34] Chien Y C, et al. Distinct decalcification process of dentin by different cariogenic organic acids: Kinetics, ultrastructure and mechanical properties. Arch Oral Biol, 2016, 63: 93–105.

[35] Cho Y S, et al. Rat odontoblasts may use glutamate to signal dentin injury. Neuroscience 3, 2016, 335: 54–63.

[36] Chung G, Jung S J, Oh S B. Cellular and molecular mechanisms of dental nociception. J Dent Res, 2013, 92: 948–955.

[37] Cook S P, et al. Distinct ATP receptors on pain-sensing and stretchsensing neurons. Nature-1997-387: 505–508.

[38] Cooper P R, Holder M, J Smith A J. Inflammation and regeneration in the dentin-pulp complex: a double-edged sword. J Endod, 2014, 40: S46–51.

[39] Couve E, Osorio R, Schmachtenberg O. The amazing odontoblast: activity, autophagy, and aging. J Dent Res 92: 765–772.

[40] Couve E, Osorio R, Schmachtenberg O. Reactionary dentinogenesis and neuroimmune response in dental caries. J Dent Res, 2014, 93: 788–793.

[41] Dahl E, Mjör I A. The structure and distribution of nerves in the pulp-dentin organ. Acta Odontol Scand, 1973, 31: 349–356.

[42] Daud S, et al. Changes in cell density and morphology of selected cells of the ageing human dental pulp Gerodontology, 2016, 33: 315–321.

[43] Dechichi P, et al. A model of the early mineralization process of mantle dentin. Micron, 2017, 38: 486–491.

[44] Do D, et al. Accelerated fatigue of dentin with exposure to lactic acid. Biomaterials, 2013, 34: 8650–8659.

[45] Dommisch H, et al. Phosphatidylinositol-3-kinase inhibitor LY 294002 blocks Streptococcus mutansinduced interleukin (IL) -6 and IL-8 gene expression in odontoblast-like cells. Int Endod J, 2008, 41: 763–771.

[46] Dommisch H, et al. Human beta-defensin (hBD-1, 2) expression in dental pulp. Oral Microbiol Immunol, 2005, 20: 163–166.

[47] Dommisch H, et al. Immune regulatory functions of human betadefensin-2 in odontoblast-like cells. Int Endod J, 2007, 40: 300–307.

[48] Durand S H, et al. Lipoteichoic acid increases TLR and functional chemokine expression while reducing dentin References 51formation in in vitro differentiated human odontoblasts. J Immunol, 2006, 176: 2880–2887.

[49] Egbuniwe O, et al. TRPA1 and TRPV4 activation in human

odontoblasts stimulates ATP release. J Dent Res, 2014, 93: 911–917.
[50] El Karim I A, et al. Human dental pulp fibroblasts express the "cold-sensing" transient receptor potential channels TRPA1 and TRPM8. J Endod, 2011, 37: 473–478.
[51] Eltit F, Ebacher V Wang R. Inelastic deformation and microcracking process in human dentin. J Struct Biol, 2013, 183: 141–148.
[52] Espina A I, Castellanos A V, Fereira J L. Age-related changes in blood capillary–endothelium of human dental pulp: an ultrastructural study. Int Endod J, 2003, 36: 395–403.
[53] Farges J C, et al. Odontoblasts in the dental pulp immune response. J Exp Zool B Mol Dev Evol, 2009, 312b: 425 36.
[54] Farge J C, et al. TGF-beta1 induces accumulation of dendritic cells in the odontoblast layer. J Dent Res, 2003, 82: 652–656.
[55] Feng J, et al. Dual origin of mesenchymal stem cells contributing to organ growth and repair. Proc Natl Acad Sci U S A, 2011, 108: 6503–6508.
[56] Franquin J C, et al. Immunocytochemical detection of apoptosis in human odontoblasts. Eur J Oral Sci, 1998, 106 Suppl 1: 384–387.
[57] Fristad I, et al. Recruitment of immunocompetent cells after dentinal injuries in innervated and denervated young rat molars: an immunohistochemical study. J Histochem Cytochem, 1995, 43: 871–879.
[58] Furseth R. A microradiographic and electron microscopic study of the cementum of human deciduous teeth. Acta Odontol Scand, 1967, 25: 613–645.
[59] Gallagher R R, et al. Optical spectroscopy and imaging of the dentinenamel junction in human third molars. J Biomed Mater Res A, 2003, 64: 372–377.
[60] Gao X, et al. Micro-CT evaluation of apical delta morphologies in human teeth. Sci Rep, 2016, 6: 36501.
[61] Gaudin A, et al. Phenotypic analysis of immunocompetent cells in healthy human dental pulp. J Endod, 2015, 41: 621–627.
[62] Georgy S R, et al. Proteinaseactivated receptor, 2 is required for normal osteoblast and osteoclast differentiation during skeletal growth and repair. Bone, 2012, 50: 704–712.
[63] Gerdes J M, Davis E E, Katsanis N. The vertebrate primary cilium in development, homeostasis, and disease. Cell ,2009, 137: 32–45.
[64] Gerli R, et al. Absence of lymphatic vessels in human dental pulp: a morphological study. Eur J Oral Sci, 2010, 118: 110–117.
[65] Gibbs J L, Hargreaves K M. Neuropeptide Y Y1 receptor effects on pulpal nociceptors. J Dent Res, 2008,87: 948–952.
[66] Gilhuus-Moe O, Kvam E. Behaviour of the epithelial remnants of malassez following experimental movement of rat molars. Acta Odontol Scand, 1972, 30: 139–149.
[67] Goga R, Chandler N P, Oginni A O. Pulp stones: a review. Int Endod J, 2008, 41: 457–468.
[68] Goldberg M, et al. Inflammatory and immunological aspects of dental pulp repair. Pharmacol Res, 2008, 58: 137–147.
[69] Goodis H E, Poon A, Hargreaves K M. Tissue pH and temperature regulate pulpal nociceptors. J Dent Res, 2006, 5: 1046–1049.
[70] Gotliv B A, Veis A. Peritubular dentin, a vertebrate apatitic mineralized tissue without collagen: role of a phospholipid-proteolipid complex. Calcif Tissue Int, 2007, 81: 191–205.
[71] Grando Mattuella L, et al. Vascular endothelial growth factor and its relationship with the dental pulp. J Endod, 2007, 33: 524–530.
[72] Gusman, H, Santana R B, Zehnder M. Matrix metalloproteinase levels and gelatinolytic activity in clinically healthy and inflamed human dental pulps. Eur J Oral Sci, 2002, 110: 353–357.
[73] Hahn C L, Liewehr F R. Innate immune responses of the dental pulp to caries. J Endod, 2007, 33: 643–651.
[74] Hahn C L, Liewehr F R. Update on the adaptive immune responses of the dental pulp. J Endod, 2007, 33: 773–781.
[75] Hahn C L, Schenkein H A, Tew J G. Endocarditis-associated oral streptococci promote rapid differentiation of monocytes into mature dendritic cells. Infect Immun, 2005, 73: 5015–5021.
[76] Hargreaves K M, Jackson D L, Bowles W R. Adrenergic regulation of capsaicin-sensitive neurons in dental pulp. J Endod, 2003, 29: 397–399.
[77] Harran Ponce E, Canalda Sahli C, Vilar Fernandez J A. Study of dentinal tubule architecture of permanent upper premolars: evaluation by SEM. Aust Endod J, 2001, 27: 66–72.
[78] Haug S R, et al. Sympathectomy causes increased root resorption after orthodontic tooth movement in rats: immunohistochemical study. Cell Tissue Res, 2003, 313: 167–175.
[79] Haug S R, Heyeraas K J. Effects of sympathectomy on experimentally induced pulpal inflammation and periapical lesions in rats. Neuroscience, 2003, 120: 827–836.
[80] Hazeki K, Nigorikawa K, Hazeki O. Role of phosphoinositide 3-kinase in innate immunity. Biol Pharm Bull, 2007, 30: 1617–1623.
[81] Heyeraas K J, et al. Nerve fibers immunoreactive to protein gene product 9.5, calcitonin gene-related peptide, substance P, and neuropeptide Y in the dental pulp, periodontal ligament, and gingiva in cats. Acta Odontol Scand, 1993, 51: 207–221.
[82] Hirsch V, et al. Inflammatory cytokines in normal and irreversibly inflamed pulps: a systematic review. Arch Oral Biol, 2017, 82: 38–46.
[83] Ho S P, et al. The tooth attachment mechanism defined by structure, chemical composition and mechanical properties

[84] Ho S P, et al. Structure, chemical composition and mechanical properties of human and rat cementum and its interface with root dentin. Acta Biomater, 2009, 5: 707–718.

[85] Horst O V, et al. Caries induced cytokine network in the odontoblast layer of human teeth. BMC Immunol, 2011, 12: 9.

[86] Horst O V, et al. TGF-beta1 inhibits TLR-mediated odontoblast responses to oral bacteria. J Dent Res, 2009, 88: 333–338.

[87] Hossain M Z, et al. Correlation between numbers of cells in human dental pulp and age: implications for age estimation. Arch Oral Biol, 2017, 80: 51–55.

[88] Huang X F, Chai Y. Molecular regulatory mechanism of tooth root development. Int J Oral Sci, 2012, 4: 177–181.

[89] Ichikawa H, et al. Voltage-dependent sodium channels and calcium-activated potassium channels in human odontoblasts in vitro. J Endod, 2012, 38: 1355–1362.

[90] Iijima T, Zhang J Q. Threedimensional wall structure and the innervation of dental pulp blood vessels. Microsc Res Tech, 2002, 56: 32–41.

[91] Ikeda H, Suda H. Odontoblastic syncytium through electrical coupling in the human dental pulp. J Dent Res, 2013, 92: 371–375.

[92] Ivancik J, et al. The reduction in fatigue crack growth resistance of dentin with depth. J Dent Res, 2011, 90: 1031–1036.

[93] Izumi T, et al. An immunohistochemical study of HLA-DR and alpha 1-antichymotrypsin-positive cells in the pulp of human non-carious and carious teeth. Arch Oral Biol, 1996, 41: 627–630.

[94] Izumi T, et al. Immunohistochemical study on the immunocompetent cells of the pulp in human non-carious and carious teeth. Arch Oral Biol, 1995, 40: 609–614.

[95] James A W, et al. Pericytes for the treatment of orthopedic conditions. Pharmacol Ther, 2017, 171: 93–103.

[96] Jang A T, et al. Adaptive properties of human cementum and cementum dentin junction with age. J Mech Behav Biomed Mater, 2014, 39: 184–196.

[97] Jarczak J, et al. Defensins: natural component of human innate immunity. Hum Immunol, 2013, 74: 1069–1079.

[98] Jiang H W, et al. Expression of Toll-like receptor 4 in normal human odontoblasts and dental pulp tissue. J Endod, 2006, 32: 747–751.

[99] Jiang J, Gu J. Expression of adenosine triphosphate P2X3 receptors in rat molar pulp and trigeminal ganglia. Oral Surg Oral Med Oral Pathol Oral Radiol Endod, 2002, 94: 622–626.

[100] Johannessen L B. Dentine apposition in the mandibular first molars of albino rats. Arch Oral Biol, 1961, 5: 81–91.

[101] Kagayama M, et al. Confocal microscopy of dentinal tubules in human tooth stained with alizarin red. Anat Embryol (Berl), 1999, 199: 233–238.

[102] Kagayama M, et al. Confocal microscopy of Tomes' granular layer in dog premolar teeth. Anat Embryol (Berl), 2000, 201: 131–137.

[103] Karashima Y, et al. TRPA1 acts as a cold sensor in vitro and in vivo. Proc Natl Acad Sci U S A, 2009, 106: 1273–1278.

[104] Karita K, et al. The blood flow in the periodontal ligament regulated by the sympathetic and sensory nerves in the cat. Proc Finn Dent Soc, 1989, 85: 289–294.

[105] Kim H Y, et al. Characterization of dental nociceptive neurons. J Dent Re, 2011, s 90: 771–776.

[106] Kim Y S, et al. Expression of transient receptor potential ankyrin 1 in human dental pulp. J Endod, 2012, 38: 1087–1092.

[107] Kim Y S, et al. Expression of metabotropic glutamate receptor mGluR5 in human dental pulp. J Endod, 2009, 35: 690–694.

[108] Kimberly C L, Byers M R. Inflammation of rat molar pulp and periodontium causes increased calcitonin gene-related peptide and axonal sprouting. Anat Rec, 1988, 222: 289–300.

[109] Kishen A, Vedantam S. Hydromechanics in dentine: role of dentinal tubules and hydrostatic pressure on mechanical stress, strain distribution. Dent Mater, 2007, 23: 1296–1306.

[110] Klonowski K D, Lefrancois L. The CD8 memory T cell subsystem: integration of homeostatic signaling during migration. Semin Immunol, 2005, 17: 219–229.

[111] Kristiansen A B, Heyeraas K J. Micropuncture measurements of interstitial fluid pressure in the rat periodontal ligament. Proc Finn Dent Soc, 1989, 85: 295–300.

[112] Kumakami-Sakano M, et al. Regulatory mechanisms of Hertwig's epithelial root sheath formation and anomaly correlated with root length. Exp Cell Res, 2014, 325: 78–82.

[113] Ladizesky M G, et al. Effect of unilateral superior cervical ganglionectomy on bone mineral content and density of rat's mandible. J Auton Nerv Syst, 2000, 78: 113–116.

[114] Lebre M C, et al. Differential expression of inflammatory chemokines by Th1-and Th2-cell promoting dendritic cells: a role for different mature dendritic cell populations in attracting appropriate effector cells to peripheral sites of inflammation. Immunol Cell Biol, 2005, 83:525–535.

[115] Levin L G, et al. Identify and define all diagnostic terms for pulpal health and disease states. J Endod, 2009, 35: 1645–1657.

[116] Levin L G, et al. Expression of IL-8 by cells of the odontoblast layer in vitro. Eur J Oral Sci, 1999, 107: 131–137.

[117] Li Y, Ikeda H, Suda H. Determination of the functional space for fluid movement in the rat dentinal tubules using fluorescent microsphere. Arch Oral Biol, 2013, 58: 780–787.

[118] Lim J C, Mitchell C H. Inflammation, pain, and pressure – purinergic signaling in oral tissues. J Dent Res, 2012, 91:

[119] Lohrberg M, Wilting J. The lymphatic vascular system of the mouse head. Cell Tissue Res, 2016, 366: 667–677.

[120] Lundquist P, et al. Na$^+$/Ca^{2+} exchanger isoforms of rat odontoblasts and osteoblasts. Calcif Tissue Int, 2000, 67: 60–67.

[121] Lundy F T, et al. PAR-2 regulates dental pulp inflammation associated with caries. J Dent Res, 2010, 89: 684–688.

[122] Maeda T, et al. The Ruffini ending as the primary mechanoreceptor in the periodontal ligament: its morphology, cytochemical features, regeneration, and development. Crit Rev Oral Biol Med, 1999, 10: 307–327.

[123] Magloire H, et al. Odontoblast primary cilia: facts and hypotheses. Cell Biol Int, 2004, 28: 93–99.

[124] Magloire H, et al. Odontoblast: a mechano-sensory cell. J Exp Zool B Mol Dev Evol, 2009, 312b: 416–424.

[125] Magloire H, et al. Expression and localization of TREK-1 K$^+$ channels in human odon toblasts. J Dent Res, 2003, 82: 542–545.

[126] Magloire H, et al. Topical review. Dental pain and odontoblasts: facts and hypotheses. J Orofac Pain, 2010, 24: 335–349.

[127] Mahdee A, et al. Complex cellular responses to tooth wear in rodent molar. Arch Oral Biol, 2016, 61: 106–114.

[128] Malone A M, et al. Primary cilia mediate mechanosensing in bone cells by a calcium-independent mechanism. Proc Natl Acad Sci U S A, 2007, 104: 13325–13330.

[129] Mannocci F, et al. Density of dentinal tubules affects the tensile strength of root dentin. Dent Mater, 2004, 20: 293–296.

[130] Marroquin T Y, et al. Age estimation in adults by dental imaging assessment systematic review. Forensic Sci Int 2, 2017, 75: 203–211.

[131] Marshall G W Jr, et al. Mechanical properties of the dentinoenamel junction: AFM studies of nanohardness, elastic modulus, and fracture. J Biomed Mater Res, 2001, 54: 87–95.

[132] Martin-De Las Heras S, Valenzuela A, Overall C M. The matrix metalloproteinase gelatinase A in human dentine. Arch Oral Biol, 2000, 45: 757–765.

[133] Martin A, Gasse H, Staszyk C. Absence of lymphatic vessels in the dog dental pulp: an immunohistochemical study. J Anat, 2010, 217: 609–615.

[134] Martinez E F, et al. Immunohistochemical localization of tenascin, fibronectin, and type III collagen in human dental pulp. J Endod, 2000, 26: 708–711.

[135] Mazzoni A, et al. A review of the nature, role, and function of dentin non-collagenous proteins. Part II: enzymes, serum proteins, and growth factors. Endodontic Topics, 2009, 21: 19–40.

[136] Menezes-Silva R, et al. Genetic susceptibility to periapical disease: conditional contribution of MMP2 and MMP3 genes to the development of periapical lesions and healing response. J Endod, 2012, 38: 604–607.

[137] Mitsiadis T A, De Bari C, About I.Apoptosis in developmental and repair-related human tooth remodeling: a view from the inside. Exp Cell Res, 2008, 314: 869–877.

[138] Mitsiadis T A, Graf D. Cell fate determination during tooth development and regeneration. Birth Defects Res C Embryo Today, 2009, 87: 199–211.

[139] Miura J, et al. Accumulation of advanced glycation end-products in human dentine. Arch Oral Biol, 2014, 59: 119–124.

[140] Mjör I A. The maxillary sinus. Human oral embryology and histology. Copenhagen: Munksgaard, 1986,

[141] Mjör I A. Dentin permeability: the basis for understanding pulp reactions and adhesive technology. Braz Dent J, 2009, 20: 3–16.

[142] Mjör I A, Nordahl I. The density and branching of dentinal tubules in human teeth. Arch Oral Biol, 1996, 41: 401–412.

[143] Mjör I A, et al. The structure of dentine in the apical region of human teeth. Int Endod J, 2001, 34: 346–353.

[144] Montoya C, et al. Effect of aging on the microstructure, hardness and chemical composition of dentin. Arch Oral Biol, 2015, 60: 1811–1820.

[145] Morgan C R, et al. Changes in proteinase-activated receptor 2 expression in the human tooth pulp in relation to caries and pain. J Orofac Pain, 2009, 23: 265–274.

[146] Murray P E, et al. Age-related odontometric changes of human teeth. Oral Surg Oral Med Oral Pathol Oral Radiol Endod, 2002, 93: 474–482.

[147] Mutoh, N, et al. Expression of Toll-like receptor 2 and 4 in dental pulp. J Endod, 2007, 33: 1183–1186.

[148] Nakatani M, et al. Mechanotransduction in epidermal Merkel cells. Pflugers Arch, 2015, 467: 101–108.

[149] Nalbandian J, Gonzales F, Sognnaes R F. Sclerotic age changes in root dentin of human teeth as observed by optical, electron, and x-ray microscopy. J Dent Res, 1960, 39: 598–607.

[150] Närhi M, et al. The neurophysiological basis and the role of inflammatory reactions in dentine hypersensitivity. Arch Oral Biol, 1994, 39 Suppl: 23s–30s.

[151] Nascimento F D, et al. Cysteine cathepsins in human carious dentin. J Dent Res, 2011, 90: 506–511.

[152] Nishiyama A, et al. Intercellular signal communication among odontoblasts and trigeminal ganglion neurons via glutamate. Cell Calcium, 2016, 60: 341–355.

[153] Ohshima H, Maeda T, Takano Y. The distribution and ultrastructure of class II MHC-positive cells in human dental pulp. Cell Tissue Res, 1999, 295: 151–158.

[154] Ohshima H, et al. Pulpal regeneration after cavity preparation, with special reference to close spatiorelationships between odontoblasts and immunocompetent cells. Microsc Res Tech,

2003, 60: 483–490.

[155] Orrego S, Xu H, Arola D. Degradation in the fatigue crack growth resistance of human dentin by lactic acid Mater Sci Eng C Mater Biol Appl, 2017, 73: 716–725.

[156] Ossovskaya V S, Bunnett N W. Protease-activated receptors: contribution to physiology and disease. Physiol Rev, 2004, 84: 579–621.

[157] Oswald R J, Byers M R. The injury response of pulpal NPY-IR sympathetic fibers differs from that of sensory afferent fibers. Neurosci Lett, 1993, 164: 190–194.

[158] Pääkköen V, et al. Mature human odontoblasts express virus-recognizing Toll-like receptors. Int Endod J, 2014, 47: 934–941.

[159] Pääkköen V, et al. Effects of TGF-beta 1 on interleukin profile of human dental pulp and odontoblasts. Cytokine, 2007, 40: 44–51.

[160] Pääkköen V, et al. Comparative gene expression profile analysis between native human odontoblasts and pulp tissue. Int Endod J, 2008, 41: 117–127.

[161] Palcanis K G. Effect of occlusal trauma on interstitial pressure in the periodontal ligament. J Dent Res, 1973, 52: 903–91s0.

[162] Pang Y W, et al. Perivascular stem cells at the tip of mouse incisors regulate tissue regeneration. J Bone Miner Res, 2016, 31:514–523.

[163] Paphangkorakit J, Osborn J W. The effect of normal occlusal forces on fluid movement through human dentine in vitro. Arch Oral Biol, 2000, 45: 1033–1041.

[164] Paqué F, et al. Tubular sclerosis rather than the smear layer impedes dye penetration into the dentine of endodontically instrumented root canals. Int Endod J, 2006, 39: 18–25.

[165] Park E S, et al. Proteomics analysis of human dentin reveals distinct protein expression profiles. J Proteome Res, 2009, 8: 1338–1346.

[166] Pashley D H, et al. State of the art etch-and-rinse adhesives. Dent Mater, 2011, 27: 1–16.

[167] Pinchi V, et al. A new age estimation procedure based on the 3D CBCT study of the pulp cavity and hard tissues of the teeth for forensic purposes: A pilot study. J Forensic Leg Med, 2015, 36: 150–157.

[168] Que K, et al. Expression of cannabinoid type 1 receptors in human odontoblast cells. J Endod, 2017, 43: 283–288.

[169] Radlanski R J, Renz H. Insular dentin formation pattern in human odontogenesis in relation to the scalloped dentino - enamel junction. Ann Anat, 2007, 189: 243–250.

[170] Reis A G, et al. Second canal in mesiobuccal root of maxillary molars is correlated with root third and patient age: a cone-beam computed tomographic study. J Endod, 2013, 39: 588–592.

[171] Ricucci D, et al. shard tissue formation in the dental pulp after the death of the primary odontoblasts a regenerative or a reparative process? J Dent, 2014, I 42: 1156–1170.

[172] Ricucci D Loghin S, Siqueira J F Jr. Correlation between clinical and histologic pulp diagnoses. J Endod, 2014, 40: 1932–1939.

[173] Ricucci D, et al. Pulp and apical tissue response to deep caries in immature teeth: A histologic and histobacteriologic study. J Dent, 2017, 56: 19–32.

[174] Roberts-Clark D J, Smith A J. Angiogenic growth factors in human dentine matrix. Arch Oral Biol, 2000, 45: 1013–1016.

[175] Roggenkamp C. Dentinal fluid transport. Loma Linda, CA: Loma Linda University Press, 2004.

[176] Sa da Bandeira D, Casamitjana J, Crisan M. Pericytes, integral components of adult hematopoietic stem cell niches. Pharmacol Ther, 2017, 171: 104–113.

[177] Saito M, Fujii K, Marumo K. Degree of mineralization-related collagen crosslinking in the femoral neck cancellous bone in cases of hip fracture and controls. Calcif Tissue Int, 2006, 79: 160–168.

[178] Salmon C R, et al. Microproteome of dentoalveolar tissues. Bone, 2017, 101: 219–229.

[179] Schell S, et al. Validity of longitudinal sections for determining the apical constriction. Int Endod J, 2017, 50: 706–712.

[180] Schubert A, Schminke B, Miosge N. Fibulins and matrilins are novel structural components of the periodontium in the mouse. Arch Oral Biol, 2017, 82: 216–222.

[181] Sessle B J. Peripheral and central mechanisms of orofacial inflammatory pain. Int Rev Neurobiol, 2011, 97: 179–206.

[182] Shibukawa Y, et al. Odontoblasts as sensory receptors: transient receptor potential channels, pannexin-1, and ionotropic ATP receptors mediate intercellular odontoblast-neuron signal transduction. Pflugers Arch, 2015, 467: 843–863.

[183] Shin S J, et al. Tissue levels of matrix metalloproteinases in pulps and periapical lesions. J Endod, 2002, 28: 313–315.

[184] Shinno Y, et al. Comprehensive analyses of how tubule occlusion and advanced glycation end-products diminish strength of aged dentin. Sci Rep, 2016, 6: 19849.

[185] Simon S, et al. Molecular characterization of young and mature odontoblasts. Bone, 2009, 45: 693–703.

[186] Sims D E. Diversity within pericytes. Clin Exp Pharmacol Physiol, 2000, 27: 842–846.

[187] Smith A J, et al. Dentine as a bioactive extracellular matrix. Arch Oral Biol, 2012, 57: 109–121.

[188] Sole-Magdalena A, et al. Human odontoblasts express transient receptor protein and acid-sensing ion channel mechanosensor proteins. Microsc Res Tech, 2011, 74: 457–463.

[189] Staquet M J, et al. Patternrecognition receptors in pulp defense. Adv Dent Res, 2011, 23: 296–301.

[190] Stenvik A, Iversen J, Mjör I A. Tissue pressure and histology of normal and inflamed tooth pulps in macaque monkeys. Arch Oral Biol, 1972, 17: 1501–1511.

[191] Su K C, et al. The effect of dentinal fluid flow during loading in various directions-simulation of fluid-structure interaction. Arch Oral Biol, 2013, 58: 575–582.

[192] Takahashi K, Kishi Y, Kim S. A scanning electron microscope study of the blood vessels of dog pulp using corrosion resin casts. J Endod, 1982, 8: 131–135.

[193] Takano Y, et al. Differential involvement of matrix vesicles during the initial and appositional mineralization processes in bone, dentin, and cementum. Bone, 2000, 26: 333–339.

[194] Takeuchi O, Akira S. Pattern recognition receptors and inflammation. Cell, 2010, 140: 805–820.

[195] Tazawa K, et al. Transient receptor potential melastatin (TRPM) 8 is expressed in freshly isolated native human odontoblasts. Arch Oral Biol, 2017, 75: 55–61.

[196] Tersariol I L, et al. Cysteine cathepsins in human dentin-pulp complex. J Endod, 2010, 36: 475–481.

[197] Tesch W, et al. Graded microstructure and mechanical properties of human crown dentin. Calcif Tissue Int, 2001, 69: 147–157.

[198] Thaler A, et al. Influence of tooth age and root section on root dentine dye penetration. Int Endod J, 2008, 41: 1115–1122.

[199] Thivichon-Prince B, et al. Primary cilia of odontoblasts: possible role in molar morphogenesis. J Dent Res, 2009, 88: 910–915.

[200] Thomas M, Leaver A G. Identification and estimation of plasma proteins in human dentine. Arch Oral Biol, 1975, 20: 217–218.

[201] Tjäderhane L. The mechanism of pulpal wound healing. Aust Endod J, 2002, 28: 68–74.

[202] Tjäderhane L. Dentin bonding: can we make it last? Oper Dent, 2015, 40: 4–18.

[203] Tjäderhane, L, et al. Matrix metalloproteinases and other matrix proteinases in relation to cariology: the era of "dentin degradomics". Caries Res, 2015, 49: 193–208.

[204] Tjäderhane L, et al. The effect of chemical inhibition of matrix metalloproteinases on the size of experimentally induced apical periodontitis. Int Endod J, 2007, 40: 282–289.

[205] Tjäderhane L, et al. Polarity of mature human odontoblasts. J Dent Res, 2013, 92: 1011–1016.

[206] Tjäderhane, L, et al. Human odontoblast culture method: the expression of collagen and matrix metalloproteinases (MMPs). Adv Dent Res, 2001, 15: 55–58.

[207] Tjäderhane L, et al. A novel organ culture method to study the function of human odontoblasts in vitro: gelatinase expression by odontoblasts is differentially regulated by TGF-beta1. J Dent Res, 1998, 77: 1486–1496.

[208] Tjäderhane L, et al. Dentin basic structure and composition-an overview. Endodontic Topics, 2009, 20: 3–29.

[209] Tjäderhane L, Haapasalo M. The dentin-pulp border: a dynamic interface between hard and soft tissues. Endodontic Topics, 2009, 20: 52–84.

[210] Tranasi M, et al. Microarray evaluation of age-related changes in human dental pulp. J Endod, 2009, 35: 1211–1217.

[211] Tsai C H, et al. The upregulation of matrix metalloproteinase-9 in inflamed human dental pulps. J Endod, 2005, 31: 860–862.

[212] Tsuchiya M, et al. The extent of odontoblast processes in the dentin is distinct between cusp and cervical regions during development and aging. Arch Histol Cytol, 2002, 65: 179–188.

[213] Tsurumachi T, et al. Scanning electron microscopic study of dentinal pulpal walls in relation to age and tooth area. J Oral Sci, 2008, 50: 199–203.

[214] Vandevska-Radunovic V. Neural modulation of inflammatory reactions in dental tissues incident to orthodontic tooth movement. A review of the literature. Eur J Orthod, 1999, 21: 231–247.

[215] Vashishth D. The role of the collagen matrix in skeletal fragility. Curr Osteoporos Rep, 2007, 5: 62–66.

[216] Vasiliadis L, Darling A I, Levers B G. The amount and distribution of sclerotic human root dentine. Arch Oral Biol, 1983, 28: 645–649.

[217] Veerayutthwilai O, et al. Differential regulation of immune responses by odontoblasts. Oral Microbiol Immunol, 2007, 22: 5–13.

[218] Virtej A, et al. Vascular endothelial growth factors signalling in normal human dental pulp: a study of gene and protein expression. Eur J Oral Sci, 2013, 121: 92–100.

[219] Wahlgren J, et al. Matrix metalloproteinase-8 (MMP-8) in pulpal and periapical inflammation and periapical root-canal exudates. Int Endod J, 2002, 35: 897–904.

[220] Wan C, et al. MMP9 deficiency mincreased the size of experimentally induced apical periodontitis. J Endod, 2014, 40: 658–664.

[221] Wang J, Feng J Q. Signaling pathways critical for tooth root formation. J Dent Res, 2017, 96: 1221–1228.

[222] Westenbroek R E, Anderson N L, Byers M R. Altered localization of Cav1.2 (L-type) calcium channels in nerve fibers, Schwann cells, odontoblasts, and fibroblasts of tooth pulp after toothinjury. J Neurosci Res, 2004, 75: 371–383.

[223] Whitfield J F. The solitary (primary, cilium-a mechanosensory toggle switch in bone and cartilage cells. Cell Signal, 2008, 20: 1019–1024.

[224] Wysolmerski J J. Osteocytes remove and replace perilacunar mineral during reproductive cycles. Bone, 2013, 54: 230–236.

[225] Xiong J, Gronthos S, Bartold P M. Role of the epithelial cell rests of Malassez in the development, maintenance and regeneration of periodontal ligament tissues. Periodontol,

2013, 2000 (63): 217–233.
[226] Xu H, et al. The effects of ageing on the biomechanical properties of root dentine and fracture. J Dent, 2014, 42: 305–311.
[227] Yamamoto T, et al. Histological review of the human cellular cementum with special reference to an alternating lamellar pattern. Odontology, 2010, 98: 102–109.
[228] Yan W, et al. Reduction in fracture resistance of the root with aging. J Endod, 2017, 43: 1494–1498.
[229] Yoshiba K, et al. Odontoblast processes in human dentin revealed by fluorescence labeling and transmission electron microscopy. Histochem Cell Biol, 2002, 118: 205–212.
[230] Yoshiba N, et al. Immunohistochemical analysis of two stem cell markers of alpha-smooth muscle actin and STRO-1 during wound healing of human dental pulp. Histochem Cell Biol, 2012, 138: 583–592.
[231] Zaslansky P, Friesem A A, Weiner S. Structure and mechanical properties of the soft zone separating bulk dentin and enamel in crowns of human teeth: insight into tooth function. J Struct Biol, 2006, 153: 188–199.
[232] Zaslansky P, Zabler S, Fratzl P. 3D variations in human crown dentin tubule orientation: a phasecontrast microtomography study. Dent Mater, 2010, 26: e1–10.
[233] Zhang Q, et al. Cloning and functional study of porcine parotid hormone, a novel proline-rich protein. J Biol Chem, 2005, 280: 22233–22244.
[234] Zhao N, Foster B L, Bonewald L F. The cementocyte-an osteocyte relative? J Dent Res, 2016, 95: 734–741.

第 3 章　牙髓病与根尖周病的病因及发病机制

Ashraf F. Fouad, Asma A. Khan

3.1　概述

本章将讨论牙髓病与根尖周炎的病因及发病机制。牙髓的微生物刺激来源多样，多数情况下来源于牙冠，也可能来源于侧支根管或根尖。微生物的刺激对牙髓组织有深远的影响，通常会导致严重的症状，但有时也只引起无症状的牙髓变性。同样，根尖周炎也可无症状或伴随严重的症状，或者可能引发扩散或者偶尔危及生命的感染。对于有着相似的病理变化的病例会出现各种各样的症状，病理改变和临床症状缺乏相关性的原因，目前尚未完全明确。虽然在以疼痛为主要症状的牙髓炎及根尖周炎中发现了大量的与疼痛相关的神经肽以及其他炎性介质，但尚不清楚在什么情况下这些因子会增多，而牙髓坏死通常不伴有明显的症状。

牙髓及根尖周疾病源于这些组织的感染，最终导致牙髓的变性坏死和根尖周骨吸收，随着根尖周病变的发展，还可能出现囊肿、严重的感染或骨髓炎。有时，正畸治疗或创伤性损伤可能会使牙根发生不同形式的吸收。一般认为，牙根吸收的发病机制与骨吸收相似，通常发生在牙骨质或内层的牙本质被破坏以后。这些病变的病理活检均为炎症反应的不同表现，由多种细胞因子、趋化因子、神经肽、蛋白酶和其他炎症相关分子所介导。目前尚未发现牙髓内发生肿瘤性变化，即使是存在颌骨肿瘤时。存在颌骨肿瘤时，根尖周骨组织可能已发生吸收，但牙髓多数仍有活力。这一表现对在临床上鉴别牙髓疾病和非牙髓起源的但表现相似的其他疾病非常重要。有趣的是，牙髓病似乎不会发展为肿瘤，通常只会发展为牙髓坏死或牙髓源性的肿瘤样疾病。

动物实验证实，一旦牙髓暴露于口腔中的细菌，牙髓坏死的牙的根尖周炎发展非常迅速，在不同的哺乳动物模型中，牙髓坏死通常在几周内发生。牙髓腔内的微生物在组织坏死后会继续向根尖进展，这取决于环境、成分和营养因素。值得注意的是，微生物刺激的持续时间决定了疾病的发病机制和机体对治疗的反应。长期的微生物刺激，无论是原发性感染还是不完善的治疗，都会影响微生物生物膜的空间分布，并可能导致其向复杂的根管环境、牙本质小管乃至根尖区域潜在扩展。在这些区域根管消毒的效果会减弱，与拔牙相比，治疗的反应可能会更慢且效果较差。

3.2　牙髓炎和根尖周炎的病因

龋病引起的微生物感染是牙髓炎和根尖周炎最常见的病因。正常情况下，已萌出牙齿的牙冠上会附着一层由共生微生物群落组成的生物膜。在高糖环境下，这些群落中的特定细菌群会产生酸使牙本质脱矿，导致龋坏。长久以来，变异链球菌被认为是龋病唯一的致病菌，但最近的研究表明龋病是由复杂微生物群引起的[39, 128, 149]。局限于牙釉质的龋损会引起牙髓内细微的变化，例如表达主要组织相容性复合体Ⅱ类（MHC Class Ⅱ）抗原细胞的增多。一旦龋损处的生物膜破坏牙釉质侵入牙本质，就会进一步引起牙髓的炎症反应[90, 91, 177, 232-234]。

除了龋损外，牙髓还可能通过其他途径直接暴露于微生物及其产物，例如外伤引起的复杂牙折或医源性牙髓暴露。牙周病在引起牙髓炎症或坏死中的作用仍存在争议[81, 152]。一些研究认为[115, 184]牙周病会引起炎症细胞侵入牙髓和牙髓钙化。然而，只有所有主根尖孔均被细菌感染时，牙髓才会发生完全坏死。一项临床前研究表明，建立边缘性牙周炎模型后，57%的患牙牙髓发生了轻微的病理改变[13]，实验组的92颗牙中只有一颗发生了牙髓坏死。其他研究则表明，牙周炎不会引起牙髓的改变。

一项关于细菌感染在牙髓及根尖周病中作用的开创性研究对比了无菌大鼠和普通大鼠在牙髓暴露后的变化。在整个实验周期中，无菌大鼠的牙髓一直有活力，根尖周组织也正常，并在牙髓暴露后的第28天观察到完整的牙本质桥形成。相反，在普通大鼠组，在实验的早期就出现牙髓坏死，并逐渐发展成根尖周脓肿和肉芽肿。另一项关于根管系统感染的开创性研究探讨了不同菌群之间的关联，这项灵长动物的研究用不同组合的细菌感染根管系统，发现当联合使用时可引发严重的炎症反应，这是首次证实不同细菌可在根尖周组织中形成多菌种群[50]。这些实验表明了牙髓及根尖周病是由能形成生物膜的多种细菌感染引起的，其他多项研究证实了这一结论[12, 50, 165, 208]。

随着先进的分子工具的发展，研究人员进一步认识了牙髓和根尖周感染的多种微生物的特性[59]。例如，一项临床观察研究收集并检测了有症状的不可复性牙髓炎深层牙本质龋坏的细菌（$N=10$）[170]，其中一半的晚期龋以乳杆菌为主，其余样本的优势菌为假分枝杆菌属、欧氏菌属、链球菌属和寡养单胞菌属。相反，其他研究发现[29, 106, 133, 182]牙本质深龋主要以普雷沃菌为主。结果不一致的主要原因可能是实验方法的差异或不同地区人群口腔微生物组成不同[11]。

将通过培养法和分子技术的研究数据整合后，发现在感染根管中已鉴定出超过460种细菌，分别隶属9门100属。其中优势菌包括了厚壁菌门、拟杆菌门、放线菌门和变形菌门[191]。这些研究还表明，感染根管中的微生物不仅限于细菌，还包括真菌、古生菌[219, 220]，以及病毒[28, 47, 82, 120, 158]。

虽然微生物感染是牙髓炎的主要病因，但诊疗过程中的操作（例如窝洞的预备和修复）也会对牙髓产生不利影响。牙釉质和牙本质是身体中最硬的组织，在窝洞预备过程中的产热可能会诱发牙髓炎症[116, 183, 197]。目前大多数的修复材料只要不直接与牙髓接触，就不会对牙髓产生不良影响，但修复体周围的微渗漏可引起牙髓炎症[73]。

3.3 牙髓和根尖周组织的炎症与感染

3.3.1 细菌刺激和侵入牙髓

冠方来源的牙髓刺激，如龋病、牙隐裂、冠折、磨损、酸蚀或牙冠的先天畸形都会引起牙髓炎症。即使是早期的窝沟龋也与牙髓炎症有关，其范围与受累的牙本质小管一致[20]。牙骨质覆盖的牙根表面暴露后，细菌从牙本质小管的外侧面侵入进而引起相应位置牙髓的轻微炎症[114]。在这种情况下，细菌可能并不存在于牙髓内，但分泌的酶、毒素或细胞壁分子会通过牙本质小管刺激牙髓。当细菌刺激物接近牙髓时，在最接近刺激的区域牙髓炎症反应最强烈，最终扩散到远处的牙髓区域。牙髓炎症的程度取决于细菌刺激物的量以及与牙髓的接近程度[140, 165]。最终，细菌感染进入牙髓并在活髓中发展，导致牙髓变性和根尖周炎。这种潜在感染引起的炎症反应最终也会发生在根尖周组织中，尤其是牙髓完全坏死之后。根尖周感染可导致急性或慢性脓肿形成，特别是当有足够数量的致病菌到达根尖区域时。因此，牙髓和根尖周组织在受到细菌侵入并感染之前都会经历一个炎症变化阶段。临床诊断的主要目的之一是确定病变的牙髓和根尖周组织是处于炎症状态还是已经感染，因为这会影响麻醉考量、应急处理、治疗方案的确定以及对预后的评估。

小鼠模型的研究表明，当牙髓暴露于口腔中的细菌时，其炎症反应及随后的退行性改变通常是由固有免疫介导的。实验结果显示：与正常组相比，适应性免疫细胞（例如T细胞和B细胞）缺乏的动物牙髓坏死发生率无明显差异[55, 222]；

而适应性免疫，特别是B细胞和免疫球蛋白，可抵御由大量致病菌引起的严重感染[212]。

强效的细菌分子，如细菌肽聚糖、革兰氏阴性菌的脂多糖（LPS，即内毒素）以及革兰氏阳性菌的脂磷壁酸（LTA）均能够引发明显的牙髓和根尖周炎症。动物实验证实，将LPS放置于无菌的根管中可导致根尖周病变[34, 45]。LPS是骨吸收的强效介质[23]，通过激活花生四烯酸途径，产生细胞因子以及补体激活发挥作用[23]。此外，研究还发现LPS可激活三叉神经痛觉感受器上的TLR4受体[221]，这与临床上龋病和感染牙髓的疼痛症状的产生有关[84, 92, 134]。然而，LPS并不是唯一参与牙髓炎和根尖周炎病程的细菌刺激物。研究验证了在LPS低反应模型中，牙髓和根尖周疾病发展进程与正常动物模型相似，这表明除LPS、肽聚糖、细菌蛋白酶、毒素以及其他毒力因子可能共同参与了这一过程[60]。

临床上，牙髓坏死时通常可在X线片上看到根尖周骨组织的丧失。一个令人惊讶的发现是在动物研究中，牙髓炎时期便可观察到根尖周炎症的病理表现。事实上，这一临床现象已被证实是根尖片对早期根尖周病变检测的灵敏度低造成的，而更先进的技术，例如CBCT在对牙髓炎中有根尖周病变的检测比根尖片灵敏[1]。因此，根尖周的骨吸收及根尖周病变的形成不需要牙髓的完全坏死。

3.4 牙髓

3.4.1 牙髓的防御系统

牙髓可以检测到入侵的病原体并建立免疫反应。与机体其他组织一样，牙髓的防御系统可分为固有免疫反应和适应性免疫反应。固有免疫反应是非抗原特异性的，包括牙本质液向外流动和小管内免疫球蛋白的沉积[130, 136, 155]，还包括常驻细胞（例如成牙本质细胞和成纤维细胞）和固有免疫细胞（例如树突状细胞，自然杀伤细胞和T细胞）。成牙本质细胞位于牙髓–牙本质交界处，其突起延伸至牙本质小管内。虽然成牙本质细胞的主要功能是在牙齿形成过程中产生前牙本质基质并控制其矿化，但它们在牙髓的免疫反应中也发挥着重要作用。据推测，它们代表了牙髓的第一道生物活性防线，其作用类似于皮肤和黏膜上皮细胞。成牙本质细胞表达Toll样受体（TLR），这是一种模式识别受体，具体来说，他们表达Toll样受体1、2、4、6和9[44, 95, 217]。刺激Toll样受体可激活MyD88依赖通路，继而激活NF-k′B和丝裂原活化蛋白激酶（MAPK），导致促炎基因和趋化因子基因的表达，例如CCL2、CCL5、CCL7、CXCL8和CXCL10[199]。成牙本质细胞还表达NLR家族蛋白，如NOD2，它能识别革兰氏阳性菌和革兰氏阴性菌共有的肽聚糖成分[198]。激活的成牙本质细胞会释放一些分子，如一氧化氮（NO）、β-防御素（BD）、脂多糖结合蛋白（LBP）、白介素-6（IL-6）、超趋化因子CXCL1、CXCL2、CXCL8、CCL2[41-42, 44, 111, 154, 217]，以及IL-10，其中一些会通过牙本质扩散至龋损部位，以达到消灭病原微生物（如NO和BD）或降低其致病力（如LBP）的目的；另一些则扩散到牙髓中，激活并调动免疫细胞[44]（图3.1）。

成纤维细胞不仅在细胞外基质的合成和转化中发挥作用，也参与了牙髓的免疫防御反应。它们表达多种模式识别受体，如TLR-2、TLR-4、TLR-5、NOD以及NOD1、NOD2[83, 103, 126, 199]，这些受体一旦被激活就会释放TNFα、CXCL8或其他介质[102]。一项研究对比了成纤维细胞和成牙本质细胞样细胞对不同TLR激动剂的反应[199]。结果发现脂磷壁酸（LTA）和TLR2特异性激动剂会使成牙本质细胞中CXCL2和CXCL10的上调，而成纤维细胞没有变化。与此同时LPS、TLR4特异性激动剂会诱导成纤维细胞中CCL7、CCL26以及CXCL11的表达增高，但未在成牙本质细胞中观察到。这说明成牙本质细胞和成纤维细胞通过影响牙髓中不同的免疫细胞建立特异性免疫应答。

牙髓内的固有免疫细胞包括白细胞、单核吞噬树突状细胞和自然杀伤细胞（NK细胞）[71]。这些细胞不断监测其所在微环境，以便探测入侵的病原微生物。一旦检测到病原体，免疫细胞的数量就会急剧增多。中性粒细胞是最早被招募到感染部位的细胞之一，接下来是单核细胞，单核细胞会进一步分化为巨噬细胞[32, 80, 90, 131]。树突状细胞和NK细胞也会在感染处聚集，它们会捕捉细菌抗原或摧毁入侵的病原体[44, 96, 101, 129, 233]。树突状细胞和NK细胞之间的相互作用会导致两者之间的双向激活，并增加细胞因子的产生。这些固有免疫细胞也会激活适应性免疫反应[107, 224]。树突状细胞会迁移至局部淋巴结，在淋巴结处向CD4+T细胞（即Th0细胞）呈递抗原并激活它们[17]。

除了上述所提到的固有免疫反应，支配牙髓的神经也能检测病原体并产生应答。一项严谨可靠的研究利用人和大鼠三叉神经以及大鼠牙髓组织清晰地展示了在牙髓感觉神经末梢中CD14和TLR4蛋白的表达[221]。后续研究表明，LPS通过激活三叉神经的TLR4从而提高TRPV1离子通道的敏感性[40, 52]。这些研究以及先前关于牙髓暴露时神经细胞反应的研究，为牙髓炎中神经源性炎症的作用提供了进一步的证据支持[105, 108, 211]。

3.4.1.1 适应性免疫

如前所述，树突状细胞激活淋巴结中的CD4+细胞，后者随后分化成效应辅助T细胞或诱导调节性T细胞（图3.2）。随着龋病病损向牙髓进展，T细胞的数量会有所增加[50, 79, 91]。健康的牙髓含有少量的B细胞，随着龋病进展和炎症发生B细胞数量会增多[71, 79]。在炎症牙髓中，主要的B细胞衍生免疫球蛋白是IgG1，其次是IgA和IgE。

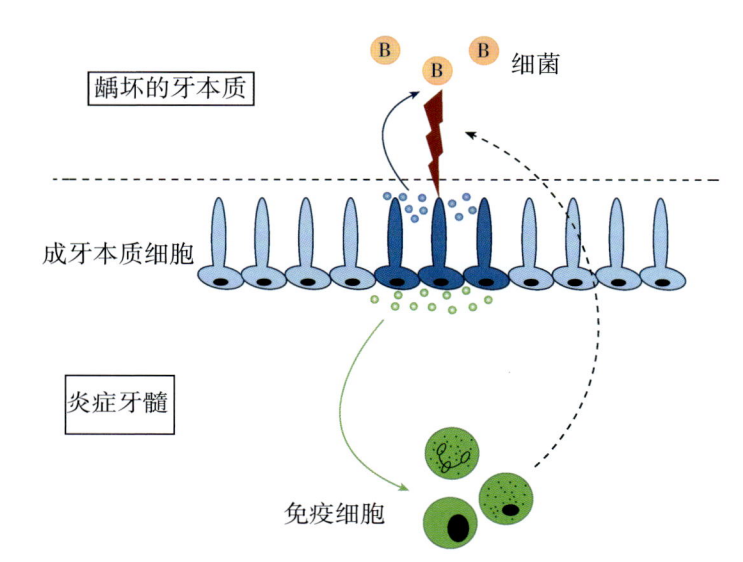

图3.1 成牙本质细胞防御机制示意图。成牙本质细胞（蓝色）对牙本质龋坏中细菌（B）刺激的应答是释放介质，如一氧化氮（NO）、防御素（BDs）、脂多糖结合蛋白（LBP）、IL-6、CXCL1、CXCL 2、CXCL 8、CCL2和IL-10。其中一些介质通过牙本质扩散到龋损处，破坏病原体以降低其致病力；另一些扩散到牙髓激活和调动免疫细胞（经许可摘自文献51）

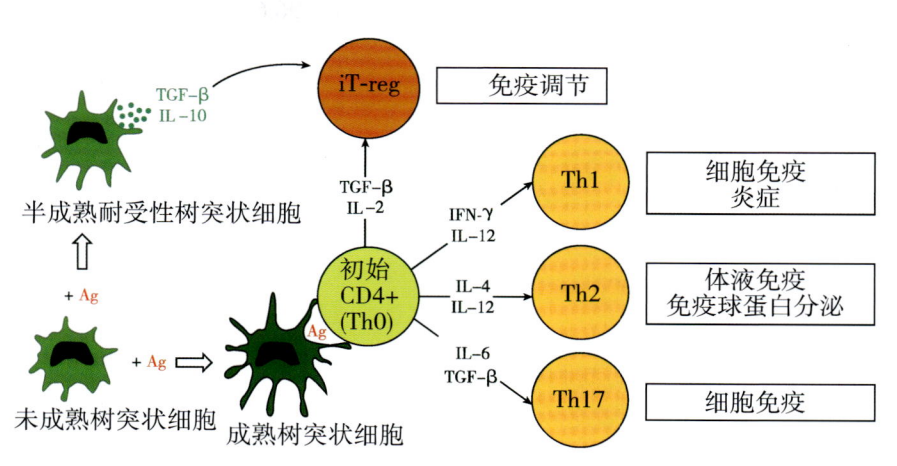

图3.2 树突状细胞(DC)在激活适应性免疫应答中的作用。未成熟的DC在遇到抗原后变成成熟的DC。DC将抗原呈递给初始CD4+细胞，接着CD4+增殖并分化成效应辅助T细胞（如Th1、Th2或Th17）或调节性T细胞(iT-reg)。此外，部分未成熟的树突状细胞形成耐受性树突细胞（Tol-DC）转而诱导iT-reg分化。TGF：转化生长因子。IL：白介素。IFN：干扰素（经许可摘自文献51）

3.4.2 牙髓炎的分类

目前，普遍接受的诊断分类是基于对治疗预后的认知。诊断主要依据患者的症状（表现、持续时间、严重程度以及类型），是否有龋病或修复体，牙髓敏感测试以及临床和影像学检查。健康的牙髓一般无症状，所有临床检查（包括探诊、叩诊、牙髓温度测试或牙髓电活力测试）结果都在正常的表现范围内，影像学表现正常，但注意正常牙髓也可能有钙化现象。

牙髓炎通常分为可复性和不可复性牙髓炎。前者是指一种可"逆转"的轻度炎症状态，换句话说，如果治疗得当，例如去除刺激因素后牙髓是可治愈的。可复性牙髓炎的病因包括龋病、创伤、近期做过治疗或存在不完善的修复治疗。临床检查探诊和叩诊无明显反应，对热刺激有一过性且不持续的反应，咬合时偶有轻微疼痛。可复性牙髓炎影像学表现正常。

当牙髓炎症比较严重，且预后不太可能恢复为正常牙髓时，牙髓状态归为"不可复性牙髓炎"。此时牙齿通常有症状，表现为自发痛和（或）在去除热刺激后持续性疼痛。牙齿可能对叩诊敏感，且通常有正常的影像学表现。病因包括深龋、深部修复体和牙隐裂。这些牙髓的又被称为"有症状的不可复性牙髓炎"。相反，相比之下一些有龋病暴露或创伤的牙齿并未表现出任何症状。基于目前的认知，这些发炎牙髓预后不良且最终可能发展为牙髓坏死。这些牙髓被划分为"无症状的不可复性牙髓炎"。

目前还没有充分的证据支持不可复性牙髓炎是真正的不可复。单纯依据患者的疼痛史和现有的诊断工具，尚不能确定退行性炎症是累及整个牙髓还是局限在部分牙髓。如本章后面所述，在对临床诊断为"不可复性炎症"的牙髓进行组织学评估后发现，在某些牙齿中，仅在一个髓角处并非全部牙髓有炎症现象[167]。随着新型盖髓材料的发展，对于不可复性牙髓炎的牙齿，进行部分或全部切髓术似乎是一种可行的治疗选择，可能不需要将整个牙髓完全摘除[8, 48]。

3.4.3 牙髓炎的组织学和分子评估

如前所述，牙髓内多种细胞都表达病源识别受体，并对微生物感染迅速反应。近期一项研究通过将大鼠牙髓暴露于磷酸盐缓冲液（PBS）或LPS，检测牙髓损伤和感染后组织学和分子学的反应[116]。分别于暴露后3h，9h和3d取材，以未处理牙牙髓作为对照。最早在暴露后9h可观察到炎细胞的浸润，3d后可见骨性牙本质基质生成。与暴露于PBS的牙髓相比，暴露于LPS的牙髓炎症细胞浸润及骨性牙本质沉积的范围更大（图3.3）。牙本质唾液磷蛋白（dspp）的表达也发生了类似的变化。流式细胞分析显示白细胞和树突状细胞增多，T细胞和NK细胞的比例不变。这项研究还检测了炎症基因的表达，LPS处理组在3h可见IL-6、IL-1β、IL-10、TNFα、iNOS、CCL2、CXCL1、CXCL2表达增高，而基质金属蛋白酶3（MMP3）在9h和3d表达上调。

另一项临床研究观察了不同牙髓的组织学状态，包括临床诊断为不可复性牙髓炎（32颗），可复性牙髓炎（59颗）以及正常牙髓（4颗）[167]。被诊断为不可复性牙髓炎的牙髓中，大部分（84.4%）在冠髓的部分区域显示出凝固性或液化性坏死，并伴有细菌定植及大量的白细胞浸润。在冠髓其余部分以及某些牙齿中，炎症/免疫反应的程度要轻得多；在对侧髓角处可见未感染的正常牙髓（图3.4）。

其余被诊断为不可复性炎症的牙髓（15.6%）可见局部的炎症细胞聚集，但无组织坏死以及细菌感染，这一组织学诊断与可复性牙髓炎相符。绝大多数（96.6%）诊断为可复性牙髓炎的组织学诊断与临床诊断一致，在这些牙髓中可见轻度至中度的慢性炎症细胞聚集及第三期牙本质形成。

另有临床研究检测了表现为轻度至重度疼痛的牙髓炎患者以及正常牙齿的基因表达[67]。与正常牙髓相比，牙髓炎组中涉及免疫应答、细胞因子受体互作和信号转导、整合素细胞表面相互作用等相关基因的表达水平升高（图3.5，图3.6）。

此外，一些已知的调节疼痛的炎症分子在无症状和轻度疼痛的患者（视觉模拟疼痛表上大于30mm）牙髓中的表达与中度到重度疼痛患者相比有差异（表3.1）。

少数临床研究已经在蛋白水平上检测了牙髓血液中的分子标记物。与健康的牙髓相比，

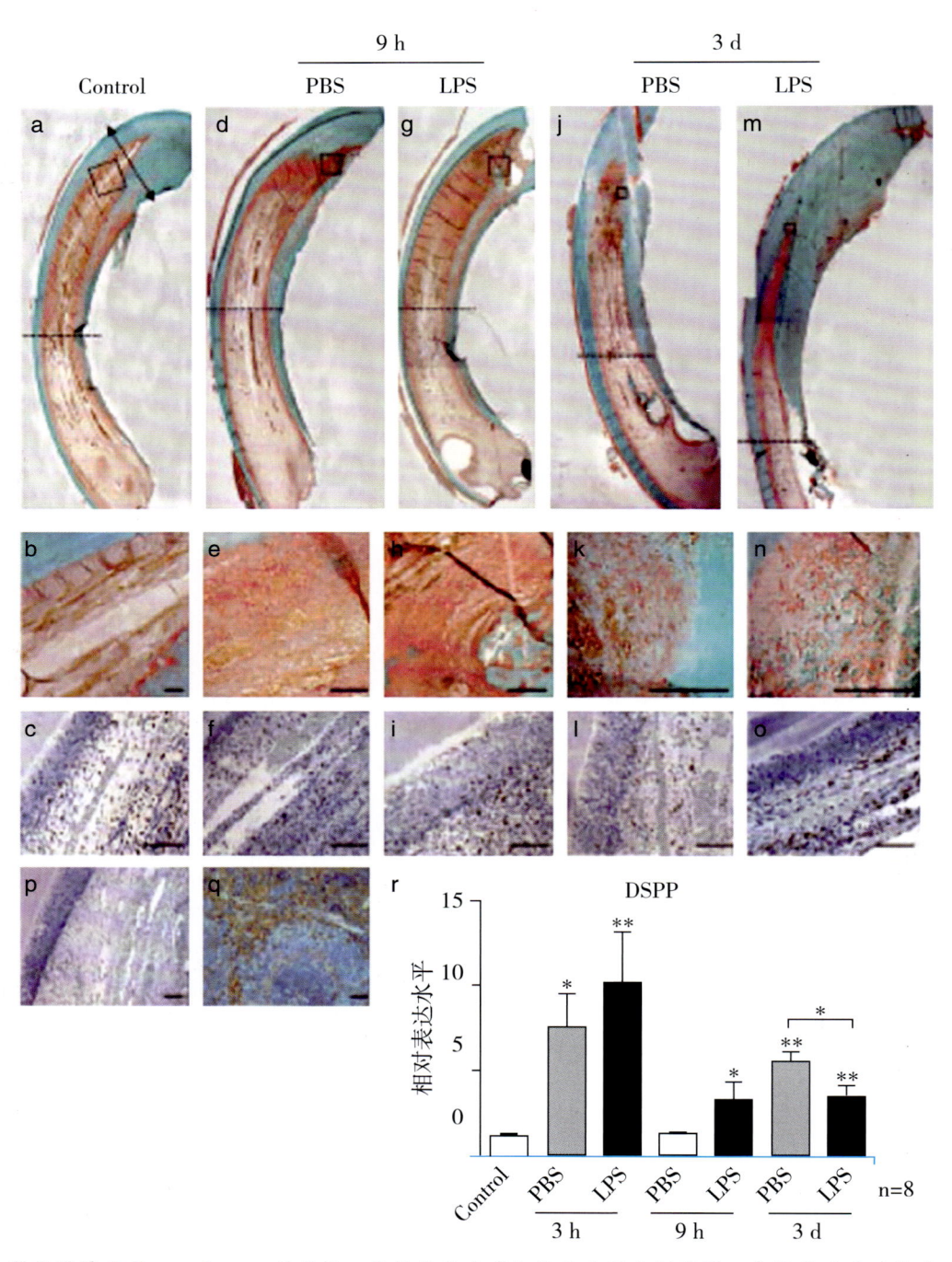

图 3.3 大鼠牙髓暴露于 LPS 和 PBS 的马松三色染色和免疫组化染色的分析结果，未暴露的牙髓作为对照组。图 a 箭头指示牙冠截断牙髓暴露处，与暴露于 PBS 的相比（d. 低倍镜；e. 高倍镜），暴露于 LPS 的大鼠牙髓表现出更明显的炎症渗出物（g. 低倍镜；h. 高倍镜）。在 PBS 组 3d 可见伤口愈合并有胶原沉积（j. 低倍镜；k. 高倍镜）。牙本质涎磷蛋白（DSPP）在 3h 和 9h 表达增高（r）（经许可摘自文献 166）。Control：对照组。PBS：磷酸盐缓冲盐水。LPS：脂多糖

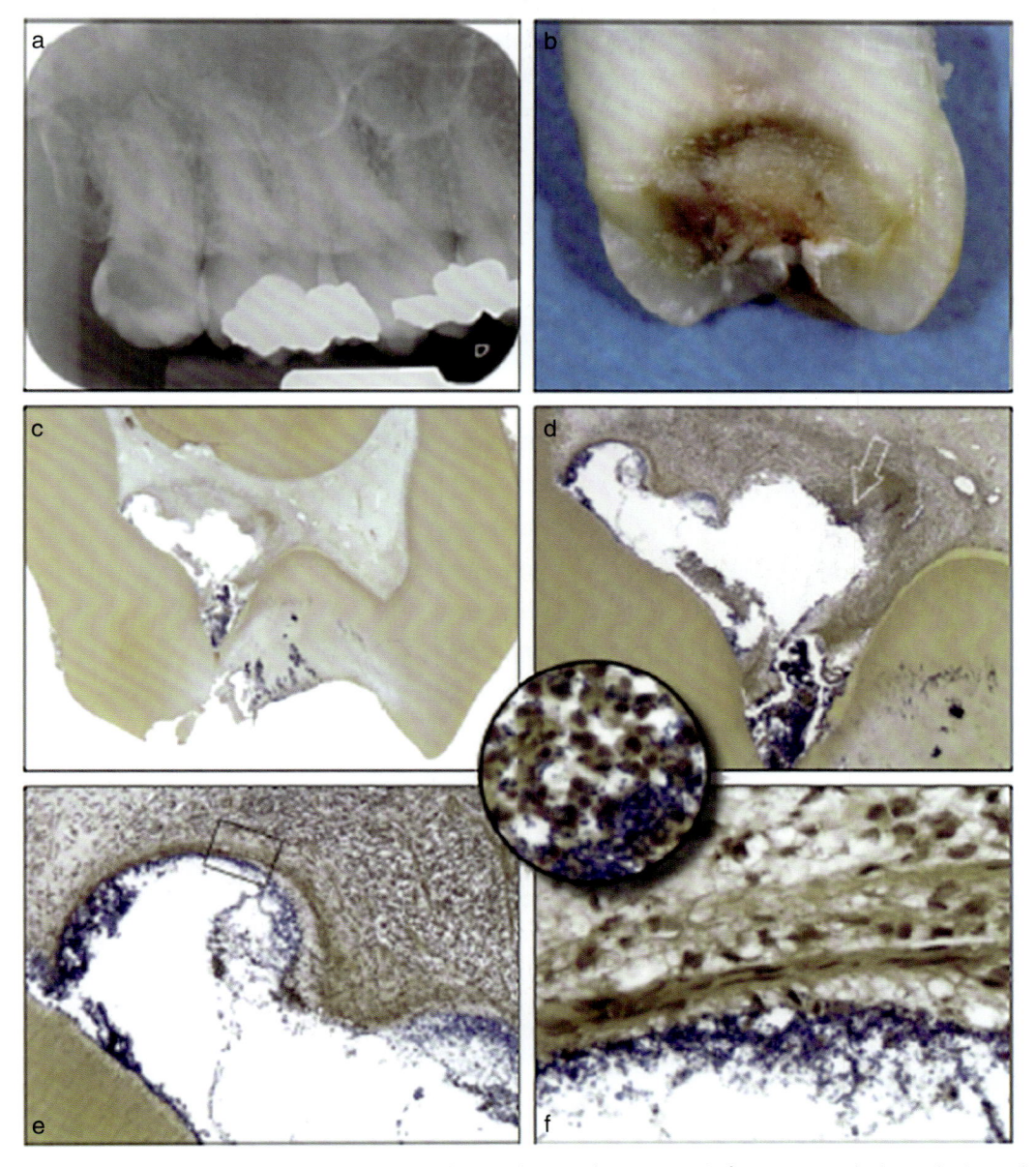

图 3.4 临床诊断为不可逆型牙髓炎的组织病理分析。患者，30岁，男，临床表现为剧烈疼痛。a. 根尖X线片。b. 准备用于切片的颊舌面。c. 冠髓的镜下大体观可见脓肿，注意对侧髓角表现正常。d. 脓肿处放大，注意坏死碎片（放大16倍）。e. 脓肿局部图（放大40倍）。f. 将E图矩形区域放大倍数（放大400倍）。插入D图中箭头所指脓肿处高倍镜图像（放大400倍），可见中性粒细胞和细菌的聚集（经许可摘自文献167）

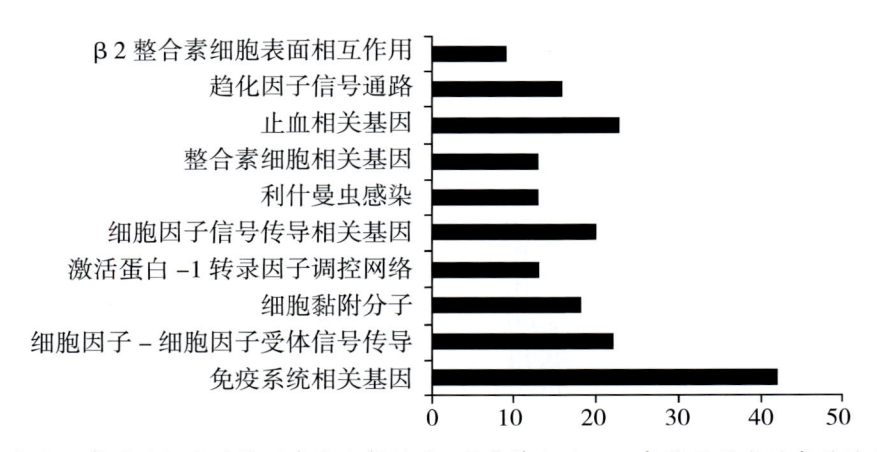

牙髓病学基础：根尖周炎的预防和治疗

功能归类	数量
β2 整合素细胞表面相互作用	
趋化因子信号通路	
止血相关基因	
整合素细胞相关基因	
利什曼虫感染	
细胞因子信号传导相关基因	
激活蛋白-1 转录因子调控网络	
细胞黏附分子	
细胞因子-细胞因子受体信号传导	
免疫系统相关基因	

图 3.5　牙髓炎标本和正常牙髓标本的基因富集分析结果。收集诊断为不可复性牙髓炎的患牙的炎症牙髓（$n=20$），因各种原因将从牙齿中取出的正常牙髓作为对照组（$n=20$），利用 Affymetrix GeneTitan 多通道仪器进行全基因组基因芯片分析。每条柱状代表两组差异基因所属不同功能归类和数量差异（经许可摘自文献 67）

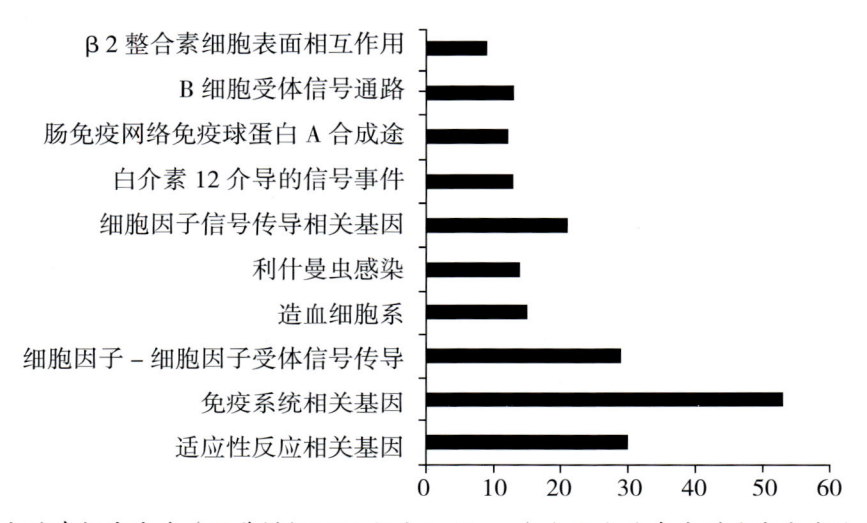

功能归类	数量
β2 整合素细胞表面相互作用	
B 细胞受体信号通路	
肠免疫网络免疫球蛋白 A 合成途	
白介素 12 介导的信号事件	
细胞因子信号传导相关基因	
利什曼虫感染	
造血细胞系	
细胞因子-细胞因子受体信号传导	
免疫系统相关基因	
适应性反应相关基因	

图 3.6　无疼痛或伴有轻度疼痛（视觉模拟 VAS 评分 ≥ 30mm）与评分为中度到重度疼痛的牙髓炎差异基因富集分析。样本收集和分析方式如图 3.5。每条柱状代表无痛、轻度疼痛与中度、重度疼痛之间的基因表达所属不同功能归类和数量差异（$q<0.05$）（经许可摘自文献 67）

表 3.1　牙髓炎患者中选出上调或下调的基因

基因符号	牙髓炎与正常牙髓	无-轻度疼痛与中-重度疼痛	基因功能 (genecards.org)
AMELX			釉质生物矿化
CALCRL			骨代谢
CCL20			趋化因子
CD14			固有免疫应答
CD163			急性期受体
CD79A			B 细胞受体功能
COL10A1			胶原形成
COL11A1			胶原形成
COL12A1			胶原形成

表 3.1（续）

基因符号	牙髓炎与正常牙髓	无 – 轻度疼痛与中 – 重度疼痛	基因功能 (genecards.org)
COL14A1			胶原形成
COL15A1			胶原形成
COL18A1			胶原形成
COL1A1			胶原形成
COL1A2			胶原形成
COL21A1			胶原形成
COL4A1			胶原形成
COL4A2			胶原形成
CXCL3			趋化因子
DEFA1B/1A			抗菌活性
DEFA3			抗菌活性
DSPP			牙本质形成
IL10RA			IL-10 信号
IL1A			炎症反应
IL1B			炎症反应
IL6			炎症，B 细胞成熟
IL8			趋化因子
LBP			固有免疫应答
MMP13			胶原降解
MMP20			釉原蛋白降解
MMP9			胶原降解
NOD2			固有免疫应答
NR5A2			抗病毒活性
PTGS2			前列腺素形成
SCN8A			钠离子通透性
TLR2			固有免疫应答
TLR2			固有免疫应答
TLR3			固有免疫应答
TLR4			固有免疫应答
TLR6			固有免疫应答
TLR8			固有免疫应答
TLR9			固有免疫应答
TNFA			炎症反应

免疫球蛋白 IgG、IgA、IgM 以及弹性蛋白酶和 PGE2 升高[2]。细胞因子 IL-8 在有症状的感染牙髓中的表达比在正常牙髓和有龋坏的无症状牙髓中高[49]。牙本质液中的内容物也会反应牙髓中的分子变化。一项有趣的临床研究对比了诊断为不可复性牙髓炎（n=19）和正常牙髓（n=12）牙本质液中 MMP9 的表达情况[235]。MMP9 是一种由中性粒细胞分泌的蛋白水解酶，可能是组织破坏的标志物。数据显示与无症状牙相比，有症状牙齿的 MMP9 水平明显升高。

表观遗传修饰在牙髓炎中作用的研究才刚刚起步。表观遗传修饰包括 DNA 甲基化、组蛋白修饰和非编码 RNA 的调控。迄今为止，只有两项研究检测了牙髓炎 DNA 甲基化。其中一项检测了感染牙髓中干扰素 γ 的甲基化状态，发现部分甲基化或非甲基化现象均存在[25]；另一项研究报道指出 CD14 和 TLR2 的甲基化在正常牙髓和炎症牙髓中没有差异[24]，最近的研究发现 H3K27 的组蛋白甲基化在牙髓炎症和修复过程中有重要作用[89,230]。

MicroRNA（miRs）是一类短小的（18~22 个核苷酸）单链非编码 RNA 核苷酸。笔者所在实验室首次报道了 miR 在炎症牙髓中的表达情况[236]。炎症牙髓来自被诊断为有症状或无症状的不可复性牙髓炎（n=18），正常牙髓来自健康的第三磨牙或因正畸拔除的健康牙（n=12）。与正常牙髓相比，炎症牙髓中有 36 个 miRs 表达异常。在另一项体外研究中，研究者证明了在牙髓炎中差异表达的 miRs 之一——miR181a。miR181a 能够调节细胞因子 IL-8 的表达[68]，从而证明了 microRNA 在调节牙髓对微生物感染的免疫应答中所发挥的作用。

3.5 根尖周组织

3.5.1 根尖周组织的防御系统

如前所述，在牙髓完全坏死之前，根尖周骨吸收和根尖周病变的形成就开始了。随着刺激物扩散至牙髓深处，根尖周骨组织吸收并被软组织替代是非常重要的，因为这一过程能够引发强大的免疫应答。根尖周病变的基本功能是保护身体免受坏死牙髓中细菌的入侵，以抵御两种严重的疾病的发生：急性扩散性感染和骨髓炎（图 3.7）。

虽然这些情况根尖周病变可能有较高的发生率，但多数情况下根尖周病变的发病率和严重程度是由根尖周免疫反应调节的。可以通过 X 线片观察到，根尖周病变的发展通常需要数周甚至数月的时间。在动物模型中，病变的大小稳步增加且随着细菌刺激和防御机制达到稳定阶段时趋于平稳[64]。在某些病例中，根尖周病变范围非常大（图 3.8）。学者们认为病变的大小与细菌刺激物的类型和数量、根尖周囊肿的形成以及病损内炎症介质的类型和浓度有关。现有证据表明，病变是一种受调控的机制，与微生物和宿主因素相关[200]。

3.5.1.1 急性感染

急性牙髓感染约占所有非创伤性牙科急诊的 56%[163]。在美国，每年约有超 40 万急诊门诊患者为急性牙髓感染[148]。一项研究报道，每年大

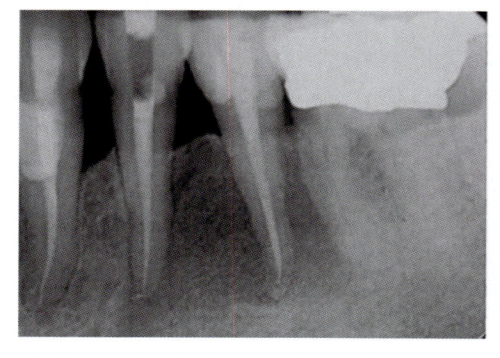

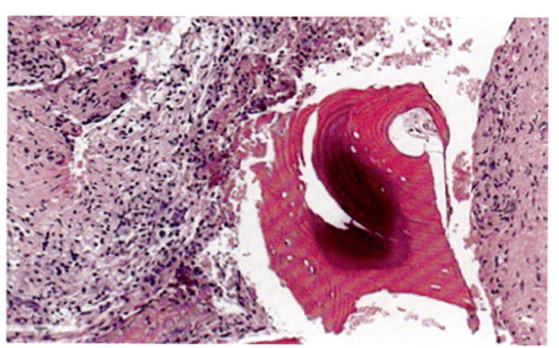

图 3.7 X 线片显示左下颌尖牙和第一、第二前磨牙进行了非手术的根管治疗，磨牙无异常。术后患者自觉此区域麻木，对前磨牙进行了根尖手术。活检结果提示有强烈的炎症反应和多个骨碎片伴空隙。诊断为骨髓炎

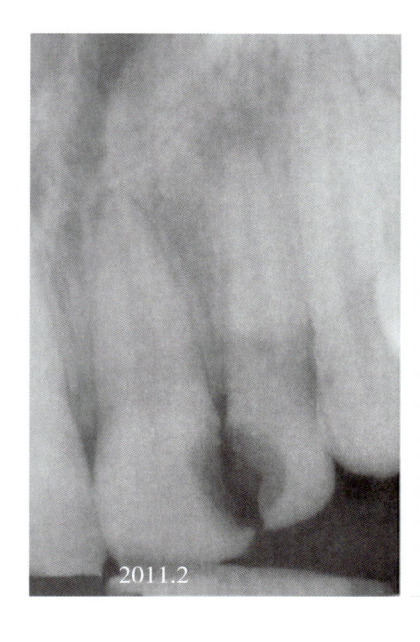

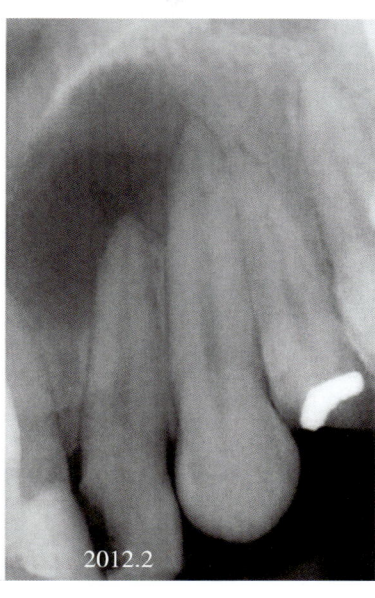

图 3.8 一个青少年患者上颌左侧侧切牙诊断为牙髓坏死和无症状的根尖周炎。患者 1 年后才进行治疗，可注意到在这期间病变显著增大（经许可摘自文献 57）

约有 8000 人因为牙髓脓肿（根尖周脓肿）住院治疗[5]，且在 8 年时间里有 66 例住院患者因此死亡[185]。在美国，27%~41% 的成年人至少有一颗牙患有根尖周炎[22]，显然，尽管数量巨大，但严重的或危及生命的牙髓感染仅限于少数病例。有症状的病例最常见的临床表现是有症状的根尖周炎伴有不可复性牙髓炎或牙髓坏死，或急性根尖周脓肿伴局部肿胀、淋巴结肿大和轻微的全身症状。根据一项研究指出，57% 有症状的不可复性牙髓炎伴有有症状的根尖周炎[151]。相反，约 40% 牙髓坏死合并慢性根尖周炎患者仅表现轻微的疼痛[139]。

目前尚不清楚哪些具体因素参与了有症状的根尖周炎或严重的根管感染的发生和发展。许多研究已经探索了特定的致病性强的牙髓病原体与牙髓感染相关的可能性。例如，多项研究证实具核梭杆菌和微小微单胞菌与牙痛之间[27, 61, 178]存在关联。此外，研究者也发现归属于普雷沃氏菌属和卟啉单胞菌属的产黑色素细菌与牙髓感染引发的疼痛症状有关[75, 77, 208-209]。通过更敏感的分子学技术研究发现，螺旋体（主要是齿垢密螺旋体）与疼痛和急性根尖周感染有密切的联系，尤其在原发性感染中[117, 176, 189]。齿垢密螺旋体（*Treponema spp.*）与急性牙髓感染之间的关联，正是分子微生物学准确性和灵敏性的体现。这是因为密螺旋体属的成员和许多其他螺旋体一样，都是非常挑剔的菌种，难以通过传统的培养法进行鉴定[58]。分子学技术还发现了与疼痛相关的其他微生物属，例如杆菌类、产丝菌属、欧陆森氏菌属，颗粒链菌属以及互养菌属[171, 192]。然而，现代深度测序技术对牙髓感染细菌样本进行分析后，清楚地揭示了其中包含数百乃至数千种不同的菌群[87, 121, 190]。此外，这些研究还显示，在感染牙髓样本中，即便最常见的单个菌群的相对丰度也非常低，没有优势菌群存在。因此，目前尚不清楚感染牙髓中的微生物群落组成如何影响症状的发展。此外，这些复杂的微生物群落在不同患者体内与宿主免疫反应的相互作用方式可能各异，这就使得准确识别真正的致病因素变得相当困难。

病毒感染可加重牙髓感染的症状，早期研究表明，人巨细胞病毒或 EB 病毒与症状明显的根尖周病变有关[174-175, 195]。然而，最近发表的一篇系统评价以及 meta 分析显示这些病毒与症状之间没有显著关联[93]。值得注意的是，水痘带状疱疹病毒感染后常继发疱疹后神经痛，临床可表现为牙痛。在一些病例报告、病例系列研究以及最新的系统评价中，这种病毒感染与牙髓病和根尖周病的发病机制有关[76, 94, 156, 187]。

3.5.1.2 慢性感染

根尖周炎似乎是牙科患者和非患者中一种非常普遍的疾病（表 3.2）。

表 3.2 在所选择的代表性研究中，成人中至少有一颗牙有根尖周病变。星号（*）代表口腔诊所患者人群

Bergström 等人，1987[15]	瑞典	48%
Odesjo 等人，1990[150]	瑞典	43%
De Cleen 等人，1993[35]	荷兰	45%*
Saunders 等人，1997[181]	苏格兰	41%*
Kirkevang 等人，2001[109]	丹麦	42%
Boucher 等人，2002[19]	法国	63%*
Kabak, Abbott, 2005[97]	白俄罗斯	80%*
Palmqvist, 1986[153]	瑞典（＞65岁）	72%
Ainamo 等人，1994[4]	芬兰（＞75岁）	41%
Caplan 等人，2006[22]	美国（＞45岁）	27%
Caplan 等人，2006[22]	美国（＞45岁）	41%

如前所述，大多数牙髓感染是无症状的，同时，微生物刺激物和宿主反应之间处于稳态关系；然而慢性或无症状的牙髓病可能会恶化，导致急性感染。这可能由于微生物群落组成或细菌载量发生了改变，也可能与宿主反应改变有关，例如免疫系统受到压力或功能损伤。由于伦理的要求，医生难以在未治疗的情况下研究病变进展，临床研究关于这一领域的客观数据十分有限。

大量的研究数据来自动物模型研究，特别是关于各种免疫因素对慢性根尖周病变大小的影响。这些动物模型大多数是慢性根尖周炎，是牙髓暴露和摘除后出现的典型病变。在某些特殊情况下，如未控制的糖尿病[62]或重度联合免疫缺陷，并且同时接种牙髓致病菌时，动物可能会发展成急性感染[212]。在正常条件下慢性根尖周病变的缓慢发展说明了免疫反应成功地防止了根尖感染向严重的弥散性感染或骨髓炎进展。这些模型中病变的大小和进展速度不同，这取决于各种微生物与宿主的反应。

在 TLR4（识别 LPS 的受体）缺陷的动物中，某些时间点的根尖周病变较小，但其他时间点并非如此[60, 85]。有趣的是，与对照组相比，识别革兰氏阳性菌脂磷壁酸的 TLR2 缺陷的动物产生的根尖周缺损较大。最近有报道称，TLR2 缺陷会增强 CD14 和 TLR4 信号，这可能解释了这些情况下根尖周病损变大的原因[169]。此外，牙髓致病菌（如具核梭杆菌）会诱导细胞因子的产生，这是由 P38 丝裂原活化蛋白激酶信号通路（MAPK）介导的，该信号传导独立于 TLRs、核苷酸结合寡聚化结构域 1（NOD-1）、NOD-2 以及 NF-kB 信号传导[162]。综上所述，这些研究表明了根尖周病变是由多种细菌和不同的识别模式导致的。

在慢性根尖周病变的发病机制中，针对正常口腔微生物，T 细胞和 B 细胞[55, 210]、补体因子 C5[86]、IL-4 [38, 180]、干扰素 γ、IL-12 或 IL-8 [179] 的缺失似乎不影响根尖周病变的发病机制。

然而，如果缺乏黏附分子 [如细胞黏附分子 1（ICAM-1）][38]、P/E 选择素[100]、IL-6[9, 88]、IL-10 [38, 180]或关键趋化因子 CCR2[70]和 CCR5 缺失[38]，则根尖周病变会变大。这些因子对于诱导循环中的炎症细胞迁移至炎症部位起着关键作用。

雌激素似乎对根尖周病变的扩大有预防作用[72, 228]，这种作用可被抗雌激素药物调节，比如雷洛昔芬[74]；相反的，像双膦酸盐类药物（如阿仑膦酸）[186, 228, 229]和二甲双胍（一种降血糖药）[127]可减少根尖周病变的骨吸收。还有许多其他药物和宿主情况可能会影响根尖周病变扩展的速度、最终病变程度以及治疗后的预后，因此这是当前研究的热点方向。

3.5.2 根尖周炎的分类

3.5.2.1 根尖周炎的组织病理学分类

根尖周炎的组织病理学分类历来都非常重要，因为它影响非手术根管治疗的预后。在这方面，根尖周炎被分为三种主要的组织病理学状态：根尖周肉芽肿、根尖周囊肿和根尖周脓肿。其他不常见的根尖部病变包括异物反应（如食物颗粒、牙科材料或封闭剂），根尖瘢痕（大的根尖病变手术治疗后纤维组织形成）或胆脂瘤（一种由胆固醇结晶伴有多核巨细胞形成的含有裂隙的病变）。

3.5.2.1.1 根尖周肉芽肿

根尖周肉芽肿因其包含诸如中性粒细胞、淋巴细胞、浆细胞、巨噬细胞和肥大细胞等多种炎症细胞而得名，这些细胞可能围绕着较大的多核巨细胞或泡沫细胞聚集，形成类似颗粒状的外观，

因此被称为"肉芽肿"。其他类似的肉芽肿性疾病还包括结核病、麻风病和结节病等。根尖周肉芽肿也含有马拉瑟上皮剩余细胞，这些是赫特维希上皮根鞘的残余，在胚胎发育过程中与牙根的发生密切相关。

即使在其他组织病理情况下（如囊肿或脓肿），病变的一部分（通常是病变周围）是根尖周肉芽肿，而且被认为是引起囊肿或脓肿的原因。根尖周肉芽肿包含上述免疫反应所涉及的细胞和分子因素。炎症细胞的数量差异可能取决于检测的技术手段、病变是否是原发性或持续性的根尖周炎，以及其来源于人类还是动物模型。人体研究表明：巨噬细胞[202,203]或淋巴细胞[14]可能在根尖肉芽肿的占主导地位。动物研究表明，辅助性T细胞普遍存在于在病变起始阶段，抑制性T细胞主要在病变后期占主导[201,225]。近期有研究表明，调节性T细胞（T-reg）在调节或控制根尖周病变扩展中发挥了重要作用。当T-reg细胞受到抑制时，会显著增加根尖周病变的严重程度，这与促炎因子、辅助性T细胞1型（Th1）和辅助性T细胞17型（Th17）表达上调有关[66]。

学者们普遍认为，根尖周肉芽肿内部包含的细菌数量极少甚至没有。动物实验显示根尖周肉芽肿中并无细菌存在[64,223]，而人类的病变（由于取样时诱导期比大多数动物实验更长）组织学检测中细菌检出率也较低[143,168]。慢性持续性病变内部含有细菌的概率可能更高[205-207]。当细菌存在时，通常被大量的炎性细胞包围，多数为中性粒细胞和巨噬细胞[64]。偶尔在肉芽肿内可见到被高度炎症细胞反应环绕的坏死区域，该病变则被称为根尖周脓肿。一项研究指出，因根尖周病变拔除的牙齿中有35%属于根尖周脓肿[146]。

3.5.2.1.2　根尖周囊肿

根尖周囊肿是由根尖肉芽肿内的马拉瑟上皮剩余增殖形成的（图3.9）。最初，上皮细胞形成条索状结构，最终这些条索状结构相互融合。上皮细胞团块的增大可能导致团块中心出现营养缺乏，进而引起组织坏死和液化，形成含有囊液的囊肿。囊中发生的另一种可能性是上皮条索状结构可能围绕部分肉芽肿组织，从而导致囊肿的形成[213]。囊肿的扩大被认为是由于囊内液体压力所致，尤其是上皮细胞可能分泌促进骨吸收的细胞因子[123,214]。临床上囊肿可能发展至非常大，导致邻牙移位。

根尖周囊肿的诊断存在差异。一些病理专家认为，只要在组织标本中看到上皮增生的迹象就认为病变是囊肿，其他专家则认为需要看到完整的上皮内衬包绕着充满液体的腔隙，其中可能含有胆固醇结晶时，才会诊断为囊肿。这种诊断上的差异性导致了对肉芽肿和囊肿患病率的研究结果存在巨大差异（表3.3）。

根尖周囊肿的进一步分类需要区分"湾形囊肿"[188]或"袋状囊肿"[164]与真正的根尖周囊肿。在湾形囊肿或袋状囊肿中，根尖深入囊肿内，且根管似乎直接开口于囊肿腔内。而在真性根尖周囊肿中，其上皮衬里和结缔组织是连续的，并与根尖分离。

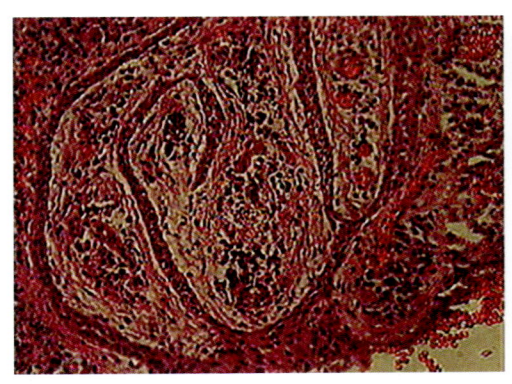

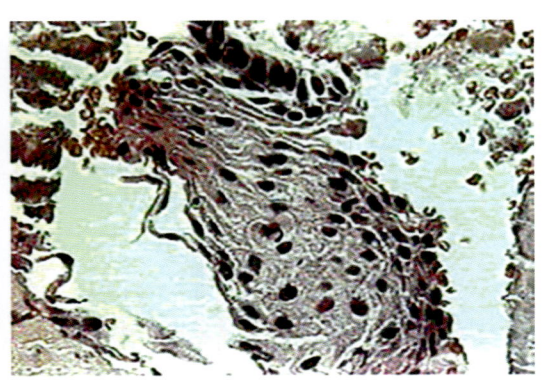

图 3.9　未愈合的根尖周炎在根尖手术中取出的组织活检标本，病理医生诊断为根尖周囊肿。a. 肉芽组织内上皮增生成束状（放大100倍）。b. 上皮增生（放大200倍）

表 3.3 在几个经常被引用的研究中囊肿和肉芽肿的患病率

	样本量	囊肿	肉芽肿
Priebe 等人, 1954[161]	101	54%	46%
Patterson 等人, 1964[157]	510	14%	20%
Bhaskar, 1966[16]	2308	42%	48%
Lalonde, Luebke 1968[113]	800	44%	45%
Mortensen 等人, 1970[142]	396	41%	59%
Block 等人, 1976[18]	230	7%	93%
Winstock, 1980[227]	9804	8%	83%
Stockdale, Chandler 1988[204]	1108	17%	77%
Spatafore 等人, 1990[196]	1659	42%	52%
Nair 等人, 1996[164]	256	15%	50%
Koivisto 等人, 2012[110]	9723	33%	40%

根尖周囊肿和肉芽肿只能通过活检或拔牙后进行组织学检查鉴别。尝试利用影像学[226]，甚至 CBCT[172]，都未能成功区分这两种根尖病变。最近，尝试用 CBCT 特殊的指标和算法在这方面可能会有一定的作用[78]。根尖部透射影有一些影像学特征提示可能是囊肿。这些特征是投射影范围较大、周围有清晰的骨皮质界，以及似乎推挤邻牙根部的现象。鉴于临床上难以准确诊断囊肿与肉芽肿，因此很难证明或否定非手术根管治疗对于治疗根尖周囊肿的有效性。在 20 世纪五六十年代，人们认为根尖周囊肿需采用与其他类型囊肿相同的治疗方法，即手术摘除。后来有人提出，囊肿在根尖周炎的诊断中相当常见，且非手术根管治疗的成功率高于根尖周肉芽肿的平均发病率，这意味着有一定数量的囊肿可通过非手术治疗得以痊愈。最近有病例报道表明，真性根尖周囊肿（相对于袋装囊肿）的患病率很低，而且非手术治疗对这些囊肿效果不佳[144-145]。这些说法还有待证实，特别是目前在术前无法准确诊断真正的根尖周囊肿。

关于根尖周囊肿作为一种病理变化的另一个重要问题是，从生物学角度来看，许多研究通过分析细胞和分子成分[21, 36-37, 132, 218]也未能明确区分肉芽肿及囊肿。最近一项研究运用当代生物信息学工具，更严谨地研究了有关根尖周肉芽肿及根尖周囊肿的基因表达[160]。这项研究发现，囊肿中主要表达的基因是 TP53（肿瘤蛋白 p53）和 EP300（E1A 结合蛋白 P300），而根尖周肉芽肿则表达 IL2R，CCL2、CCL4、CCL5、CCR1、CCR3 和 CCR5 基因[160]。

3.5.2.2 根尖周炎的临床分类

多年来，不同地区根尖周炎的临床分类发生了很多变化。通过临床体征和症状基本上可诊断为根尖周炎。在没有组织病理学诊断的情况下，可根据临床诊断制定治疗计划、判断预后和是否需要进一步检查。

根尖周炎的患者可能没有症状，也可能主诉为轻度或中度的咬合痛，有可能会出现强烈疼痛，伴有或者不伴有患牙处的肿胀。影像学特征包括患牙根尖处（或边缘处）的低密度影，牙周膜间隙增宽，在透射区有硬骨板影像缺失。在 X 线片上低密度影边界可呈弥散性或边界清晰，且被骨皮质边界包围。有时，在透射区的边缘有一个高密度影像区。根尖周炎还有一些其他表现，如指向根尖透射区的窦道。

根据患者的主观症状、临床检查以及影像学特点，临床医生可以初步对根尖周炎做出临床诊断。确切的术语将在其他章节进一步讨论。经过数十年的研究，关于根尖周炎的发病机制和诊断的关系已有了一些已知的发现。如前所述（关于牙髓感染微生物学的详细讨论请见第 4 章），临床症状可能与某些细菌或病毒有关，也可能与根管内细菌细胞壁的成分有关[84, 92]，如 LPS 或内毒素；根尖周疼痛可能与几种降低疼痛阈值的炎症介质有关，如神经肽、缓激肽、白细胞三烯和二十烷类[26,138,215]；病变的大小可能与骨吸收细胞因子的水平有关，如 IL-1β[112]。

3.5.3 根尖周炎症的免疫调节和骨吸收

根尖周病变是一个骨吸收与沉积的动态过程，伴随含有多种免疫和结构细胞的软组织病变发展（图 3.10）。免疫细胞主要包括淋巴细胞、巨噬细胞、中性粒细胞、浆细胞和肥大细胞。结构细胞主要包括成纤维细胞和成骨细胞。此外，内皮细胞和破骨细胞在炎症进程中发挥着重要作用。偶尔也会出现上皮细胞，如前所述，上皮细胞可能与囊肿形成有关。

根尖周病变初始发生阶段，固有免疫细胞和因子似乎发挥关键作用。根尖损伤动物模型实验显示，在根尖处可见中性粒细胞，它们似乎在抑制微生物进入病损部位的环节发挥着关键作用（图 3.11）。

动物实验发现，抑制中性粒细胞可以有效阻断病变形成[147,231]。中性粒细胞减少症患者即使有轻度龋损，也会有自发性坏死和脓肿形成[159]。当宿主接触到大量致病性强的口腔细菌时，适应

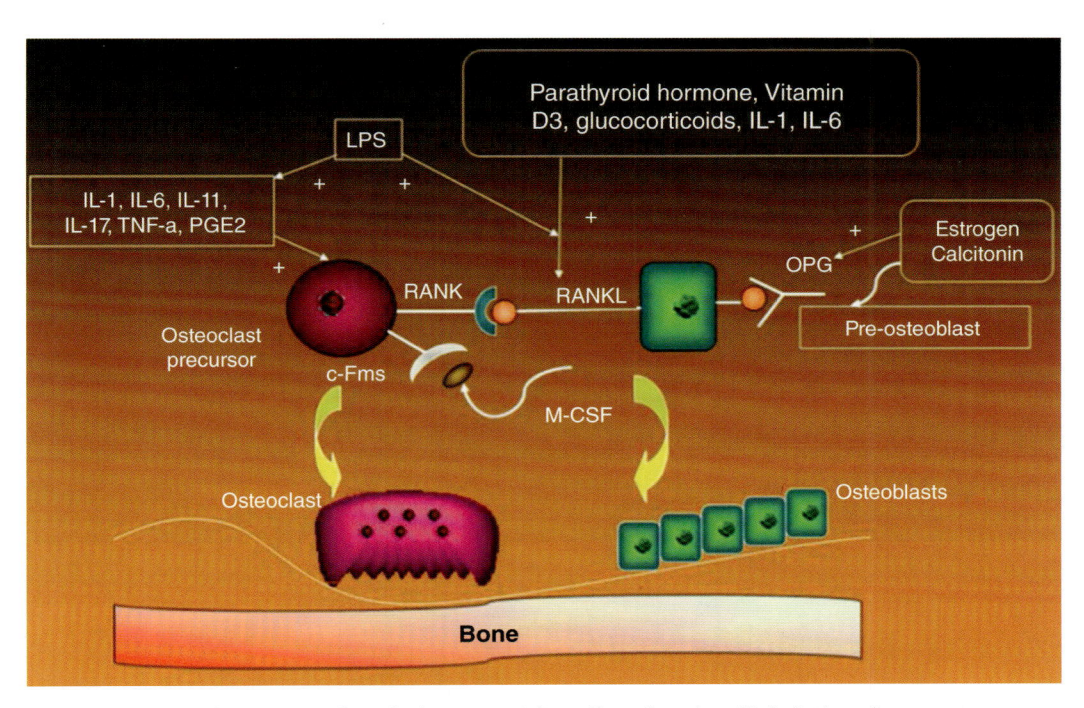

图 3.10 骨重建过程中成骨细胞与破骨细胞前体之间的相互作用（经许可摘自文献 59）。LPS:lipopolysaccharide，脂多糖。Parathyroid hormone：甲状旁腺激素。Vitamin D3：维生素 D3。Glucocorticoids：糖皮质激素。IL-1：白介素 -1。IL-6：白介素 -6。IL-11：白介素 -11。IL-17：白介素 -17。TNF-α：肿瘤坏死因子 -α。PGE2：前列腺素 E2。Estrogen：雌激素。Calcitonin：降钙素。Pre-osteoblast：前成骨细胞。OPG：骨保护素。Osteoclast precursor：破骨细胞前体。RANK：破骨细胞分化因子受体。RNAKL：破骨细胞分化因子。Osteoclast：破骨细胞。c-Fms：集落刺激因子 -1 受体。M-CSF：巨噬细胞集落刺激因子。Osteoblast：成骨细胞。Bone：骨

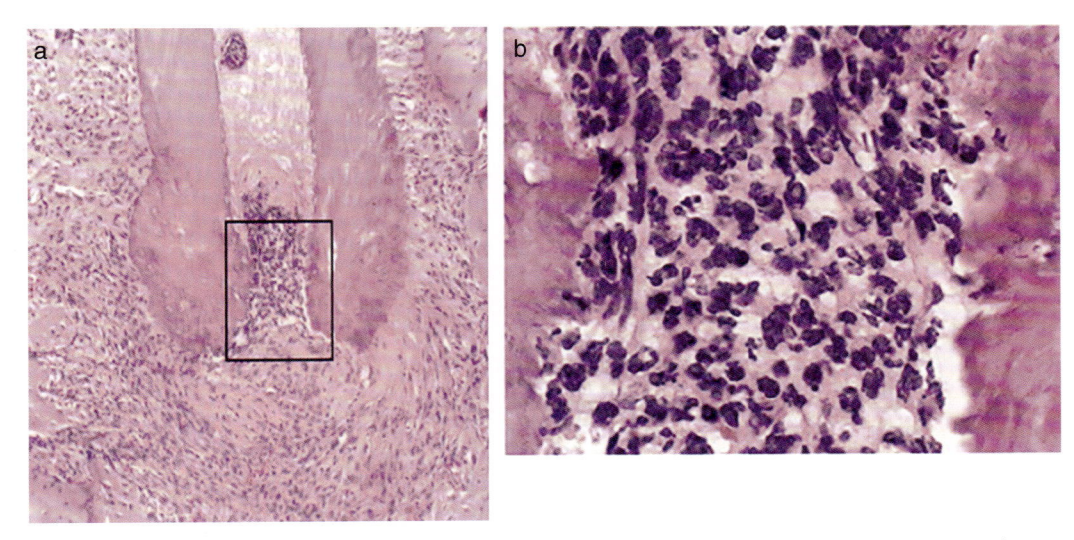

图 3.11 小鼠根尖周病变模型。a. 牙髓坏死，根尖孔和和病变区域内不规则分布的强烈炎症反应（放大 100 倍）。b.a 图中矩形框中的高倍镜视野可见大多数炎细胞是中性粒细胞（放大 400 倍）

性免疫的作用就显现出来。研究发现将 T 细胞和 B 细胞缺乏的小鼠（免疫缺陷小鼠）暴露于每毫升 10^{10} 个细胞的中间普氏菌、具核梭杆菌、微小消化链球菌（现在也称为微小微单胞菌）、中间链球菌[212]或齿垢密螺旋体[54]环境中，这些免疫缺陷小鼠会出现严重的肿胀和弥散性感染。

在大多数情况下，细菌刺激并不严重，机体的免疫反应能够在不引发严重疾病的情况下有效控制感染。各种免疫因子和微生物刺激之间的相互作用决定了根尖周病变的实际大小。在大多数动物实验中，病变的大小在 4~6 周达到特定的影像学或病理学水平，然后趋于稳定[10,55,60]。这种平衡是由促炎细胞、抗炎细胞以及分子介质维持的，它们协同作用来调节产生的免疫反应强度。这对于根尖周炎至关重要，就如同在牙髓炎以及其他类型的炎症中一样，这种机制限制了炎症带来的副作用。这一过程确保了炎症的保护功能得以发挥，同时也限制了其对机体造成的破坏性影响。

正如前面所提到的，活跃的骨吸收与根尖周病变的发展有关。根尖周病变中普遍表达的 NF-kB 与骨吸收有关[173]，具体来说，破骨细胞及其前体细胞上的 NF-kB 受体与成骨细胞上的 RANK 配体（RANKL）相互作用引发骨吸收。RANKL 对骨调节至关重要，在动物模型中，阻断这一分子活性会导致骨坏死[3]。同时，当刺激物和宿主反应达到平衡时，骨保护素（OPG）作为诱饵来阻断 RANK/RANKL 反应并维持骨结构（图 3.10），限制骨吸收，使病变大小维持稳定。病变超出必要程度后停止发展，这可能由 T-reg 细胞[66]以及其他多种细胞因子、激素和其他因素协同调控的（图 3.10）。

由此可知，研究者可以直接检测坏死牙髓的根管或者根尖周病变，以判断病变是在活跃发展期、稳定期还是愈合期。这方面已有一些初步研究成果，在一项研究中，发现活跃期和非活跃期的病变可以根据 RANKL/OPG 的比值来判定，这个比值在 5 或者更高[69]。这与 83 个肉芽肿和 25 个对照组样本中的 84 个愈合相关基因的表达情况有关。此研究发现，活跃性病变与 TNF（一种促炎细胞因子）和 CXCL11（一种趋化因子）的上调有关，而非活跃性病变则与 SERPINE1（纤溶酶原激活物抑制因子）、TIMP1、COL1A1（细胞外基质成分）、TGF-beta1（生长因子），以及 ITGA4（细胞黏附分子）上调有关[69]。在另一项研究中，将活跃性病变与非活跃性病变的区分依据是临床诊断结果，其中活跃性病变诊断为慢性根尖周脓肿，而非活跃性病变则诊断为无症状（慢性）根尖周炎[119]。研究者对这两种病变中的基质金属蛋白酶（MMP）及其抑制剂（TIMP）进行了检测。结果发现，活跃性病变中 MMP2、MMP7，以及 MMP9 的表达上调，而 TIMP1 在非活跃性病变中表达上调[119]。

3.5.4 根尖周炎的愈合

一旦通过拔牙的方式消除了微生物刺激，或通过非手术或手术治疗大幅减少微生物刺激，根尖周组织即开始愈合。愈合过程表现为血管增多，胶原纤维形成，骨岛发展及融合，细胞性牙骨质的沉积（图 3.12）[65]。根尖周病变处含有多种促进伤口愈合以及矿化的生长因子，其中包括转化生长因子（TGF-α 和 TGF-β）[69,216]、表皮生长因子[124]、血管内皮生长因子[53,118]和骨形态发生蛋白 2（BMP-2）[135]。

多种宿主相关因素影响根尖周病变的愈合速度。例如，在队列研究中发现，糖尿病[7,63]和吸烟[43]均与根尖周愈合能力降低有关。全身因素对根尖周病变愈合的研究存在一些干扰因素，这是由于患者服用的药物可能会改变病变区域的骨代谢动力学。结果表明，常用于治疗 2 型糖尿病的二甲双胍[127]、用于治疗骨质疏松的双磷酸盐[99]以及

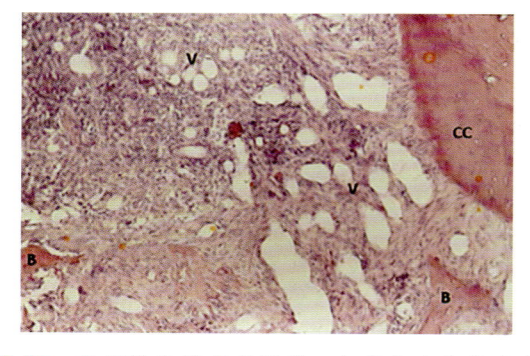

图 3.12 雪貂根尖周病变模型，尖牙在非手术治疗后 4 个月的愈合情况。愈合主要包括骨（B）、血管增殖（V）以及细胞牙骨质（CC）生成（经许可摘自文献 65）

许多老年人使用的他汀类药物[122, 125]，在动物模型中已被证实减小了根尖周炎的病损大小。

IL-1β 等位基因 2 或某些 FC-γ 受体的遗传多态性[193-194]与根尖周炎愈合能力下降有关。FC-γ 受体广泛分布于许多炎症细胞上，特别是巨噬细胞，其能够结合免疫球蛋白的 Fc 部分，以促进对抗体 Fab 部分附着抗原的吞噬。然而现阶段将愈合不良归因于遗传多态性还为时过早，因为有些研究结果尚未得到其他研究的支持[6]。

3.6 结语

目前认为，轻度的牙髓炎症可以促进组织再生，即第三期牙本质的形成，而更严重的炎症则会导致牙髓坏死[31,91]。在这方面，关于创伤后或大量修复后的牙齿中出现的牙髓过度钙化的确切机制尚不完全清楚。减少牙髓炎症反应的治疗方法可能有利于保持牙髓的活力和进行有效免疫的反应。在犬牙髓炎模型中，使用 MMP3 治疗可降低促炎因子 IL-6 的表达，并减少了巨噬细胞和抗原呈递细胞的数量[46]，从而逆转牙髓炎症。提高对分子机制在组织再生和维持健康的活髓中作用的理解，可能对牙科患者改善口腔健康状况带来极大的益处。

非手术和手术牙髓治疗后的根尖周炎愈合速度通常比拔除患牙慢，这可能与拔牙能更有效地消除微生物因素有关，根管治疗后的愈合延迟问题会影响医生对治疗效果的随访及在必要时提供额外的治疗。在根管治疗后，使用市售的生长因子（如釉基质蛋白）或其他蛋白来增强根尖周组织愈合能力可能成为可行的方法，从而能在较短的时间判断预后。此外，如前所述，评价根尖周病变的活跃水平可以帮助制定治疗计划和预测症状的发展。要最终理解牙髓病和根尖周病的发病机制和愈合，就需要更深入地了解牙髓菌群，患者的基因组，表观遗传学以及健康状况等因素。

参考文献

[1] Abella F, et al. Evaluating theperiapical status of teeth with irreversible pulpitis by using cone-beam computed tomography scanning and periapical radiographs. J Endod, 2012, 38: 1588–1591.

[2] Adachi T, et al. Caries-related bacteria and cytokines induce CXCL10 in dental pulp. J Dent Res, 2007, 86: 1217–1222.

[3] Aghaloo T L, et al. RANKL inhibitors induce osteonecrosis of the jaw in mice with periapical disease. J Bone Miner Res, 2014, 29: 843–854.

[4] Ainamo A, et al. Dental radiographic findings in the elderly in Helsinki, Finland. Acta Odontol Scand, 1994, 52: 243–249.

[5] Allareddy V, et al. Outcomes in patients hospitalized for periapical abscess in the United States: an analysis involving the use of a nationwide inpatient sample. J Am Dent Assoc, 2010, 141: 1107–1116.

[6] Aminoshariae A, Kulild J C. Association of functional gene polymorphism with apical periodontitis. J Endod, 2015, 41: 999–1007.

[7] Arya S, et al. Healing of apical periodontitis after nonsurgical treatment in patients with type 2 diabetes. J Endod, 2017, 43: 1623–1627.

[8] Asgary S, Eghbal M J, Ghoddusi J. Two-year results of vital pulp therapy in permanent molars with irreversible pulpitis: an ongoing multicenter randomized clinical trial. Clinical Oral Investigations, 2014, 18: 635–641.

[9] Balto K, Sasaki H, Stashenko P. Interleukin-6 deficiency increases inflammatory bone destruction. Infect Immun, 2001, 69: 744–750.

[10] Balto K, et al. A mouse model of inflammatory root resorption induced by pulpal infection. Oral Surg Oral Med Oral Pathol Oral Radiol Endod, 2002, 93: 461–468.

[11] Baumgartner J C, et al. Geographical differences in bacteria detected in endodontic infections using polymerase chain reaction. Journal of endodontics, 2004, 30: 141–144.

[12] Bergenholtz G. Micro-organisms from necrotic pulp of traumatized teeth. Odontol Revy, 1974, 25: 347–358.

[13] Bergenholtz G, Lindhe J. Effect of experimentally induced marginal periodontitis and periodontal scaling on the dental pulp. J Clin Periodontol, 1978, 5(1): 59–73.

[14] Bergenholtz G, et al. Morphometric analysis of chronic inflammatory periapical lesions in root-filled teeth. Oral Surg Oral Med Oral Pathol, 1983, 55: 295–301.

[15] Bergström J, Eliasson S, Ahlberg K F. Periapical status in subjects with regular dental care habits. Community Dent Oral Epidemiol, 1987, 15: 236–239.

[16] Bhaskar S N. Periapical lesions-types, incidence, and clinical features. Oral Surg Oral Med Oral Pathol, 1966, 21: 657–671.

[17] Bhingare A C, et al. Dental pulp dendritic cells migrate to regional lymph nodes. Journal of Dental Research, 2014, 93: 288–293.

[18] Block R M, et al. A histopathologic, histobacteriologic, and radiographic study of periapical endodontic surgical specimens. Oral Surgery, Oral Medicine, Oral Pathology, Oral Radiology, 1976, 42: 656–678.

[19] Boucher Y, et al. Radiographic evaluation of the prevalence and technical quality of root canal treatment in a French subpopulation. Int Endod J, 2002, 35: 229–238.

[20] Brannstrom M, Lind P O. Pulpal response to early dental caries. J Dent Res, 1965, 44: 1045–1050.

[21] Campos K, et al. Methylation pattern of IFNG in periapical granulomas and radicular cysts. J Endod, 2013, 39: 493–496.

[22] Caplan D J, et al. Lesions of endodontic origin and risk of coronary heart disease. J Dent Res, 2006, 85: 996–1000.

[23] Cardoso F G, et al. Correlation between volume of apical periodontitis determined by cone-beam computed tomography analysis and endotoxin levels found in primary root canal infection. J Endod, 2015, 41: 1015–1019.

[24] Cardoso F P, et al. Methylation pattern of the CD14 and TLR2 genes in human dental pulp. Journal of Endodontics, 2014, 40: 384–386.

[25] Cardoso F P, et al. Methylation pattern of the IFN-gamma gene in human dental pulp. Journal of Endodontics, 2010, 36: 642–646.

[26] Caviedes-Bucheli J, et al. Neuropeptides in dental pulp: the silent protagonists. J Endod, 2008, 34: 773–788.

[27] Chavez de Paz, Villanueva L E. Fusobacterium nucleatum in endodontic flare-ups. Oral Surg Oral Med Oral Pathol Oral Radiol Endod, 2002, 93: 179–183.

[28] Cheung G S, Ho M W. Microbial flora of root canal-treated teeth associated with asymptomatic periapical radiolucent lesions. Oral microbiology and immunology, 2001, 16: 332–337.

[29] Chhour K L, et al. Molecular analysis of microbial diversity in advanced caries. Journal of clinical microbiology, 2005, 43: 843–849.

[30] Cooper P R, Holder M J, Smith A J. Inflammation and regeneration in the dentin-pulp complex: a double-edged sword. J Endod, 2014, 40: S46–51.

[31] Cooper P R, et al. Mediators of inflammation and regeneration. Adv Dent Res, 2011, 23: 290–295.

[32] Cooper P R, et al. Inflammationregeneration interplay in the dentine-pulp omplex. Journal of Dentistry, 2010, 38: 687–697.

[33] da Silva R A, et al. Toll-like receptor 2 knockout mice showed increased periapical lesion size and osteoclast number. J Endod, 2012, 38: 803–813.

[34] Dahlén G, Magnusson B C, Möller, A. Histological and histochemical study of the influence of lipopolysaccharide extracted from Fusobacterium nucleatum on the periapical tissues in the monkey Macaca fascicularis. Arch Oral Biol, 1981, 26: 591–598.

[35] De Cleen M J, et al. Periapical status and prevalence of endodontic treatment in an adult Dutch population. Int Endod J, 1993, 26: 112–119.

[36] de Oliveira Rodini C, Batista A C, Lara V S. Comparative immunohistochemical study of the presence of mast cells in apical granulomas and periapical cysts: possible role of mast cells in the course of human periapical lesions. Oral Surg Oral Med Oral Pathol Oral Radiol Endod, 2004, 97: 59–63.

[37] de Oliveira Rodini C, Lara V S. Study of the expression of CD68+ macrophages and CD8+ T cells in human granulomas and periapical cysts. Oral Surg Oral Med Oral Pathol Oral Radiol Endod, 2001, 92: 221–227.

[38] De Rossi A, Rocha L B, Rossi M A. Interferon-gamma, interleukin-10, Intercellular adhesion molecule-1, and chemokine receptor 5, but not interleukin-4, attenuate the development of periapical lesions. J Endod, 2008, 34: 31–38.

[39] de Soet J J, et al. A comparison of the microbial flora in carious dentine of clinically detectable and undetectable occlusal lesions. Caries research, 1995, 29: 46–49.

[40] Diogenes A, et al. LPS sensitizes TRPV1 via activation of TLR4 in trigeminal sensory neurons. Journal of Dental Research, 2011, 90: 759–764.

[41] Dommisch H, et al. Human beta-defensin (hBD-1, -2) expression in dental pulp. Oral Microbiology and Immunology, 2005, 20: 163–166.

[42] Dommisch H, et al. Immune regulatory functions of human betadefensin-2 in odontoblast-like cells. Int Endod J, 2007, 40: 300–307.

[43] Doyle S L, et al. Factors affecting outcomes for single-tooth implants and endodontic restorations. J Endod, 2007, 33: 399–402.

[44] Durand S H, et al. Lipoteichoic acid increases TLR and functional chemokine expression while reducing dentin formation in in vitro differentiated human odontoblasts. J Immunol, 2006, 176: 2880–2887.

[45] Dwyer T G, Torabinejad M Radiographic and histologic evaluation of the effect of endotoxin on the periapical tissues of the cat. J Endod, 1980, 7: 31–35.

[46] Eba H, et al, 2012, The anti-inflammatory effects of matrix metalloproteinase-3 on irreversible pulpitis of mature erupted teeth. PLoS One 7: e52523.

[47] Egan M W, et al. Prevalence of yeasts in saliva and root canals of teeth associated with apical periodontitis. International endodontic journal, 2002, 35: 321–329.

[48] Eghbal M J, et al. MTA pulpotomy of human permanent molars with irreversible pulpitis. Australian Endodontic Journal, 2009, 35: 4–8.

[49] ElSalhy M, Azizieh F, Raghupathy R Cytokines as diagnostic markers of pulpal inflammation. International Endodontic Journal, 2013, 46: 573–580.

[50] Fabricius L, et al. Influence of combinations of oral bacteria on periapical tissues of monkeys. Scandinavian journal of dental research, 1982, 90: 200–206.

[51] Farges J C, et al. Dental pulp defence and repair mechanisms in dental caries. Mediators Inflamm, 2015: 230251.

[52] Ferraz C C R, et al. Lipopolysaccharide from porphyromonas gingivalis sensitizes capsaicin-sensitive nociceptors. Journal of Endodontics, 2011, 37: 45–48.

[53] Fonseca-Silva T, et al. Detection an quantification of mast cell, vascular endothelial growth factor, and microvessel density in human inflammatory periapical cysts and granulomas. Int Endod J, 2012, 45: 859–864.

[54] Foschi F, et al. Treponema denticola in disseminating endodontic infections. J Dent Res, 2006, 85: 761–765.

[55] Fouad A F. IL-1 alpha and TNFalpha expression in early periapical lesions of normal and immunodeficient mice. J Dent Res, 1997, 76: 1548–1554.

[56] Fouad A F. Molecular mediators of pulpal inflammation// Hargreaves K M, Goodis H E.Seltzer and Bender's Dental Pulp. 2ed. Chicago IL: Quintessence Publishing Co Inc, 2012: 241–276

[57] Fouad A F. Infections of the dental Pulp// Hupp J R F, Ferneine E M. Head/Neck/Orofacial Infections: A Multidisciplinary Approach. St Louis MO: Elsevier, 2016: 175–188.

[58] Fouad A F. Treponema spp. shown to be important pathogens in primary endodontic infections. J Evid Based Dent Pract, 2016, 16: 50–52.

[59] Fouad A F. Endodontic microbiology and pathobiology: current state of knowledge. Dental clinics of North America, 2017, 61: 1–15.

[60] Fouad A F, Acosta A W. Periapical lesion progression and cytokine expression in an LPS hyporesponsive model. Int Endod J, 2001, 34: 506–513.

[61] Fouad A F, et al. PCR-based identification of bacteria associated with endodontic infections. J Clin Microbiol, 2002, 40: 3223–3231.

[62] Fouad A F, et al. Periapical lesion progression with controlled microbial inoculation in a type I diabetic mouse model. J Endod, 2002, 28: 8–16.

[63] Fouad A F, Burleson J. Theeffect of diabetes mellitus on endodontic treatment outcome: data from an electronic patient record. J Am Dent Assoc, 2003, 134: 43–51; quiz 117–118.

[64] Fouad A F, Walton R E, Rittman B R. Induced periapical lesions in ferret canines: histologic and radiographic evaluation. Endod Dent Traumatol, 1992, 8: 56–62.

[65] Fouad A F, Walton R E, Rittman B R. Healing of induced periapical lesions in ferret canines. J Endod, 1993, 19: 123–129.

[66] Francisconi C F, et al. Characterization of the protective role of regulatory T cells in experimental periapical lesion development and their chemoattraction manipulation as a therapeutic tool. J Endod, 2016, 42: 120–126.

[67] Galicia J C, et al. Gene expression profile of pulpitis. Genes and Immunity, 2016, 17: 239–243.

[68] Galicia J C, et al. MiRNA-181a regulates Toll-like receptor agonistinduced inflammatory response in human fibroblasts. Genes Immun, 2014, 15: 333–337.

[69] Garlet G P, et al. Expression analysis of wound healing genes in human periapical granulomas of progressive and stable nature. J Endod, 2012, 38: 185–190.

[70] Garlet T P, et al. CCR2 deficiency results in increased osteolysis in experimental periapical lesions in mice. J Endod, 2010, 36: 244–250.

[71] Gaudin A, et al. Phenotypic analysis of immunocompetent cells in healthy human dental pulp. Journal of Endodontics, 2015, 41: 621–627.

[72] Gilles J A, et al. Oral bone loss is increased in ovariectomized rats. J Endod, 1997, 23: 419–422.

[73] Goldman M, Laosonthorn P, White R R. Microleakage-full crowns and the dental pulp. Journal of endodontics, 1992, 18:473–475.

[74] Gomes-Filho J E, et al. Raloxifene nmodulates regulators of osteoclastogenesis and angiogenesis in an oestrogen deficiency periapical lesion model. Int Endod J, 2015, 48: 1059–1068.

[75] Gomes B P, Drucker D B, Lilley J D. Associations of specific bacteria with some endodontic signs and symptoms. Int Endod J, 1994, 27: 291–298.

[76] Goon W W, Jacobsen P L. Prodromal odontalgia and multiple devitalized teeth caused by a herpes zoster infection of the trigeminal nerve: report of case. J Am Dent Assoc, 1988, 116: 500–504.

[77] Griffee M B, et al. The relationship of Bacteroides melaninogenicus to symptoms associated with pulpal necrosis. Oral Surg Oral Med Oral Pathol, 1980, 50: 457–461.

[78] Guo J, et al. Evaluation of the reliability and accuracy of using cone-beam computed tomography for diagnosing periapical cysts from granulomas. J Endod, 2013, 39: 1485–1490.

[79] Hahn C L, Falkler W A, Siegel M A. A study of T-cell and B-cell in pulpal pathosis. Journal of Endodontics, 1989, 15: 20–26.

[80] Hahn C L, Liewehr F R. Update on the adaptive immune responses of the dental pulp. Journal of Endodontics, 2007, 33: 773–781.

[81] Harran Ponce E, et al. Consequences of crown fractures with pulpal exposure: histopathological evaluation in dogs. Dental traumatology: official publication of International Association for Dental Traumatology, 2002, 18: 196–205.

[82] Hernandez Vigueras S, et al. Viruses in pulp and periapical inflammation: a review. Odontology, 2016, 104: 184–191.

[83] Hirao K, et al. Roles of TLR2, TLR4, NOd2, and NOd1 in Pulp Fibroblasts. Journal of Dental Research, 2009, 88:

[84] Horiba N, et al. Correlations between endotoxin and clinical symptoms or radiolucent areas in infected root canals. Oral Surg Oral Med Oral Pathol, 1991, 71: 492–495.

[85] Hou L, Sasaki H, Stashenko P. Toll-like receptor 4-deficient mice have reduced bone destruction following mixed anaerobic infection. Infect Immun, 2000, 68: 4681–4687.

[86] Hou L, Sasakj H, Stashenko P. B-Cell deficiency predisposes mice to disseminating anaerobic infections: protection by passive antibody transfer. Infect Immun, 2000, 68: 5645–5651.

[87] Hsiao W W, et al. Microbial transformation from normal oral microbiota to acute endodontic infections. BMC Genomics, 2012, 13: 345.

[88] Huang G T, et al. Effect of interleukin-6 deficiency on the formation of periapical lesions after pulp exposure in mice. Oral Surg Oral Med Oral Pathol Oral Radiol Endod, 2001, 92: 83–88.

[89] Hui T Q, et al. EZH2, a Potential regulator of dental pulp inflammation and regeneration. Journal of Endodontics, 2014, 40: 1132–1138.

[90] Izumi T, et al. An immunohistochemical study of HLA-DR and alpha 1-antichymotrypsin-positive cells in the pulp of human non-carious and carious teeth. Archives of oral biology, 1996, 41: 627–630.

[91] Izumi T, et al. Immunohistochemical study on the immunocompetent cells of the pulp in human non-carious and carious teeth. Archives of oral biology, 1995, 40: 609–614.

[92] Jacinto R C, et al. Quantification of endotoxins in necrotic root canals from symptomatic and asymptomatic teeth. J Med Microbio, 2005, 54: 777–783.

[93] Jakovljevic A, Andric M. Human cytomegalovirus and Epstein-Barr virus in etiopathogenesis of apical periodontitis: a systematic review. J Endod, 2014, 40: 6–15.

[94] Jakovljevic A, et al. The role of varicella zoster virus in the development of periapical pathoses and root resorption: a systematic review. J Endod, 2017, 43: 1230–1236.

[95] Jiang H W, et al. Expression of Toll-like receptor 4 in normal human odontoblasts and dental pulp tissue. J Endod, 2006, 32: 747–751.

[96] Jontell M, et al. Immune defense mechanisms of the dental pulp. Crit Rev Oral Biol Med, 1998, 9: 179–200.

[97] Kabak Y, Abbott P V. Prevalence of apical periodontitis and the quality of endodontic treatment in an adult Belarusian population. Int Endod J, 2005, 38: 238–245.

[98] Kakehashi S, Stanley H R, Fitzgerald R J. The effects of surgical exposures of dental pulps in germ-free and conventional laboratory rats. Oral Surgery, Oral Medicine, Oral Pathology, Oral Radiology, 1965, 20: 340–349.

[99] Kang B, et al. Periapical disease and bisphosphonates induce osteonecrosis of the jaws in mice. J Bone Miner Res, 2013, 28: 1631–1640.

[100] Kawashima N, et al, Infectionstimulated infraosseus inflammation and bone destruction is increased in P-/Eselectin knockout mice. Immunology, 1999 97: 117–123.

[101] Kawashima N, et al. NK and NKT cells in the rat dental pulp tissues. OralSurgery Oral Medicine Oral Pathology Oral Radiology and Endodontics, 2006, 102: 558–563.

[102] Keller J F, et al. Toll-like receptor 2 activation by lipoteichoic acid induces differential production of pro-inflammatory cytokines in human odontoblasts, dental pulp fibroblasts and immature dendritic cells. Immunobiology, 2010, 215: 53–59.

[103] Keller J F, et al. Expression of NOD2 is increased in inflamed human dental pulps and lipoteichoic acidstimulated odontoblast-like cells. Innate Immunity, 2011, 17: 29–34.

[104] Khabbaz M G, Anastasiadis P L, Sykaras S N. Determination of endotoxins in caries: association with pulpal pain. Int Endod, 2000, J 33: 132–137.

[105] Khayat B G, et al. Responses of nerve-fibers to pulpal inflammation and periapical lesions in rat molars demonstrated by calcitonin gene-related peptide immunocytochemistry. Journal of Endodontics, 1988, 14: 577–587.

[106] Kianoush N, et al. Bacterial profile of dentine caries and the impact of pH on bacterial population diversity. PloS one, 2014, 9: e92940.

[107] Kikuchi T, et al. Dendritic cells stimulated with Actinobacillus actinomycetemcomitans elicit rapid gamma interferon responses by natural killer cells. Infection and Immunity, 2004, 72: 5089–5096.

[108] Kimberly C L, Byers M R. Inflammation of rat molar pulp and periodontium causes increased calcitonin gene-related peptide and axonal sprouting. Anatomical Record, 1988, 222: 289–300.

[109] Kirkevang L L, et al. Frequency and distribution of endodontically treated teeth and apical periodontitis in an urban Danish population. Int Endod J, 2001, 34: 198–205.

[110] Koivisto T, Bowles W R, Rohrer M. Frequency and distribution of radiolucent jaw lesions: a retrospective analysis of 9, 723 cases. J Endod, 2012, 38: 729–732.

[111] Korkmaz Y, et al. Irreversible inflammation is associated with decreased levels of the alpha, 1)-, beta, 1)-, and alpha, 2)-subunits of sGC in human odontoblasts. Journal of Dental Research, 2011, 90: 517–522.

[112] Kuo M L, Lamster I B, Hasselgren. Host mediators in endodontic exudates. I. Indicators of inflammation and humoral immunity. J Endod, 1998, 24: 598–603.

[113] Lalonde E R, Luebke R G. The frequency and distribution of periapical cysts and granulomas. An evaluation of 800 specimens. Oral Surg Oral Med Oral Pathol, 1968, 25:

861–868.

[114] Langeland K. Tissue response to dental caries. Endod Dent Traumatol, 1987, 3: 149–171.

[115] Langeland K, Rodrigues H, Dowden W. Periodontal disease, bacteria, and pulpal histopathology. Oral Surgery, Oral Medicine, Oral Pathology, Oral Radiology, 1974, 37: 257–270.

[116] Lawton F E, Myers G E. The control of frictional heat in cavity preparation. British dental journal. 1947, 83: 75–77.

[117] Leite F R, et al. Prevalence of treponema species detected in endodontic infections: systematic review and metaregression analysis. J Endod, 2015, 41: 579–587.

[118] Leonardi R, et al. Detection of vascular endothelial growth factor/ vascular permeability factor in periapical lesions. J Endod, 2003, 29: 180–183.

[119] Letra A, et al. MMP-7 and TIMP-1, new targets in predicting poor wound healing in apical periodontitis. J Endod, 2013, 39: 1141–1146.

[120] Li H, et al. Herpesviruses in endodontic pathoses: association of Epstein-Barr virus with irreversible pulpitis and apical periodontitis. Journal of endodontics, 2009, 35: 23–29.

[121] Li L, et al. Analyzing endodontic infections by deep coverage pyrosequencing. J Dent Res, 2010, 89: 980–984.

[122] Lin L D, et al. Simvastatin suppresses osteoblastic expression of Cyr61 and progression of apical periodontitis through enhancement of the transcription factor Forkhead/winged helix box protein O3a. J Endod, 2013, 39: 619–625.

[123] Lin L M, Huang G T, Rosenberg P A. Proliferation of epithelial cell rests, formation of apical cysts, and regression of apical cysts after periapical wound healing. J Endod, 2007, 33: 908–916.

[124] Lin L M, et al. Detection of epidermal growth factor receptor in inflammatory periapical lesions. Int Endod J, 1996, 29: 179–184.

[125] Lin S K, et al. Simvastatin as a novel strategy to alleviate periapical lesions. J Endod, 2009, 35: 657–662.

[126] Lin Z M, et al. Expression of nucleotide-binding oligomerization domain 2 in normal human dental pulp cells and dental pulp tissues. Journal of Endodontics, 2009, 35: 838–842.

[127] Liu L, et al. Protective effect of metformin on periapical lesions in rats by decreasing the ratio of receptor activator of nuclear factor kappa B ligand/ osteoprotegerin. J Endod, 2012, 38: 943–947.

[128] Loesche W J. Role of Streptococcus mutans in human dental decay. Microbiological reviews, 1986, 50: 353–380.

[129] Maghazachi A A. Compartmentalization of human natural killer cells. Molecular Immunology, 2005, 42: 523–529.

[130] Maita E, et al. Fluid and protein flux across the pulpodentine complex of the dog in vivo. Arch Oral Biol, 1991, 36: 103–110.

[131] Mangkornkarn C, et al. Flow cytometric analysis of human dental-pulp tissue. Journal of Endodontics, 1991, 17: 49–53.

[132] Marcal J R, et al. T-helper cell type 17/regulatory T-cell immunoregulatory balance in human radicular cysts and periapical granulomas. J Endod, 2010, 36: 995–999.

[133] Martin F E, et al. Quantitative microbiological study of human carious dentine by culture and real-time PCR: association of anaerobes with histopathological changes in chronic pulpitis. Journal of clinical microbiology, 2002, 40: 1698–1704.

[134] Martinho F C, et al. Clinical investigation of bacterial species and endotoxin in endodontic infection and evaluation of root canal content activity against macrophages by cytokine production. Clin Oral Investig., 2014,

[135] Matsumoto N, et al. Histologic evaluation of the effects of Emdogain gel on injured root apex in rats. J Endod, 2014, 40: 1989–1994.

[136] Matthews B, Vongsavan N. Interactions between neural and hydrodynamic mechanisms in dentine and pulp. Arch Oral Biol, 1994, 39 Suppl: 87s–95s.

[137] Mazur B, Massler M. Influence of periodontal disease of the dental pulp. Oral surgery, oral medicine, and oral pathology, 1964, 17: 592–603.

[138] McNicholas S, et al. The concentration of prostaglandin E2 in human periradicular lesions. J Endod, 1991, 17:97–100.

[139] Michaelson P L, Holland G R. Is pulpitis painful? Int Endod J, 2002, 35: 829–832.

[140] Mjör I A, Tronstad L. Experimentally induced pulpitis. Oral Surg Oral Med Oral Pathol, 197234: 102–108.

[141] Morsani J M, et al. Genetic predisposition to persistent apical periodontitis. J Endod, 2011, 37: 455–459.

[142] Mortensen H, Winther J E, Birn H. Periapical granulomas and cysts. An investigation of 1, 600 cases. Scandinavian Journal of Dental Research, 1970, 78: 241–250.

[143] Nair P. ight and electron microscopic studies of root canal flora and periapical lesions. J Endod, 1987, L 13: 29–39.

[144] Nair P N. New perspectives on radicular cysts: do they heal? Int Endod J, 1998, 31: 155–160.

[145] Nair P N. On the causes of persistent apical periodontitis: a review. Int Endod J, 2006, 39: 249–281.

[146] Nair P N, et al. Radicular cyst affecting a root-filled human tooth: a long-term post-treatment follow-up. Int Endod J, 1993, 26: 225–233.

[147] Nakamura K, et al. Effect of methotrexate-induced neutropenia on pulpal inflammation in rats. J Endod, 2002, 28: 287–290.

[148] Nalliah R P, et al. Hospital emergency department visits attributed to pulpal and periapical disease in the United States in 2006. J Endod, 2011, 37: 6–9.

[149] Neves B G, et al. Molecular detection of bacteria associated to caries activity in dentinal lesions. Clinical oral

[150] Odesjo B, et al. Prevalence of previous endodontic treatment, technical standard and occurrence of periapical lesions in a randomly selected adult, general population. Endod Dent Traumatol, 1990, 6: 265–272.

[151] Owatz C B, et al. The incidence of mechanical allodynia in patients with irreversible pulpitis. J Endod, 2007, 33:552–556.

[152] Ozcelik B, et al. Histopathological evaluation of the dental pulps in crownfractured teeth. Journal of endodontics, 2000, 26: 271–273.

[153] Palmqvist S. Oral health patterns in a Swedish county population aged 65 and above. Swed Dent J Suppl, 1986, 32: 1–87.

[154] Paris S, et al. Gene expression of human beta-defensins in healthy and inflamed human dental pulps. Journal of Endodontics, 2009, 35: 520–523.

[155] Pashley D H. The influence of dentin permeability and pulpal blood flow on pulpal solute concentrations. J Endod, 1979, 5: 355–361.

[156] Patel K, et al. Multiple apical radiolucencies and external cervical resorption associated with varicella zoster virus: a case report. J Endod, 2016, 42: 978–983.

[157] Patterson S S, Shafer W G, Healey H J. Periapical lesions associated with endodontically treated teeth. J Am Dent Assoc, 1964, 68: 191–194.

[158] Peciuliene V, et al. Isolation of yeasts and enteric bacteria in root-filled teeth with chronic apical periodontitis. International endodontic journal, 2001, 34: 429–434.

[159] Pernu H E, Pajari U H, Lanning M. The importance of regular dental treatment in patients with cyclic neutropenia. Follow-up of 2 cases. J Periodontol, 1996, 67: 454–459.

[160] Poswar F de O, et al. Bioinformatics, interaction network analysis, and neural networks to characterize gene expression of radicular cyst and periapical granuloma. J Endod, 2015, 41: 877–883.

[161] Priebe W A, Lazansky J P, Wuehrmann A H. The value of the roentgenographic film in the differential diagnosis of periapical lesions. Oral Surg Oral Med Oral Pathol, 1954, 7: 979–983.

[162] Quah S Y, Bergenholtz G, Tan K S. Fusobacterium nucleatum induces cytokine production through Toll-likereceptor-independent mechanism. Int Endod J, 2013.

[163] Qui onez C, et al. Emergencydepartment visits for dental care of nontraumatic origin. Community Dent Oral Epidemiol, 2009, 37: 366–371.

[164] Ramachandran Nair P N, Pajarola G, Schroeder H E. Types and incidence of human periapical lesions obtained with extracted teeth. Oral Surg Oral Med Oral Pathol Oral Radiol Endod, 1996, 81: 93–102.

[165] Reeves R, Stanley H R. The relationship of bacterial penetration and pulpal pathosis in carious teeth. Oral surgery, oral medicine, and oral pathology, 1966, 22: 59–65.

[166] Renard E, et al. Immune cells and molecular networks in experimentally induced pulpitis. J Dent Res, 2016, 95: 196–205.

[167] Ricucci D, Loghin S, Siqueira J F. Correlation between clinical and histologic pulp diagnoses. Journal of Endodontics, 2014, 40: 1932–1939.

[168] Ricucci D, et al. Epithelium and bacteria in periapical lesions. Oral Surg Oral Med Oral Pathol Oral Radiol Endod, 2006, 101: 239–249.

[169] Rider D, et al. Elevated CD14 (cluster of differentiation 14) and Toll-like receptor (TLR) 4 signaling deteriorate periapical inflammation in TLR2 deficient mice. Anat Rec (Hoboken), 2016, 299: 1281–1292.

[170] Rôças I N, et al. Microbiome of deep dentinal caries lesions in teeth with symptomatic irreversible pulpitis. PloS one, 2016, 11: e0154653.

[171] Rôças I N, Siqueira J F Jr. Detection of novel oral species and phylotypes in symptomatic endodontic infections including abscesses. FEMS Microbiol Lett, 2005, 250: 279–285.

[172] Rosenberg P A, et al. Evaluation of pathologists (histopathology) and radiologists (cone beam computed tomography) differentiating radicular cysts from granulomas. J Endod, 2010, 36: 423–428.

[173] Sabeti M, et al. Detection of receptor activator of NF-kappa beta ligand in apical periodontitis. J Endod, 2005, 31: 17–18.

[174] Sabeti M, Simon J H, Slots J. Cytomegalovirus and Epstein-Barr virus are associated with symptomatic periapical pathosis. Oral Microbiol Immunol, 2003, 18: 327–328.

[175] Sabeti M, et al. Cytomegalovirus and Epstein-Barr virus DNA transcription in endodontic symptomatic lesions. Oral Microbiol Immunol, 2003, 18: 104–108.

[176] Sakamoto M, et al. Diversity of spirochetes in endodontic infections. J Clin Microbiol, 2009, 47: 1352–1357.

[177] Sakurai K, Okiji T, Suda H. Co-increase of nerve fibers and HLA-DRand/ or factor-XIIIa-expressing dendritic cells in dentinal caries-affected regions of the human dental pulp: an immunohistochemical study. J Dent. Res, 1999, 78: 1596–1608.

[178] Santos A L, et al. Comparing the bacterial diversity of acute and chronic dental root canal infections. PLoS One, 2011, 6: e28088.

[179] Sasaki H, et al. Gamma interferon (IFN-gamma) and IFN-gamma-inducing cytokines interleukin-12 (IL-12) and IL-18 do not augment infection-stimulated bone resorption in vivo. Clin Diagn Lab Immunol, 2004, 11: 106–110.

[180] Sasaki H, et al. IL-10, but not IL-4, suppresses infection-

stimulated bone resorption in vivo. J Immunol, 2000, 165: 3626–3630.
[181] Saunders W P, et al. Technical standard of root canal treatment in an adult Scottish sub-population. Br Dent J, 1997, 182: 382–386.
[182] Schulze-Schweifing K, Banerje A, Wade W G. Comparison of bacterial culture and 16S rRNA community profiling by clonal analysis and pyrosequencing for the characterization of the dentine cariesassociated microbiome. Frontiers in cellular and infection microbiology, 2014, 4: 164.
[183] Searls J C. Light and electron microscope evaluation of changes induced in odontoblasts of the rat incisor by the high-speed drill. Journal of dental research, 1967, 46: 1344–1355.
[184] Seltzer S, Bender I B, Ziontz M. The interrelationship of pulp and periodontal disease. Oral surgery, oral medicine, and oral pathology, 1963, 16: 1474–1490.
[185] Shah A C, et al. Outcomes of hospitalizations attributed to periapical abscess from 2000 to 2008: a longitudinal trend analysis. J Endod, 2013, 39: 1104–1110.
[186] Shelton F, Romberg E, Fouad A F. The effects of bisphosphonate treatment on the pathogenesis of endodontic pathosis. J Endod, 2010, 36: 556.
[187] Sigurdsson A, Jacoway J R. Herpes zoster infection presenting as an acute pulpitis. Oral Surg Oral Med Oral Pathol Oral Radiol Endod, 1995, 80: 92–95.
[188] Simon J H. Incidence of periapical cysts in relation to the root canal. J Endod, 1980, 6: 845–848.
[189] Siqueira J F Jr, Rôcas I N. PCR-based identification of Treponema maltophilum, T amylovorum, T medium, and T lecithinolyticum in primary root canal infections. Arch Oral Biol, 2003, 48: 495–502.
[190] Siqueira J F Jr, Rôcas I N. Community as the unit of pathogenicity: an emerging concept as to the microbial pathogenesis of apical periodontitis. Oral Surg Oral Med Oral Pathol Oral Radiol Endod, 2009, 107: 870–878.
[191] Siqueira J F Jr, Rôças I N. Diversity of endodontic microbiota revisited. Journal of dental research, 2009, 88: 969–981.
[192] Siqueira J F Jr, Rôças I N. Microbiology and treatment of acute apical abscesses. Clin Microbiol Rev, 2013, 26:255–273.
[193] Siqueira J F Jr, et al. Relationship between Fcgamma receptor and interleukin-1 gene polymorphisms and post-treatment apical periodontitis. J Endod, 2009, 35: 1186–1192.
[194] Siqueira J F Jr, et al. Polymorphism of the Fcgamma RIIIa gene and post-treatment apical periodontitis. J Endod, 2011. 37: 1345–1348.
[195] Slots J, Nowzari H, Sabeti M. Cytomegalovirus infection in symptomatic periapical pathosis. Int Endod J, 2004, 37: 519–524.
[196] Spatafore C M, et al, Periapical biopsy report: an analysis of over a 10-year period. J Endod, 1990, 16: 239–241.
[197] Stanley H R. Pulpal response to dental techniques and materials. Dental clinics of North America, 1971, 15: 115–126.
[198] Staquet M J, et al. Patternrecognition receptors in pulp defense. Adv Dent Res, 2011, 23: 296–301.
[199] Staquet M J, et al. Different roles of odontoblasts and fibroblasts in immunity. J Dent Res, 2008, 87: 256–261.
[200] Stashenko P, Teles R D, Souza R. Periapical inflammatory responses and their modulation. Crit Rev Oral Biol Med, 1998, 9: 498–521.
[201] Stashenko P, Yu S M, Wang C Y. Kinetics of immune cell and bone resorptive responses to endodontic infections. J Endod, 1992, 18: 422–426.
[202] Stern M H, et al. Isolation and characterization of inflammatory cells from the human periapical granuloma. Journal of Dental Research, 1982, 61: 1408–1412.
[203] Stern M H, et al. Quantitative analysis of cellular composition of human periapical granuloma. J Endod, 1981, 7: 117–122.
[204] Stockdale C R, Chandler N P. The nature of the periapical lesion-a review of 1108 cases. Journal of Dentistry, 1988, 16: 123–129.
[205] Subramanian K, Mickel A K. Molecular analysis of persistent periradicular lesions and root ends revealsa diverse microbial profile. J Endod, 2009, 35: 950–957.
[206] Sunde P T, et al. Microbiota of periapical lesions refractory to endodontic therapy. J Endod, 2002, 28: 304–310.
[207] Sunde P T, et al. Fluorescence in situ hybridization (FISH) for direct visualization of bacteria in periapical lesions of asymptomatic root-filled teeth. Microbiology, 2003, 149: 1095–1102.
[208] Sundqvist G. Ecology of the root-canal flora. Journal of Endodontics, 1992, 18: 427–430.
[209] Sundqvist G, Johansson E, Sjögren U. Prevalence of black-pigmented Bacteroides species in root canal infections. J Endod, 1989, 15: 13–19.
[210] Tani N, et al. Effect of T-cell deficiency on the formation of periapical lesions in mice: histological comparison between periapical lesion formation in BALB/c and BALB/c nu/nu mice. J Endod, 1995, 21: 195–199.
[211] Taylor P E, Byers M R. An immunocytochemical study of the morphological reaction of nerves containing calcitonin gene-related peptide to microabscess formation and healing in rat molars. Archives of Oral Biology, 1990, 35: 629–638.
[212] Teles R, Wang C Y, Stashenko P. Increased susceptibility of RAG-2 SCID mice to dissemination of endodontic infections. Infect Immun, 1997, 65: 3781–3787.
[213] Ten Cate A R. The epithelial cell rests of Malassez and the genesis of the dental cyst. Oral Surg Oral Med Oral Pathol, 1972, 34: 956–964.

[214] Torabinejad M. The role of immunological reactions in apical cyst formation and the fate of epithelial cells after root canal therapy: a theory. Int J Oral Surg, 1983, 12: 14–22.

[215] Torabinejad M, Cotti E, Jung T. Concentrations of leukotriene B4 in symptomatic and asymptomatic periapical lesions. J Endod, 1992, 18: 205–208.

[216] Tyler L W, et al. Eosinophilderived transforming growth factors (TGF-alpha and TGF-beta 1) in human periradicular lesions. J Endod, 1999, 25: 619–624.

[217] Veerayutthwilai O, et al. Differential regulation of immune responses by odontoblasts. Oral Microbiol, 2007, Immunol 22: 5–13.

[218] Velickovic M, et al. Expression of interleukin-33 and its receptor ST2 inperiapical granulomas and radicular cysts. J Oral Pathol Med, 2016, 45: 70–76.

[219] Vianna M E, et al. Identification and quantification of archaea involved in primary endodontic infections. Journal of clinical microbiology, 2006, 44: 1274–1282.

[220] Vickerman M M, et al. Phylogenetic analysis of bacterial and archaeal species in symptomatic and asymptomatic endodontic infections. Journal of medical microbiology, 2007, 56: 110–118.

[221] Wadachi R, Hargreaves K M. Trigeminal nociceptors express TLR-4 and CD14: a mechanism for pain due to infection. J Dent Res, 2006, 85: 49–53.

[222] Wallstrom J B, et al. Role of T cells in the pathogenesis of periapical lesions. A preliminary report. Oral Surg Oral Med Oral Pathol, 1993, 76: 213–218.

[223] Walton R E, Ardjmand K. Histological evaluation of the presence of bacteria in induced periapical lesions in monkeys. J Endod, 1992, 18: 216–227.

[224] Walzer T, et al. Natural-killer cells and dendritic cells: "l'union fait la force". Blood, 2005, 106: 2252–2258.

[225] Wang C Y, Stashenko P. Kinetics of bone-resorbing activity in developing periapical lesions. Journal of Dental Research, 1991, 70: 1362–1366.

[226] White S C, et al. Absence of radiometric differentiation between periapical cysts and granulomas. Oral Surg Oral Med Oral Pathol, 1994, 78: 650–654.

[227] Winstock D. Apical disease: an analysis of diagnosis and management with special reference to root lesion resection and pathology. Annals of the Royal College of Surgeons of England, 1980, 62: 171–179.

[228] Xiong H, et al. Effect of an estrogen-deficient state and alendronate therapy on bone loss resulting from experimental periapical lesions in rats. J Endod, 2007, 33: 1304–1308.

[229] Xiong H, et al. Effect of alendronate on alveolar bone resorption nd angiogenesis in rats with experimental periapical lesions. Int Endod J, 2010, 43: 485–491.

[230] Xu J, et al. KDM6B epigenetically regulates odontogenic differentiation of dental mesenchymal stem cells. International Journal of Oral Science, 2013, 5: 200–205.

[231] Yamasaki M, et al. Effect of methotrexate-induced neutropenia on rat periapical lesion. Oral Surg Oral Med Oral Pathol, 1994, 77: 655–661.

[232] Yoshiba K, Yoshiba N, Iwaku M. Class II antigen-presenting dendritic cell and nerve fiber responses to cavities, caries, or caries treatment in human teeth. Journal of dental research, 2003, 82: 422–427.

[233] Yoshiba N, et al. Immunohistochemical localizations of class II antigens and nerve fibers in human carious teeth: HLA-DR immunoreactivity in Schwann cells. Archives of histology and cytology, 1998, 61: 343–352.

[234] Yoshiba N, et al. Immunohistochemical localization of HLA-DR-positive cells in unerupted and erupted normal and carious human teeth. Journal of dental research, 1996, 75: 1585–1589.

[235] Zehnder M, Wegehaupt F J, Attin T. A first study on the usefulness of matrix metalloproteinase 9 from dentinal fluid to indicate pulp inflammation. Journal of Endodontics, 2011, 37: 17–20.

[236] Zhong S, et al. Differential expression of MicroRNAs in normal and inflamed human pulps. Journal of Endodontics, 2012, 38: 746–752.

第 4 章　根尖周炎的微生物学

José F. Siqueira Jr, Isabela N. Rôças

4.1　概述

牙齿根管系统的感染是根尖周炎的主要原因（图 4.1）。尽管化学和物理因素也可以诱发根尖周组织炎症，但大量科学研究证据表明微生物在根尖周炎的发展和持续存在起着至关重要的作用[99, 137, 291]。科学家们已经证实了真菌、古生菌以及病毒与根尖周炎的发生有关，但细菌仍是根尖周炎病因学中的主要微生物。

根管感染仅发生在部分或全部牙髓坏死的牙齿，或者先前已行去髓治疗的根管中。牙髓坏死是龋齿、创伤、牙周病，也是部分医源性手术的后果。这些情况为口腔细菌创造了进入根管系统的通路。坏死的牙髓缺乏有效的血液循环，因此不能再引发炎症反应保护自身免遭细菌侵袭和定植。牙髓一经感染，细菌将通过根尖孔和侧支根管与根尖周组织接触。根尖周组织将发生炎症变化，并引起各种形式的根尖周炎。

根尖周炎被认为是由发生在根管系统的细菌感染引起的感染性疾病，这种疾病的成功治疗取决于感染微生物的完全消除或有效控制。充分了解该病的病因是成功治疗的关键。在这种背景下，建立在坚实科学基础上的根尖周炎微生物学方面的知识对高质量的牙髓治疗是至关重要的。

本章讨论了与牙髓感染的微生物学以及根尖周炎发病机制相关的多个方面的内容。为了更好地理解文中所使用的术语，表 4.1 列举了其中许多术语的定义。

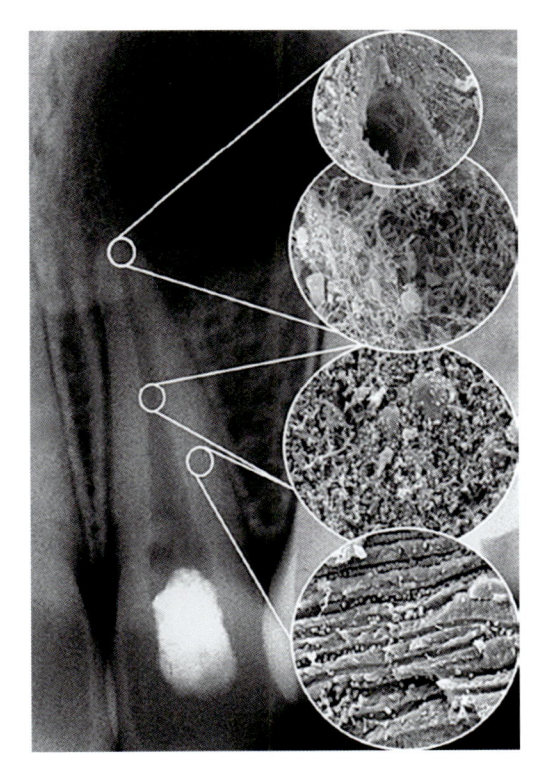

图 4.1　定植在根管系统的细菌是根尖周炎病变的主要病原体

表 4.1　本章所用术语的定义

术语	定义
16S rRNA	较小的（30S）原核核糖体亚单位的组成部分。编码这种结构的基因具有包含物种特异性特征序列的高变区，这对于在物种水平上鉴别细菌和古生菌非常有用。它还包含保守的通用区域，允许来自几乎所有细菌和古生菌的部分或全部 16S rRNA 基因进行扩增
偏害共栖	两种生物之间的关系，表现为当其中一种受到抑制时，另一种不受影响的现象
古生菌	一个包含与细菌不同的原核微生物的领域，而细菌组成另一个领域。真核生物（包含了有核细胞的生物体）是生命的第三个领域
糖酵解	一种不能代谢碳水化合物的微生物，需要其他碳源（如肽）来获取能量（在无氧条件下，葡萄糖在细胞质中被分解成为丙酮酸的过程，期间每分解一分子葡萄糖会产生两分子丙酮酸以及两分子 ATP，属于糖代谢的一种类型）
生物膜	一种固着的多细胞微生物群落，其特征是细胞牢牢地附着在表面，并嵌入其自身产生的细胞外聚合物基质中
群落	一个相互作用的生物群体
群落特征	群落中的生物种类丰富度和数量丰富度
群落结构	群落中的生物种类丰富度和数量丰富度
密度	单位面积上的细胞数量（个体）
多样性	群落中物种丰富度和相对丰富度的度量
生态学	生物与其生长环境之间相互关系的研究
内源性感染	由正常人体微生物组分引起的感染
外源性感染	由不属于人体正常微生物群而是被引入宿主的微生物引起的感染
食物链	群落中的生物通过营养物质和能量的转移而相互联系，呈线性排列的关系
食物网	相互连接的食物链网络。它显示了不同物种是如何通过不同的代谢途径连接起来的
水平（或横向）基因转移	遗传物质在同时代生物之间的交换，与代表着从祖先那里获得遗传物质的垂直转移相反，水平转移允许一个物种将其遗传物质转移给另一个物种
感染	微生物在原来不应存在的地方入侵和增殖。感染并不一定会导致疾病
感染性疾病	微生物感染并对宿主组织损伤后，症状和体征逐渐显现
嗜炎细菌	与炎症组织接触时生长旺盛的细菌种类，从炎症渗出物和组织分解产物中获取营养
负载	细胞数（个体）
宏蛋白质组学	对直接从环境或临床样本中回收的所有蛋白质的研究
微生物区	在特定结构区域形成复杂多样群落的微生物的总称
调控蛋白	具有调节宿主免疫反应能力，特别是刺激细胞因子的合成和释放的细菌结构成分或释放产物
小生境	个体在社群落中的功能角色（代谢功能）
条件致病菌	一种只在宿主防御系统受损时才引起疾病的微生物
病原体	引起疾病的微生物
病原性	引起疾病的能力
种系型	作为未经培育的物种，仅通过 16S rRNA 基因序列被识别，而非表型特征
多重微生物感染	由几种不同微生物引起的感染

表 4.1（续）

术语	定义
种群	一组生长中的细胞（微菌落）
原发性或真病原体	一种在特定宿主体内经常引起疾病的微生物
假定或候选病原体	横断面研究中发现的与疾病相关的微生物，但缺乏纵向观察的证据
相对丰度	群落中每个物种的比例
丰度	群落中不同物种的数量（组成）
协同作用	两个或两个以上物种或因素之间的相互作用，其影响大于其各自影响的总和
毒力	致病度
毒力因子	有助于致病的微生物产物、结构成分或机制

4.2 根尖周炎的微生物病因

首次对根管内细菌的观察报告可追溯到 17 世纪，荷兰的业余显微镜制造者安东尼·范·列文虎克（Antony van Leeuwenhoek，1632—1723 年）写道："这颗牙齿的牙冠几乎完全腐烂，而它的牙根由两个根组成，因此，牙根非常中空，牙根上的孔洞里塞满了一种柔软的物质。我把这些东西拿出来，与干净的雨水混合，放在放大镜下，看看里面是否像我之前发现的那样有许多的微生物，我必须承认，在我看来，所有的东西都是有生命的[38]。"在当时，列文虎克所发现的微生物作为感染源的作用尚不清楚。200 多年后，列文虎克的观察结果才得到证实，人们开始提出细菌与根尖周炎之间的因果关系。

1894 年，受德国柏林 Robert Koch 的启发，美国牙医 Willoughby Dayton Miller 开展了开创性的口腔微生物学实验。在分析了从根管内收集的样本材料后，他发表了一项里程碑式的研究，报告了细菌与根尖周炎的关系[131]。通过对根管样本进行细菌学检查，Miller 发现了三种基本的细菌，即球菌、杆菌和螺旋菌（图 4.2）。他写道："一般情况下，我们认为，细菌在某种程度上一定与这些过程有关（牙髓疾病）……那么，正如我已经指出的，在病变牙髓中存在不同种类的细菌，这些细菌尚未在人工培养基上培养出来，且其致病机制我们还不清楚。这些细菌在某些牙髓中大量存在，尤其是螺旋体的反复出现，证明了在某些情况下，它们可能在化脓过程中发挥重要作用。"

Miller 提出了以下假说：细菌是根尖周炎的致病因素；根管冠部、中部和根尖部的微生物群落的物种组成明显不同。在光学显微镜下观察到的根管样本中的一些细菌无法通过当时可用的方法进行培养。这些细菌中的大多数都是厌氧菌。20 世纪，尽管学者们在细菌培养方面取得了相当大的技术进步，但人们普遍认识到，还有许多种微生物无法培养[3,179]。

Miller 的发现虽然具有开创性，但仅仅提示了细菌和根尖周炎之间可能存在因果关系。两个事件同时发生并不一定意味着存在因果关系。直到 Miller 的经典发现近 70 年后，Kakehashi 等人对无菌大鼠进行的一项出色的研究才明确证明了细菌与根尖周炎之间的因果关系[99]。这些学者将普通大鼠和无菌大鼠的牙髓暴露在口腔中，观察牙髓和根周组织的反应。在术后 1~42d 的时间间

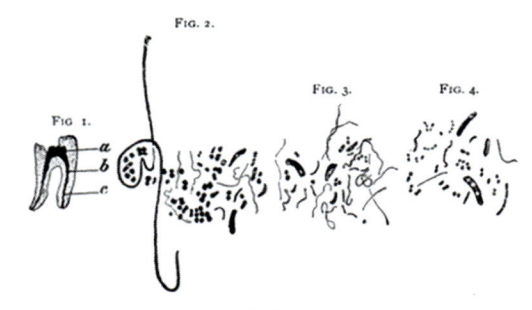

图 4.2 Miller 经典文章[131]中显示了通过显微镜观察到的根管样本中不同的细菌

隔内进行的组织学评估显示：在常规饲养的动物中，所有时间较久的标本均显示牙髓完全坏死和根尖周炎性病变。无菌动物的牙髓通过形成牙本质桥进行自我修复，这一变化在14d时已经明显可见；到21d和28d，新形成的硬组织完全封闭了先前暴露的区域，且与暴露的角度和严重程度无关。在每个案例，牙本质桥下方的牙髓组织依然保持活性。

1976年，Sundqvist使用厌氧培养方法来评估创伤后失去活力的人类完整牙齿的牙髓细菌学情况[291]。他的研究结果显示，没有根尖周炎病变的牙齿，其坏死牙髓是无菌的；而有根尖周炎病变的牙齿，其牙髓几乎都是受到感染的。分离出的细菌中厌氧菌占主导地位，占比超过90%。从他的发现也可以推断，坏死的牙髓组织本身以及根管内淤积的组织液并不能诱发和维持根尖周炎。

Möller等人也提供了细菌与根尖周炎之间存在因果关系的有力证据[137]。一项针对猴子牙齿的研究发现：只有感染的失活牙髓才会引起根尖周炎，而仅仅失活却未感染的牙髓则没有显示根周组织中有病理变化的存在。除了佐证细菌在根尖周炎发展中的重要性，该研究还表明，在没有感染的情况下，坏死的牙髓组织无法导致根尖周炎的发生发展。

与根尖周炎相关的定植在根管系统的细菌主要以生物膜结构实现聚集。一些形态学研究报告了[138, 148, 233, 276]根管感染中存在类似生物膜的细菌结构，但Ricucci和Siqueira的研究[183]结果发现：存在于根尖部分的细菌生物膜与原发性以及治疗后的根尖周炎密切相关。鉴于大多数牙髓微生物学研究的片面性，目前尚不清楚细菌生物膜这种存在形式对根尖周炎的发展是否是必要的。然而，从临床角度来看，必须认识到，细菌生物膜不论在未经治疗还是治疗过后的患有根尖周炎的牙齿根尖根管中都普遍存在，并且可能对合理的抗菌治疗构成挑战。

4.3 牙髓生物膜和病原体群落的概念

生物膜可以定义为一种固着的多细胞微生物群落，其特征是细胞牢牢附着在一个表面上，并被细胞外多聚体（EPS）基质所包裹[28, 39]（图4.3）。自然界中绝大多数微生物物种都生活在代谢整合的生物膜群落中，人体也不例外[28, 126]。

大多数需要快速诊断和干预以避免严重损伤或死亡的急性医疗感染是由浮游细菌引起的，而与持续性炎症和渐进性组织损伤相关的慢性感染通常与生物膜有关[168, 273, 330]。细菌生物膜感染导致了65%~80%的人类感染性疾病，包括心内膜炎、中耳感染（中耳炎）、骨髓炎、前列腺炎和骨科器械相关感染[27, 30, 168]。在口腔中，龋病、牙龈炎以及边缘性牙周炎是由细菌生物膜引起疾病的典型例子[125]。最近，根尖周炎也被纳入由生物膜诱发的口腔疾病的范畴[183]。

4.3.1 结构

细菌生物膜中的细胞通常聚集在微菌落中，这些微菌落嵌入并非随机分布在整个细胞外多聚体（EPS）基质中[29, 39, 283, 286]。这些群体生物膜结构中的分布取决于多种因素，包括到达时间、群落成员之间积极的代谢相互作用以及与便捷营养源的接近程度。贯穿生物膜结构的水通道将种群分隔开，这些水通道输送水和营养物质并排出代谢废物。细胞数量最多的聚集区通常在生物膜结构的底部，即靠近生物膜黏附的表面。

细胞外多聚体基质由生物膜群落中的微生物自己产生，并且在生物膜干重的占比最大（>90%）；细胞成分不到生物膜干重的10%[58]。EPS基质主要由多糖构成，但也存在蛋白质、核

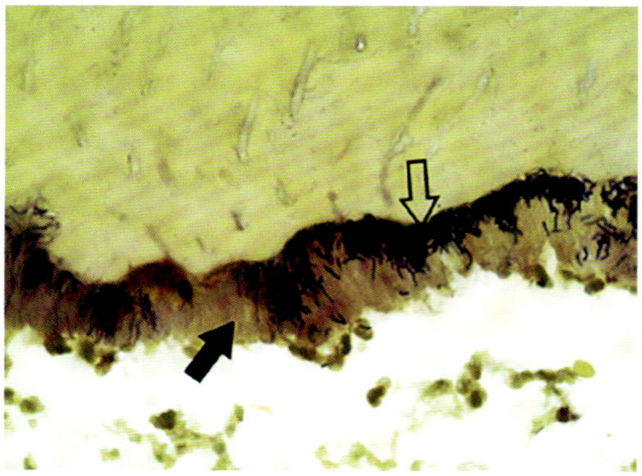

图4.3 原发性根尖周炎牙齿中的细菌生物膜中细菌细胞黏附在牙本质上（空箭头）并嵌入在厚的细胞外基质中（黑色箭头）(Brown和Brenn染色，原始放大400倍)

酸和脂质[28]。EPS为生物膜群落提供了许多基本功能，介导了细菌与表面的黏附，提供了群落机械稳定性，允许生物膜群落积累参与营养获取和抗生素防御的细胞外酶，还能通过保持细胞接近的状态以利于细胞间的积极相互作用；同时作为群落营养储备，保持水分，保护群落对抗抗菌剂和宿主防御[58, 239]。生物膜中的细菌对中性粒细胞[94]和巨噬细胞[297]的吞噬作用表现出更强的抵抗力。

与浮游状态下的细胞相比，生物膜中的细胞表现出不同的表型。这在很大程度上是由于两种状态之间的差异性基因表达[16, 154, 228]。生物膜表型的基因表达的改变和低生长率通常也会增强生物膜对抗菌剂、环境压力和宿主防御的抵抗力[120]。

4.3.2 生物膜中的细菌相互作用和相互交流

在多菌种生物膜中，细胞彼此紧密接触，这有利于它们之间的相互作用和交流。这些相互作用会影响生物膜群落的整体功能和生理特性，同时影响它们对外部威胁的抵抗力的毒力[20]。生物膜细菌之间的相互作用可以使它们作为一个群体协同行动。

细菌之间的交流通常被称为群体感应，可能发生在革兰氏阳性和革兰氏阴性菌种[44, 59, 329]。群体感应涉及一种被称为自诱导分子的化学信号分子的产生、释放和随后的检测。产生和释放自诱导分子的细菌种群进行繁殖时，细胞外自诱导分子的浓度也会增加。当自诱导分子的浓度达到关键阈值水平时，菌群将通过改变基因表达来应答[159]。这是因为细菌只有在群体中才能执行特定的行为和功能。已知交流信号在同一群体成员之间的作用比在不同群体之间重要得多，但存在这样一种可能性，即存在于不同群体中的细胞释放的信号也可能相互影响[20]。群体感应系统对于毒力调节、对饥饿和宿主防御的抗性、次级代谢产物的产生和生物膜的形成都非常重要。例如，一些机会性病原体通过检测自身细胞密度来表达毒力因子。一些候选牙髓病病原体已被证实能产生群体感应信号分子[61, 167, 324, 334]。

多物种生物膜中细菌之间的交流可导致相互的转录组学和蛋白质组学反应，从而调节营养素的获取、代谢过程和毒力因子的表达[81, 144]。基于生物膜群落成员之间众多可能的互动，可以推断群落多样性越高，其复杂性越高。

生物膜中较高的细胞密度和稳定的细胞间接触条件也有利于群落成员之间的水平基因转移[20]。因此，与抗药性或与毒力特性相关的基因可能会转移至群落的其他成员。

群落成员之间的共营养关系（一个菌种依赖于另一个菌种释放的产物）有助于形成整个生物膜结构中的种群组织。从这个意义上讲，分解复杂基质的协同作用也很重要（详见4.5节）。

4.3.3 病原体群落的概念

与大多数内源性感染相关的生物膜通常由多种菌种组成。因此，科学家们提出了这些疾病的多种微生物病因。基于生物膜的概念，目前的趋势是将细菌群落作为一个整体看作这些疾病的致病单位[93, 109, 273]。因此，致病单位与其说是一种或几种定植微生物释放的特定因子，不如说是生物膜群落中物种的总体组成和相对丰度，以及无数细菌间的相互作用。

似乎根尖周炎的发病机制有赖于多菌种群落中细菌的协同作用[273]。群落微生物的种类和水平，以及它们之间的相互作用导致生物膜基质中多种毒力因子的累积[269]。当生物膜到达根管系统的根尖区域时，其中的毒力因子扩散引发并维持根尖周组织炎症[258]。

生物膜感染通常相当于对组织的持续性侵害源。在根管感染中，宿主防御难以进入感染的解剖部位，加重了感染的持久性。细菌生物膜与根尖周组织相邻，可引发破坏性炎症反应。

生物膜的集群致病性受群落成员之间协同相互作用的影响，其结果可能比单个成分的预期结果更加严重。如前所述，协同相互作用增强了细菌对宿主防御行为和抗菌剂的抵抗，并且增加了多菌种群落的毒力。此外，在某些情况下，炎症环境中细菌生物膜的生存和持续存在或将变得更具优势。事实上，有人提出：与长期存在的炎症过程相关的口腔细菌群落可被视为"嗜炎性群落"[80]。这意味着群落成员不仅有能力在炎症反应的攻击中幸存下来，而且还可以利用这种情况。

炎症是对抗感染的重要过程，但在生物膜感染中，它通常不能成功根除感染，而是在感染源未被清除的情况下导致组织损伤。炎症可能是根尖部根管生物膜中某些细菌的重要营养来源。营养物质以糖蛋白形式存在于渗出液的糖蛋白和组织分解产物，例如降解的胶原蛋白和含血红素的化合物（结合珠蛋白、血红素结合蛋白和血红蛋白）[80, 258]。已有研究表明，牙周生物膜中的细菌载量随着炎症的加剧而增高[1]，并且与牙周炎相关的微生物群落表现出与铁摄取和蛋白水解活性相关的基因表达的增加[45]。

根尖周炎进展后，炎症衍生产物成为根管内细菌的主要营养来源。因此，获取铁并利用这些产物（肽和氨基酸）作为主要能量来源的糖酵解和蛋白水解的细菌在根尖根管系统中占据主导地位[258]。

炎症就像一把双刃剑。一方面，持续的根管内生物膜感染同时激活先天性和适应性免疫应答，防止根管感染扩散到骨甚至身体其他部位。另一方面，这两种免疫应答都不能消除根管内生物膜，并且最终导致组织损伤（见下文细菌致病机制）。此外，持续性炎症为根尖根管中嗜炎性细菌的生长和存活提供了新的和可持续的底物来源。

基于群落作为病原体的概念，致病性牙髓细菌群落富含毒力因子，这些因子在生物膜中积累并逐渐释放，以刺激和维持根尖周组织炎症。该群落还在炎症环境下适于生存，并且能够从炎症中获得维持其生存的重要营养。

4.3.4　根尖周炎患牙的细菌生物膜

几项形态学研究描述了在患有根尖周炎的牙齿根管中存在类似于悬浮生物膜结构的细菌组织[22, 138, 148, 186, 229, 276]。在主根管腔内，许多细菌细胞悬浮在液体中或被包裹在牙髓坏死组织中（浮游状态）（图4.4），但研究者还观察到密集的细菌生物膜群落不同程度地黏附在根管壁上[148, 276]（图4.5）。主根管中的浮游细菌可能是新进入的，也可能是从附着在根管壁上的生物膜结构中分离出来的。生物膜不仅存在于主根管中，还可以扩散到根尖分支、侧支根管、根管峡部和根管系统的凹陷处[22, 147, 182, 184]。偶尔，它们也可以到达根尖孔并延伸到牙根外表面，形成根管外生物膜[54, 185, 298]。

Ricucci 和 Siqueira 的一项组织细菌学研究证明了根尖部根管中生物膜的高发生率及其与根尖周炎的强相关性[183]。在80%的患有原发性根尖周炎的牙齿和74%的治疗后发生根尖周炎的牙齿的根尖根管内发现了生物膜。牙髓病相关的生物膜通常较厚且呈多层，基质-细胞相对比例差异很大（图4.5）。虽然大多数根管壁都被生物膜定植，但仍有部分区域生物膜很少定植甚至没有。

生物膜在具有较大范围病变的牙齿和组织病理学诊断为囊肿的牙齿中更常见[183]。这可能与较大病变和囊肿代表了长期病理过程有关。在这些病例中，作为病变原因的根管内感染甚至更"久"。预计参与以上过程的细菌有足够的时间和条件在成熟的生物膜群落中自我规划。根尖周炎范围会影响治疗的结果，这是因为由大量细胞和多物种组成的复杂感染[196, 291]难以控制。这些感染通常以生物膜的形式存在[183]。

Ricucci 和 Siqueira 的研究[183]发现一些临床标本中有细菌絮状物。细菌絮状物是被 EPS 基质包围的大型细菌菌落。这些结构可能源自浮游细胞的团聚体/共团聚体的生长，或者是从附着在表面的生物膜脱落的[82]。

细菌对牙本质小管的侵袭常见于生物膜结构之下[183]。牙本质小管直径足够大，允许绝大多数口腔细菌的入侵。牙本质小管感染可以发生在

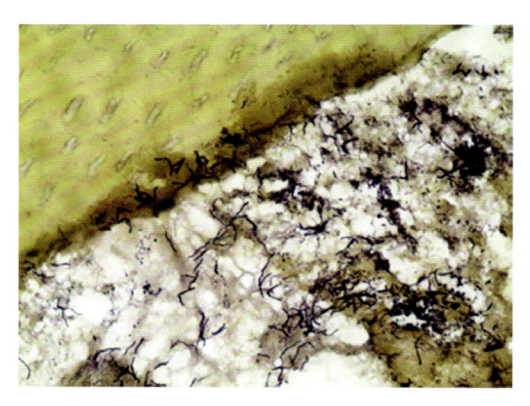

图4.4　出现在管腔内的浮游细菌。细胞通常悬浮在液体中并与坏死组织交织（Brown 和 Brenn 染色，原始放大400倍）

50%~80% 有根尖周炎的牙齿[79, 130]。浅层细菌入侵更为常见，但有时可以在牙本质 300μm 深处观察到细菌[276]。一项对猴子的研究表明这种感染甚至可能波及整个牙本质小管的长度和引起牙周膜的变化，特别是当牙骨质被吸收而丢失时[302]。即使有些牙本质小管感染严重，但邻近牙本质小管也有可能未被感染（图 4.6）。能动性似乎不是细菌侵入牙本质的必要特征，因为迄今为止在小管中发现的大多数细菌都是无能动性的物种[130, 165]。在原位研究中，小管内经常观察到分裂细胞[276]（图 4.7），这表明细菌可以在小管内获取营养，可能通过降解的成牙本质突、变性的胶原、感染过程中死亡的细菌细胞以及通过毛细血管进入小管的管内液体获得营养。事实上，在体外[116, 163, 260]和体内研究[130, 165]中，一些候选牙髓致病菌已被证明能够穿透牙本质小管。

生物膜附着在根尖孔或侧孔周围的牙根外表面是相当罕见的。然而，当其存在时，牙根外生物膜通常与症状或窦道相关（见"根外感染"部分）。

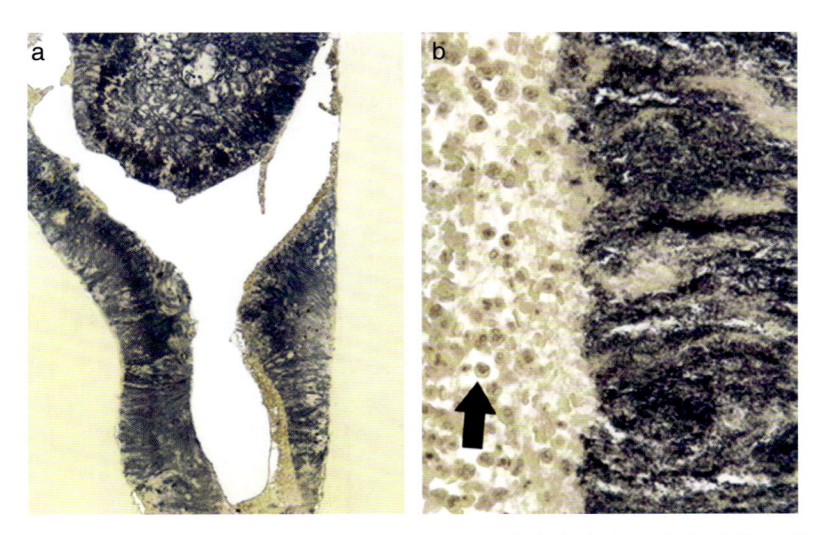

图 4.5　a. 有广泛冠状破坏和根尖周炎的牙齿，向口腔开放，拔牙前有多次加重史的厚细菌生物膜（改良革兰氏染色，放大 50 倍）。b. 高倍镜显示密集的细菌细胞群面临着炎症细胞的聚集，特别是多形核中性粒细胞（箭头）（放大 400 倍）（由 Domenico Ricucci 博士提供）

图 4.6　a. 细菌侵入根尖周炎牙齿的牙本质小管（改良革兰氏染色，放大 100 倍）。b. 放大倍数更高（400 倍）（由 Domenico Ricucci 博士提供）

4.3.5 牙髓动力学：生物膜形成理论

生物膜在自然界不同表面的形成机制与牙菌斑相似。这个过程开始于漂浮在液体中的浮游细菌细胞定植于固体表面。最初，由于唾液中的大分子（蛋白质和糖蛋白）被吸附到牙齿表面，牙齿表面形成了一层条件膜。浮游状态下的细菌通过非特异性和特异性的方式接近并附着在表面。EPS基质产生并允许更强的黏附。最后，这些先锋物种生长并共同聚集其他物种，包括新物种，形成一个多物种群落——生物膜。

当无髓根管对口腔开放，唾液渗入时，这些机制可能有助于生物膜的形成。然而，在大多数情况下，根管内生物膜的形成过程可能遵循一个不同的过程。牙髓炎症、坏死和感染通常是龋病的后果，龋齿也是由生物膜引起的[127]。随着龋病对牙本质的破坏，与龋相关的生物膜逐渐向牙髓推进。当牙髓组织暴露于龋生物膜时，炎症的严重程度会加剧，并可能导致局部组织坏死（图 4.8）。随着细菌细胞沿牙本质管壁黏附生长，生物膜向前占据这些区域，并沿根尖方向移动。从生物膜脱落的细胞和来自口腔的晚期浮游细胞也会出现在有坏死组织的管腔内。细菌侵袭、炎症、坏死和感染等在牙髓组织进一步发生，并逐渐向根尖移动。因此，随着感染前端的生物膜向根尖移动，坏死根管内生物膜的逐渐形成。

4.3.6 根尖周炎是一种由生物膜引起的疾病

根尖周炎符合通常用于建立感染性疾病和生物膜之间因果关系的标准[82, 160, 183]，具体如下。

· 感染根管的细菌通常以群落的形式存在，附着在主根管的牙本质壁以及根管系统的其他部位[22, 138, 148, 183, 186, 229, 276]。

· 对感染组织的直接检查显示，细菌形成了包裹在细胞外基质中的群体。组织细菌学研究表明，黏附在根管壁上的细菌群落包裹在一种无定形的细胞外基质中，其厚度各不相同[183, 186, 239]，这种结构类似于在其他人体部位（包括牙菌斑）报道的生物膜。

· 感染一般局限于特定部位，虽然可能发生播散，但为次要事件。在牙髓感染中，生物膜通常局限于根管系统（根管内生物膜）[183]。在极少数情况下，发现生物膜延伸到牙根外表面，但在

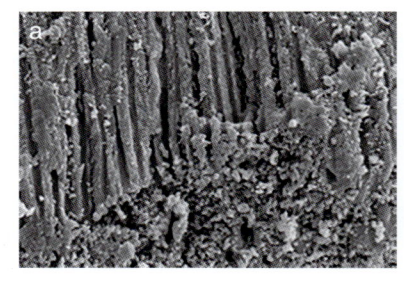

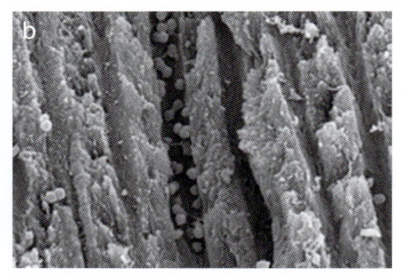

图 4.7 根尖周炎患牙的根管细菌感染扫描电子显微镜照。a. 密集的细菌聚集在根管壁，部分细菌侵入牙本质小管内（原始放大 1800 倍）。b. 小管内细菌分裂（5500 倍）

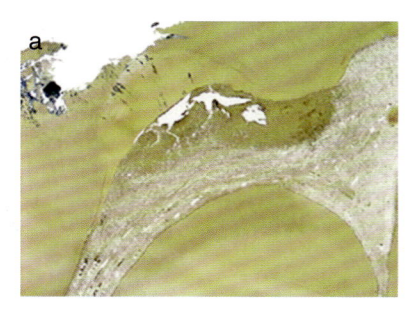

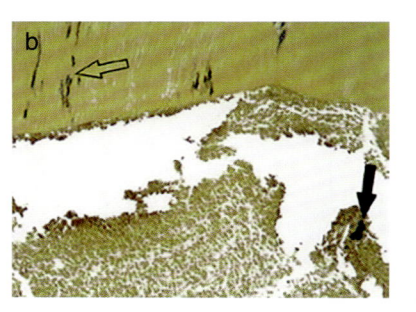

图 4.8 a. 龋生物膜到达牙髓并引起广泛炎症（改良革兰氏染色，放大 16 倍）。b. 高倍镜显示细菌侵入三层牙本质（空箭头）。细菌也可见于严重发炎的牙髓（黑色箭头）（100 倍）。由 Domenico Ricucci 博士提供

慢性病例中，很少有生物膜扩散到这一区域或根尖周炎病变之外的报道。

· 尽管致病微生物在浮游细胞状态下容易被杀死，但用抗生素很难或不可能根除感染。全身性抗生素并不能成功治疗牙髓感染。抗生素通常是在细菌有扩散迹象的情况下使用。使用抗生素无效的原因是细菌位于无血管坏死腔内，抗生素不能达到足够的浓度而起作用。此外，据报道，生活在生物膜中的细菌细胞对抗生素的耐药性是其浮游状态的100~1000倍[153]。

· 宿主清除无效，其证据可能是细菌菌落位于与炎症细胞相关的宿主组织区域。炎症细胞（主要是多形核中性粒细胞）堆积在牙髓生物膜上[183]。

· 消除或显著破坏生物膜结构和生态可导致疾病进程缓解。如果根管充填时根管内未检出细菌，则根尖周炎的治疗成功率显著提高[50]。在根管治疗过的根尖周炎牙齿中经常观察到生物膜，而在根尖健康区域的牙齿中则缺乏生物膜[183, 187]，这表明生物膜有可能满足这一标准。

4.3.7 牙髓病致病性细菌群落的要求

生物膜群落应满足以下必要条件才能引起疾病并导致病情发展。

1）群落密度必须足够高，以达到致病负荷。

2）根管感染时，菌群中存在大量抗原和毒力因子，这些抗原和毒力因子在菌群中表达，在菌群中积累并释放到环境中。

3）该菌群必须位于根管系统中，这样细胞和（或）毒力因子与抗原才能进入根尖周组织。

4）该群落必须包含与其他生物膜物种有良好整合和协同关系的致病物种。

5）宿主必须在根尖周组织建立防御策略，抑制感染扩散到骨骼和其他部位，但这也会导致损伤。

4.4 细菌致病机制

微生物引起疾病的能力被称为致病性。毒力表示微生物致病性的强弱，而毒力因子是有助于致病的微生物产物、结构成分或策略。

细菌群落的集体致病性取决于总体种群密度、物种组成以及它们之间的协同作用。生物膜中的细菌不断蓄积毒力因子，并将其从EPS基质中逐渐释放，从而影响邻近的宿主组织。不同的病毒因子常在感染的不同阶段联合作用，单个因子在不同阶段也可能具有多种功能。毒力因子可能参与细菌附着宿主表面组织、入侵宿主细胞、在宿主组织的扩散、直接和间接的组织损伤以及生存策略，包括逃避宿主防御反应。

细菌通过直接和（或）间接机制破坏宿主组织来发挥其致病性。细菌引起直接有害的物质通常涉及其分泌产物，包括酶（蛋白酶、肽酶、透明质酸酶等）、外毒素和代谢产物（丁酸、丙酸、铵、多胺、吲哚、挥发性含硫化合物等）[245]。在根尖周炎中，间接机制在组织损伤的发展中占主导地位。最终导致根尖周炎典型组织破坏的是宿主对细菌刺激产生的免疫反应。宿主免疫反应的刺激和激活是由细菌抗原和结构成分（调节素）引起的，包括脂多糖（LPS或内毒素）、肽聚糖、脂磷壁酸、菌毛、鞭毛、外膜蛋白和胞外多糖[86, 303]。

骨吸收就是一个例子。细菌成分刺激炎症和非炎症宿主细胞释放细胞因子和前列腺素等化学介质，这些介质参与诱导慢性根尖周炎病变中的特征性骨吸收[226]。细菌DNA还激活巨噬细胞和树突状细胞，并引发促炎细胞因子的释放[108]。促炎细胞因子通过促进破骨细胞前体的增殖和分化或通过促进成熟破骨细胞的活化，或同时通过上述两种方式来刺激破骨细胞性骨吸收[213]。

细菌间接损伤的另一个例子是急性根尖周脓肿中的脓液形成。尽管一些细菌产物可能会导致组织损伤并在脓液的生成中发挥直接作用，但结缔组织破坏和液化的主要原因是多形核嗜中性粒细胞（PMNs）在感染反应中释放的产物。过度活跃、多余或失调的PMNs通过释放有毒物质（如氧自由基或组织降解溶酶体酶）引起组织损伤。

根管微生物群在隐蔽位置时，细菌要发挥其致病性就必须侵入根周组织，或其产物和（或）结构成分必须穿透组织并引起宿主组织的反应。细菌通过运动或生长侵入组织。运动细菌（如密螺旋体）可以通过快速运动逃离吞噬细胞。然而，大多数牙髓细菌是不动的，通过生长入侵组织需要繁殖速度能克服宿主防御机制。根周组织的明显侵犯是相当罕见的，因为侵犯一旦发生，细菌通常迅速被清除。在某些情况下，细菌对根周组织的大量侵袭会导致严重的炎症和脓肿形成。有毒菌种或毒株的存在，以及强毒力多物种群落容易导致脓肿形成。

据推测，口腔微生物群仅少数真正致病，且其中大多数均表现为低毒力。这与根尖周炎最常见的形式为慢性进行性这一本质相一致。从根内生物膜中扩散出来的或到达根周组织的细菌释放的分泌产物或结构引起根周组织的直接或间接损伤，但致病物质又很快被破坏，因此，根周组织很少发生细菌感染（脓肿除外）。

几乎所有毒力因子都受到严格调控，它们的表达与环境信号或线索有关。影响毒力因子调节的生化和物理因素包括饥饿、人口密度、pH、温度、铁可用性、氧张力和氧化还原电位等。因此，在接收到适当的环境信号后，不同组的毒力基因可以被表达或抑制，这使细菌能够适应不同的环境条件。

饥饿等应激条件可能会刺激某些病原体的毒力装置[110, 129]。活的细菌在自然环境中通常会经历饥饿期。一旦饥饿基因被表达出来，细菌就会改变它们的行为，以便在养分耗尽的情况下生存。主要的诱导机制包括控制饥饿期间的能量生成和增强对稀缺养分的摄取能力。这些机制可能允许细菌在接受根管治疗的牙齿中存活，并诱发治疗后的根尖周炎病变。

4.4.1 根管环境中释放的细菌毒性因子

多物种生物膜群落的致病能力与 EPS 基质中不同成分的毒力因子和抗原的积累和逐渐释放有关。因此，对多物种感染过程中释放的细菌物质进行评估，可以为生理和致病行为提供有价值的信息。

脂多糖（LPS）是大多数革兰氏阴性细菌外膜的主要成分之一，由亲水性多糖和疏水性糖脂成分（脂质 A）组成[193]。大多数生物学效应与细胞死亡后或增殖期间暴露的脂质 A 部分有关。LPS 与宿主细胞的相互作用会产生多种生物学效应，包括激活巨噬细胞/单核细胞，进而合成和释放促炎细胞因子、前列腺素、一氧化氮和氧自由基[86, 303, 328]；补体系统的激活[96, 332]；刺激破骨细胞分化和骨吸收[345]；激活三叉神经传入神经元上表达的模式识别受体，触发细胞内信号级联，导致神经肽的外周释放和中枢伤害性神经传递[316]。在有原发感染、有症状的根尖周炎、大面积根周骨破坏和持续渗出的牙齿中，感染根管中的 LPS 含量较高[31, 69, 91–92, 230, 231]。牙髓病原体产生的 LPS 被认为在脓肿[142]和骨吸收[32]相关的组织损伤中起着重要作用。

虽然 LPS 已被广泛研究，并被视为革兰氏阴性菌在根尖周炎发病中的重要毒力因子，但将与根尖周炎病因相关的牙髓感染的所有生物学效应都归因于这种物质似乎过于简单。在像牙髓生物膜这样的多物种群落中，预计会产生许多其他毒力因子，这些因子在疾病发病机制中发挥作用。事实上，在感染过程中，许多其他潜在的毒力因子被释放到根管环境中。

脂磷壁酸（LTA）是一种阴离子聚合物，是革兰氏阳性细胞壁的主要成分。鉴于其生物学效应，LTA 可被视为革兰氏阳性细菌 LPS 的对应物。LTA 刺激巨噬细胞/单核细胞释放促炎细胞因子[303, 321]并激活补体系统[66]。一项研究量化了治疗后根尖周炎患者牙齿中的 LTA，并在所有受检病例中发现了这种分子[9]。

细菌代谢的几种最终产物释放到细胞外环境中，可能对宿主细胞有毒，导致结缔组织细胞外基质成分降解，并干扰宿主防御过程[46, 73, 304]。短链脂肪酸（SCFAs）是众所周知的厌氧菌代谢终产物，被视为潜在的毒力因子[150, 175]。Provenzano 等人[172]评估了治疗前后原发感染根管中 SCFAs 的出现情况，发现丁酸和丙酸是最常见的。在化学机械操作后也发现了这两种 SCFAs。SCFAs 在治疗前未达到可检测的水平，但在氢氧化钙治疗后的检测中频繁出现。

多胺是由细菌在氨基酸酶解脱羧后产生的。多胺的例子包括腐胺、亚精胺、精胺和尸体胺。多胺可以调节中性粒细胞的凋亡，导致细胞过早死亡[122]。一项研究发现，与无症状牙齿相比，自发性疼痛和肿胀的牙齿根管中含有更多的多胺[121]。

群落分析研究表明,在根管感染的细菌多样性方面,个体间有高度差异[225, 238],无数细菌组合导致相同的疾病。在这些情况下,尽管个体之间的物种组成存在差异,但细菌群落可能表现出类似的生理和致病行为。尽管物种组成中受试者之间的变异性很高,但疾病相关生物膜群落显示出保守的代谢基因表达谱[97]。尽管与特定疾病相关的群落在物种组成上有所不同,但它们对宿主组织的行为可能类似。这表明,在疾病相关群落中,细菌生理学和功能方面存在一些冗余,释放的细菌产物的总体多样性低于物种多样性。在这种功能冗余的情况下,对群落的生理学或致病性至关重要的特定产物可能由不同物种的不同个体提供。这有助于解释患有相同疾病(无症状根尖周炎、急性根尖周脓肿)的不同个体的群落物种组成的高度多样性。

元蛋白质组学技术已被用于在给定时间点大规模表征微生物群落的整个蛋白质补体[327]。因此,基因表达产物(蛋白质)直接在样品中鉴定。一些研究已经使用元蛋白质组学来评估牙髓感染。Nandakumar 等人[149]在原发性或持续性感染的病例中鉴定了细菌蛋白质,并发现了蛋白酶、毒力因子、自溶蛋白,以及与黏附、接合、抗生素耐药性有关的蛋白质。Provenzano 等人[171]评估了与急性根尖周脓肿和无症状根尖周炎相关的原发性感染的元蛋白质组,并发现急性根尖周脓肿在总体上有更多的蛋白质。大多数微生物蛋白质与代谢和管家基因表达过程有关,包括蛋白质合成、能量代谢和 DNA 过程,表明有活力和活性的细胞的存在。已鉴定出几种与致病性和耐药性/存活相关的蛋白质,包括与黏附、生物膜形成和抗生素耐药性相关的蛋白质、应激蛋白、外毒素、侵袭素、蛋白酶和内肽酶(主要在脓肿中),以及一种与甲烷生成相关的古细菌蛋白质。

在另一项研究中,Provenzano 等人[173]评估了根尖周炎治疗后的牙齿根尖及其相关炎症病变中的细菌元蛋白质组。在顶端和相关病变中均检测到来自活性和代谢活性细菌细胞的蛋白质。在根尖和病变中发现了几种与致病性和耐药性/存活率相关的细菌蛋白质,包括与抗生素耐药性、蛋白水解功能、应激反应、黏附和毒力相关的蛋白质。

4.5 微生物生态学与根管生态系统

由于坏死组织中缺乏有效的血液循环,基本上不受宿主免疫的影响,因此含有坏死牙髓组织的根管会为细菌提供一个定殖空间,以及一个潮湿、温暖、营养和厌氧的环境。根管壁是非脱落表皮,有利于持续定植和形成复杂的固着生物膜群落。

直觉上,根管系统可以被认为是细菌生长的一个相当繁茂的环境。因此,有人可能会认为,几乎所有口腔细菌物种都很容易定植。据报道,口腔中存在超过 700 多种不同的细菌,有 100~300 种细菌可构成一个人的口腔微生物群[37, 106]。理论上这些细菌都有同样的机会入侵和定植根管。然而,在感染的根管中仅发现了 10~30 个物种的相对优势。事实上,即使没有宿主防御因子的显著存在,坏死的根管也为细菌适应和定植提供了一个相当有选择性的环境。根管内的环境压力必然有利于某些物种的建立,而抑制其他物种。

4.5.1 生态决定因素

在大多数环境中,影响定殖微生物群建立的生态因素包括:氧张力、氧化还原电位(Eh)、有效营养素、细菌相互作用、宿主防御因素、温度、pH 和细菌黏附受体。

4.5.1.1 氧张力和氧化还原电位

根管感染是一个动态过程,在感染过程的不同阶段,群落中占主导地位的细菌种类不同。在根管感染的早期,定植于根管系统的细菌种类和细胞数量较少。牙髓感染通常是龋齿的后遗症,因此龋齿生物膜最前端的细菌物种常是最先到达牙髓的细菌。除乳酸杆菌外,与牙髓暴露和不可逆牙髓炎相关的晚期龋损中经常检测到的大多数细菌也存在于牙髓感染中[209-210](图 4.9)。早期定植菌或先锋菌为其他物种的进一步定植奠定了基础。

随着时间的推移,可以观察到微生物群组成的变化。主要是由于环境条件的变化,包括氧张力和氧化还原电位。一项针对猴子的研究表明,在牙髓感染过程的最初阶段,兼性细菌占优势[49]。几天或几周后,由于牙髓坏死和兼性细菌的消耗,根管内的氧气耗尽;另外,由于坏死牙髓组织的

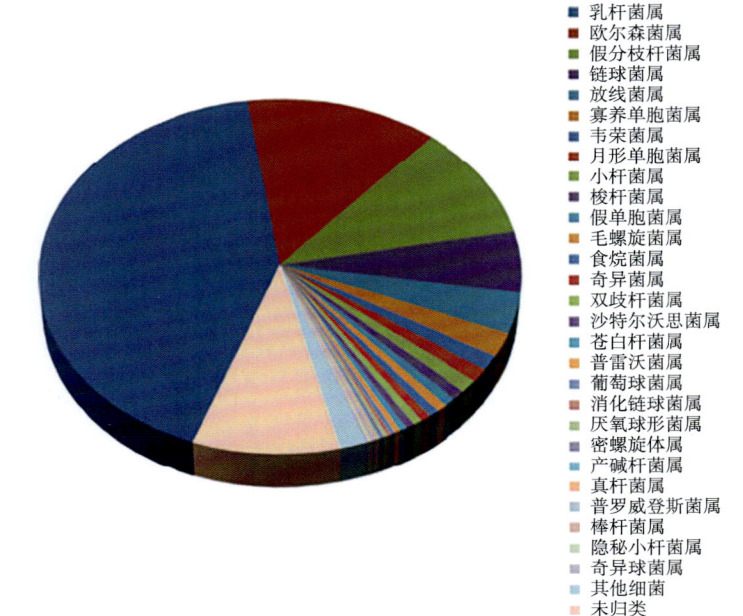

图4.9 有症状的不可逆牙髓炎牙齿深龋病变中细菌属的平均相对丰度。根据Rôas等人的数据总结[210]

血液循环丧失，进一步的氧气供应被中断，形成了一个低氧化还原电位的厌氧环境，这非常有利于专性厌氧细菌的生存和生长。随着时间的推移，厌氧条件变得更加明显，尤其是在根尖段。在患有原发性根尖周炎的牙齿的根尖段，已经发现了几种厌氧细菌[12, 207]。

4.5.1.2 有效营养素

显而易见，根管系统的选择性物理环境能使细菌很好地获得营养，具体取决于特定细菌种群的空间位置和感染阶段。牙髓细菌的绝大多数营养素都来自宿主。然而，某些物种的某些必需营养素并非由宿主提供，而是由感染部位的其他物种提供（见"细菌相互作用"）。由于根管系统可能不富含营养素，因此会存在细菌对可利用量的竞争。口腔细菌的营养需求和获取及清除营养的能力都不同。因此，利用和竞争根管系统中营养素能力最好的细菌将更容易成功定植。

在根管系统中，细菌可以利用以下营养来源：①坏死的牙髓组织，含有坏死牙髓细胞的残余物和牙髓结缔组织的其他变性成分；②通过根尖孔和侧支根管渗入根管系统的组织液和渗出液成分（通常为蛋白质和糖蛋白）；③唾液，可沿冠方渗入根管内；④其他细菌代谢产物。由于大量的营养素存在于根管系统中体积最大的主管腔中，因此预计大多数感染微生物群位于该区域，尤其是严格厌氧菌群。

微生物利用营养物的动力学也会导致根管系统感染微生物群的变化，在感染的早期阶段，糖解物种占主导地位，但很快会被抗糖物种所超过，后者将占主导地位。为了更好地理解，可以在血清营养利用研究的基础上进行类比[295]。在感染过程的初始阶段，血清中可用的少量碳水化合物被糖解细菌迅速消耗。在中间阶段，碳水化合物从糖蛋白中分离出来，其含量被完全消耗。蛋白质被水解，一些氨基酸发生发酵。这表明从糖水解群落向蛋白水解群落的转变。在这一阶段，普氏菌属、卟啉单胞菌属和梭杆菌属的物种占优势。在最后阶段，观察到渐进的蛋白质降解和广泛的氨基酸发酵，此时，细小单胞菌、普雷沃菌、卟啉单胞菌和核梭杆菌占主导地位[295]。

占据根管系统的组织体积较小，故而坏死的牙髓组织是细菌生长的有限基质来源；但根周炎症的发展确保了蛋白质、糖蛋白、降解的胶原蛋白和含铁化合物等营养物质的可持续来源。这些营养物质通过炎性渗出物经由根尖孔和侧支根管的渗出被带入根管。在这一阶段，具有蛋白水解能力的细菌，或者那些与代谢中能够利用这种底物的细菌建立合作关系的细菌开始在群落中占主导作用。当感染过程发展到诱导牙根周围炎症的阶段，蛋白质成为氮和碳的主要来源，根尖处有利于在代谢中利用肽和（或）氨基酸的厌氧物种的建立。因此，未经治疗的坏死牙齿的根管环境为细菌提供了一种营养可用性随时间变化的模式，这将影响微生物群的组成。

4.5.1.3 细菌相互作用

根管微生物群的结构也可以由侵入根管系统的物种之间的生态关系决定。牙髓感染具有生物多样性的特点，因此不同种类的细菌彼此非常接近，并且不可避免地会发生多种相互作用。这些相互作用可以是积极的，也可以是消极的。

正相互作用增强了相互作用物种的生存能力。有时，不同的物种共存于栖息地中，但两者都不能单独存在。多物种群落中的正细菌相互作用包括细菌间营养相互作用（食物链/网，分解复杂基质的协同行动）；当环境改变时共同抵御外部威胁；细胞间的信号传导（群体感应系统）；基因的水平转移。

细菌间营养相互作用主要表现为食物链/食物网。这包括一个物种对另一个物种代谢终产物的利用，形成互惠或共生关系（图4.10）。当两种物种都从这种关系中受益时，例如双向使用代谢物，就会出现两种物种之间的互利共生关系。共生是细菌之间的单向关系，其中一个物种受益，另一个物种不受影响。

一些物种可以改变环境，从而为其他物种提供有利的生长条件。例如，先锋兼性细菌可以通过降低环境中的氧张力，有利于厌氧菌的定植。此外，通过在环境中释放蛋白酶或抗生素失活酶，一些物种可以独自保护整个系统免受宿主防御（如抗体和补体）和抗生素的影响。

负相互作用作为反馈机制，可限制细菌密度。在牙髓环境中可能发生的例子包括竞争和无营养状态。当两个物种争夺相同的资源，并专注于可用的养分和殖民空间时，就会发生竞争。当一个物种产生一种抑制另一个物种的物质（细菌素或代谢终产物）时，就会发生偏害共生（拮抗作用）。拓殖栖息地的先锋物种可能会抑制竞争性后来者的生长定植。避免一种细菌释放抑制因子的最简单方法是找到不被拮抗细菌定植的位点。还有一个方法是通过产生抑制或杀死因子来反击拮抗物种。

4.5.1.4 其他生态决定因素

宿主防御因素。在牙髓感染的初始过程中，入侵的细菌会受到炎症牙髓中宿主免疫防御系统的攻击。只有那些耐受的物种才能成功地在根管定植。当整个牙髓坏死时，由于缺乏活跃的血运循环，根管微生物群在一定程度上受到保护，不受宿主防御系统的攻击。在根尖区，微生物群仍然可能受到特定宿主防御成分的影响，这些成分随炎症渗出物进入根管内。只有能够抵御这些防御机制的菌种才能生存。形成生物膜的能力是细菌的一个重要生存策略。

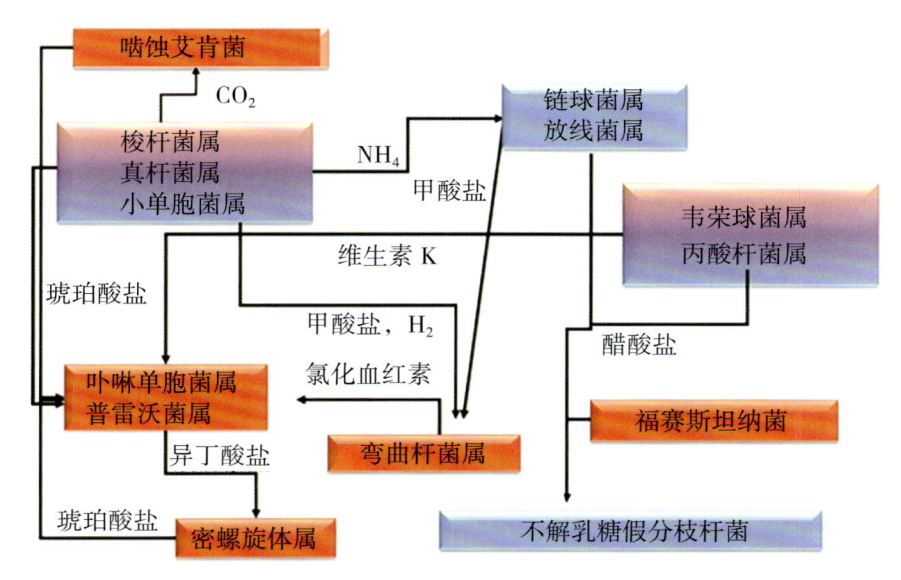

图4.10　牙髓多物种群落中细菌物种之间可能发生的营养关系

温度。根管内的温度可能在35℃~38℃，这几乎有利于所有口腔细菌和许多环境细菌定植。

pH。坏死牙髓中的pH范围为6.4~7.0[299]，但由于一些菌种的蛋白质代谢，pH可能会略有升高。一些假定的牙髓病原体在弱碱性pH下生长更好，在这种条件下酶谱出现显著变化。例如，牙龈卟啉单胞菌中的胰蛋白样酶活性在pH 8.0时最大[128]。细菌对pH耐受性各不相同，大多数物种在pH为6.0~9.0时生长最好[7]。真菌通常表现出略宽的pH范围，在5.0~9.0的范围内生长[7]。

细菌黏附素受体。黏附素是与特定宿主组织识别和黏附以及参与细菌之间细胞与细胞特异性结合的细菌分子，它们通常是菌毛、菌丝、细胞壁和荚膜的化学成分，在细菌黏附到宿主表面形成初始生物膜方面发挥重要作用。细胞与细胞结合也有利于后来者的附着，从而建立复杂的多物种细菌群落。由于黏附素与宿主表面的特定互补受体结合，宿主分子表达的类型将影响黏附和定植于表面的物种。虽然这一因素是定植于牙齿表面形成牙菌斑的细菌种类的重要决定因素，但与根管内生物膜形成有关的细菌黏附素受体类型的相关信息很少。纤溶酶原是一种主要的血浆蛋白，从组织液渗入根管后可以覆盖牙本质壁，同时来自前牙本质和牙本质的I型胶原蛋白可能作为牙髓坏死根管[107,117,139]中细菌黏附的受体。在唾液漏入根管的情况下，可以在管壁上形成由唾液蛋白组成的调节膜，有利于细菌黏附和生物膜的形成[65]。

4.5.2 牙髓生物膜群落生态学

如前所述，在坏死的根管系统中有一个动态的细菌生物膜群落，该群落随着时间的推移逐渐形成物种演替[49,294]。先锋物种会影响根管内细菌演替的模式。随着时间的推移，物种数量逐渐变化和增加，群落变得更加复杂。群落成员可能会被其他物种加入或取代。

牙髓生物膜内细菌种群的空间组织不太可能是随机的。相互依存的物种很可能彼此靠近。

在牙髓感染过程的后期，某些厌氧菌开始控制微生物群。最终，可能会达到一个稳定的局面和高水平的群落组，所有细菌与环境和谐平衡地共存。这意味着群落在成熟度和组织方面达到了顶峰[124, 284]。生物膜联盟中可能存在多种生态位（代谢功能）。因此，生理上不同的物种可以无限期共存，只要它们在功能上兼容。

根管系统内环境条件的差异将影响感染群落的组成和不同生态位的建立。可以想象，牙髓群落中的种群组成由根管系统不同部分的生态决定因素决定。根管系统整个范围内的环境条件可能不同，两端（冠部和根尖部）的差异更为明显。在暴露于口腔环境的根管中可以建立氧气和营养梯度[285]。由于离口腔很近，在牙髓腔的冠方，氧张力高于根管系统其他区域。因此，兼性厌氧菌和耐氧厌氧菌有望在这一领域占主导地位，而顶端（根尖）段的厌氧条件极有利于建立几乎完全由专性厌氧菌控制的微生物群[49]。类似地，位于根管最冠方的细菌可以利用宿主饮食和唾液中通过冠部缺损渗入根管的碳水化合物。根管系统根尖区的细菌利用通过根尖孔和侧支根管渗透到根管中的富含蛋白质和糖蛋白的组织液和渗出液。因此，在根管系统的不同部位，生物膜结构的优势菌群可以根据耐氧性和营养需求进行预测。

4.6 牙髓感染的类型

根管感染可根据其解剖位置（根内或根外感染）和获得性感染细菌进入根管的时机（原发性、继发性或持续性感染）进行分类[245]。不同类型的感染和不同形式的根尖周炎，其微生物群的组成可能有所不同。

4.6.1 根内感染

根内感染是由细菌定植根管系统引起的。它可以分为三类。

4.6.1.1 原发性根内感染

原发性根内感染是由侵入和定植坏死牙髓组织的细菌引起的，也被称为初始感染，是原发性根尖周炎的原因。原发性感染的特点是每个根管内由10~30种细菌[140, 180, 196, 267, 272, 277]组成混合群落。单个感染根管中的细菌细胞数量可能是10^3~10^8 [18, 222, 250, 291, 311]。有窦道和（或）大型根尖周炎病变的牙齿中含有的微生物群的种类（丰富度）和细胞（密度）更为复杂[196, 251, 291]，感染的微生物群大多数由厌氧菌控制，尤其是梭杆菌属、密螺旋体属、坦纳菌属、双歧杆菌属、卟啉单胞菌属、普雷沃菌属和弯曲菌属的革兰氏阴性菌。在原发性根内感染中也常见来自细小单胞菌属、丝状菌属、放线菌属、奥尔森菌属和假分枝杆菌属的革兰氏阳性厌氧菌，以及兼性或微需氧性链球菌。

4.6.1.2 继发性根内感染

继发性根内感染是由原发感染中不存在的微生物引起的，在专业干预期间或之后的某个时间被引入根管系统。在任何情况下，如果渗透性微生物成功存活并定植根管，则会产生继发感染。

治疗期间继发感染的主要来源包括牙菌斑，牙石或牙冠上的龋齿残留物，橡皮障渗漏，牙髓器械污染，冲洗溶液的污染。

在干预期间，微生物也可以进入根管系统。这可能发生在临时修复材料渗漏后，临时修复体损坏、断裂或丢失，牙齿结构断裂，开放引流导致根管系统暴露在口腔环境中。

在放置根管充填物后，微生物仍可以穿透根管系统的情况如下：通过临时或永久性修复材料渗漏，临时/永久修复体破裂、断裂或丢失，牙齿结构断裂，暴露根管充填材料的复发性龋齿，因永久修复延迟而导致临时材料封闭性丧失。

引起继发感染的物种取决于污染源。可能发现非口腔菌种，包括铜绿假单胞菌、葡萄球菌、肠杆菌、念珠菌和粪肠球菌[77, 176–177, 262, 279, 318]。如果继发感染的原因是牙冠渗漏或使根管暴露于唾液的任何其他情况，那么所涉及的物种将来自受试者自己的口腔。

4.6.1.3 持续性根内感染

持续性根内感染是由那些通过某种方式抵抗了体内抗菌程序，并在感染的根管治疗期间耐受营养缺乏的细菌引起的。与持续感染相关的可培养微生物区系通常由比原发感染更少的物种组成，革兰氏阳性兼性细菌[135, 169, 266, 271, 272, 292]是最常见的。与原发感染相比，治疗后患牙中真菌的出现概率明显更高[278]。

持续感染和继发感染在临床中很难区分，并可能导致一些临床问题，包括持续渗出、持续症状、治疗期间恶化和继发根尖周炎（图4.11）。

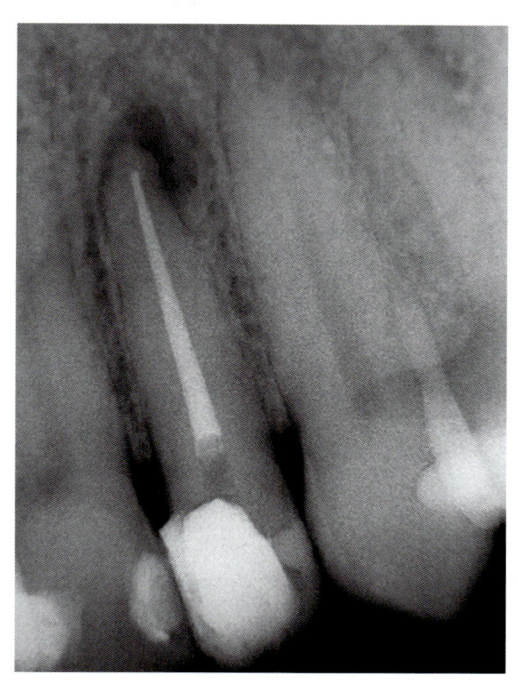

图 4.11 治疗后患有根尖周炎的牙齿持续性或继发性根内感染是这种疾病的主要病原体

4.6.2 根外感染

根外感染的特点是细菌侵入发炎的根周组织。虽然它几乎都是根内感染的后遗症，但已确定的根外感染可能依赖或独立于根内感染。最常见的依赖根内感染的根外感染是急性根尖周脓肿。有人认为，由放线菌或丙酸杆菌引起的根尖放线菌病可能是一种独立于根内感染的根外感染[145]。这种情况占根尖周病变的2%~4%，但其独立性尚未得到证实[257]。从治疗角度来看，关于根外感染是否依赖或独立于根内感染的问题具有特殊的相关性，因为依赖型感染可以通过根管治疗来成功治疗，而独立型感染可能必须通过根周手术来治疗。

4.7 牙髓细菌的鉴定

尽管最终的致病性在很大程度上取决于细菌群落生物膜，但识别与特定传染病相关的菌种对于理解疾病的病因和发病机制以及制定更好的治疗和预防疾病的策略仍然是必要的。根据所使用的不同战略方法及其对知识的贡献，用于鉴定参与牙髓感染的微生物学研究可以按时间顺序分为五代[272, 275]。

·第一代：表现为使用开放式培养方法对牙髓微生物群进行研究，以检测根管中几乎所有可培养物种。这一代的巨大贡献主要为发现许多与根尖周炎密切相关的可培养物种，包括有核梭杆菌、普雷沃菌属、卟啉单胞菌属、微小弧菌和链球菌属。

·第二代：包括采用封闭式（物种或群体特异性）基于DNA的分子微生物学方法的研究，如聚合酶链反应（PCR）和传统棋盘杂交法，主要针对可培养的细菌物种。这些研究的结果通常表明，许多可培养细菌的患病率较高，并有助于加强其与根尖周炎的联系。此外，来自福赛斯坦纳菌属、小杆菌属、产丝菌属和密螺旋体属的一些难以生长的物种也包括在候选牙髓病原体中。

·第三代：涉及基于开放式DNA的分子研究，使用大范围PCR，然后进行克隆和Sanger测序，末端限制性片段长度多态性（T-RFLP）或变性梯度凝胶电泳（DGGE）被用于检测牙髓感染中的可培养物种和尚未培养的系统类型。这些分子方法通常费力、耗时且昂贵，每次研究仅可分析少数样本。然而，第三代方法允许对根尖菌群中可培养和尚未培养/未鉴定的部分进行编目，从而完善了与根尖周炎相关的细菌多样性知识。

·第四代：这些研究使用封闭的分子方法，如物种或群体特异性PCR和反向捕获棋盘法，大规模调查牙髓感染中可培养和未培养细菌的患病率和水平。这一代的研究结果证实了几种可培养细菌与根尖周炎的相关性，并包括在成组候选牙髓病原体中的一些尚未培养的系统型。

·第五代：高通量（通常为"下一代"）测序（HTS）方法已经引入，与传统的Sanger测序方法相比，该方法允许从样本进行DNA测序，覆盖范围更广，通量更高[88,315]。因此，研究了样本中的细菌多样性，以揭示群落中较低丰度的成分。这些方法，特别是高温淬火和Illumina技术已用于牙髓样本的开放式分析，并大大丰富了与根尖周炎相关的细菌多样性的知识。

4.7.1 牙髓感染的分类

目前的证据表明，在牙髓感染中已鉴定出500多种不同的细菌；这些物种属于13个具有口腔代表性的菌属中的9个，即拟杆菌属、厚壁菌属、螺旋体属、梭杆菌属、放线菌属、变形菌属、协同菌属、糖化假丝酵母菌属（前身为TM7）和

常见代表物种/表型

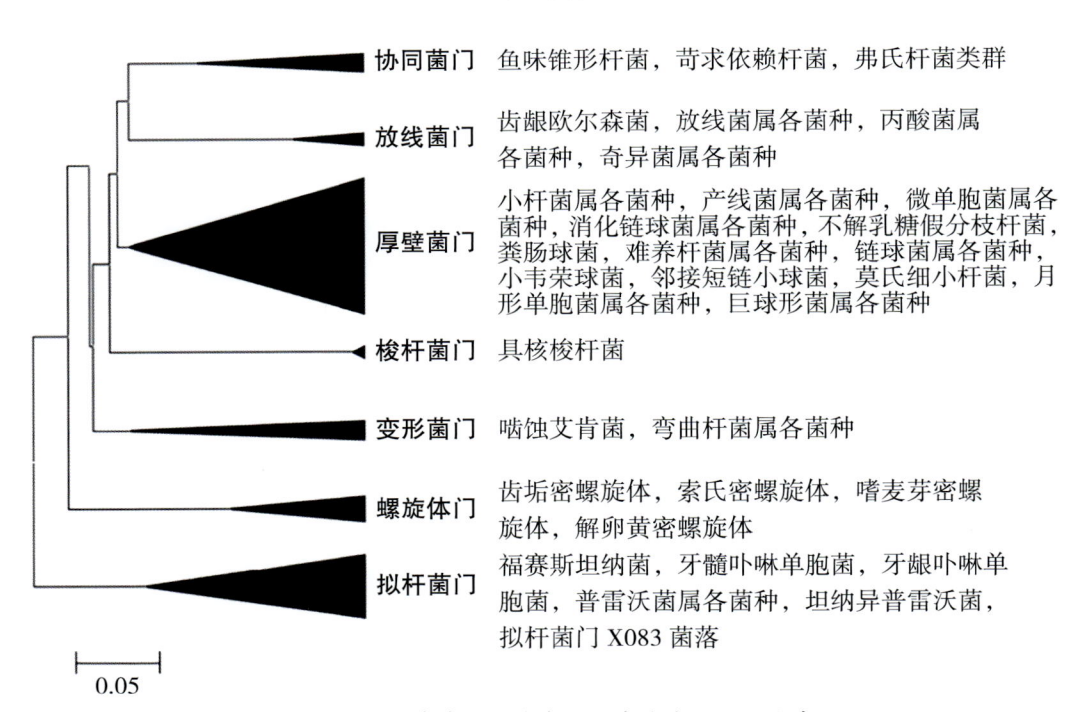

菌门	常见代表物种/表型
协同菌门	鱼味锥形杆菌，苛求依赖杆菌，弗氏杆菌类群
放线菌门	齿龈欧尔森菌，放线菌属各菌种，丙酸菌属各菌种，奇异菌属各菌种
厚壁菌门	小杆菌属各菌种，产线菌属各菌种，微单胞菌属各菌种，消化链球菌属各菌种，不解乳糖假分枝杆菌，粪肠球菌，难养杆菌属各菌种，链球菌属各菌种，小韦荣球菌，邻接短链小球菌，莫氏细小杆菌，月形单胞菌属各菌种，巨球形菌属各菌种
梭杆菌门	具核梭杆菌
变形菌门	啮蚀艾肯菌，弯曲杆菌属各菌种
螺旋体门	齿垢密螺旋体，索氏密螺旋体，嗜麦芽密螺旋体，解卵黄密螺旋体
拟杆菌门	福赛斯坦纳菌，牙髓卟啉单胞菌，牙龈卟啉单胞菌，普雷沃菌属各菌种，坦纳异普雷沃菌，拟杆菌门X083菌落

0.05

图4.12 细菌菌属及其在牙髓感染中的主要代表

SR1[272]（图 4.12）。然而，正如 HTS 方法所揭示的那样，牙髓感染中可能有至少 10 个其他菌属的表达[90, 114, 156, 225, 255, 259, 301, 308, 339]。已被视为候选牙髓致病菌的物种包括来自革兰氏阴性菌的梭杆菌属、卟啉单胞菌属、普雷沃菌属、双歧杆菌属、密螺旋体属、坦纳菌属、锥杆菌属和弯曲菌属，以及来自革兰氏阳性菌的细小单胞菌属、假分枝杆菌属、链球菌属、肠球菌属、奥尔森氏菌属、纤丝因子属、放线菌属和丙酸杆菌属[12, 64, 68, 104, 140, 180, 196, 221, 224, 268, 272, 291]（表 4.2）。

表 4.2 牙髓感染中的细菌属和各自常见的代表物种

菌属	常见菌	原发感染（无症状根尖周炎）	原发感染（急性根尖周脓肿）	持续/继发感染（治疗后根尖周炎）
革兰氏阴性菌				
厌氧棒状菌属				
小杆菌属	D. invisus, D. 肺炎球菌, 未经培养的系统型[a]	+++	+++	+
卟啉单胞菌属	牙髓 P. 牙龈 P.	+++	+++	+
坦纳菌属	T. forsythia	+++	+++	+
普雷沃菌属	P. intermedia, P. nigrescens, P. multissacharivorax, P. baroniae, P. denticola, 未经培养的系统型[a]	+++	+++	+
拟普雷沃菌属	A. tannerae	++	++	−
梭菌属	F. nucleatum, 未经培养的系统型[a]	+++	+++	+
弯曲菌属	C. rectus, C. gracilis, C. showae	++	+	+
弗氏菌属	F. fastidiosum 未经培养的系统型[a]	++	++	−
锥形菌属	P. piscolens	++	++	+
月形单胞菌属	S. sputigena, S. noxia, 未经培养的系统型[a]	++	+	−
厌氧球菌				
韦荣球菌属	V. parvula, 未经培养的系统型[a]	++	+	−
巨球形菌属	未经培养的系统型[a]	+	+	−
厌氧螺旋菌属				
密螺旋体属	T. denticola, T. socranskii, T. parvum, T. maltophilum, T. lecithinolyticum	+++	+++	−

表 4.2（续）

菌属	常见菌	原发感染（无症状根尖周炎）	原发感染（急性根尖周脓肿）	持续/继发感染（治疗后根尖周炎）
兼性棒状菌属				
嗜二氧化碳噬细胞菌	C. gingivalis C. ochracea	+	−	−
艾肯菌属	E. corrodens	++	++	−
革兰氏阳性菌 **厌氧杆菌属**				
放线菌属	A. israelii A. gerencseriae, A. meyeri, A. odontolyticus	++	+	++
假分枝杆菌属	P. alactolyticus	+++	+	++
产丝菌属	F. alocis	++	+	+
消化链球菌属（真杆菌属）	P. infirmum P. saphenum, P. nodatum, P. brachy, P. sulci	+	+	+
艰难杆菌属	M. timidum M. pumilum, M. neglectum, M. vescum	+	+	+
丙酸菌属	P. acnes, P. propionicum	++	+	++
埃氏菌属	E. lenta	+	+	−
欧氏菌属	O. uli, O. profusa	++	+	+
阿托波氏菌属	A. parvulum A. minutum, A. rimae	+	−	+
Solobacterium 菌属	S. moorei 未经培养的系统型 [a]	+	−	+
厌氧球菌				
细小单胞菌属	P. micra	+++	+++	++
消化链球菌属	P. stomatis P. anaerobius, 未经培养的系统型 [a]	+	+	−
厌氧球菌属	A. prevotii	+	−	−
链球菌属	S. anginosus, 星形链球菌，中间链球菌	+++	+++	+++
孪生球菌属	G. morbillorum	+	+	+
兼性棒状菌属				
放线菌属	A. naeslundii	+	−	+

表 4.2（续）

菌属	常见菌	原发感染（无症状根尖周炎）	原发感染（急性根尖周脓肿）	持续/继发感染（治疗后根尖周炎）
兼性球菌属				
链球菌属	S. mitis, S. sanguinis S. gordonii, S. oralis	++	+	+++
肠球菌	粪肠球菌	+	−	+++
颗粒链菌属	G. adiacens	+	−	−

a 表示未培养的系统类型，革兰氏染色模式，细胞形态和与氧的关系是根据该属的一般特征估计的
+++，在大量研究中频繁发现
++，在许多研究中经常发现
+，在许多研究中发现
−，很少发现

4.7.2 尚未培育的系统类型

系统类型是一个术语，用于表示那些仅通过第三代、第四代和第五代分子微生物学方法鉴定的 16S rRNA 基因序列已知的尚未培育物种。第三代牙髓细菌多样性研究表明，40%~60% 的物种级分类群（丰富度）仍有待培养和有效命名[140, 180, 221-222, 313]。就相对丰度而言，尚未培育的系统类型可能代表 30%~40% 的牙髓细菌群落[221]。在牙髓感染中检测到的未经培养的系统类型已被划分为几个已知属，包括小杆菌属、密螺旋体属、普雷沃菌属、索氏菌属、欧氏菌属、梭杆菌属、巨球形菌属、韦荣菌属和月形单胞菌属[140, 195, 212, 219, 221, 224, 248, 268]。在第四代研究中，牙髓感染中最常见的尚未培养的系统类型之一是类杆菌科 HOT-272（类杆菌口腔克隆 X083）[196-197]。在感染的根管中发现了协同菌属的几个成员；其中的大多数仍未培养[195, 208, 268, 270]。然而，最近使用特殊策略对其中一些细菌进行了培养，从而对其进行了表征，并将其正式命名为鱼味锥形杆菌[41] 和苛求依赖杆菌[307]。

4.8 牙髓生物膜群落概况

细菌群落结构由物种丰富度和数量决定。基于 DNA 的分子方法已用于分析与不同类型牙髓感染和根尖周炎相关的生物膜群落。这些研究表明，与原发性根尖周炎[26, 119, 277] 和治疗后根尖周炎[18, 26, 114, 194, 205, 223, 266] 相关的牙髓细菌群落是混合的，由几个不同的物种组成，包括尚未培养的细菌[118, 248]。与不同临床条件相关的牙髓细菌群落会表现不同的特征，包括无症状根尖周炎、急性根尖周脓肿和治疗后根尖周炎[205, 221, 277, 301]。

牙髓感染群落在丰富度和数量方面是各不相同的，因此个体间的变异性很高[26, 114, 151, 225, 277]。即使是同一个体中的两颗受感染的牙齿也显示出不同的菌落组成[2]。这表明根尖周炎具有异质性病因，多物种组合可导致类似的疾病结果。尽管个体间存在差异，但与生活在远距离的个体间相比，生活在同一地理位置的个体间的样本更为相似[64, 119, 205, 252, 277]。这种菌群分布特征中与地域相关的模式，引发了人们对在全球范围内使用的特定抗生素治疗的效果提出质疑。

4.9 根尖根管内的微生物群

根管系统的根尖段是宿主、感染菌群和临床医生的关键区域。由于顶孔是细菌及其毒力因子的主要出口，宿主的防御必须在这些区域附近安装和集中，以防止感染进入骨骼和扩散到其他身体区域。在根尖区根管内中，细菌位

于获取根管周围营养物质和对根管周围组织造成损伤的重要位置。为了根管治疗的成功,临床医生必须控制感染,尤其是该部位的感染,同时创造条件防止再感染。

根管提供了不同的生态条件,即氧分压和可利用的营养物质类型,这有利于建立与根管系统最冠状部分显著不同的微生物群[2, 12, 49, 131, 296]。根尖管细菌计数为 10^4~10^6 个 [12]。

在该区域发现的细菌种类很可能是根尖周炎病因中最重要的细菌种类,它们与受累组织有密切的接触。大多数研究评估了整个根管系统的微生物群,也有少数研究只观察了根尖根管内的细菌种类。这样的研究只能在拔除的牙齿或根尖切除的牙齿中进行。在根尖管段已鉴定出几种候选的牙髓致病菌[12,40,207,247,253],包括普雷沃菌属、卟啉单胞菌属、假枝杆菌属、链球菌属、*Olsenella uli*、*F. nucleatum*、*P.micra*、福赛坦纳菌和密螺旋体属。

分子研究发现,在根尖区和根中/冠部根管样本中平均有 28 个物种;然而,平均共享微生物物种只有 54%,范围为 2%~79%[2]。因此,尽管细菌物种组成相似,根尖区和冠部根管内细菌组成还是存在一定的差异的。在根尖区根管微生物群的组成方面,受试者之间也存在高度的变异性[2, 259]。

有些菌种则常见于根管的根尖部分,包括巴氏普雷沃菌(*Prevotella baroniae*)、连翘菌(*T. forsythia*)和具核梭菌(*F. nucleatum*),而其他菌种(如链球菌属)则更常见于根中部和冠部根管[207]。使用高通量测序(HTS)方法的研究已经证实了根尖部微生物群的复杂性[156,259]。

根尖管内的细菌是导致治疗失败的主要原因。对经过充分治疗的持续性根尖周炎牙的根尖根管系统进行的分子分析揭示了高度复杂的细菌群落[255](图 4.13)。群落组成具有显著的个体间差异。根尖周炎患者冷冻根尖管标本的平均细菌载量约为 10^4 个 [5]。

4.10 症状性感染

4.10.1 症状发展的主要原因

在某些情况下,根管细菌感染可引起急性根尖周炎,包括有症状的根尖周炎和急性根尖周脓肿(图 4.14)。牙髓微生物学研究人员长期以来一直在寻找特定细菌种类与症状性疾病之

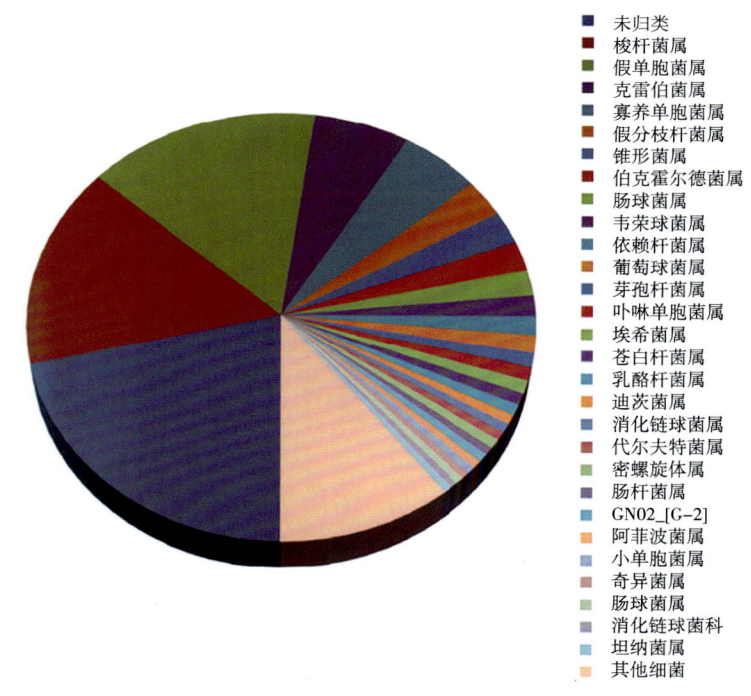

图 4.13 难治性根尖周炎牙齿根尖样本中细菌属的平均相对丰度(根据 Siqueira 等人的数据整理)

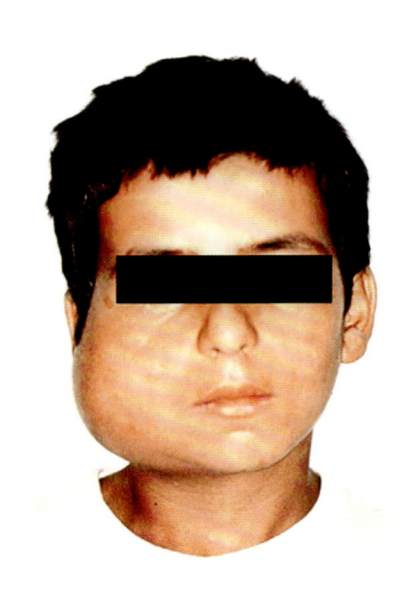

图 4.14 急性根尖周脓肿伴面部肿胀。在这一病例中，根外感染肯定存在

间的联系。虽然有人认为一些革兰氏阴性厌氧菌可能与症状有关[71, 74, 204, 274, 291, 305, 335]，但几项研究发现，在无症状自动病例中，相同物种的患病率相似度低[15, 60, 78, 98, 196, 242, 243]。这表明，除了仅仅存在一个特定的致病物种外，其他因素可以影响症状的发展。实际上，根尖周炎的症状表现的是多种因素相互作用的结果[245, 275]。

4.10.1.1　同一致病菌不同克隆类型的毒力能力差异

同一致病菌不同克隆类型在致毒力能力上存在显著差异[8, 56, 75, 143, 155]。一种属于病原体的疾病实际上是由该物种[143]的特定毒性克隆类型引起的。因此，在根管中存在的候选根管病原体的强毒性克隆型可能是疼痛的一个易感因素。这有助于解释为什么在有症状和无症状的病例中都发现了相同的物种。

4.10.1.2　细胞数量或感染负荷

导致症状性感染发展的其他重要因素是总体和特定的细菌负荷。总细菌负荷是指群落中的细胞总数，而特定负荷与某些致病物种的计数和相对丰度有关。群落中细菌细胞的总数导致了宿主需要应对沉重的传染性生物负担，其特征是毒力因子的大量积累。急性根尖周脓肿的细菌总数，每个样本[104, 112, 325]可有 10^4~10^9 个细胞。某些特定毒性种的水平对群落的致病性也很重要。有症状和无症状感染中，有症状感染的细胞数量的可能性更大。一项分子研究发现连翘在有症状根管感染中的密度明显高于无症状根管感染[227]。另一项分子研究表明，虽然根管内存在目标物种/系统类型，但可能没有症状，而有症状的感染根管中一些类群的数量（卟啉单胞菌、巴氏普雷沃菌、密螺旋体和链球菌）明显高于无症状病例[201]。因此，潜在的毒性病原体大量存在可能会增加整个微生物群落的毒性，并引起症状。

4.10.1.3　细菌相互作用和集体致病性

大多数根管病原体只有在与其他物种相关时才能引起疾病[13, 55, 101, 241, 293, 333]。这是因为在一个群落中，不同的物种之间发生了协同作用。相互作用可能影响毒性，并在症状的病因中发挥作用。研究显示有症状和无症状的感染根管的群落中的优势种不同，有症状的牙齿[220, 221, 225, 277, 337]的物种丰富度明显较高。有症状的感染牙齿多样性的增加预计会影响生物膜的集体致病性，导致社区成员之间不可估量的协同作用。多微生物感染的每一个组成部分，即使是在群落中被认为是无毒和（或）数量较少的物种，都会影响整个生物膜群落[42, 43, 164, 236]的毒力。细菌群落成员之间的交流可以改变某些致病物种的毒力因子的表达，并影响集体致病性[42]。

4.10.1.4　毒力因子表达的环境线索

致病物种在其一生中并不总是表达其毒力因子。环境在诱导毒力基因[10, 57, 105, 329]的开启或关闭中起着重要作用。细菌可以感知环境的变化，并通过有利于适应和生存的基因表达来做出相应的反应。一些根管病原体（如密螺旋体、核梭菌、牙龈卟啉和中间普雷沃菌）已被证明具有受环境影响[61, 102, 103, 336, 343]的基因表达和毒力。这些症状也可能是由有利于细菌毒力基因表达的根管环境条件引起的。

4.10.1.5　宿主抗性和疾病修饰剂

个体应对感染的能力存在显著差异，差异甚至可能贯穿每个个体的一生[132]。那些对感染的抵抗力降低的人可能更容易出现临床症状。此外，疾病修饰因子（如遗传多态性和糖尿病）可能会影响疾病的严重程度，并容易导致症状[4,36,59]。

4.10.1.6 伴随的疱疹病毒感染

疱疹病毒感染可能是一种疾病调节剂，通常与宿主抵抗力减弱有关。人巨细胞病毒（HCMV）和（或）EB病毒（EBV）在与症状相关的根尖周炎病变标本中被检测到[215,217]。其他疱疹病毒，如人类疱疹病毒（HHV）-8、水痘带状疱疹病毒（VZV）和HHV-6也在急性根尖周脓肿样本中被发现[52-53]。然而，仍然需要确定疱疹病毒颗粒是否参与急性感染，或者它们只是细菌诱导的炎症吸引到该区域的旁观者。

4.10.2 症状出现前微生物群的变化

症状性根管感染，包括急性根尖周脓肿可在有或没有根管周围放射透光性的牙齿中发生。在没有放射透光性的牙齿中，初始感染被认为达到显著的毒性，在骨吸收发展之前，感染引起快速发展的急性牙根周围炎症。这是因为骨吸收通常是一个缓慢的慢性过程，与长期的根管感染有关。当脓肿发生在放射学上可见的牙根周围病变的牙齿上时，这表明脓肿是由先前存在的慢性病变加重引起的。在这些情况下，宿主-病原体关系的改变容易恶化。脓肿可能是宿主免疫抵抗的暂时或最终的下降，例如由应激或病毒感染（如流感、感冒、疱疹病毒）引起的；脓肿也可能是由根管微生物群结构变化引起的。

横断面研究表明，有症状牙的牙髓细菌群落的结构（丰富度和相对丰度）与无症状牙的有显著差异[225,277]，在优势种类型、物种总数（丰富度）和细菌负荷等方面存在明显差异。这可能表明，细菌群落结构中的生态重排先于症状的出现。从无症状到有症状状态的生态演替可能与新优势群落成员的出现有关，这可能是由容易导致某些特定成员生长的环境变化引起的，甚至是因为新物种的到来引起的。优势种的类型和负荷的差异以及由此产生的细菌相互作用可能是导致整个生物膜群落致病性程度差异的原因，并引起相应症状。

4.11 持续性/继发性根管感染

鉴于细菌在根尖周炎的病因学中所起的重要作用，根管治疗应集中在消除根管系统定植的细菌和预防再感染。灭菌是治疗的理想目标，但目前可用的技术和现实目标是消毒。因此，细菌必须被消除到与牙根周围组织愈合的[271]相兼容的水平。如果在填充时允许细菌留在根管中，那么不良治疗结果[50,281,317]的风险就会增加。治疗过程中根管污染引起的继发性感染或治疗后冠方渗漏可能是治疗后根尖周炎的原因，但细菌持续感染是治疗失败[271]的最常见原因。值得注意的是，即使抗菌根管治疗不能完全根除根内感染，大量的细菌也会被消除，根管环境也会受到明显的干扰。细菌要想生存，它们需要抵抗或逃脱根管内消毒程序，并迅速适应急剧变化的环境。

大多数根管内细菌对标准治疗程序很敏感。然而，一些细菌可能经受住治疗过程，特别是如果它们位于仪器和抗菌物质无法到达的区域。当治疗低于可接受的标准时，细菌持续存在的风险明显很高。峡部、牙本质小管、牙槽、外侧管和根尖分叉等区域很难用器械和冲洗剂到达，在这些部位的细菌可不受治疗的影响[6, 22, 147, 181, 186, 309, 314]。

治疗后持续存在于根管内的细菌并不总是保持感染并引起治疗后的根尖周炎[50,281]。其可能的原因见表4.3。实际上，残留的细菌导致持续感染并影响治疗结果，需要满足表4.4中所示的某些要求。

几乎所有根尖周炎的牙齿经过根管治疗后都被证明存在根管内感染[115,186,200,266]。这个指数表明残留的细菌可以通过某种方式在填充的根管内获取营养。由于没有任何封闭技术或填充材料可以促进根管系统的可预测的抗菌和完全紧密的冠状、外侧和根尖密封[76]，持续存在的细菌可以从唾液（冠状渗漏到根管中）或根管周围的炎症渗出物（根尖或外侧渗漏到根管中）中获取营养[256]。即使大多数坏死的牙髓组织在化学机械过程中被移除，残留的细菌可以利用一些坏死组织残留物作为营养来源。这些组织残留物可能局限于峡部、牙槽、牙本质小管和外侧管，这些部位通常不受器械和冲洗剂的影响[35, 240, 320, 346]。此外，即使在主根管管腔中，一些牙本质壁在器械治疗后也可能未处理到[240,331]，不同的器械治疗技术使高达50%的根管表面积未处理[123, 158, 166, 254]。

表 4.3 残留细菌不会影响治疗效果的情况

下列情况中残留细菌不会引发难治性根尖周炎

1）放置根管封闭剂后，细菌死亡

2）细菌仍保持一定数量并具有毒性，但在引发根尖周炎的临界值以下

3）细菌存在区域与根尖周组织不相通

表 4.4 残留细菌影响治疗效果的必要条件

残留细菌引发难治性根尖周炎需要以下条件

1）能够耐受寡营养条件，可以利用极少的营养物质并（或）可以将代谢维持在较低水平

2）有可供生存和增殖所需的稳定营养来源

3）能够抵抗治疗对菌群生态环境的影响，如群体感应系统被扰乱、食物网/链断裂和基因交流

4）能够达到引起组织损伤的细菌数量

5）能够通过根尖孔、侧/副根管、医源性穿孔到达根尖周组织，引发损伤

6）能够在受治疗影响的根管环境内分泌毒力因子，并达到致病浓度

如果残余细菌位于根管的最顶端或分叉处，它们可以无限制地获取富含蛋白质和糖蛋白的组织液和渗出物的营养物质。对治疗后根尖周炎的牙齿进行的组织学分析发现[6, 146, 182, 186]：在根尖分叉区域和侧根管区域[181, 186]存在持续感染。与原发感染不同，在根管治疗后的根尖周炎相关的牙齿中发现了一组更有限的菌种。粪肠球菌是根尖周炎患者经过根管治疗后的牙齿样本中最常见的菌种之一[48, 83, 87, 135, 141, 161, 169–170, 203, 206, 232, 266, 292, 326, 344]（图4.15）。使用实时定量 PCR（聚合酶链式反应）分析的第四代研究报告称，在处理过的根管中，该菌种占总细菌负荷的中位数约为1%（范围为0.1%~100%）[200, 232]。

粪肠球菌[17, 48, 203, 244, 342]在原发性感染中并不常见，并且经过根管治疗的牙齿中含有粪肠球菌的可能性大约是未经治疗牙齿的9倍[203]（图4.16）。

在评估治疗的抗菌效果和填充时根管的微生物条件[21, 211, 222, 261, 264–265, 281, 312, 338]的研究中，粪肠状菌很少作为持续存在的细菌被发现。据报道，肠球菌经常发生在多次就诊和（或）牙齿引流的病例[279]。它们也被发现在根管治疗的冠状修复[170]中高流行。因为肠球菌可以是在食物中传播的定植者，并且已经在各种奶酪[63]中被发现，它们在口腔中的出现被认为与食物摄入[178, 340]有关。

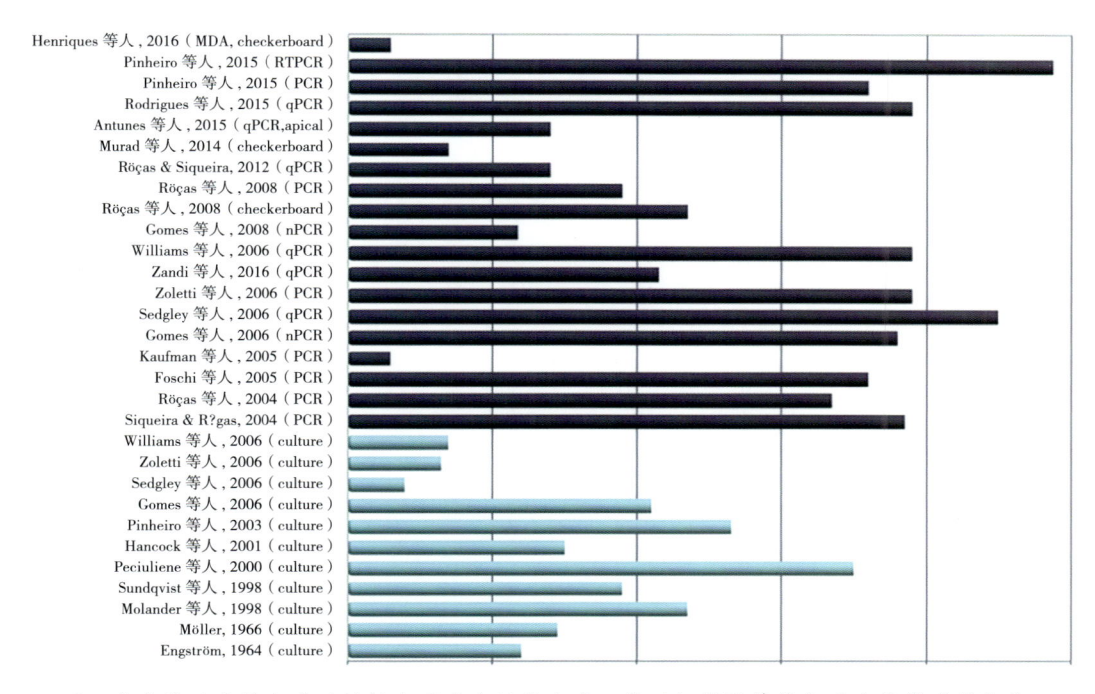

图 4.15 不同研究中粪肠球菌在难治性根尖周炎中的检出率，使用细菌培养或分子生物学手段鉴定。apical：根尖区域。checkerboard：棋盘法。culture：细菌培养。qPCR：定量 PCR。RTPCR：反转录 PCR。MOA：多重置换扩增

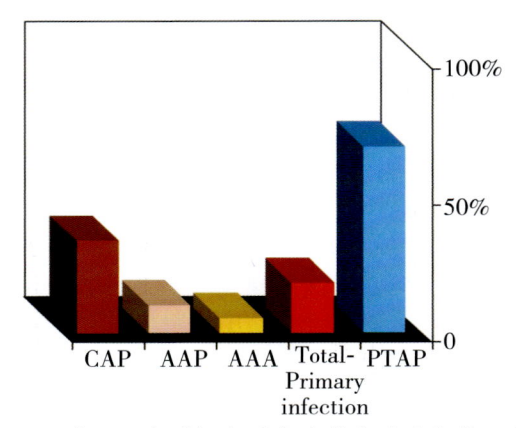

图4.16 伴不同类型根尖周炎的感染牙髓中粪肠球菌的检出率。CAP：慢性根尖周炎。AAP：急性根尖周炎。AAA：急性根尖周脓肿。PTAP：难治性根尖周炎。Total-Primarg infection：原发感染（数据来自 Rôças 等人的研究[203]）

根据许多横断面研究，如图4.15所示，粪肠球菌被认为可能是治疗后根尖周炎的主要病原体。然而，最近它的地位受到以下研究结果的质疑：①在评估根管治疗后疾病的牙齿微生物群的所有研究中均未检测到粪肠球菌[25, 212]。②当存在时，粪肠球菌在群落中很少是最优势种[87, 194, 205, 223, 255]。③粪肠球菌在有或没有根尖周炎病变的根管治疗过的牙齿中有相似的患病率[100, 344]。

链球菌属也常常见于根尖周炎治疗后的根管内[5, 23, 169, 206, 266]。正如第四代和第五代研究所示[5, 200, 338, 339]：链球菌在经过治疗的根管中的检出率和相对丰度甚至可能高于粪肠球菌。在患有治疗后疾病的牙齿中发现的其他细菌包括苛养厌氧菌，如非解乳糖卟啉单胞菌、丙酸杆菌属、牙龈纤毛菌、小杆菌属、梭杆菌属、微小消化链球菌、消化链球菌以及普雷沃菌属[2, 135, 194, 200, 205, 223, 266, 268, 339]。

在治疗后的根尖牙炎的牙齿中也发现了未培养的细菌。就丰富度和相对丰度而言，未培养的细菌类群均占细菌群落的一半[223]。一些未培养的系统类型，如拟杆菌科 HOT-272（拟杆菌门口腔克隆 X083）是在治疗过的根管中发现的最常见的未培养类群之一。尚未培养出来的细菌可能是细菌群落中的优势成员，这一事实有助于解释为什么一些培养研究未能在经过治疗的根管中检测到细菌。

与原发性感染一样，根管治疗后患牙根管内的细菌群落特征因个体而异，这表明在根管治疗后的患牙感染中起作用的是不同的细菌组合[205, 223, 255]。与治疗失败相关的感染的特征是菌群混杂，但其多样性不如原发性感染。

据报道，铜绿假单胞菌、肠杆菌和葡萄球菌的继发感染会导致牙髓治疗周期延长[77, 177, 262]。这些细菌很可能是因为治疗期间无菌环境被破坏而进入根管的。

4.12　根管外感染

根尖周炎是一种炎症性疾病，是由根管内细菌感染而发展的，通常也是防止感染扩散到牙槽骨和其他身体部位的有效屏障（将感染局限在根尖周区域）。然而，细菌有时可能会突破这种防御屏障并引起根管外感染。与根尖周脓肿不同，还有其他形式的根管外感染，其特征可能是轻度甚至无症状的。这种感染被认为是根管治疗后根尖周炎的可能原因。通过形成黏附在根管外表面的生物膜[152, 189, 190, 298]，或者通过在炎性病变体内定植的黏性放线菌菌落[85]。

根管外感染可能有以下途径。

1）根管外感染可能是根管内感染过程的延伸，由直接侵入根周组织并克服局部宿主防御的细菌引起。在牙髓感染病例中发现的大多数口腔细菌是机会致病菌，缺乏使其能够侵入根周组织、破坏宿主防御、并在严酷的炎症环境中存活的毒力因子。然而，一些候选口腔致病菌，如密螺旋体、牙髓卟啉单胞菌、牙龈卟啉单胞菌、连翘曲霉、普雷沃菌和具合梭杆菌已被证明具有这种毒力因子[19, 51, 89, 95, 306, 341]。

2）细菌可能通过穿透"湾"状囊肿的空腔而到达根尖周组织，该囊肿与根尖孔直接连通（图4.17）。

3）急性根尖周脓肿缓解后，细菌可能会持续存在于根外间隙。然后，这些持续存在的感染源将导致介于与慢性炎症相关的可引流的窦道及慢性根尖周脓肿之间的根外感染。

4）在化学机械预备过程中感染的碎屑被挤出根尖孔是细菌可能到达根尖周组织的另一种方式。一旦进入其中，嵌入其中的细菌可以受到宿主防御机制的物理保护，并持续存在于发炎的组织中。

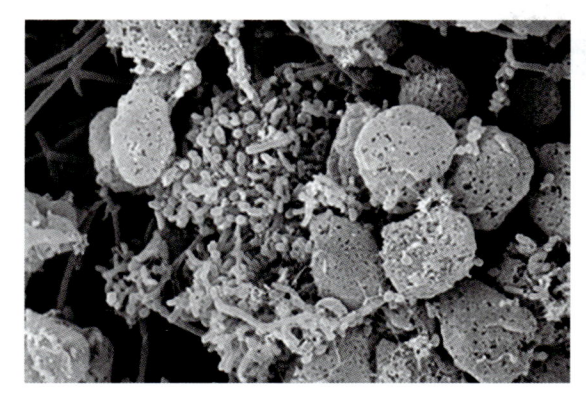

图 4.17 袋状囊肿囊腔内吞噬细胞攻击大型菌落（原始放大 3300 倍，由 Siqueira 拍摄）

5）位于根管系统根尖部的细菌菌落或生物膜可能在根尖段再吸收后暴露在根外。

6）根管内生物膜中的细菌可能通过根表面牙骨质被吸收区域的牙本质小管到达根尖外表面，然后形成根管外生物膜。

据推测，根管外感染可能依赖或独立于根管内感染[257]。依赖性感染是由根管内细菌群落引起的。因此，如果临床医生能成功控制根管内感染，宿主就可以控制根管外感染。独立的根管外感染反过来不受根内感染的影响，因此非手术牙髓治疗无效。由放线菌属和丙酸丙酸杆菌引起的根尖放线菌病被认为是另一种独立的根管外感染（图 4.18）[85, 280]。然而，它是否能作为一种自我维持的病理实体成为治疗失败的唯一原因，仍有待通过使用现代检测方法和评估根尖根管系统细菌学状况的研究来证明。

目前已发现大约 6% 的根尖周炎牙齿中存在根管外生物膜[183]（图 4.19）。在大多数情况下，根管外生物膜与根管内生物膜相关，提示依赖性感染[183, 288]。然而，根管外生物膜可能偶尔独立于根管内感染并导致治疗失败。根管外生物膜实际上总是与未经治疗的患牙症状有关，并且可能是已接受根管治疗的牙齿症状持续或炎性渗出的原因。

一项评估慢性根尖周脓肿和窦道患牙感染分布的组织细菌学研究显示，83% 的病例出现了根管外细菌感染。在 71% 的检测患牙中，细菌正在形成黏附于根管外表面的生物膜。这些结构中的大多数都显示出一定程度的矿化现象，这表明有牙结石的形成[191]。

除了有窦道的病例外，无症状的慢性根尖周炎病变是否可以在最初的组织侵袭之后长期残留细菌，或者不受伴随的根管感染的影响仍然存在争议[111, 82]。有研究指出根管治疗后病变中厌氧菌混合感染在根管外发生[62, 84, 214, 237, 288–290, 300, 323, 337]。与根尖放线菌病一样，除了讨论在根尖周炎的手术取样过程中是否能有效预防污染外，没有证据表明这些根管外感染病例与根管内感染无关。

未经治疗的无症状根尖周炎患牙的根管外感染率较低[148, 183, 263]，这与非手术牙髓治疗的高成

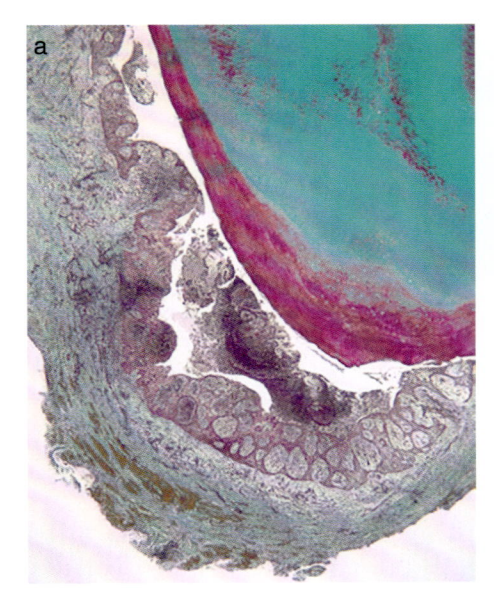

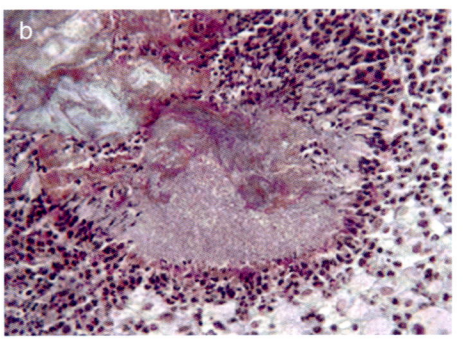

图 4.18 根尖周放线菌病。a. 上皮化根尖周炎病变内的细菌聚合物，提示放线菌病（Masson 三色染色法，放大 25 倍）。b. 高倍数下观察放线菌聚合物，可见其被炎症细胞包围（400 倍）（感谢 Domenico Ricucci 医生供图）

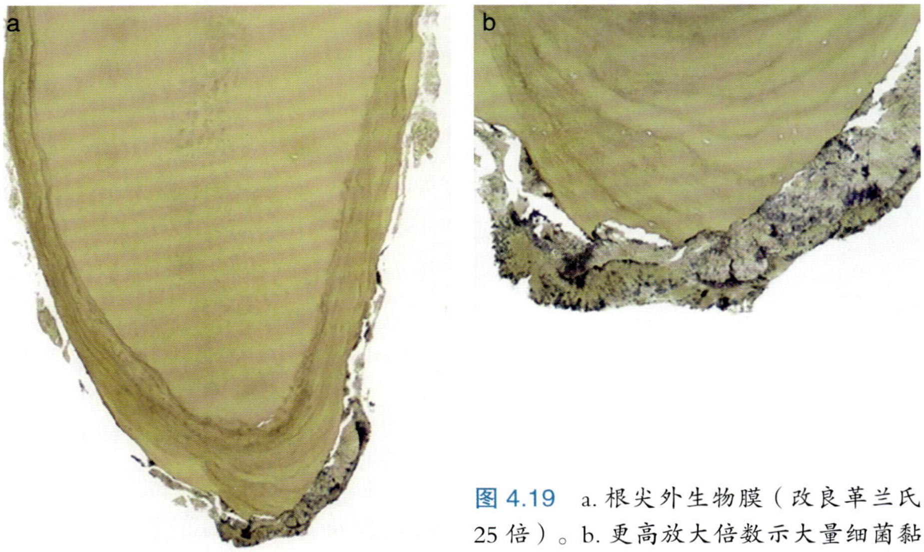

图 4.19 a. 根尖外生物膜（改良革兰氏染色，放大 25 倍）。b. 更高放大倍数示大量细菌黏附于牙骨质（100 倍）（感谢 Domenico Ricucci 医生供图）

功率相一致[33, 188]。在已行根管治疗的病例中，根管外细菌被认为是失败的可能原因，组织细菌学研究显示没有病例提示独立的根管外感染[186]。实际上，据报道只有少数治疗后根尖周炎病例可能是由与根管系统感染无关的根管外感染引起的[189, 192]。此外，再治疗后根尖周炎的高愈合率[34, 188]也表明根管治疗后疾病的主要原因位于根管内，可通过非手术治疗方式治疗。微生物学研究证实，几乎所有根管治疗后根尖周炎的患牙都与根内细菌感染有关[115, 186, 200, 205, 266]。

4.13 牙髓感染中的其他微生物

细菌是牙髓感染中发现的主要微生物。然而，也发现有其他微生物零星存在，包括真菌、古菌和病毒。

4.13.1 真菌

真菌是以两种基本形式出现的真核微生物：霉菌（由分支的圆柱形小管组成的多细胞丝状真菌）和酵母（具有球形或椭圆形细胞的单细胞真菌）。真菌偶尔在原发性根管感染中被发现。然而，一些研究已经在约 20% 的原发性根管感染样本中检测到念珠菌[14, 133]。研究之间存在差异的原因尚不明确，但可能包括所用鉴定方法和患者一般健康状况的差异。

在评估根管治疗患牙微生物状况的研究中，真菌被更频繁地检测到。持续性/继发性感染中念珠菌的检测频率[25, 47, 135-136, 162, 169, 194, 266, 292]为 3%~18%。真菌可以通过牙髓治疗过程中的污染进入根管，或者在导致微生物群失衡的无效根管内抗菌治疗后过度繁殖。到目前为止，白念珠菌是根管治疗后患牙中最常见的真菌种类。该物种由于其定植和侵入牙本质的能力而被认为是嗜牙本质微生物[234-235, 246]（图 4.20）。除了入侵能力外，白念珠菌也被证明对一些根管内封药（如氢氧化钙）[319]具有抗性。真菌是否参与根尖周炎的发病机制仍有待澄清。

4.13.2 古细菌

古细菌与细菌和真核生物一起代表了生命的三个主要进化领域之一。该结构域包含与细菌

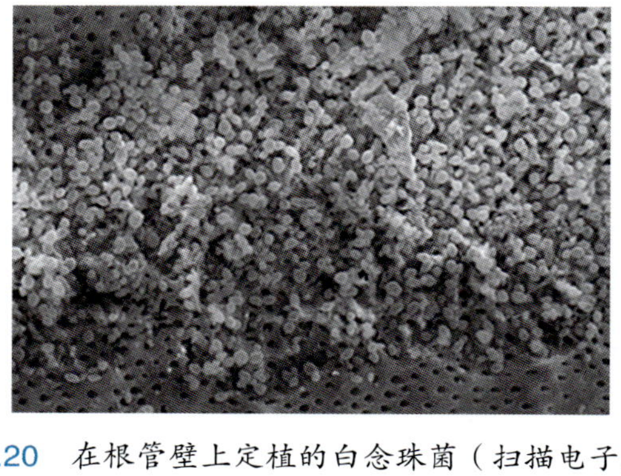

图 4.20 在根管壁上定植的白念珠菌（扫描电子显微镜，原始放大倍数 600 倍）

不同的高度多样化的原核生物群。迄今为止，古细菌结构域的任何成员都没有被描述为人类病原体。在与牙周病相关的龈下菌斑样本中检测到产甲烷古细菌。虽然许多研究未能在原发性牙髓感染中检测到古细菌[198, 199, 249]，但其他研究发现产甲烷古细菌的患病率较低[156-157, 313]，一个值得注意的例外是一项研究在25%的原发感染根管中检测到古细菌[310]。在该研究中，古细菌的多样性仅限于口腔甲烷短杆菌类群，古菌种群的相对丰度[310]占原核群落（即细菌加古菌）总数的2.5%。鉴于大多数研究报道古细菌总体患病率较低，古细菌不太可能在根尖周炎中发挥重要的致病作用。

4.13.3 病毒

病毒不是细胞，而是由核酸分子（DNA或RNA）和蛋白质外壳结构组成的颗粒。它们在细胞外环境中是惰性的；作为专性细胞内寄生生物，病毒完全依赖活细胞来执行生命功能。当它们感染活细胞时，病毒核酸分子介导完整病毒的复制，并控制宿主细胞的代谢活动。因为病毒需要活的宿主细胞来感染并利用细胞成分复制病毒基因组，所以它们不能在含有坏死牙髓组织的根管内繁殖。据报道，病毒仅在牙髓有活力的根管中发生。例如，在HIV血清阳性患者的感染牙髓中检测到人类免疫缺陷病毒（HIV）[67]，并且在非感染和重度感染的牙髓中都发现过一些疱疹病毒[113]。在根尖周炎病变处检测到了不同的疱疹病毒，因为那里存在大量的活细胞[52, 53, 215-217]。

有人提出，疱疹病毒，特别是人巨细胞病毒和EBV可能与根尖周炎的发病机制有关。这可能是病毒感染和复制的直接结果，也可能是病毒诱导的局部宿主防御受损，从而导致根尖段病原菌过度繁殖。已经有研究者提出了疱疹病毒参与根尖周炎发病机制的假说[282]。根管内细菌感染会导致被疱疹病毒感染的细胞进入根尖周组织。细菌引起的组织损伤使这些疱疹病毒被重新激活，可能会导致根尖周微环境中宿主免疫防御的局部损伤，从而影响对感染的反应。此外，疱疹病毒感染的炎症细胞被刺激，从而释放促炎细胞因子并导致炎症增重[134, 282, 322]。

在有症状的根尖周炎病变[215, 217]、急性根尖周脓肿[24, 52]、根尖周大面积病损[216-217]和HIV阳性患者病变[218]的样本中均已检出疱疹病毒。然而，单纯在根尖周炎样本中发现疱疹病毒并不一定意味着其在疾病原因中发挥作用。感染炎性细胞的疱疹病毒可能在人体内长期存在。由于这些病毒感染的炎性细胞被吸引并积聚在发炎的牙根周围神经组织中，因此这些病毒也能被检测到。如果在病变样品中检测到高病毒滴度和（或）病毒RNA转录物或蛋白质，或者在抗病毒治疗后临床状况得以改善且病变愈合，则可以推断疱疹病毒参与疾病病因。在相关文献报道之前，疱疹病毒在根尖周炎发病机制中的作用仍然未知。

参考文献

[1] Abusleme L, et al. The subgingival microbiome in health and periodontitis and its relationship with community biomass and inflammation. ISME J, 2013, 7: 1016–1025.

[2] Alves F R, et al. Bacterial community profiling of cryogenically ground samples from the apical and coronal root segments of teeth with apical periodontitis. J Endod, 2009, 35: 486–492.

[3] Amann R I, Ludwig W, Schleifer K H. Phylogenetic identification and in situ detection of individual microbial cells without cultivation. Microbiol Rev, 1995, 59: 143–169.

[4] Amaya M P, et al. Polymorphisms of pro-inflammatory cytokine genes and the risk for acute suppurative or chronic nonsuppurative apical periodontitis in a Colombian population. Int Endod J, 2013, 46: 71–78.

[5] Antunes H S, et al. Total and specific bacterial levels in the apical root canal system of teeth with post-treatment apical periodontitis. J Endod, 2015, 41: 1037–1042.

[6] Arnold M, Ricucci D, Siqueira J F Jr. Infection in a complex network of apical ramifications as the cause of0 persistent apical periodontitis: a case report. J Endod, 2013, 39: 1179–1184.

[7] Atlas R M. Principles of Microbiology. 2nd. Dubuque I A: W C B Publishers, 1997.

[8] Baker P J, et al. Heterogeneity of Porphyromonas gingivalis strains in the induction of alveolar bone loss in mice. Oral Microbiol Immunol, 2000, 15: 27–32.

[9] Barbosa-Ribeiro M, et al. Quantification of lipoteichoic acid contents and cultivable bacteria at the different phases of the endodontic retreatment. J Endod, 2016, 42: 552–556.

[10] Bassler B L. How bacteria talk to each other: regulation of gene expression by quorum sensing. Curr Opin Microbiol, 1999, 2: 582–587.

[11] Baumgartner J C. Microbiologic aspects of endodontic

[12] Baumgartner J C, Falkler W A Jr. Bacteria in the apical 5 mm of infected root canals. J Endod, 1991, 17: 380–383.

[13] Baumgartner J C, Falkler W A Jr, Beckerman T. Experimentally induced infection by oral anaerobic microorganisms in a mouse model. Oral Microbiol Immunol, 1992, 7: 253–256.

[14] Baumgartner J C, Watts C M, Xia T. Occurrence of Candida albicans in nfections of endodontic origin. J Endod, 2000, 26: 695–698.

[15] Baumgartner J C, et al. Association of black-pigmented bacteria with endodontic infections. J Endod, 1999, 25: 413–415.

[16] Beloin C, et al. Global impact of mature biofilm lifestyle on Escherichia coli K-12 gene expression. Mol Microbiol, 2004, 51: 659–674.

[17] Bergenholtz G. Micro-organisms from necrotic pulp of traumatized teeth. Odontol Revy, 1974, 25: 347–358.

[18] Blome B, et al. Molecular identification and quantification of bacteria from endodontic infections using real-time polymerase chain reaction. Oral Microbiol Immunol, 2008, 23: 384–390.

[19] Bolstad A I, Jensen H, Bakken V. Taxonomy, biology, and periodontal aspects of Fusobacterium nucleatum. Clin Microbiol Rev, 1996, 9: 55–71.

[20] Burmolle M, et al. Interactions in multispecies biofilms: do they actually matter? Trends Microbiol, 2014, 22: 84–91.

[21] Bystrm A, Sundqvist G. The antibacterial action of sodium hypochlorite and EDTA in 60 cases of endodontic therapy. Int Endod J, 1985, 18: 35–40.

[22] Carr G B, et al. Ultrastructural examination of failed molar retreatment with secondary apical periodontitis: an examination of endodontic biofilms in an endodontic retreatment failure. J Endod, 2009, 35: 1303–1309.

[23] Chavez de Paz L, et al. Streptococci from root canals in teeth with apical periodontitis receiving endodontic treatment. Oral Surg Oral Med Oral Pathol Oral Radiol Endod, 2005, 100: 232–241.

[24] Chen V, et al. Herpesviruses in abscesses and cellulitis of endodontic origin. J Endod, 2009, 35: 182–188.

[25] Cheung G S, Ho M W. Microbial flora of root canal-treated teeth associated with asymptomatic periapical radiolucent lesions. Oral Microbiol Immunol, 2001, 16: 332–337.

[26] Chugal N, et al. Molecular characterization of the microbial flora residing at the apical portion of infected root canals of human teeth. J Endod, 2011, 37: 1359–1364.

[27] Costerton B. Microbial ecology comes of age and joins the general ecology community. Proc Natl Acad Sci U S A, 2004, 101: 16983–16984.

[28] Costerton J W. The Biofilm Primer Berlin. Heidelberg: Springer-Verlag, 2007.

[29] Costerton J W, Stewart P S, Greenberg E P. Bacterial biofilms: a common cause of persistent infections. Science, 1999, 284: 1318–1322.

[30] Costerton J W, et al. New methods for the detection of orthopedic and other biofilm infections. FEMS Immunol Med Microbiol, 2011, 61: 133–140.

[31] Dahlén G, Bergenholtz G. Endotoxic activity in teeth with necrotic pulps. J Dent Res, 1980, 59: 1033–1040.

[32] Dahlén G, Magnusson B C, Möller A. Histological and histochemical study of the influence of lipopolysaccharide extracted from Fusobacterium nucleatum on the periapical tissues in the monkey Macaca fascicularis. Arch Oral Biol, 1981, 26: 591–598.

[33] de Chevigny C, et al. Treatment outcome in endodontics: the Toronto study-phase 4: initial treatment. J Endod, 2008, 34: 258–263.

[34] de Chevigny C, et al. Treatment outcome in endodontics: the Toronto study-phases 3 and 4: orthograde retreatment. J Endod, 2008, 34: 131–137.

[35] De-Deus G, Garcia-Filho P. Influence of the NiTi rotary system on the debridement quality of the root canal space. Oral Surg Oral Med Oral Pathol Oral Radiol Endod, 2009, 108: e71–76.

[36] de Sá A R, et al. Association of CD14, IL1B, IL6, IL10 and TNFA functional gene polymorphisms with symptomatic dental abscesses. Int Endod J, 2007, 40: 563–572.

[37] Dewhirst F E, et al. The human oral microbiome. J Bacteriol, 2010, 192: 5002–5017.

[38] Dobell C. Antony van Leeuwenhoek and his "Little Animals". London: Staples Press Limited, 1932.

[39] Donlan R M, Costerton J W. Biofilms: survival mechanisms of clinically relevant microorganisms. Clin Microbiol Rev, 2002, 15: 167–193.

[40] Dougherty W J, Bae K S, Watkins B J, et al. Blackpigmented bacteria in coronal and apical segments of infected root canals. J Endod, 1998, 24: 356–358.

[41] Downes J, et al. Pyramidobacter piscolens gen. nov, sp. nov, a member of the phylum "Synergistetes" isolated from the human oral cavity. Int J Syst Evol Microbiol, 2009, 59: 972–980.

[42] Duan K, et al. Modulation of Pseudomonas aeruginosa gene expression by host microflora through interspecies communication. Mol Microbiol, 2003, 50: 1477–1491.

[43] Duan K, et al. Chemical interactions between organisms in microbial communities. Contrib Microbiol, 2009, 16: 1–17.

[44] Dunny G M, Leonard B A. Cell-cell communication in Gram-positive bacteria. Annu Rev Microbiol, 1997, 51: 527–564.

[45] Duran-Pinedo A E, et al. Community-wide transcriptome of the oral microbiome in subjects with and without periodontitis. ISME J, 2014, 8: 1659–1672.

[46] Eftimiadi C, et al. Divergent effect of the anaerobic

bacteria by-product butyric acid on the immune response: suppression of T-lymphocyte proliferation and stimulation of interleukin-1 beta production. Oral Microbiol Immunol, 1991, 6: 17–23.

[47] Egan M W, et al. Prevalence of yeasts in saliva and root canals of teeth associated with apical periodontitis. Int Endod J, 2002, 35: 321–329.

[48] Engström B. The significance of enterococci in root canal treatment. Odontol Revy, 1964, 15: 87–106.

[49] Fabricius L, et al. Predominant indigenous oral bacteria isolated from infected root canals after varied times of closure. Scand J Dent Res, 1982, 90: 134–144.

[50] Fabricius L, et al. Influence of residual bacteria on periapical tissue healing after chemomechanical treatment and root filling of experimentally infected mo-nkey teeth. Eur J Oral Sci, 2006, 114: 278–285.

[51] Fenno J C, McBride B C. Virulence factors of oral treponemes. Anaerobe, 1998, 4: 1–17.

[52] Ferreira D C, et al. Identification of herpesviruses types 1 to 8 and human papillomavirus in acute apical abscesses. J Endod, 2011, 37: 10–16.

[53] Ferreira D C, et al. Viral-bacterial associations in acute apical abscesses. Oral Surg Oral Med Oral Pathol Oral Radiol Endod, 2011, 112: 264–271.

[54] Ferreira F B, et al. Resolution of persistent periapical infection by endodontic surgery. Int Endod J, 2004, 37: 61–69.

[55] Feuille F, et al. Mixed infection with Porphyromonas gingivalis and Fusobacterium nucleatum in a murine lesion model: potential synergistic effects on virulence. Infect Immun, 1996, 64: 2095–2100.

[56] Finlay B B, Falkow S. Common themes in microbial pathogenicity. Microbiol Rev, 1989, 53: 210–230.

[57] Finlay B B, Falkow S. Common themes in microbial pathogenicity revisited. Microbiol Mol Biol Rev, 1997, 61: 136–169.

[58] Flemming H C, Wingender J. The biofilm matrix. Nat Rev Microbiol, 2010, 8: 623–633.

[59] Fouad A F. Diabetes mellitus as a modulating factor of endodontic infections. J Dent Educ, 2003, 67: 459–467.

[60] Fouad A F, et al. PCR-based identification of bacteria associated with endodontic infections. J Clin Microbiol, 2002, 40: 3223–3231.

[61] Frias J, Olle E, Alsina M. Periodontal pathogens produce quorum sensing signal molecules. Infect Immun, 2001, 69: 3431–3434.

[62] Gatti J J, et al. Bacteria of asymptomatic periradicular endodontic lesions identified by DNA-DNA hybridization. Endod Dent Traumatol, 2000, 16: 197–204.

[63] Gelsomino R, et al. Source of enterococci in a farmhouse raw-milk cheese. Appl Environ Microbiol, 2002, 68: 3560–3565.

[64] George N, et al. Oral microbiota species in acute apical endodontic abscesses. J Oral Microbiol, 2016, 8: 30989.

[65] George S, Kishen A. Effect of tissue fluids on hydrophobicity and adherence of enterococcus faecalis to dentin. J Endod, 2007, 33: 1421–1425.

[66] Ginsburg I. Role of lipoteichoic acid in infection and inflammation. Lancet Infect Dis, 2002, 2: 171–179.

[67] Glick M, et al. Human immunodeficiency virus infection of fibroblasts of dental pulp in seropositive patients. Oral Surg Oral Med Oral Pathol, 1991, 71: 733–736.

[68] Gomes B P, Drucker D B, Lilley J D. Associations of specific bacteria with some endodontic signs and symptoms. Int Endod J, 1994, 27: 291–298.

[69] Gomes B P, Endo M S, Martinho F C. Comparison of endotoxin levels found in primary and secondary endodontic infections. J Endod, 2012, 38: 1082–1086.

[70] Gomes B P, Lilley J D, Drucker D B. Associations of endodontic symptoms and signs with particular combinations of specific bacteria. Int Endod J, 1996, 29: 69–75.

[71] Gomes B P, Lilley J D, Drucker D B. Clinical significance of dental root canal microflora. J Dent, 1996, 24: 47–55.

[72] Gomes B P, et al. Microbial analysis of canals of root-filled teeth with periapical lesions using polymerase chain reaction. J Endod, 2008, 34: 537–540.

[73] Grenier D, Mayrand D. Cytotoxic effects of culture supernatants of oral bacteria and variou ative gram-negative enteric rods in persistent periapical infections. Acta Odontol Scand, 1983, 41: 19–22.

[78] Haapasalo M, et al. Black-pigmented Bacteroides spp. in human apical periodontitis. Infect Immun, 1986, 53: 149–153.

[79] Haapasalo M, et al. Eradication of endodontic infection by instrumentation and irrigation solutions. Endod Topics, 2005, 10: 77–102.

[80] Hajishengallis G. The inflammophilic character of the periodontitis-associated microbiota. Mol Oral Microbiol, 2014, 29: 248–257.

[81] Hajishengallis G. Periodontitis: from microbial immune subversion to systemic inflammation. Nat Rev Immunol, 2015, 15: 30–44.

[82] Hall-Stoodley L, Stoodley P. Evolving concepts in biofilm infections. Cell Microbiol, 2009, 11: 1034–1043.

[83] Hancock H H, et al. Bacteria isolated after unsuccessful endodontic treatment in a North American population. Oral Surg Oral Med Oral Pathol Oral Radiol Endod, 2001, 91: 579–586.

[84] Handal T, et al. Bacterial diversity in persistent periapical lesions on root-filled teeth. Journal of Oral Microbiology, 2009, 1: 1–7.

[85] Happonen R P. Periapical actinomycosis: a follow-up study of 16 surgically treated cases. Endod Dent Traumatol, 1986, 2: 205–209.

[86] Henderson B, Poole S, Wilson M. Bacterial modulins: a novel class of virulence factors which cause host tissue pathology by inducing cytokine synthesis. Microbiol Rev, 1996, 60: 316–341.

[87] Henriques L C, et al. Microbial Ecosystem Analysis in Root Canal Infections Refractory to Endodontic Treatment. J Endod, 2016, 42: 1239–1245.

[88] Higuchi R, Gyllensten U, Persing D H. Next-generation DNA sequencing and microbiology// Persing D H, et al. Molecular Microbiology. Diagnostic, Principles and Practice. Washington DC: ASM Press, 2011: 301–312.

[89] Holt S C, Ebersole J L. Porphyromonas gingivalis, Treponema denticola and Tannerella forsythia: the "red complex", a prototype polybacterial pathogenic consortium in periodontitis. Periodontol, 2005, 2000 (38): 72–122.

[90] Hong B Y, et al. Microbial analysis in primary and persistent endodontic infections by using pyrosequencing. J Endod, 2013, 39: 1136–1140.

[91] Horiba N, et al, 1991, Correlations between endotoxin and clinical symptoms or radiolucent areas in infected root canals. Oral Surg Oral Med Oral Pathol 71: 492–495.

[92] Jacinto R C, et al, 2005, Quantification of endotoxins in necrotic root canals from symptomatic and asymptomatic teeth. J Med Microbiol 54: 777–783.

[93] Jenkinson H F, Lamont R J. Oral microbial communities in sickness and in health. Trends Microbiol, 2005, 13: 589–595.

[94] Jesaitis A J, et al. Compromised host defense on Pseudomonas aeruginosa biofilms: characterization of neutrophil and biofilm interactions. J Immunol, 2003, 171: 4329–4339.

[95] Ji S, Choi Y S, Choi Y. Bacterial invasion and persistence: critical events in the pathogenesis of periodontitis? J Periodontal Res, 2015, 50: 570–585.

[96] Joiner K A, et al. A quantitative analysis of C3 binding to O-antigen capsule, lipopolysaccharide, and outer membrane protein of E. coli O111B4. J Immunol, 1984, 132: 369–375.

[97] Jorth P, et al. Metatranscriptomics of the human oral microbiome during health and disease. MBio, 2014, 5: e01012–01014.

[98] Jung I Y, et al. Molecular epidemiology and association of putative pathogens in root canal infection. J Endod, 2000, 26: 599–604.

[99] Kakehashi S, Stanley H R, Fitzgerald R J. The effects of surgical exposures of dental pulps in germ-free and conventional laboratory rats. Oral Surg Oral Med Oral Pathol, 1965, 20: 340–349.

[100] Kaufman B, et al. Enterococcus spp. in endodontically treated teeth with and without periradicular lesions. J Endod, 2005, 31: 851–856.

[101] Kesavalu L, Holt S C, Ebersole J L. Virulence of a polymicrobic complex, Treponema denticola and Porphyromonas gingivalis, in a murine model. Oral Microbiol Immunol, 1998, 13: 373–377.

[102] Kesavalu L, Holt S C, Ebersole J L. Environmental modulation of oral treponeme virulence in a murine model. Infect Immun, 1999, 67: 2783–2789.

[103] Kesavalu L, Holt S C, Ebersole J L. In vitro environmental regulation of Porphyromonas gingivalis growth and virulence. Oral Microbiol Immunol, 2003, 18: 226–233.

[104] Khemaleelakul S, Baumgartner J C, Pruksakorn S. Identification of bacteria in acute endodontic infections and their antimicrobial susceptibility. Oral Surg Oral Med Oral Pathol Oral Radiol Endod, 2002, 94: 746–755.

[105] Kievit T R, Iglewski B H. Bacterial quorum sensing in pathogenic relationships. Infect Immun, 2000, 68: 4839–4849.

[106] Kilian M, et al. The oral microbiome-an update for oral healthcare professionals. Br Dent J, 2016, 221: 657–666.

[107] Kinnby B, Chavez de Paz L E. Plasminogen coating increases initial adhesion of oral bacteria in vitro. Microb Pathog, 2016, 100: 10–16.

[108] Krieg A M, Hartmann G, Yi A-K. Mechanism of action of CpG DNA. Curr Top Microbiol Immunol, 2000, 247: 1–21.

[109] Kuramitsu H K, et al. Interspecies interactions within oral microbial communities. Microbiol Mol Biol Rev, 2007, 71: 653–670.

[110] Lazazzera B A. Quorum sensing and starvation: signals for entry into stationary phase. Curr Opin Microbiol, 2000, 3: 177–182.

[111] Lepp P W, et al. Methanogenic Archaea and human periodontal disease. Proc Natl Acad Sci USA, 2004, 101: 6176–6181.

[112] Lewis M A, MacFarlane T W, McGowan D A. Quantitative bacteriology of acute dento-alveolar abscesses. J Med Microbiol, 1986, 21: 101–104.

[113] Li H, et al. Herpesviruses in endodontic pathoses: association of Epstein-Barr virus with irreversible pulpitis and apical periodontitis. J Endod, 2009, 35: 23–29.

[114] Li L, et al. Analyzing endodontic infections by deep coverage pyrosequencing. J Dent Res, 2010, 89: 980–984.

[115] Lin L M, Skribner J E, Gaengler P. Factors associated with endodontic treatment failures. J Endod, 1992, 18: 625–627.

[116] Love R M, Jenkinson H F. Invasion of dentinal tubules by oral bacteria. Crit Rev Oral Biol Med, 2002, 13: 171–183.

[117] Love R M, McMillan M D, Jenkinson H F. Invasion of dentinal tubules by oral streptococci is associated with collagen recognition mediated by the antigen I/II family of polypeptides. Infect Immun, 1997, 65: 5157–5164.

[118] Machado de Oliveira J C, Rôças I N, Peixoto R S, et al. On the use of denaturing gradient gel electrophoresis approach for bacterial identification in endodontic infections. Clin Oral Investig, 2007, 11: 127–132.

[119] Machado de Oliveira J C, et al. Bacterial community profiles of endodontic abscesses from Brazilian and USA subjects

as compared by denaturing gradient gel electrophoresis analysis. Oral Microbiol Immunol, 2007, 22: 14–18.
[120] Mah T F, O'Toole G A. Mechanisms of biofilm resistance to antimicrobial agents. Trends Microbiol, 2001, 9: 34–39.
[121] Maita E, Horiuchi H. Polyamine analysis of infected root canal contents related to clinical symptoms. Endod Dent Traumatol, 1990, 6: 213–217.
[122] Mariggiò M A, et al. In vitro effects of polyamines on polymorphonuclear cell apoptosis and implications in the pathogenesis of periodontal disease. Immunopharmacol Immunotoxicol, 2004, 26: 93–101.
[123] Markvart M, et al. Micro-CT analyses of apical enlargement and molar root canal complexity. Int Endod J, 2012, 45: 273–281.
[124] Marsh P, Martin M V. Oral Microbiology. 4th ed. Oxford: Wright, 1999.
[125] Marsh P D. Are dental diseases examples of ecological catastrophes? Microbiology, 2003, 149: 279–294.
[126] Marsh P D. Dental plaque as a microbial biofilm. Caries Res, 2004, 38: 204–211.
[127] Marsh P D. Microbiology of dental plaque biofilms and their role in oral health and caries. Dent Clin North Am, 2010, 54: 441–454.
[128] Marsh P D, McKee A S, McDermid A S. Continuous culture studies// Shah H N, Mayrand D, Genco R J. Biology of the Species Porphyromonasgingivalis. Boca Raton: CRC Press, 1993, 105–123.
[129] Matin A. Physiology, molecular biology and applications of the bacterial starvation response. J Appl Bacteriol, 1992, 73 (Symposium supplement,: 49S–57S.
[130] Matsuo T, et al. An immunohistological study of the localization of bacteria invading root pulpal walls of teeth with periapical lesions. J Endod, 2003, 29: 194–200.
[131] Miller W D. An introduction to the study of the bacterio-pathology of the dental pulp. Dent Cosmos, 1894, 36: 505–528.
[132] Mims C, Nash A, Stephen J. Mims' Pathogenesis of Infectious Diseases. 5 ed. San Diego: Academic Press, 2001.
[133] Miranda T T, et al. Diversity and frequency of yeasts from the dorsum of the tongue and necrotic root canals associated with primary apical periodontitis. Int Endod J, 2009, 42: 839–844.
[134] Mogensen T H, Paludan S R. Molecular pathways in virus-induced cytokine production. Microbiol Mol Biol Rev, 2001, 65: 131–150.
[135] Molander A, et al. Microbiological status of root-filled teeth with apical periodontitis. Int Endod J, 1998, 31: 1–7.
[136] Möller Å J R. Microbial examination of root canals and periapical tissues of human teeth. Odontol Tidskr 74(supplement), 1966: 1–380.
[137] Möller Å J R, et al, Influence on periapical tissues of indigenous oral bacteria and necrotic pulp tissue in monkeys. Scand J Dent Res, 1981, 89: 475–484.
[138] Molven O, Olsen I, Kerekes K. Scanning electron microscopy of bacteria in the apical part of root canals in permanent teeth with periapical lesions. Endod Dent Traumatol, 1991, 7: 226–229.
[139] Moses P J, Vickerman M M. Streptococcus gordonii collagen-binding domain protein CbdA may enhance bacterial survival in instrumented root canals ex vivo. J Endod, 2013, 39: 39–43.
[140] Munson M A, et al. Molecular and cultural analysis of the microflora associated with endodontic infections. J Dent Res, 2002, 81: 761–766.
[141] Murad C F, et al. Microbial diversity in persistent root canal infections investigated by checkerboard DNA-DNA hybridization. J Endod, 2014, 40: 899–906.
[142] Murakami Y, et al. A possible mechanism of maxillofacial abscess formation: involvement of Porphyromonas endodontalis lipopolysaccharide via the expression of inflammatory cytokines. Oral Microbiol Immunol, 2001, 16: 321–325.
[143] Musser J M. Molecular population genetic analysis of emerged bacterial pathogens: selected insights. Emerg Infect Dis, 1996, 2: 1–17.
[144] Nadell C D, et al. Spatial structure, cooperation and competition in biofilms. Nat Rev Microbiol, 2016, 14: 589–600.
[145] Nair P N. Pathogenesis of apical periodontitis and the causes of endodontic failures. Crit Rev Oral Biol Med, 2004, 15: 348–381.
[146] Nair P N, et al. Intraradicular bacteria and fungi in root-filled, asymptomatic human teeth with therapyresistant periapical lesions: a long-term light and electron microscopic follow-up study. J Endod, 1990, 16: 580–588.
[147] Nair P N, et al. Microbial status of apical root canal system of human mandibular first molars with primary apical periodontitis after "one-visit" endodontic treatment. Oral Surg Oral Med Oral Pathol Oral Radiol Endod, 2005, 99: 231–252.
[148] Nair P N R. Light and electron microscopic studies of root canal flora and periapical lesions. J Endod, 1987, 13: 29–39.
[149] Nandakumar R, Madayiputhiya N, Fouad A F. Proteomic analysis of endodontic infections by liquid chromatography-tandem mass spectrometry. Oral Microbiol Immunol, 2009, 24: 347–352.
[150] Niederman R, et al. Short-chain carboxylic acid concentration in human gingival crevicular fluid. J Dent Res, 1997, 76: 575–579.
[151] Nobrega L M, et al. Bacterial diversity of symptomatic primary endodontic infection by clonal analysis. Braz Oral Res, 2016, 30: e103.
[152] Noiri Y, et al. Participation of bacterial biofilms in refractory and chronic periapical periodontitis. J Endod, 2002, 28:

679–683.

[153] Olsen I. Biofilm-specific antibiotic tolerance and resistance. Eur J Clin Microbiol Infect Dis, 2015, 34: 877–886.

[154] Oosthuizen M C, et al. Proteomic analysis reveals differential protein expression by Bacillus cereus during biofilm formation. Appl Environ Microbiol, 2002, 68: 2770–2780.

[155] Özmeri N, Preus H R, Olsen I. Genetic diversity of Porphyromonas gingivalis and its possible importance to pathogenicity. Acta Odontol Scand, 2000, 58: 183–187.

[156] Ozok A R, et al. Ecology of the microbiome of the infected root canal system: a comparison between apical and coronal root segments. Int Endod J, 2012, 45: 530–541.

[157] Paiva S S, et al. Supplementing the antimicrobial effects of chemomechanical debridement with either passive ultrasonic irrigation or a final rinse with chlorhexidine: a clinical study. J Endod, 2012, 38: 1202–1206.

[158] Paqué F, Zehnder M, De-Deus G. Microtomography-based comparison of reciprocating single-file F2 ProTaper technique versus rotary full sequence. J Endod, 2011, 37: 1394–1397.

[159] Parsek M R, Greenberg E P. Sociomicrobiology: the connections between quorum sensing and biofilms. Trends Microbiol, 2005, 13: 27–33.

[160] Parsek M R, Singh P K. Bacterial biofilms: an emerging link to disease pathogenesis. Annu Rev Microbiol, 2003, 57: 677–701.

[161] Peciuliene V, et al. Isolation of Enterococcus faecalis in previously rootfilled canals in a Lithuanian population. J Endod, 2000, 26: 593–595.

[162] Peciuliene V, et al. Isolation of yeasts and enteric bacteria in root-filled teeth with chronic apical periodontitis. Int Endod J, 2001, 34: 429–434.

[163] Perez F, et al. Migration of a Streptococcus sanguis strain through the root dentinal tubules. J Endod, 1993, 19: 297–301.

[164] Peters B M, et al. Polymicrobial interactions: impact on pathogenesis and human disease. Clin Microbiol Rev, 2012, 25: 193–213.

[165] Peters L B, et al. Viable bacteria in root dentinal tubules of teeth with apical periodontitis. J Endod, 2001, 27: 76–81.

[166] Peters O A, Arias A, Paqué F. A micro-computed tomographic assessment of root canal preparation with a novel instrument, TRUShape, in mesial roots of mandibular molars. J Endod, 2015, 41: 1545–1550.

[167] Petersen F C, Pecharki D, Scheie A A. Biofilm mode of growth of Streptococcus intermedius favored by a competence-stimulating signaling peptide. J Bacteriol, 2004, 186: 6327–6331.

[168] Peyyala R, Ebersole J L. Multispecies biofilms and host responses: "discriminating the trees from the forest". Cytokine, 2013, 61: 15–25.

[169] Pinheiro E T, et al. Microorganisms from canals of root-filled teeth with periapical lesions. Int Endod J, 2003, 36: 1–11.

[170] Pinheiro E T, et al. RNA-based Assay Demonstrated Enterococcus faecalis Metabolic Activity after Chemomechanical Procedures. J Endod, 2015, 41: 1441–1444.

[171] Provenzano J C, et al. Metaproteome analysis of endodontic infections in association with different clinical conditions. PLoS One, 2013, 8: e76108.

[172] Provenzano J C, et al. Short-chain fatty acids in infected root canals of teeth with apical periodontitis before and after treatment. J Endod, 2015, 41: 831–835.

[173] Provenzano J C, et al. Hostbacterial interactions in post-treatment apical periodontitis: a metaproteome analysis. J Endod, 2016, 42: 880–885.

[174] Qi Z, et al. Combinations of bacterial species associated with symptomatic endodontic infections in a Chinese population. Int Endod J, 2016, 49: 17–25.

[175] Qiqiang L, Huanxin M, Xuejun G. Longitudinal study of volatile fatty acids in the gingival crevicular fluid of patients with periodontitis before and after nonsurgical therapy. J Periodontal Res, 2012, 47: 740–749.

[176] Ranta H, et al. Bacteriology of odontogenic apical periodontitis and effect of penicillin treatment. Scand J Infect Dis, 1988, 20: 187–192.

[177] Ranta K, Haapasalo M, Ranta H. Monoinfection of root canal with Pseudomonas aeruginosa. Endod Dent Traumatol, 1988, 4: 269–272.

[178] Razavi A, et al. Recovery of Enterococcus faecalis from cheese in the oral cavity of healthy subjects. Oral Microbiol Immunol, 2007, 22: 248–251.

[179] Relman D A. Microbial genomics and infectious diseases. N Engl J Med, 2011, 365: 347–357.

[180] Ribeiro A C, et al. Exploring bacterial diversity of endodontic microbiota by cloning and sequencing 16S rRNA. J Endod, 2011, 37: 922–926.

[181] Ricucci D, Loghin S, Siqueira J F Jr. Exuberant biofilm infection in a lateral canal as the cause of short-term endodontic treatment failure: report of a case. J Endod, 2013, 39: 712–718.

[182] Ricucci D, Siqueira J F Jr. Apical actinomycosis as a continuum of intraradicular and extraradicular infection: case report and critical review on its involvement with treatment failure. J Endod, 2008, 34: 1124–1129.

[183] Ricucci D, Siqueira J F Jr. Biofilms and apical periodontitis: study of prevalence and association with clinical and histopathologic findings. J Endod, 2010, 36: 1277–1288.

[184] Ricucci D, Siqueira J F Jr. Fate of the tissue in lateral canals and apical ramifications in response to pathologic conditions and treatment procedures. J Endod, 2010, 36: 1–15.

[185] Ricucci D, et al. Calculus-like deposit on the apical external root surface of teeth with post-treatment apical periodontitis: report of two cases. Int Endod J, 2005, 38: 262–271.

[186] Ricucci D, et al. Histologic investigation of root canal-treated teeth with apical periodontitis: a retrospective study from twenty-four patients. J Endod, 2009, 35: 493–502.

[187] Ricucci D, et al. Wound healing of apical tissues after root canal therapy: a long-term clinical, radiographic, and histopathologic observation study. Oral Surg Oral Med Oral Pathol Oral Radiol Endod, 2009, 108: 609–621.

[188] Ricucci D, et al. A prospective cohort study of endodontic treatments of 1, 369 root canals: results after 5 years. Oral Surg Oral Med Oral Pathol Oral Radiol Endod, 2011, 112: 825–842.

[189] Ricucci D, et al. Extraradicular infection as the cause of persistent symptoms: a case series. J Endod, 2015, 41: 265–273.

[190] Ricucci D, et al. Complex apical intraradicular infection and extraradicular mineralized biofilms as the cause of wet canals and treatment failure: report of 2 cases. J Endod, 2016, 42: 509–515.

[191] Ricucci D, et al. Histobacteriologic conditions of the apical root canal system and periapical tissues in teeth associated with sinus tracts. J Endod, 2018, 44: 405–413.

[192] Ricucci D, et al. Large bacterial floc causing an independent extraradicular infection and posttreatment apical periodontitis: a case report. J Endod, 2018, 44: 1308–1316.

[193] Rietschel E T, Brade H. Bacterial endotoxins. Sci Am, 1992, 267: 26–33.

[194] Rôças I N, Hülsmann M, Siqueira J F Jr. Microorganisms in root canal-treated teeth from a German population. J Endod, 2008, 34: 926–931.

[195] Rôças I N, Siqueira J F Jr. Detection of novel oral species and phylotypes in symptomatic endodontic infections including abscesses. FEMS Microbiol Lett, 2005, 250: 279–285.

[196] Rôças I N, Siqueira J F Jr. Root canal microbiota of teeth with chronic apical periodontitis. J Clin Microbiol, 2008, 46: 3599–3606.

[197] Rôças I N, Siqueira J F Jr, Prevalence of new candidate pathogens Prevotella baroniae, Prevotella multisaccharivorax and as-yetuncultivated Bacteroidetes clone X083 in primary endodontic infections. J Endod, 2009, 35: 1359–1362.

[198] Rôças I N, Siqueira J F Jr. Comparison of the in vivo antimicrobial effectiveness of sodium hypochlorite and chlorhexidine used as root canal irrigants: a molecular microbiology study. J Endod, 2011, 37: 143–150.

[199] Rôças I N, Siqueira J F Jr. In vivo antimicrobial effects of endodontic treatment procedures as assessed by molecular microbiologic techniques. J Endod, 2011, 37: 304–310.

[200] Rôças I N, Siqueira J F Jr. Characterization of microbiota of root canal-treated teeth with posttreatment disease. J Clin Microbiol, 2012, 50: 1721–1724.

[201] Rôças I N, Siqueira J F Jr. Frequency and levels of candidate endodontic pathogens in acute apical abscesses as compared to asymptomatic apical periodontitis. PLoS One, 2018, 13: e0190469.

[202] Rôças I N, Siqueira J F Jr, Debelian G J. Analysis of symptomatic and asymptomatic primary root canal infections in adult Norwegian patients. J Endod, 2011, 37: 1206–1212.

[203] Rôças I N, Siqueira J F Jr, Santos K R. Association of Enterococcus faecalis with different forms of periradicular diseases. J Endod, 2004, 30: 315–320.

[204] Rôças I N, et al. Identification of selected putative oral pathogens in primary root canal infections associated with symptoms. Anaerobe, 2002, 8: 200–208.

[205] Rôças I N, et al. Denaturing gradient gel electrophoresis analysis of bacterial communities associated with failed endodontic treatment. Oral Surg Oral Med Oral Pathol Oral Radiol Endod, 2004, 98: 741–749.

[206] Rôças I N, et al. Polymerase chain reaction identification of microorganisms in previously root-filled teeth in a South Korean population. J Endod, 2004, 30: 504–508.

[207] Rôças I N, et al. Apical root canal microbiota as determined by reversecapture checkerboard analysis of cryogenically ground root samples from teeth with apical periodontitis. J Endod, 2010, 36: 1617–1621.

[208] Rôças I N, et al. Susceptibility of as-yet-uncultivated and difficult-toculture bacteria to chemomechanical procedures. J Endod, 2014, 40: 33–37.

[209] Rôças I N, et al. Advanced caries microbiota in teeth with irreversible pulpitis. J Endod, 2015, 41: 1450–1455.

[210] Rôças I N, et al. Microbiome of deep dentinal caries lesions in teeth with symptomatic irreversible pulpitis. PLoS One, 2016, 11: e0154653.

[211] Rodrigues R C, et al. Infection control in retreatment cases: in vivo antibacterial effects of 2 instrumentation systems. J Endod, 2015, 41: 1600–1605.

[212] Rolph H J, et al. Molecular identification of microorganisms from endodontic infections. J Clin Microbiol, 2001, 39: 3282–3289.

[213] Roodman G D. Role of cytokines in the regulation of bone resorption. Calcif Tissue Int 53 Suppl, 1993, 1: S94–98.

[214] Saber M H, et al. Bacterial flora of dental periradicular lesions analyzed by the 454-pyrosequencing technology. J Endod, 2012, 38: 1484–1488.

[215] Sabeti M, Simon J H, Slots J. Cytomegalovirus and Epstein-Barr virus are associated with symptomatic periapical pathosis. Oral Microbiol Immunol, 2003, 18: 327–328.

[216] Sabeti M, Slots J. Herpesviralbacterial coinfection in periapical pathosis. J Endod, 2004, 30: 69–72.

[217] Sabeti M, et al. Cytomegalovirus and Epstein-Barr virus DNA transcription in endodontic symptomatic lesions. Oral Microbiol Immunol, 2003, 18: 104–108.

[218] Saboia-Dantas C J, et al. Herpesviruses in asymptomatic apical periodontitis lesions: an immunohistochemical approach. Oral Microbiol Immunol, 2007, 22: 320–325.

[219] Saito D, et al. Identification of bacteria in endodontic infections by sequence analysis of 16S rDNA clone libraries. J Med Microbiol, 2006, 55: 101–107.

[220] Saito D, et al. Assessment of intraradicular bacterial composition by terminal restriction fragment length polymorphism analysis. Oral Microbiol Immunol, 2009, 24: 369–376.

[221] Sakamoto M, et al. Molecular analysis of bacteria in asymptomatic and symptomatic endodontic infections. Oral Microbiol Immunol, 2006, 21: 112–122.

[222] Sakamoto M, et al. Bacterial reduction and persistence after endodontic treatment procedures. Oral Microbiol Immunol, 2007, 22: 19–23.

[223] Sakamoto M, et al. Molecular analysis of the root canal microbiota as sociated with endodontic treatment failures. Oral Microbiol Immunol, 2008, 23: 275–281.

[224] Sakamoto M, et al. Diversity of spirochetes in endodontic infections. J Clin Microbiol, 2009, 47: 1352–1357.

[225] Santos A L, et al. Comparing the bacterial diversity of acute and chronic dental root canal infections. PLoS One, 2011, 6: e28088.

[226] Sasaki H, Stashenko P. Interrelationship of the pulp and apical Periodontitis// Hargreaves K M, Goodis H E, Tay F R. Seltzer and Bender's Dental Pulp. Chicago IL: Quintessence Publishing, 2012:277–299

[227] Sassone L M, et al. A microbiological profile of symptomatic teeth with primary endodontic infections. J Endod, 2008, 34: 541–545.

[228] Sauer K, et al. Pseudomonas aeruginosa displays multiple phenotypes during development as a biofilm. J Bacteriol, 2002, 184: 1140–1154.

[229] Schaudinn C, et al. Imaging of endodontic biofilms by combined microscopy (FISH/cLSM-SEM). J Microsc, 2009, 235: 124–127.

[230] Schein B, Schilder H. Endotoxin content in endodontically involved teeth. J Endod, 1975, 1: 19–21.

[231] Schonfeld S E, et al. Endotoxin activity in periapical lesions. Oral Surg Oral Med Oral Pathol, 1982, 53: 82–87.

[232] Sedgley C, et al. Real-time quantitative polymerase chain reaction and culture analyses of Enterococcus faecalis in root canals. J Endod, 2006, 32: 173–177.

[233] Sen B H, Piskin B, Demirci T. Observation of bacteria and fungi in infected root canals and dentinal tubules by SEM. Endod Dent Traumatol, 1995, 11: 6–9.

[234] Sen B H, Safavi K E, Spångberg L S. Colonization of Candida albicans on cleaned human dental hard tissues. Arch Oral Biol, 1997, 42: 513–520.

[235] Sen B H, Safavi K E, Spångberg L S. Growth patterns of Candida albicans in relation to radicular dentin. Oral Surg Oral Med Oral Pathol Oral Radiol Endod, 1997, 84: 68–73.

[236] Sibley C D, et al. Discerning the complexity of community interactions using a Drosophila model of polymicrobial infections. PLoS Pathog, 2008, 4: e1000184.

[237] Signoretti F G, et al. Investigation of cultivable bacteria isolated from longstanding retreatment-resistant lesions of teeth with apical periodontitis. J Endod, 2013, 39: 1240–1244.

[238] Siqueira J F, Rôças I N. Present status and future directions in endodontic microbiology. Endod Topics, 2014, 30: 3–22.

[239] Siqueira J F, Rôças I N, Ricucci D. Biofilms in endodontic infection. Endod Topics, 2010, 22: 33–49.

[240] Siqueira J F, et al. Histological evaluation of the effectiveness of five instrumentation techniques for cleaning the apical third of root canals. J Endod, 1997, 23: 499–502.

[241] Siqueira J F, et al. Pathogenicity of facultative and obligate anaerobic bacteria in monoculture and combined with either Prevotella intermedia or Prevotella nigrescens. Oral Microbiol Immunol, 1998, 13: 368–372.

[242] Siqueira J F, et al. Checkerboard DNA-DNA hybridization analysis of endodontic infections. Oral Surg Oral Med Oral Pathol Oral Radiol Endod, 2000, 89: 744–748.

[243] Siqueira J F, et al. Microbiological evaluation of acute periradicular abscesses by DNA-DNA hybridization. Oral Surg Oral Med Oral Pathol Oral Radiol Endod, 2001, 92: 451–457.

[244] Siqueira J F, et al. Actinomyces species, streptococci, and Enterococcus faecalis in primary root canal infections. J Endod, 2002, 28: 168–172.

[245] Siqueira J F, et al. Endodontic infections: concepts, paradigms, and perspectives. Oral Surg Oral Med Oral Pathol Oral Radiol Endod, 2002, 94: 281–293.

[246] Siqueira J F, et al. Fungal infection of the radicular dentin. J Endod, 2002, 28: 770–773.

[247] Siqueira J F, et al. Selected endodontic pathogens in the apical third of infected root canals: a molecular investigation. J Endod, 2004, 30: 638–643.

[248] Siqueira J F, et al. Novel bacterial phylotypes in endodontic infections. J Dent Res, 2005, 84: 565–569.

[249] Siqueira J F, et al. Searching for Archaea in infections of endodontic origin. J Endod, 2005, 31: 719–722.

[250] Siqueira J F, et al. Bacteriologic investigation of the effects of sodium hypochlorite and chlorhexidine during the endodontic treatment of teeth with apical periodontitis. Oral Surg Oral Med Oral Pathol Oral Radiol Endod, 2007, 104: 122–130.

[251] Siqueira J F, et al. Cultivable bacteria in infected root canals as identified by 16S rRNA gene sequencing. Oral Microbiol Immunol, 2007, 22: 266–271.

[252] Siqueira J F, et al. Profiling of root canal bacterial communities associated with chronic apical periodontitis

from Brazilian and Norwegian subjects. J Endod, 2008, 34:1457–1461.
[253] Siqueira J F, et al. Bacteria in the apical root canal of teeth with primary apical periodontitis. Oral Surg Oral Med Oral Pathol Oral Radiol Endod, 2009, 107: 721–726.
[254] Siqueira J F, et al. Correlative bacteriologic and micro-computed tomographic analysis of mandibular molar mesial canals prepared by selfadjusting file, Reciproc, and Twisted File systems. J Endod, 2013, 39: 1044–1050.
[255] Siqueira J F, et al. Microbiome in the apical root canal system of teeth with post-treatment apical periodontitis. PLoS One, 2016, 11: e0162887.
[256] Siqueira J F Jr. Aetiology of root canal treatment failure: why well-treated teeth can fail. Int Endod, 2001, J 34: 1–10.
[257] Siqueira J F Jr. Periapical actinomycosis and infection with Propionibacterium propionicum. Endod Topics, 2003, 6: 78–95.
[258] Siqueira J F Jr. Treatment of endodontic infections. London: Quintessence Publishing, 2011:403.
[259] Siqueira J F Jr, Alves F R, Rôças I N. Pyrosequencing analysis of the apical root canal microbiota. J Endod, 2011, 37: 1499–1503.
[260] Siqueira J F Jr, de Uzeda M, Fonseca M E. A scanning electron microscopic evaluation of in vitro dentinal tubules penetration by selected anaerobic bacteria. J Endod, 1996, 22: 308–310.
[261] Siqueira J F Jr, Guimarães-Pinto T, Rôças I N. Effects of chemomechanical preparation with 2.5% sodium hypochlorite and intracanal medication with calcium hydroxide on cultivable bacteria in infected root canals. J Endod, 2007, 33: 800–805.
[262] Siqueira J F Jr, Lima K C. Staphylococcus epidermidis and Staphylococcus xylosus in a secondary root canal infection with persistent symptoms: a case report. Aust Endod J, 2002, 28: 61–63.
[263] Siqueira J F Jr, Lopes H P. Bacteria on the apical root surfaces of untreated teeth with periradicular lesions: a scanning electron microscopy study. Int Endod J, 2001, 34: 216–220.
[264] Siqueira J F Jr, Magalhães K M, Rôças I N. Bacterial reduction in infected root canals treated with 2.5% NaOCl as an irrigant and calcium hydroxide/camphorated paramonochlorophenol paste as an intracanal dressing. J Endod, 2007, 33: 667–672.
[265] Siqueira J F Jr, Paiva S S, Rôças I N. Reduction in the cultivable bacterial populations in infected root canals by a chlorhexidine-based antimicrobial protocol. J Endod, 2007, 33: 541–547.
[266] Siqueira J F Jr, Rôças I N. Polymerase chain reaction-based analysis of microorganisms associated with failed endodontic treatment. Oral Surg Oral Med Oral Pathol Oral Radiol Endod, 2004, 97: 85–94.
[267] Siqueira J F Jr, Rôças I N. Exploiting molecular methods to explore endodontic infections: Part 2-redefining the endodontic microbiota. J Endod, 2005, 31: 488–498.
[268] Siqueira J F Jr, Rôças I N. Uncultivated phylotypes and newly named species associated with primary and persistent endodontic infections. J Clin Microbiol, 2005, 43: 3314–3319.
[269] Siqueira J F Jr, Rôças I N. Bacterial pathogenesis and mediators in apical periodontitis. Braz Dent J, 2007, 18: 267–280.
[270] Siqueira J F Jr, Rôças I N. Molecular detection and identification of Synergistes phylotypes in primary endodontic infections. Oral Dis, 2007, 13: 398–401.
[271] Siqueira J F Jr, Rôças I N. Clinical implications and microbiology of bacterial persistence after treatment procedures. J Endod, 2008, 34: 1291–1301 e1293.
[272] Siqueira J F Jr, Rôças I N. Diversity of endodontic microbiota revisited. J Dent Res, 2009, 88: 969–981.
[273] Siqueira J F Jr, Rôças I N. Community as the unit of pathogenicity: an emerging concept as to the microbial pathogenesis of apical periodontitis. Oral Surg Oral Med Oral Pathol Oral Radiol Endod, 2009, 107: 870–878.
[274] Siqueira J F Jr, Rôças I N. The microbiota of acute apical abscesses. J Dent Res, 2009, 88: 61–65.
[275] Siqueira J F Jr, Rôças I N. Microbiology and treatment of acute apical abscesses. Clin Microbiol Rev, 2013, 26: 255–273.
[276] Siqueira J F Jr, Rôças I N, Lopes H P. Patterns of microbial colonization in primary root canal infections. Oral Surg Oral Med Oral Pathol Oral Radiol Endod, 2002, 93: 174–178.
[277] Siqueira J F Jr, Rôças I N, Rosado A S. Investigation of bacterial communities associated with asymptomatic and symptomatic endodontic infections by denaturing gradient gel electrophoresis fingerprinting approach. Oral Microbiol Immunol, 2004, 19: 363–370.
[278] Siqueira J F Jr, Sen B H. Fungi in endodontic infections. Oral Surg Oral Med Oral Pathol Oral Radiol Endod, 2004, 97: 632–641.
[279] Siren E K, et al. Microbiological findings and clinical treatment procedures in endodontic cases selected for microbiological investigation. Int Endod J, 1997, 30: 91–95.
[280] Sjögren U, et al. Survival of Arachnia propionica in periapical tissue. Int Endod J, 1988, 21: 277–282.
[281] Sjögren U, et al. Influence of infection at the time of root filling on the outcome of endodontic treatment of teeth with apical periodontitis. Int Endod J, 1997, 30: 297–306.
[282] Slots J, Sabeti M, Simon J H. Herpesviruses in periapical pathosis: an etiopathogenic relationship? Oral Surg Oral Med Oral Pathol Oral Radiol Endod, 2003, 96: 327–331.
[283] Socransky S S, Haffajee A D. Dental biofilms: difficult therapeutic targets. Periodontol, 2002, 2000 (28): 12–55.
[284] Socransky S S, Haffajee A D. Periodontal microbial ecology.

Periodontol, 2005, 2000 (38): 135–187.
[285] Spratt D A, Pratten J. Biofilms and the oral cavity. Rev Environ Science Biotechnol, 2003, 2: 109–120.
[286] Stoodley P, et al. Biofilms as complex differentiated communities. Annu Rev Microbiol, 2002, 56: 187–209.
[287] Strindberg L Z. The dependence of the results of pulp therapy on certain factors. Acta Odontol Scand 1956, 14, (suppl 21): 1–175.
[288] Subramanian K, Mickel A K. Molecular analysis of persistent periradicular lesions and root ends reveals a diverse microbial profile. J Endod, 2009, 35: 950–957.
[289] Sunde P T, et al. Assessment of periradicular microbiota by DNA-DNA hybridization. Endod Dent Traumatol, 2000, 16: 191–196.
[290] Sunde P T, et al. Fluorescence in situ hybridization (FISH) for direct visualization of bacteria in periapical lesions of asymptomatic root-filled teeth. Microbiology, 2003, 149: 1095–1102.
[291] Sundqvist G. Bacteriological Studies of Necrotic Dental Pulps. Odontological Dissertation 7. Umea, Sweden: University of Umea, 1976.
[292] Sundqvist G, et al. Microbiologic analysis of teeth with failed endodontic treatment and the outcome of conservative re-treatment. Oral Surg Oral Med Oral Pathol Oral Radiol Endod, 1998, 85: 86–93.
[293] Sundqvist G K, et al. Capacity of anaerobic bacteria from necrotic dental pulps to induce purulent infections. Infect Immun, 1979, 25: 685–693.
[294] Tani-Ishii N, et al. Changes in root canal microbiota during the development of rat periapical lesions. Oral Microbiol Immunol, 1994, 9: 129–135.
[295] Ter Steeg P F, van der Hoeven J S. Development of periodontal microflora on human serum. Microb Ecol Health Dis, 1989, 2: 1–10.
[296] Thilo B E, Baehni P, Holz J. Dark-field observation of the bacterial distribution in root canals following pulp necrosis. J Endod, 1986, 12: 202–205.
[297] Thurlow L R, et al. Staphylococcus aureus biofilms prevent macrophage phagocytosis and attenuate inflammation in vivo. J Immunol, 2011, 186: 6585–6596.
[298] Tronstad L, Barnett F, Cervone F. Periapical bacterial plaque in teeth refractory to endodontic treatment. Endod Dent Traumatol, 1990, 6: 73–77.
[299] Tronstad L, et al. pH changes in dental tissues after root canal filling with calcium hydroxide. J Endod, 1981, 7: 17–21.
[300] Tronstad L, et al. Extraradicular endodontic infections. Endod Dent Traumatol, 1987, 3: 86–90.
[301] Tzanetakis G N, et al. Comparison of bacterial community composition of primary and persistent endodontic infections using pyrosequencing. J Endod, 2015, 41: 1226–1233.
[302] Valderhaug J. A histologic study of experimentally induced periapical inflammation in primary teeth in monkeys. Int J Oral Surg, 1974, 3: 111–123.
[303] Van Amersfoort E S, van Berkel T J C, Kuiper J. Receptors, mediators, and mechanisms involved in bacterial sepsis and septic shock. Clin Microbiol Rev, 2003, 16: 379–414.
[304] Van Steenbergen T J M, van der Mispel L M S, de Graaff J. Effect of ammonia and volatile fatty acids produced by oral bacteria on tissue culture cells. J Dent Res, 1986, 65: 909–912.
[305] Van Winkelhoff A J, Carlee A W, de Graaff J. Bacteroides endodontalis and others black-pigmented Bacteroides species in odontogenic abscesses. Infect Immun, 1985, 49: 494–498.
[306] Van Winkelhoff A J, van Steenbergen T J, de Graaff J. Porphyromonas (Bacteroides endodontalis: its role in endodontal infections. J Endod, 1992, 18: 431–434.
[307] Vartoukian S R, et al. Fretibacterium fastidiosum gen. nov, sp. nov, isolated from the human oral cavity. Int J Syst Evol Microbiol, 2013, 63: 458–463.
[308] Vengerfeldt V, et al. Highly diverse microbiota in dental root canals in cases of apical periodontitis (data of illumina sequencing). J Endod, 2014, 40: 1778–1783.
[309] Vera J, et al. One-versus twovisit endodontic treatment of teeth with apical periodontitis: a histobacteriologic study. J Endod, 2012, 38: 1040–1052.
[310] Vianna M E, et al. Identification and quantification of archaea involved in primary endodontic infections. J Clin Microbiol, 2006, 44: 1274–1282.
[311] Vianna M E, et al. In vivo evaluation of microbial reduction after chemo-mechanical preparation of human root canals containing necrotic pulp tissue. Int Endod J, 2006, 39: 484–492.
[312] Vianna M E, et al. Effect of root canal procedures on endotoxins and endodontic pathogens. Oral Microbiol Immunol, 2007, 22: 411–418.
[313] Vickerman M M, et al. Phylogenetic analysis of bacterial and archaeal species in symptomatic and asymptomatic endodontic infections. J Med Microbiol, 2007, 56: 110–118.
[314] Vieira A R, Siqueira J F Jr, Ricucci D, et al. Dentinal tubule infection as the cause of recurrent disease and late endodontic treatment failure: a case report. J Endod, 2012, 38: 250–254.
[315] Voelkerding K V, Dames S A, Durtschi J D. Next-generation sequencing: from basic research to diagnostics. Clin Chem, 2009, 55: 641–658.
[316] Wadachi R, Hargreaves K M. Trigeminal nociceptors express TLR-4 and CD14: a mechanism for pain due to infection. J Dent Res, 2006, 85: 49–53.
[317] Waltimo T, et al. Clinical efficacy of treatment procedures in endodontic infection control and one year follow-up of periapical healing. J Endod, 2005, 31: 863–866.

[318] Waltimo T M, et al. Fungi in therapy-resistant apical periodontitis. Int Endod J, 1997, 30: 96–101.

[319] Waltimo T M, et al. Susceptibility of oral Candida species to calcium hydroxide in vitro. Int Endod J, 1999, 32: 94–98.

[320] Walton R E. Histologic evaluation of different methods of enlarging the pulp canal space. J Endod, 1976, 2: 304–311.

[321] Wang J E, et al. Peptidoglycan and lipoteichoic acid in gram-positive bacterial sepsis: receptors, signal transduction, biological effects, and synergism. Shock, 2003, 20: 402–414.

[322] Wara-Aswapati N, Boch J A, Auron P E. Activation of interleukin 1beta gene transcription by human cytomegalovirus: molecular mechanisms and relevance to periodontitis. Oral Microbiol Immunol, 2003 18: 67–71.

[323] Wayman B E, et al. A bacteriological and histological evaluation of 58 periapical lesions. J Endod, 1992, 18: 152–155.

[324] Wen Z T, Burne R A. LuxS-mediated signaling in Streptococcus mutans is involved in regulation of acid and oxidative stress tolerance and biofilm formation. J Bacteriol, 2004, 186: 2682–2691.

[325] Williams B L, McCann G F, Schoenknecht F D. Bacteriology of dental abscesses of endodontic origin. J Clin Microbiol, 1983, 18: 770–774.

[326] Williams J M, et al. Detection and quantitation of Enterococcus faecalis by real-time PCR (qPCR), reverse transcription-PCR (RT, PCR), and cultivation during endodontic treatment. J Endod, 2006, 32: 715–721.

[327] Wilmes P, Bond P L. The application of two-dimensional polyacrylamide gel electrophoresis and downstream analyses to a mixed community of prokaryotic microorganisms. Environ Microbiol, 2004, 6: 911–920.

[328] Wilson M, Reddi K, Henderson B. Cytokine-inducing components of periodontopathogenic bacteria. J Periodontal Res, 1996, 31: 393–407.

[329] Withers H, Swift S, Williams P. Quorum sensing as an integral component of gene regulatory networks in Gram-negative bacteria. Curr Opin Microbiol, 2001, 4: 186–193.

[330] Wolcott R, Dowd S. The role of biofilms: are we hitting the right target? Plast Reconstr Surg, 2011, 127 Suppl 1: 28S–35.

[331] Wu M-K, van der Sluis L W M, Wesselink P R. The capability of two hand instrumentation techniques to remove the inner layer of dentine in oval canals. Int Endod J, 2003, 36: 218–224.

[332] Ying S C, et al. C1q peptides bind endotoxin and inhibit endotoxin-initiated activation of the classical complement pathway. J Immunol, 1993, 150: 304A.

[333] Yoneda M, et al. Mixed infection of Porphyromonas gingivalis and Bacteroides forsythus in a murine abscess model: involvement of gingipains in a synergistic effect. J Periodontal Res, 2001, 36: 237–243.

[334] Yoshida A, et al. LuxS-based signaling affects Streptococcus mutans biofilm formation. Appl Environ Microbiol, 2005, 71: 2372–2380.

[335] Yoshida M, et al. Correlation between clinical symptoms and microorganisms isolated from root canals of teeth with periapical pathosis. J Endod, 1987, 13: 24–28.

[336] Yuan L, Hillman J D, Progulske-Fox A. Microarray analysis of quorum-sensing-regulated genes in Porphyromonas gingivalis. Infect Immun, 2005, 73: 4146–4154.

[337] Zakaria M N, et al. Microbial community in persistent apical periodontitis: a 16S rRNA gene clone library analysis. Int Endod J, 2015, 48: 717–728.

[338] Zandi H, et al. Antibacterial effectiveness of 2 root canal irrigants in root-filled teeth with infection: a randomized clinical trial. J Endod, 2016, 42: 1307–1313.

[339] Zandi H, et al. Microbial analysis of endodontic infections in root-filled teeth with apical periodontitis before and after irrigation using pyrosequencing. J Endod, 2018, 44: 372–378.

[340] Zehnder M, Guggenheim B. The mysterious appearance of enterococci in filled root canals. Int Endod J, 2009, 42: 277–287.

[341] Zenobia C, Hajishengallis G. Porphyromonas gingivalis virulence factors involved in subversion of leukocytes and microbial dysbiosis. Virulence, 2015, 6: 236–243.

[342] Zhang C, Du J, Peng Z. Correlation between Enterococcus faecalis and Persistent Intraradicular Infection Compared with Primary Intraradicular Infection: A Systematic Review. J Endod, 2015, 41: 1207–1213.

[343] Zhang Y, et al. Differential protein expression by Porphyromonas gingivalis in response to secreted epithelial cell components. Proteomics, 2005, 5: 198–211.

[344] Zoletti G O, Siqueira J F Jr, Santos K R. Identification of Enterococcus faecalis in root-filled teeth with or without periradicular lesions by culturedependent and-independent approaches. J Endod, 2006, 32: 722–726.

[345] Zou W, Bar-Shavit Z. Dual modulation of osteoclast differentiation by lipopolysaccharide. J Bone Miner Res, 2002, 17: 1211–1218.

[346] Zuolo M L, Walton R E, Imura N. Histologic evaluation of three endodontic instrument/preparation techniques. Endod Dent Traumatol, 1992, 8: 125–129.

第5章 根尖周炎的流行病学、疗效和风险因素

Lise-Lotte Kirkevang, Michael Vaeth

5.1 概述

根尖周炎是一种常见的疾病。在一些人群中，大约一半的成年人至少有一颗发生根尖周炎的患牙。如果不加以治疗，根尖周炎可能引起疼痛，咀嚼功能降低，并最终导致牙齿脱落。预防和治疗根尖周炎已成为牙医工作的核心部分和牙齿保健计划的一个重要方面。因此，确定合适的预防措施和最佳治疗策略变得非常重要。

寻求牙科治疗的患者主要关注的是消除疼痛和不适。患者期望治疗决策是基于现有的最佳证据所得，并希望了解不同治疗方案的优点和风险。牙医必须能够与患者分享基于循证的信息，以便患者能够根据其个人价值观和偏好选择治疗方法。通过互联网，患者可以轻易获得有关现有治疗方法的更多信息，并利用这些信息来质疑临床医生的建议。因此，牙医必须掌握向患者介绍能支持治疗程序的最新知识。

为了选择最适合患者的治疗方法，医生需要了解不同治疗方法的预后。治疗成功的可能性有多大？回答这个问题所需的信息只能由临床和流行病学研究提供[51]。根尖周炎通常是无症状的、慢性的，对根管治疗的评价主要是基于根尖周结构的影像学资料，而临床症状和体征可能有助于提供有关临床功能和患者满意度的额外信息。来自临床研究的信息代表了利用现有知识和治疗原则可以实现的最佳情况，而流行病学研究可以阐明牙科专业在控制和消除根尖周炎方面的成就。

此外，为了确定最佳治疗方法，必须确定"最佳"的含义。什么是相关结果，如何定义成功的结果？牙髓治疗结果研究通常集中在根尖周炎，并将成功定义为根尖周病变影像消失或减少。然而，对于患者来说，无痛、咀嚼功能恢复或保留牙齿可能是成功治疗的最重要方面。此外，在比较牙髓治疗和种植治疗的相对成功率时，还会出现其他并发症，因此需要可比较的疗效评估指标，但这些指标很少使用。"成功的治疗"有不同的含义，不同的研究可能难以比较结果。

本章节描述了目前关于根尖周炎预后的知识。这些知识来自使用临床和流行病学方法的研究。研究主要关注在严格控制的实验室条件下的患病机制或对技术设备的评估，这些结果很少直接适用于现实生活情况。传统的流行病学研究是调查疾病如何在不同人群或群体中发生和持续的，而临床研究则关注个体患者及其健康问题的治疗。流行病学方法也可用于分析疾病模式和确定预后因素。因此，流行病学信息对预防性医疗保健的规划和评估以及患者的指导和管理都是非常重要的。此外，在临床中，流行病学方法越来越多地被用于根据相似患者群体的研究结果对健康结果进行预测。临床流行病学在循证医学中发挥着核心作用，因此，需要对流行病学研究方法有基本的了解，从而了解不同研究的优缺点。基本流行病学术语解释见表5.1。

表 5.1　常见的流行病学术语

人口	一群人在一个特定的环境中
样本	人口中选定的一部分
选择偏差	由于样本的失真，系统性地高估或低估了结果
长度偏差	由于病程长的人所占比例过高，导致样本失真
信息偏差	由于不适当的数据收集或记录，高估或低估了结果
混杂因素	由与结果和相关研究因素相关的变量引起的系统性高估或低估结果
适应证的混杂因素	由于治疗程序不是随机选择的，而是由疾病的性质或调查诊所的标准程序所指导的，从而造成了混杂现象
暴露因素	一个被认为能引起疾病的研究因素
结果	衡量当前疾病的一个标准
患病率	在某一特定时间点，某种疾病的病例数量/比例
发病率	在一段时期内发生的新病例的数量/比例
风险	在特定时期内与结果相关的概率

5.2　流行病学的一般情况

世界卫生组织将流行病学定义为"研究健康相关状态或事件（包括疾病）的分布和决定因素，并将该研究应用于控制疾病和其他健康问题"[184]。流行病学调查根据研究目的分为描述性流行病学和分析性流行病学；更详细的解释见框表 5.1。

> **框表 5.1　定义**
>
> 世界卫生组织对流行病学的定义如下："流行病学是研究与健康有关的状态或事件（包括疾病）的分布和决定因素，并将这种研究用于控制疾病和其他健康问题。可以使用各种方法来进行流行病学调查：监测和描述性研究可以用来研究分布；分析性研究可以用来研究决定因素"[184]。
>
> 传统上，流行病学被划分为描述性流行病学和分析性流行病学。描述性流行病学涉及与健康有关的状态或事件的分布，其主要方面是人（何人）、地点（何地）和时间（何时）。分析性流行病学的重点是决定因素，即影响与健康有关的状态和事件发生的原因和其他条件（为什么，如何）。在这两种情况下，与健康有关的状态或事件（什么）必须被识别和适当地定义，这些事件被用来确定研究的结果。

传统上，牙科的重点是治疗牙齿，牙医可能认为流行病学研究的结果与他们的日常牙科实践不太相关。然而，许多重要问题的正确答案除了来自临床研究的信息外，还取决于流行病学数据。流行病学研究中不同的设计反映了所考虑问题的类型。框表 5.2 简要介绍了流行病学中最常用的设计方法。

> **框表 5.2　流行病学设计**
>
> 随机对照试验（RCT）：通常为比较两种治疗方法的效果而进行的试验，患者被随机分配到其中一个治疗组。
>
> 队列研究：一组人/患者从一个特定的时间点开始被追踪。起点可以定义为一个给定的日期，或一些事件，如治疗。在基于人群的队列研究中，参与者是从普通人群中选出的。在基于患者的队列研究中，参与者是来自一个或几个诊所的患者。在历史队列研究中，有时被称为回顾性队列研究，参与者在过去被确定，并跟踪到现在。
>
> 病例控制研究：一组病例，即患病的人或有不利结果的患者，将其过去的暴露史与从源人口（确定病例的人口）中选出的对照组的暴露史进行比较。许多不同类型的病例对照设计已经被开发出来。病例对照研究有时被称为回顾性研究；它们在牙髓病研究中很少使用。
>
> 横断面研究：在横断面研究中，在一个特定的时间点收集一组人的信息。这种设计可以估计疾病的流行率和某一条件在所选人群中的分布。在横断面研究中不能评估因果关系。

5.2.1　患病率

诸如"根尖周炎的发病率是多少，它与年龄、性别和其他个人特征有何关系？"和"哪些特异性因素和条件与根尖周炎的发生有关？"这样的问题与根尖周炎在人群中的患病率以及与疾病存在相关的因素有关，也与医疗保健规划和资源分配有关，通常通过横断面研究来解决，包括参与单次检查的个体样本。这可以快速了解该疾病在人群中的分布情况。结果通常是没有或存在根尖周炎，由二元变量或多个有序类别的评分系统来定义，这些类别反映了疾病的严重程度。

对健康和病变的根尖周牙槽骨进行分类的指标源自 1956 年 Strindberg 的一项研究[169]。Strindberg 对与牙髓治疗结果相关的因素进行了全面的纵向研究。牙周韧带的宽度、硬骨板的完整性和根尖周透射影的存在被当作根尖周疾病的主要指标。1967年，Brynolf通过比较人类尸检样本中根尖周病变的组织学和放射学表现，研究了组织学变化程度与放射线照片反映的关系[21]。该研究非常详细地描述了不同程度的根尖周炎的特征。Brynolf的研究为制定用于确定根尖周炎的五级指数，即根尖周指数（PAI）奠定了基础[128]。

为了提供有效信息，研究样本中的年龄、性别和其他相关因素的分布应反映人口的分布。随机抽样或分层随机抽样通常是满足这一要求的最佳方式。其他抽样方法可能会导致研究数据受到选择偏差的影响，其结果对社会或医疗保健规划人员的作用有限。1997至1998年，丹麦有两项研究的比较凸显了这一问题[87-88]；详情见框表5.3。

牙髓病学文献包括大量的横断面研究报告，其中许多报告是基于牙科学校或专科诊所的患者样本。表5.2给出了牙髓病学横断面研究的概要信息。图5.1显示了患有根尖周炎的个体比例、牙齿比例、根管充填的牙齿比例的长期趋势。

> **框表5.3**
>
> 1997至1998年，对居住在丹麦奥胡斯市的参与者进行了两项横断面研究。其中一项研究是基于对1935至1975年出生人群的随机抽样样本。在这个样本中，人群平均年龄为42.3岁，42%的人至少有一颗牙齿患有根尖周炎，52%的人至少有一颗根管充填的牙齿。另一项研究是基于1997至1998年在奥胡斯大学牙科学院征集的患者样本；该研究报告了患者在牙科学院接受治疗之前的牙髓状况。患者样本年龄稍大，平均年龄为45.8岁，但90%的患者至少有一颗牙齿患有根尖周炎，99%的患者至少有一颗根管充填过的牙齿。在牙科学院寻求治疗的患者的牙髓病状况和治疗需求与普通人群明显不同[87-88]。

5.2.2 发病率

"哪些因素和条件会影响根尖周炎的发病率？"这个问题涉及健康牙齿的疾病发展。横断面研究不能回答这个问题，因为它不包括时间维度，而且临床研究的重点是治疗而不是预防。制定适当的预防措施取决于对影响根尖周炎发病率的因素和条件的了解。这些知识只能从基于人群的队列研究中获得。基于人群的队列研究是观察性研究，可以研究疾病的自然发展及其在普通人群中的治疗情况。在特定时间内，对一组定义明确的人和（或）牙齿的疾病状况进行定期检查。健康和患病的人或牙齿都包括在内并被跟踪，对数据的分析可以确定从一次检查到下一次检查的与疾病状态变化有关的因素。检查的时间可能与治疗的时间不一致，因此，研究人员无法得知牙齿术前的确切状态，只能根据先前检查获得的信息进行估计。此外，关于术中因素的信息，如临床记录中的冲洗剂类型也很少体现。基于人群的队列研究通常依赖对疾病状态和根管充填质量的影像学评估。

基于人群的队列研究需要长时间的随访，而且通常成本高昂。此外，队列研究的成功与否取决于队列成员是否愿意继续参加检查。在牙髓病学文献中，该类型研究相对较少（表5.3）。

5.2.3 预后

一些重要问题与治疗预后有关，例如"疾病对特定治疗有反应的概率是多少？"或"哪些因素和条件影响治疗的预后？"目前，我们的知识主要来自临床研究。这些研究通常是一系列的病例，所有这些病例都接受了相同的治疗。有些研究通过随机/非随机分配对不同的治疗方法进行比较。

牙髓病学中的主要临床研究描述了对患者和（或）牙齿的治疗，这些患者和（或）牙齿从治疗开始一直被跟踪。在预定的时间段后或在共同的截止日期观察结果，因此，这种临床研究可以被视为基于患者的队列研究。基于患者的队列研究通常是由单个诊所的专家按照详细的方案进行，因此，结果可能无法直接解释其他机构或普遍情况。换句话说，外部有效性可能很低。

临床环境确保了患者档案的可用性，从而可以获取相关的临床信息，但基于患者的队列研究的成本高昂且耗时。有时，基于患者的队列研究依赖于从患者档案中检索到的前期治疗的信息；随后，新的检查可以提供结果信息，不需要等待随访信息，因此可以快速进行研究。然而，来自历史记录的信息可能因缺乏标准化和经常出现数据缺失而受限，这可能会影响研究的质量。这些研究通常被称为回顾性队列研究，或更准确地说是历史前瞻性队列研究；这样的研究在牙髓病学文献中很常见。表5.4给出了基于患者的队列研究的结果摘要。

表 5.2　以发生根尖周炎为结局的横断面研究的信息摘要

作者	国家	年份	人群	年龄	方法	人数	有根尖周炎的人群	牙齿数量	平均牙齿数量	有根尖周炎的牙齿	根管充填的牙齿	根管充填后仍有根尖周炎的牙齿
Bergenholtz 等人 (1973) [15] [42]	瑞典	1973	DSP	20~70+	F+P	240	57	5472	22.8	6%	12.5%	31%
Kerekes, Bervell (1976) [83]	挪威	1976	DSP	19~81	F	200	34.5	4832	24.2	2.8%	5.7%	25.4%
Allard, Palmqvist (1986) [5]	瑞典	1986	GP	>65	F	183	72	2567	14	9.8%	17.6%	27%
Petersson 等人 (1986) [141]	瑞典	1986	GP	–	I	861	–	4985	–	6.6%	13.3%	33.8%
Bergström 等人 (1987) [16]	瑞典	1987	GP[a]	21~60	F	250	46.8	6600	26.4	3.5%	6.5%	28.8%
Eckerbom 等人 (1987) [36]	瑞典	1987	PP	20~60+	F	200	63	4889	24.4	4.6%	13%	26.4%
Eriksen 等人 (1988) [43]	挪威	1988	GP	35	P+I	141	29.8	3917	27.8	1.4%	3.4%	25.6%
Petersson 等人 (1989) [140]	瑞典	1989	PP	–	F	567	76.5	11497	20.3	8.7%	22.2%	26.5%
Ödesjö 等人 (1990) [123]	瑞典	1990	GP	20~80+	F	967	33.2	17430	18.2	2.9%	8.6%	24.5%
Eriksen, Bjertness (1991) [42]	挪威	1991	GP	50	P+I	119	–	2940	24.7	3.5%	6%	36.6%
Imfeld (1991) [75]	瑞士	1991	GP	66	P+I	143	–	2004	14	8%	20.3%	31%
De Cleen 等人 (1993) [32]	荷兰	1993	PP	20~59+	P	184	44.6	4196	–	6%	2.3%	39.2%
Buckley, Spångberg (1995) [22]	美国	1995	DSP	–	F	208	–	5272	25.3	4.1%	5.5%	31.3%
Eriksen 等人 (1995) [41]	挪威	1995	GP	35	P	118	14.4	3282	27.8	0.5%	1.3%	38.1%
Soikkonen (1995) [168]	芬兰	1995	GP	76~86	P+I	169	41.4	2355	13.9	6.6%	21.5%	16.8%
Saunders 等人 (1997) [154]	英格兰	1997	DSP	20~59+	F	340	67.7	8420	–	4.6%	5.6%	58.1%
Weiger 等人 (1997) [182]	德国	1997	PP	12~89	P+I	323	–	7897	24.4	3.1%	2.7%	60.9%
Marques 等人 (1998) [107]	葡萄牙	1998	GP	30~39	P+I	179	26	4446	–	2%	1.6%	21.7%
Sidaravicius 等人 (1999) [161]	立陶宛	1999	GP	25~44	P+I	147	70	3892	26.5	7.2%	15.1%	35%
De Moor 等人 (2000) [33]	比利时	2000	DSP	18~59+	P	206	63.1	4617	–	6.6%	6.8%	40.4%
Kirkevang 等人 (2001) [88]	丹麦	2001	GP	20~60+	F	614	42.3	15984	26	3.4%	4.8%	52.3%
Boucher 等人 (2002) [20]	法国	2002	DSP	18~70+	F	208	–	5373	–	7.4%	19.1%	29.6%
Lupi-Pegurier 等人 (2002) [105]	法国	2002	DSP	>20	P	344	–	7561	22	7.3%	18.9%	31.5%

表 5.2（续）

作者	国家	年份	人群	年龄	方法	人数	有根尖周炎的人群	牙齿数量	平均牙齿数量	有根尖周炎的牙齿	根管充填的牙齿	根管充填后仍有根尖周炎的牙齿
Ridell 等人 (2006)[148]	瑞典	2006	GP	19	-	-	-	-	-	-	-	-
Dugas 等人 (2003)[35]	加拿大	2003	DSP	25~40	F+P+I	610	-	16 148	26.5	3.1%	2.5%	45.4%
Jiménez-Pinzón 等人 (2004)[78]	西班牙	2004	DSP	-	F	180	61.1	4453	-	4.2%	2.1%	64.5%
Georgopoulou 等人 (2005)[56]	希腊	2005	PP	16~77	F	320	85.9	7664	24	13.6%	8.9%	60%
Kabak, Abbott (2005)[80]	白俄罗斯	2005	DSP	15~65+	P	1423	80	31 212	-	11.7%	20.3%	45.2%
Loftus 等人 (2005)[103]	I 爱尔兰	2005	DSP	16~75+	P	302	33.1	7424	24.6	2%	2%	25%
Tsuneishi 等人 (2005)[177]	日本	2005	DSP	20~89	F	672	69.8	16 232	-	9.4%	20.5%	40%
Peciuliene 等人 (2006)[133]	立陶宛	2006	DSP	-	F	83	-	2186	26.3	-	12.9%	43.1%
Skudutyte-Rysstad 等人 (2006)[165]	挪威	2006	GP	35	P	146	16	3971	27.2	1.1%	1.5%	42.6%
Chen 等人 (2007)[25]	美国	2007	GP	-	P	244	-	3533	14.5	5.1%	4.8%	35.5%
Sunay 等人 (2007)[171]	土耳其	2007	DSP	-	P	375	-	8863	-	4.2%	5.3%	51.1%
Touré 等人 (2008)[175]	塞内加尔	2008	F	-	F	208	-	6234	30	4.7%	2.6%	-
Gulsahi 等人 (2008)[60]	土耳其	2008	DSP	-	P	1000	23.8	24 344	-	1.4%	3.3%	18.2%
Hollanda 等人 (2008)[68]	巴西	2008	PP	48[b]	P	1401	-	29 467	-	-	21.4%	-
Da Silva 等人 (2009)[30]	澳大利亚	2009	DSP	-	P	243	-	5647	23.24	-	8.8%	21.6%
Al-Omari 等人 (2011)[3]	约旦	2011	DSP	16~59	P	294	83.7	7390	-	11.6%	5.7%	71.9%
Matijevic 等人 (2011)[109]	克罗地亚	2011	PP	-	P	1462	76.9	38 440	-	8.5%	8.5%	54%
Peters 等人 (2011)[134]	荷兰	2011	PP	18~59+	P	178	36.5	4594	25.8	2.6%	4.9%	24.1%
Gumru 等人 (2011)[61]	土耳其	2011	DSP	19	P	1077	-	28 974	26.9	2.2%	-	42%
Lopez-Lopez 等人 (2012)[104]	西班牙	2012	DSP	19~70	P	397	34	9390	-	2.8%	6.4%	23.8%
Kalender 等人 (2012)[81]	巴西	2012	DSP	18~50	P+I	1006	68	24 730	-	7%	8.9%	62%
Huumonen 等人 (2012)[73]	芬兰	2012	GP	30~95	P	5244	-	120 250	22.9	-	7%	-

表 5.2（续）

作者	国家	年份	人群	年龄	方法	人数	有根尖周炎的人群	牙齿数量	平均牙齿数量	有根尖周炎的牙齿	根管充填的牙齿	根管充填后仍有根尖周炎的牙齿
Jersa, Kundzina (2013)[77]	拉脱维亚	2013	PP	35~44	P	312	72	7 065	—	7%	18%	30.5%
Hebling 等人 (2014)[67]	巴西	2014	GP	60~94	F	98	42.9	942	11.6%	12.1%	13.4%	65.1%
Berlinck 等人 (2015)[18]	巴西	2015	DSP	0~60+	F	1126	—	25 292	—	7.9%	6.9%	16.7%
Oginni 等人 (2015)[124]	尼日利亚	2015	DSP	—	F	756	67.2	21 468	—	—	12.2%	41%
Huumonen 等人 (2017)[72]	芬兰	2017	GP	30~95	P	5335	27	120 635	—	—	—	39%
Kielbassa 等人 (2017)[85]	澳大利亚	2017	PP	18~70	P	1000	60.5	22 586	—	6.4%	11%	42.6%

DSP：牙科学院患者。GP：一般人群。PP：患者人群。P：全景照片。I：口内X线片。F：全面口腔检查。a. 普通诊所患者。b. 平均年龄

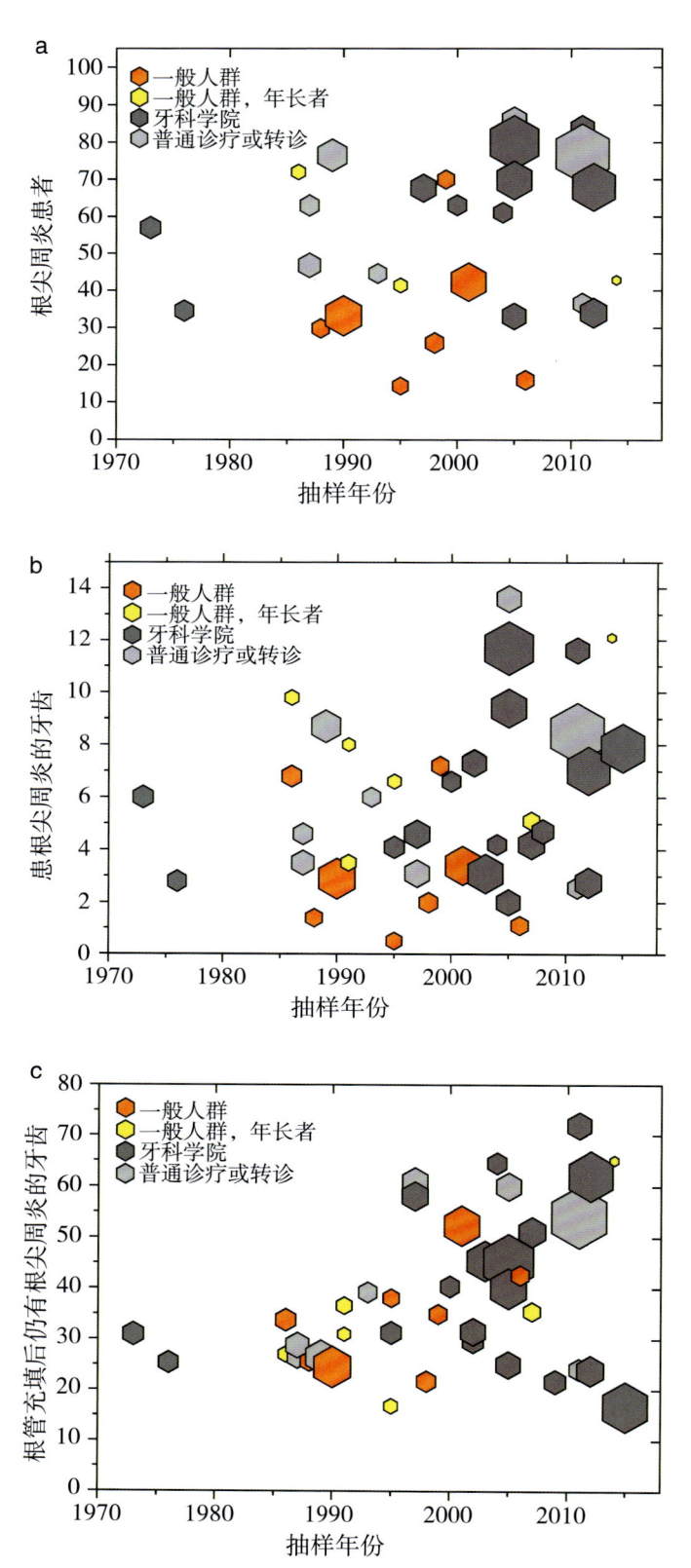

牙髓病学基础：根尖周炎的预防和治疗

图 5.1 a. 拥有一至多颗患根尖周炎牙齿的人的比例。b. 患根尖周炎的牙齿的比例。c. 根管充填牙齿患根尖周炎的比例。泡泡的大小反映出研究规模的大小

表 5.3 关于人群队列研究的信息摘要

研究人员	年份	国家	患者数	随访时间/月	有根尖周炎的人群	AP 占比	根管充填人群	RF 占比	牙齿数	平均牙齿数	AP 牙齿数	AP 牙占比	RF 牙齿数	RF 牙占比	RF 后有 AP 牙齿数	RF 后 AP 牙占比
Petersson 等人 (1991/1993)[137, 139] [a]	1974	瑞典	351	—	—	25%	—	46%	2100	6	107	5.1%	258	12.3%	82	31.8%
	1985	瑞典	345	120	—	29%	—	52%	1962	5.7	121	5.9%	323	16.5%	94	29.1%
Frisk 等人 (2005)[53]	1968	瑞典	1220	—	—	41.9%	—	18.3%	24156	19.8	—	0.7%[b]	—	3.4%	—	—
	1980	瑞典	1023	144	—	41.9%	—	22.1%	20255	19.8	—	0.6%[b]	—	4%	—	—
	1992	瑞典	867	288	—	31.1%[c++]	—	21.9%	17253	19.9	—	0.5%[b]	—	3.8%	—	—
Eckerbom 等人 (2007)[38][c]	1975	瑞典	200	—	126	63%	—	83.5%	4889	24.4	255	5.2%	636	13%	168	26.4%
	1980	瑞典	(200)	60	44	61.7%	98	85.2%	2825	24.6	97	3.3%	393	13.9%	68	17.3%
	2002	瑞典	115	240	42	63.2%	100	87%	2461	21.4	168	6.8%	598	24.3%	93	21.4%
Kirkevang 等人 (2012)[92]	1997	丹麦	616	—	259	42%	319	51.8%	16016	26.0	534	3.3%	776	4.8%	402	51.8%
	2003	丹麦	473	60	236	49.9%	279	58.4%	12345	26.1	461	3.7%	705	5.7%	311	44.4%
	2008	丹麦	360	120	189	52.5%	214	59.4%	9360	26.0	395	4.2%	543	5.8%	233	42.9%

AP: 根尖周炎。RF: 根管充填。a: 磨牙和前磨牙。b: 均数。c: 早期患者未源于影像检查

表 5.4 以根尖周炎愈合为结果的患者队列研究信息摘要

研究	年份	国家	设计	患者数	牙齿数	根管数	随访月份	根尖周炎比例	愈合 无根尖周炎	愈合 根尖周炎	总体情况
Strindberg[169]	1956	瑞典	ClinCoh	254	529	—	6~120	42%	93%	88%	90%
Seltzer 等人[158]	1963	美国	ClinCoh	2784	2921	—	6	—	94%	76%	84%
Engström[40]	1964	美国	ClinCoh	—	306	—	48~60	53	88%	76%	82%
Harty 等人[65]	1970	英国	HistProsp	—	1139	1139	24+/6~24	—	—	—	90%
Jokinen 等人[79]	1978	芬兰	HistProsp	1199	1782	2459	24~84	33	61%	38%	53%
Kerekes 等人[82]	1979	挪威	HistProsp	—	—	501	36~60	34	92%	89%	90%
Barbakow 等人[10]	1980	南非	HistProsp	—	332	—	12+	—	—	—	87%
Oliet[125]	1983	美国	ClinCoh	—	153	—	18	—	—	—	89%[a]
Swartz 等人[172]	1983	美国	HistProsp	—	1007	1770	12+	—	—	—	88%[a]
Byström 等人[24]	1987	瑞典	HistProsp	53	—	79	24~60	100	—	85%	84%
Ørstavik 等人[129]	1987	挪威	ClinCoh	102	—	546	12	29	—	—	82%
Eriksen 等人[44]	1988	挪威	ClinCoh	67	—	121	36	100	—	82%	90%
Sjögren 等人[164]	1990	瑞典	HistProsp	356	—	849	96~120	24	96%	86%	53%
Smith 等人[167]	1993	英国	HistProsp	—	821	—	60+	—	—	75%	90%
Ørstavik[126]	1996	挪威	HistProsp	—	—	599	48	—	94%	75%	87%
Sjögren 等人[163]	1997	瑞典	ClinCoh	53	—	—	60+	100	—	—	89%[a]
Trope 等人[176]	1999	美国	RCT	102	—	—	12	—	—	—	88%[a]
Weiger 等人[183]	2000	德国	RCT	67	894	—	12~60	100	—	—	74%
Benenati 等人[13]	2002	美国	HistProsp	—	—	—	6~72	—	—	—	62%(91%[a])
Hoskinson 等人[69]	2002	英国	HistProsp	167	200	489	48~60	70	88%	74%	77%
Peters 等人[135]	2002	荷兰	RCT	38	—	—	12~54	100	—	—	76%
Huumonen 等人[70]	2003	芬兰	RCT	156	—	—	12	100	—	—	76%
Peters 等人[136]	2004	瑞士	HistProsp	179	233	—	12~36	44	95%	76%	87%

根尖周炎的流行病学、疗效和风险因素 | 第 5 章

表 5.4（续）

研究	年份	国家	设计	患者数	牙齿数	根管数	随访月份	根尖周炎比例	愈合 无根尖周炎	愈合 根尖周炎	总体情况
Marending 等人[106]	2005	瑞士	ClinCoh	66	—	—	30	52	—	—	88%
Negishi 等人[115]	2005	日本	HistProsp	57	114	—	12+	—	—	—	85%
Marquis 等人[108]	2006	加拿大	HistProsp	325	373	—	48~72	57	93%	80%	85%
Doyle 等人[34]	2007	美国	HistProsp	—	196	—	12+	65	87%	75%	82%
Gilbert 等人[58]	2010	美国	PracBased	—	115	—	14~343	49	81%	60%	71%
Riccucci 等人[147]	2011	意大利	ClinCoh	470	816	1369	60	53	92%	83%	89%
Ng 等人	2011	英国	ClinCoh	534	702	1170	24~48	66	—	—	87%
Ng 等人[118]	2011	英国	ClinCoh	—	1617	—	24~48	—	—	—	95b%
Setzer 等人[159]	2011	美国	HistProsp	42	50	—	48+	36	—	—	52%(96%[b])
Bernstein 等人[19]	2012	美国	ClinCoh	1312	—	—	36~60	—	—	—	89[b]%
Arya 等人[7]	2017	—	ClinCoh	46	200	—	12	100	—	—	62%
Barborka 等人[11]	2017	美国	HistProsp	—	100	—	60~72	—	—	—	72%
Pirani 等人[143]	2017	加拿大	HistProsp	94	193(213)	—	60	83	—	—	85%(88%[b])
He 等人[66]	2017	美国	ClinCoh	54	54	—	12	—	—	—	69%

ClinCoh: 临床队列。HistProsp: 历史前瞻性。RCT: 随机对照试验。PracBased: 基于实践。a. 治愈。b. 存留

5.2.4 患病率与发病率

上述描述表明，研究设计和研究环境的选择取决于所要解决的问题。此外，必须认识到患病率和发病率之间的区别。患病率描述了特定时间内人群中疾病的状况，因此给出了疾病分布的静态图像。发病率与疾病的动态有关；在目前情况下，它描述了根尖周炎在人群中随时间推移的发生情况，通常被量化为发生率或在特定时间间隔内新增病例的比例。愈合和拔牙描述了疾病动态的其他方面。在讨论与根尖周炎有关的情况时，区分患病率和发病率也很重要。某一群体的高患病率可能反映了发病率的增加，但愈合延迟或不愿意寻求治疗也是可能的原因。因此，与疾病流行相关的条件不一定是降低发病率的预防措施的潜在目标。

众所周知，横断面抽样会导致样本长度偏差，因为采用这种抽样方法时，患病时间较长的个体会占比过高。图 5.2 说明了这种现象。水平线代表了一些牙齿从治疗到痊愈的时间段。图中显示了两种恢复类型，一组牙齿恢复速度较慢；另一组牙齿迅速愈合。这两种类型的发生率相同，但在横断面样本中，在垂直线表示的图中，恢复缓慢的牙齿占主导地位。根尖周组织中超填的根管充填材料可能会延长愈合期，因此在患有根尖周炎的根管充填后牙齿的横断面样本中，此类牙齿的占比过高，根管超填的影响会被高估。

系统评价和 meta 分析经常被用来获取关于特定研究问题的更多信息，例如年龄对根管治疗结果的影响[160]。如果这种评价和（或）meta 分析所包括的研究是同质的，病例的积累可能会提高评估的确定性。然而，研究结果往往相差甚远，难以获得有效的结论[119]。图 5.3 概述了不同类型的研究和证据在提供证据的强度方面的差别。

5.3 流行病学研究的要素

对患者或牙齿的牙髓病学研究通常侧重于根尖周炎的治疗或预防，因此其典型的结果描述是从根尖片上观察到的根尖病损的缺失、减轻或消除。尽管已有具有精确分类的指数系统或量表用于描述疾病范围和严重程度[113, 128, 149]，但在已发表的研究中，通常只是根据结果量表上的合适分界点将治疗结果划分为"成功"或"失败"。对不同研究的成功率进行有效比较需要使用具有相同分界点的结果量表来定义成功，并且采用相同类型的影像学照片来评估结果。此外，治疗结果评价的时机也很重要，随访时间的长度应该反映出所选择的结果。对于愈合来说，1 年到数年的随访时间可能是合适的；对于牙齿保存来说，则需要更长的随访时间（可能是 5~10 年）。在报告横断面研究的结果时，使用"成功-失败"的术语可能产生进一步的混淆。为了得出治疗成功的结论，必须观察疾病状态的改善情况，因此需要对病例、患者或牙齿进行反复的随访评价。

即使由经过培训和标准校准的观察者按照定义明确的量表进行评估，其结果也会出现错误分

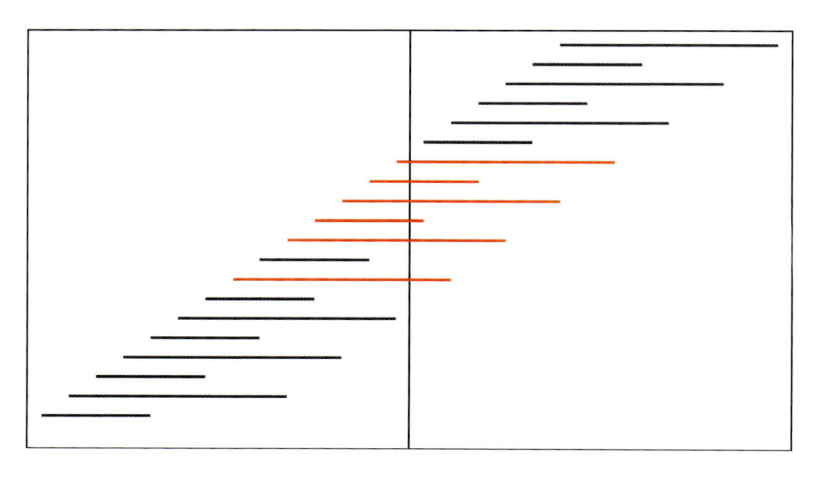

图 5.2 横断面样本的长度偏差。水平线代表一些牙齿从治疗到愈合的时间段。显示了两种同样频次的恢复类型：一组牙齿的恢复速度很慢，另一组则很快愈合。垂直线代表横断面研究的取样时间。包括在横断面样本中的牙齿的水平线为红色。这个样本中，恢复缓慢的牙齿占多数

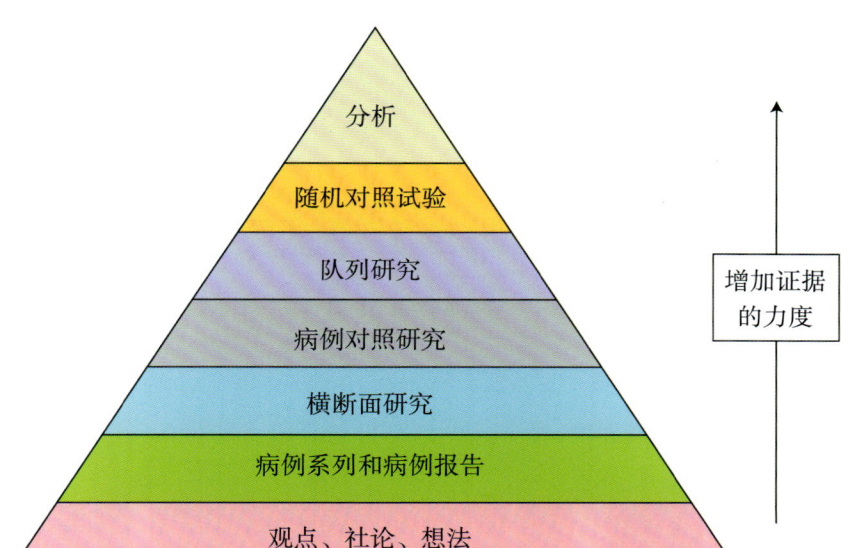

图 5.3 证据金字塔显示了不同研究设计和信息来源的证据的相对强度

类或测量误差（图 5.4）。因此，评分系统的可靠性和有效性也很重要。可靠性主要与测量的可重复性有关：如果对同一图像进行多次评估，经过培训的观察者是否总是给出相同的分数？训练有素的观察者出现意见不一致的频率是多少？有效性主要是衡量评价的真实性。尽管在临床环境中，真实值是未知的，但体外实验可以对来源于不同成像技术的结果进行组织学评估，从而确定测量方法的有效性。遗憾的是，用于描述测量方法的术语并不统一；同一属性有多个名称，而给定的名称也可能具有不同的含义。因此，近年来，为了在测量特性术语和定义方面形成国际共识而设立了 COSMIN 清单[110-111]，表 5.5 展示了该清单和其他常用的术语。

当确定相关结果后，下一个问题是如何获得或评估结果以及希望纳入研究的决定因素。同样，答案取决于研究目的。如果研究目的是对大量人群的牙齿健康情况进行全面描述，采用全景片可能比较方便，并且能够提供足够的信息，如根管充填的牙齿的数量。如果研究的重点是根尖周炎的愈合，以根尖指数作为结果，根管填充质量为可能的决定因素，则需要使用根尖 X 线片。此外，如果是以患者的症状或者满意度作为治疗结果，则可以不需要任何影像学信息。

5.4 流行病学数据的评估

5.4.1 数据结构

统计学评价在流行病学中至关重要。标准的统计学方法假设各观测值之间相互独立，但在牙科研究中，所谓的多级数据很常见，因此通常需要对此进行特殊考虑。"多级"一词反映了用于描述患者的信息是统一的，如年龄、性别和吸烟习惯；而与患者牙齿相关的信息存在差异，如牙齿类型、冠修复情况。在牙髓病学研究中，研究数据通常来源于个体、牙齿、牙根，偶尔还会来源于根管；而在数据分析时，通常选择个体和牙齿作为分析单位。当在个体层面评估结果时，通常应假设研究具有独立性。以牙齿为分析单位时，通常预期从同一个体获得的结果之间存在正

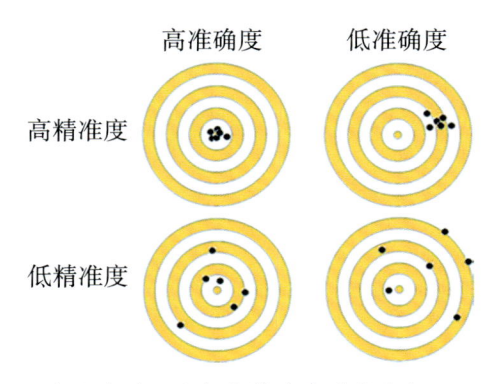

图 5.4 准确度（效度）和精确度（信度）

表 5.5 常见的测量性质相关术语

测量误差和错误分类	
有效性	COMSIN 专家组[110]将"有效性"定义为"测量工具或手段能够测出所需测量的事物的准确程度"。"准确性"是该属性的另一个常用名称。在统计学中则使用"无偏性"。
可靠性	COMSIN 专家组[110]将"可靠性"定义为"测量结果不存在测量误差的程度"。其他常用名称包括"可重复性""可再现性"。在统计学中通常表示为精度。
与疾病状态测量相关的术语，如存在或不存在	
灵敏度	对患病个体进行正确分类的概率
特异度	对健康个体进行正确分类的概率
阳性预测值	被分类为患病的个体被正确分类的概率
阴性预测值	被分类为健康的个体被正确分类的概率
ROC 曲线	是受试者工作特征曲线，是以灵敏度和 1- 特异度反映诊断阈值变化的图

相关；而不同个体的牙齿则被认为是相互独立的。部分依赖性可以用已知的因素和条件解释，如果有可用的数据，可以根据其影响调整统计分析。但如果在统计分析中忽略了结果之间的正相关性，数据的不确定性将被低估，置信区间将变窄，从而高估了研究的准确性。在以牙齿为单位的分析中，在诸如吸烟者与非吸烟者个体之间更容易受到这种偏倚的影响，而在诸如有冠修复体与没有冠修复体的个体之间的比较受到的影响较小。Strindberg（1956）[169] 在其统计学附录部分仔细研究了同一牙齿的两个牙根和同一患者的两个牙齿之间治疗结果的相互依赖性，他的分析数据表明这两种情况下得到的数据确实具备一定的相关性，但这种相关性并不是很强。框表 5.4 中的示例说明了同一患者口腔内牙齿治疗结果之间的关联性。

框表 5.4

一项基于丹麦人群开展的队列研究中，比较了吸烟和非吸烟患者 5 年内根尖周炎的发病率。以牙齿作为单位的 Logistic 回归分析结果显示吸烟患者相较于非吸烟患者的优势比（OR）为 1.77。当忽略来源于同一个体的牙齿数据的相关性时，优势比的 95% 可信区间为（1.40，2.23），而当将数据相关性纳入考虑后，可信区间变宽为（1.32，2.35）[91]。

关于决定因素、潜在风险因素或预后因素相关的数据同样是多层次的。当分析单位是牙齿，即在牙齿水平上测量时，有关根管和牙根水平的信息会汇聚到牙齿层面上；对于多根牙而言，根管充填的质量不是以每个牙根的分数表示，而是汇总为一个分数。同样，当以个体作为分析单位时，牙齿层面的风险因素会汇总到个体层面，如根管填充牙齿的数量或去牙冠的数量。

5.4.2 观察性研究中混杂因素的校正

实验性研究中，研究者在设计时可以确保实验的平衡性，即分配到不同治疗组的实验个体是相似的。而在流行病学研究中，大多数研究是观察性的；研究者是观察者，不能影响治疗或干预的分配。

牙髓病学的流行病学研究通常是观察性研究，因此，为了准确评估某一特定因素对结果的影响，有必要对混杂偏倚的影响进行校正，即与研究结果和所研究的因素相关的因素。在对混杂偏倚不校正或校正不完全的情况下对每个因素进行单独分析，可能会导致对风险因素与结果之间关联的估计出现偏差。因此，为了确定某一特定因素的影响，必须在分析中纠正所有已知的混杂因素。此外，对于校正程度不同的研究结果可能无法进行有效的比较。框表 5.5 中提供的示例说明了上述问题的重要性。

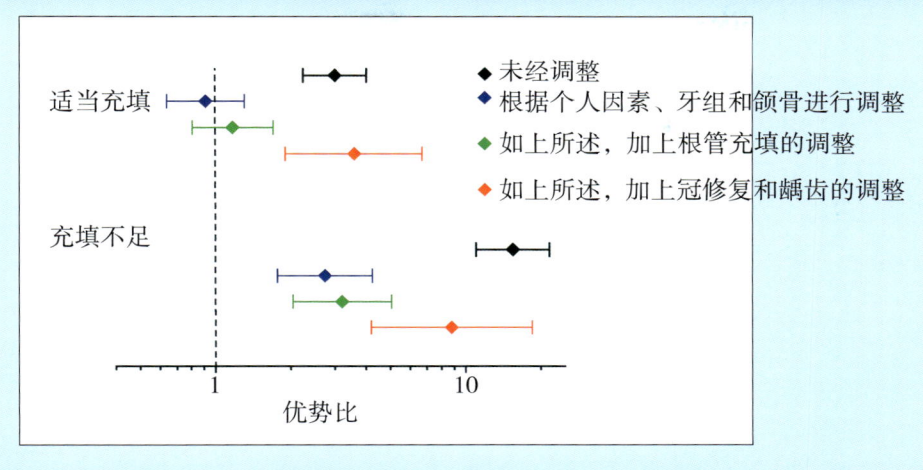

框表 5.5 不同混杂因素校正的比较

上图显示了校正混杂因素对冠部充填质量与根尖周炎发病率之间关联的影响。该关联用优势比来描述，并根据 5 年内根尖周炎发病率数据的 Logistic 回归分析结果进行估计。图中菱形代表相对于无冠部充填的牙齿，冠部充填良好的牙齿（顶部）和冠部充填不良的牙齿（底部）根尖周炎的优势比估计值，95% 可信区间与估计值一起显示为条形图。

如图所示的结果来自四种不同的分析。这四种分析对其他风险因素的校正程度有报不同。第一个结果是一个简单的未经校正的分析，第二个结果包括对个体特定因素（性别、年龄、吸烟习惯）、牙齿因素（前牙、前磨牙、磨牙）和颌骨因素的校正。校正后的估计值大大降低，冠部封闭良好的优势比与 1 无显著差异。第三次分析中估计值略有增加，其中包含了对存在牙根充填的校正。在最后的分析中，纳入了对牙冠和龋病的校正，对 OR 估计值的大小有很大影响。这一变化说明牙冠的存在增加了患根尖周炎的风险，而在之前的分析中，这些牙齿被归类为没有冠部填充物的牙齿，导致低估了与冠部填充物相关的风险。这个例子说明了在分析中对所有混杂因素校正的重要性，以及对不同校正程度的研究的估计值之间无法进行正确比较（数据来源于文献 91）

5.4.3 回归模型

回归分析常用于混杂因素的校正，而选取何种类型的回归模型则取决于所选结果的类型。详见框表 5.6。

框表 5.6

结果数据的类型和其相对应的回归模型

数据类型	回归模型
二分类资料	Logistic 回归
多分类资料	多元 Logistic 回归
等级资料	有序 Logistic 回归
计数资料	泊松回归，负二项回归
计量资料、正态误差	多元回归

先进的统计软件包含上述各种回归模型数据分析的模块（如 SAS、Stata、R 语言等）。需要注意的是，校正混杂因素的回归分析和具备多个预测因子的预测模型可能需要大样本数据才能产生可靠的结果。从计算机模拟中得出的经验法则表明，对于 Logistic 回归，其模型中拟合的每个参数的记录数至少应有 15 个样本。类似的原则同样适用于其他回归模型，有关回归分析策略选择问题的更全面的讨论请参阅 Harrell 的著作的第 4 章[64]。

许多统计软件包都包含一些选项，允许校正来自同一个体的样本结果之间的相关性。由于相关的方法策略众多，超出了本章节涉及的范围，在此不做详细描述。Kirkwood 和 Sterne 的著作（2003）[95] 简要概述了可用的方法。

在关于根尖周炎发病率的队列研究中，以是否存在根尖周炎作为每颗牙齿的结果时，一种更简单的方法可能有用。如果研究主要关注牙齿的特异性风险因子，那么个体的特异性风险因子就是混杂偏倚，需要对其影响进行校正。通过条件性 Logistic 回归分析对同一个体牙齿比较的分析可能是一种更为方便的选择，其可以自动校正已测量的和未测量的个体特异性因素。

了解治疗结果的总体成功率很有意义，因为它为我们提供了在不同环境和不同人群中取得的成果的信息。但是，为了准确评价不同个体治疗的预后，应将患者个体、患牙以及治疗术前、术中、术后的因素都纳入考虑。

5.5 与治疗结果相关的因素和条件

当牙齿出现根尖周炎时，医生必须决定是否对患牙进行处理以及应当采取何种治疗手段。不同治疗手段的预后一方面取决于患牙，另一方面取决于患者。在不同的治疗方案中，医生必须具体评估治疗过程的各个方面是否会影响最终的治疗成功。目前可用于评估预后的信息主要来自探究牙齿因素和患者个体因素与牙髓疾病关联的队列研究。由于不同的因素是相互关联的，因此病情和治疗结果之间的明显关联实际上可能混杂了其他因素的效应。因此，单因素分析可能无法提供有效的预后判断。与预后相关的因素和条件通常被称为预后因素，如果关注的是治疗失败相关的因素，则称为风险因素。接下来，我们将列举一些与预防和治疗根尖周炎相关的个体或牙齿的预后因素。值得一提的是，关注的重点是根尖周炎愈合的结果，但是基于牙齿存活率以及患者相关结果的信息同样很重要。

5.5.1 治疗效果

5.5.1.1 根尖周疾病

大多数牙髓病学研究的重点都是通过传统的 X 线片评估根尖周炎的存在，有时还辅以有关临床症状的信息，但很少有研究报道与治疗后牙齿存活率和患者满意度相关的结果。

根据报道，初次根管治疗的成功率从70%到90%以上[12, 98, 119, 181]。这些信息主要来源于过往的前瞻性队列研究，如 Ng 等人[119]的综述。尽管综述被认为是循证医学中最高等级的证据，但综述的准确性主要取决于所纳入研究的质量，而回顾性研究结果的准确性是值得怀疑的。

在以患者为基础的队列研究中，初次根管治疗的成功率为70%至90%以上（图5.5）。这些研究通常是在具备高度质量控制的环境下进行的，由来自专科诊所或牙科学校的学生、研究生或教师等人进行临床操作，其代表了在理想条件下对选定的患者进行治疗所能取得的结果。

大多数已发表的研究结果主要针对初次根管治疗的成功率，或者没有区分初次治疗和再治疗。根据一项针对根管再治疗成功率的综述报道，再治疗成功率为78%~82%[118]。

在基于人群的队列研究中，由于研究人群的不同，估计的治疗成功率的差异较大。在美国私立机构，治疗成功率可高达89%[185]，然而在该人群中，治疗前的根尖周炎发生率仅有13%。而在丹麦开展的一项研究发现，治疗成功率仅

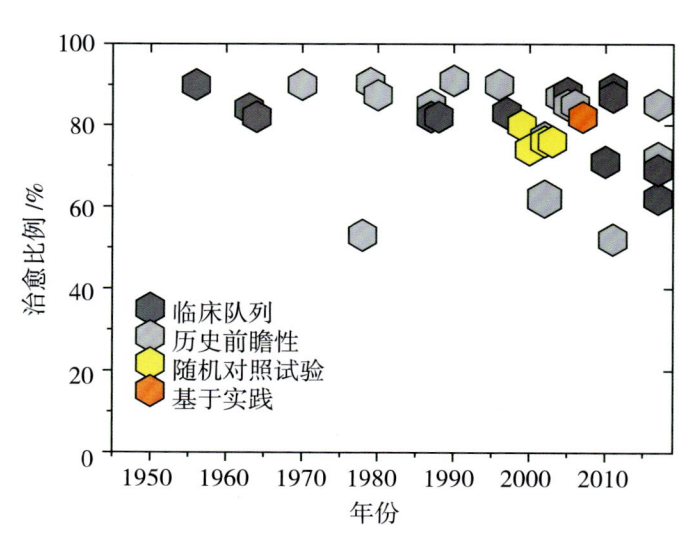

图 5.5 基于患者队列研究的根管治疗结果。根据研究进行的年份绘制成功治疗的比例，并根据研究的类型分层

有59%，而根尖周炎在该人群中的发生率高达42%[92]。在瑞典的一项研究中，32%的牙齿治疗前存在根尖周炎，这些患牙的成功率为33%。而当治疗前没有根尖周炎时，83%的患牙在10年后也没有发生根尖周炎[137]。近来，瑞典一家公立医院的研究报告指出，根尖周炎的发病率约为61%，治疗后3年的成功率为58%[97]。很少有基于人群的队列研究对再治疗结果进行评估。在丹麦开展的一项研究中，26%的患者根尖周病损在5年内痊愈，但10年后，治疗成功率达到50%[92]。

基于人群的队列研究结果表明，在综合医院进行的牙髓治疗的成功率低于专科医院。尽管横断面研究不能用于准确估计治疗成功率，但这些研究中发现的根尖周炎患病率能够反映人群的总体治疗结果和治疗策略（表5.2，图5.1a~c）。

5.5.1.2 与患者相关的结果

根据综述报告，术后1周患者牙齿疼痛的发生率约为14%[132]。最近的一项研究证实了这一点，其中90%的患者在牙髓治疗后7d没有或几乎没有疼痛[114]，而在随访6个月后，疼痛发生率降低到5%左右[122]，这一结果与近期开展的一项基于患者的队列研究一致，该研究还指出，少于5%的患者在根管治疗后3~5年内会出现持续性疼痛[19, 179]。

5.5.1.3 根管充填后牙齿的保存情况

根管治疗的目的是消除牙髓疾病，以帮助患者在无痛的状态下保存牙齿功能。尽管根管治疗后的牙齿相较于未治疗牙齿的存留率更低（表5.6），但在部分人群中治疗后牙齿的存留率可以达到较高水平。

一项为期2~10年的关于根管治疗后牙齿存活率的回顾研究发现，在以患者为基础的队列研究中，根管治疗后牙齿的存留率为86%~93%[117]，近期的类似研究也证实了该结果，报告显示患牙的十年生存率分别为86%和81.5%[23, 100]。与此同时，保险数据显示约90%的经过根管治疗的牙齿在5~10年后仍保留在口腔内[52, 150, 151]。

在一项基于普通人群的观察性研究中，大约90%根管充填后的牙齿在治疗后10年内得以在口腔内留存[93, 139]；而在另一项长达20年的研究中，留存率约为70%[38]。牙齿保存与否同样取决于人群，如在瑞典人群中开展的调查指出接受高成本牙科护理的人群，20年后患牙留存率只有65%[138]。总体而言，大多数根管治疗后的患牙在10~20年内得以保留。

表5.6 5年（A组）和10年（B组）后非根管充填牙和根管充填牙的损失情况。百分比和相对风险[92]

A组					
根管充填与否	丢失与否（2003）				
1997*	是	否	总计	百分比	相对风险
否	65	11 754	11 819	0.50%	
是	42	579	621	6.80%	12.3
合计	107	12 333	12 440	0.90%	

*473例

B组					
根管充填与否	丢失与否（2008）				
1997**	是	否	总计	百分比	相对风险
否	122	8952	9074	1.30%	
是	57	398	455	12.50%	9.3
合计	179	9350	9529	1.90%	

**360例

5.5.2 个体特异性风险因素

5.5.2.1 性别

大部分研究指出，性别对于根管治疗的结果影响微乎其微，一些研究表明女性的成功率略高，而另一些研究则相反[69, 91,116,118,120,147]。

总体而言，牙髓治疗的结果与性别无关这一结论似乎更稳妥。

5.5.2.2 年龄

横断面研究显示，老年人中根管治疗牙齿和根尖周炎的患病率较高。此外，老年人有根管治疗后的牙齿的概率更高[63]。

然而，在以人群为基础的队列研究中，根管治疗牙齿的根尖周炎的发生似乎与年龄或研究人群无关[53, 91, 137]。一些研究表明，至少有一颗牙齿存在根管充填物的比例随着年龄的增长而增加。这可能会影响根尖周炎的总体发病率，因为根管充填后的牙齿比正常牙齿更容易发生根尖周炎。如果不拔牙，根尖周炎的发病率就会累积，形成年龄依赖性。其他研究表明，年龄对根尖周炎患者影响不大，甚至随着年龄增长而略有下降[37, 53]。最近一项以患者为基础的队列研究得出结论，患者的年龄不是非手术根管治疗的预后因素[160]。

总之，老年人也许比年轻人更有可能患有根尖周炎，特别是在很少拔牙的情况下，但患者的年龄不应被视为根管治疗结果的预后因素。

5.5.2.3 吸烟

横断面研究和队列研究都曾调查过吸烟对根尖周炎的影响，但结果相互矛盾。6项横断面研究中有5项发现根尖周炎的存在与吸烟之间存在显著的正相关关系；一项基于人群的队列研究表明接受根管治疗的风险增加，而一项基于人群和一项基于患者的队列研究发现吸烟对根尖周炎的发展没有统计学意义上的显著影响[180]。

吸烟可能会延迟愈合，吸烟习惯可能与不良的生活方式选择有关。但在决定是否进行根管治疗时，不应将吸烟视为风险因素。

5.5.2.4 社会经济状况

在以患者为基础的队列研究中，尚未对社会经济状况对治疗结果的影响进行探究。横断面研究表明，在对牙齿状况进行调整后，个人的社会经济状况并不能提供更多有关根尖周状况的信息[4, 54, 94]。

总之，患者的社会经济状况与根尖周炎的发生无关，也不太可能影响根管治疗的预后。

5.5.2.5 全身健康状况

大多数以患者为基础的队列研究排除了患有一般疾病的患者。因此，很难对患者的全身健康状况对治疗效果的影响进行可靠的评估。在Strindberg（1956年）的研究中[169]，没有发现患者全身健康状况对治疗效果的影响。2005年进行的一项基于患者的前瞻性队列研究发现，免疫系统受损与预后较差有关[106]。

有研究调查了糖尿病对根尖周炎的影响，但尽管有些研究表明糖尿病与牙髓治疗效果不佳有关，但目前的证据尚无定论，不足以证明两者之间存在关联[6, 84]。

有学者对牙髓病变与心血管疾病之间的关联进行了研究，结果并不一致。然而，只有4项研究是队列研究，其中3项研究报告称根尖周炎的存在可能会影响心血管系统[17]。

横断面研究中关于全身健康状况与根尖周炎之间关联的发现并不一致[4, 54]。

谨慎起见，我们似乎可以得出这样的结论，即缺乏关于全身健康状况与牙髓治疗结果之间关联的相关信息。

5.5.2.6 牙齿健康状况

基于患者和普通人群的队列研究显示，牙齿健康状况不佳和丰富的牙科治疗经历与牙髓治疗结果不佳的风险增高有关[54, 91, 137, 169]。

横断面研究的调查结果同样支持这一观点。既往牙科治疗的程度和质量以及当前或既往牙科疾病的症状均与根尖周炎的发生有关[59, 131]。以往牙科治疗的程度和质量以及以前牙科疾病的症状可以用于预测未来治疗的成功率。这些信息可能反映了患者个人的习惯和牙科治疗的质量。

总体而言，与牙齿特定变量相比，个体相关的风险因素对于预测牙髓治疗结果的意义不是很大。

5.5.3 牙齿特异性风险因素

5.5.3.1 术前风险因素

术前诊断

术前诊断（牙髓炎、牙髓坏死、根尖周炎）是研究最多的术前因素之一。患者的队列研究[19, 118, 147, 169]、人群队列研究[91, 93, 139]和综述表明，术前根尖周病损的存在与治疗效果不佳有关。

研究发现，与术前没有根尖病变的牙齿相比，存在根尖病变可能会使治疗成功率降低10%~20%（表5.2）[12]。此外，一些研究表明，根尖病变的大小同样会影响治疗的成功率，病变越大，治疗结果越不乐观[27, 118, 147, 169]。这可能是由于较大的阴影需要的愈合时间更久，因此需要更长的随访时间。1998年，Weiger等人的研究就强调了随访时间的重要性，研究结果指出：如果在计算成功率时不把随访时间纳入考虑将会导致严重的信息误导[181]。然而，Ng等人在2011年开展的一项基于患者的队列研究指出，即使在校正随访时间这一偏倚因素后，较大的根尖病变还是会降低根管治疗的成功率[118]。近来，有研究指出，以PAI评分划分的不同等级的根尖周炎预后同样不同，炎症程度越严重预后越差[71, 89-90]。

总的来说，术前诊断确实会显著影响治疗的结果，与术前没有根尖病变的牙齿相比，术前即存在根尖周病变的患牙预后较差。

牙齿类型

大多数临床研究和基于人群的队列研究指出，磨牙根管治疗的失败率更高[10, 26, 55, 82, 91, 172]。一项综述表明，下颌前磨牙治疗失败的风险最低[120]。

由于有的研究以牙齿作为基本单位而另一些研究以牙根作为基本单位，因此，对牙齿类型与根尖周炎关系的研究结论进行比较较为困难，这至少可以部分解释研究结果之间的差异性。即使以牙齿作为研究单位，多根牙患根尖周炎的风险更高，更不用说以牙根为研究单位了。假设同一牙齿的各牙根治疗结果独立，那么如果一个根管治疗的成功率为80%，那么有三个根管的牙齿治疗的成功率（任何根管均无根尖周炎）约为50%。类似地，如果一个根管治疗成功率为70%，则具有三根管的牙齿治疗成功概率为30%。当然，这种粗略的估计没有考虑牙根的形态和其他相关因素。

总体而言，多根牙的根管治疗成功率可能低于单根牙。

窦　道

尽管尚无定论，但一些研究表明窦道会导致来自口腔的细菌定植在根尖周附近，增加根尖外感染的风险。两项以患者为基础的队列研究发现，术前的窦道不会影响治疗结果[27,147]，但另一项研究认为术前的窦道对治疗有负面影响[118]。

目前尚不能完全明确术前的窦道对根管治疗结果的影响。但现有的研究表明，即便存在关联，也是负面影响。

术前疼痛

术前的长期疼痛以及患者的负面期望可能是术后疼痛的预测因素。据报道，5%~10%的接受初次根管治疗的患者即使在6个月后仍可能出现术后疼痛。然而，术前疼痛并未被证明与根管治疗的不良结果有关[24, 47, 127, 130, 147, 164]。

牙槽骨水平

许多研究发现了边缘性牙周炎和根尖周炎之间的联系，牙周病变会对治疗结果产生负面影响[19, 84, 90, 145, 166]。牙周支持不良会导致根管治疗的成功率降低。

牙根充填

基于患者的队列研究的综述指出，根管再治疗的成功率在70%以上，根据随访时间分层时，随访2~4年的成功率为70%[116, 178]，而随访4~6年的成功率为83%[174]。

在基于人群的队列研究中，与再治疗结果相关的数据很少。一项丹麦的研究指出，26%的再治疗牙齿在5年内愈合，而10年后，愈合率达50%[92]。Petersson等人的研究同样指出，再治疗10年后的愈合率约为66%[139]。

当医生能够重新建立进入根尖区域的通路并有效清洁根管时，原有的根充物可能不会影响治疗结果。然而基于人群的研究结果表明，上述条件并不容易满足。因此，原有的根管充填可能会增加治疗失败的风险。

5.5.3.2 术中风险因素

治疗程序和治疗决策是医生在治疗过程中采取的行动、干预和选择，通常是指对根管清理、预备和充填过程中发生的事件的反应。在病例研究和基于患者队列研究中，研究者很难，甚至不可能区分所选反映的影响与触发事件对根管治疗结果的影响。在流行病学中，这种情况被称为混杂指征（表 5.1）。对治疗程序的有效评估需要进行随机对照试验，但不幸的是，这些试验在根管研究中并不常见。现有的观察性研究有时会得到相背离的结论。

无菌操作

微生物感染是牙髓病的主要原因，因此在进行牙髓治疗时，尽可能地减少或消除工作区域的污染至关重要。橡皮障在牙科的应用已有百年历史，在此期间，大学和牙髓病专家一直在教授和推荐使用橡皮障。研究表明，不使用橡皮障多与临床治疗时应用低效率（毒性小）的根管冲洗剂有关，此外，还会使患者面临误吞材料和器械的风险[2, 45]。一项历史性前瞻性人群队列研究表明，使用橡皮障可以有效提升初次根管治疗后牙齿的存留率[102]。还有研究表明，在根管治疗时使用过橡皮障的患者在未来的治疗过程中也更愿意使用橡皮障[2]。

总而言之，无菌操作有利于提高根管治疗的成功率。

器械选择

根管治疗的目的是尽可能彻底有效地清理和预备根管系统，同时避免形成台阶、侧穿、根管壁撕裂或根管过度拉直的情况。根管的机械预备被认为是根管治疗中最重要的步骤之一，在过去的十年间，我们已经见证了许多新技术、新器械的引入。许多体外研究表明，相较于不锈钢器械，镍钛器械能更好地保持原始根管的解剖结构，有助于根管预备，尤其是在弯曲根管的预备中[74]。

到目前为止，关于不同种类的器械或技术对于治疗结果影响的研究相对较少。一项体内研究证实，对于缺乏经验的操作者，使用更先进的技术时出现的操作失误更少[142]。然而，根据现有证据，尚不能得出使用不同类型的器械和系统会导致根管治疗结果差异的确切结论。

一些社区试验指出，从 X 线片评估的结果来看，相较于传统的治疗器械和程序，选用更新的器械和仪器有利于提高治疗质量，且这种改善能够随着时间的推移而长期保持[31, 96, 112]。但 Kock 等人（2013 年）开展的社区试验中的结果显示，尽管新器械可以提高根管恰填的比例，但遗憾的是并没有改善根尖周的病损状态。

目前，对于不同器械和技术对治疗结果的影响还知之甚少。尽管使用镍钛器械可以让操作简化，更好地维持根管原有的形态，使根管预备更为可控，但这些并不意味着使用这些器械就能获得更好的根管治疗效果。

根尖预备的尺寸

根管内的细菌以生物膜的形式黏附于根管壁上，甚至可以渗透进牙本质小管内，这导致细菌难以被消毒剂清理。为了消除这些细菌，有学者主张通过机械方法清除根尖部分感染的牙本质。一些以患者为基础的队列研究调查了不同根尖预备尺寸对于根管治疗结果的影响，但结果尚无定论。大部分研究认为增大根尖预备尺寸并不能改善治疗结果[69, 82, 118, 130, 135]，甚至有研究认为，过度的根尖预备会对治疗产生负面影响[169]。

由于研究结果均来自基于患者的队列研究，且不能排除适应证的混杂因素。因此，需要进行更多的研究来确定最佳的根尖预备尺寸，从而确保在保存根部牙本质的同时彻底清除感染。

通畅性

在根管预备过程中，关于使用细锉反复疏通根尖孔以保持根管通畅的观点已经争论了几十年。一些研究表明，疏通至根尖会对治疗结果产生负面影响[1, 12, 14]，而另一些研究则认为根管通畅有利于提高疗效[65, 118]。Strindberg 等人于 1956 年研究发现，如果根管堵塞且根尖段不能进行机械预备，治疗的失败率会增加[169]。同样，由于根管通畅性对疗效影响的研究仅限于基于患者的队列研究，没有随机化，因此不同治疗理念下开展的研究会出现相互矛盾的结果。

治疗并发症

根管治疗期间可能发生与根管阻塞或穿孔相关的各种并发症。根管阻塞多是由于冲洗不足导致的牙本质碎屑在根尖部堆积，或是器械分离所致。这两种并发症都会导致根管内部分区域的清理不够彻底,从而导致问题的发生,尤其是在感染的根管内。基于患者的队列研究结果显示根管阻塞会引起一系列问题[29, 115, 164, 169],尤其是发生器械分离时,可能会对治疗结果产生负面影响[76, 169]。牙本质穿孔同样会对疗效产生负面影响[29, 76, 118, 164],尤其是当穿孔的位置邻近牙槽骨嵴时[48, 118, 144]。此外,穿孔部位的术前病变可能会对愈合产生负面影响[99, 144]。

总的来说,治疗并发症会对治疗结果产生负面影响。

冲洗

根管预备期间,彻底的根管冲洗是至关重要的,许多实验室研究比较了不同种类和浓度的冲洗液的效果[74]。瑞典牙科协会 SBU 报告（2010）指出尚无足够的证据支持使用特定的根管冲洗液可以确保良好的治疗效果[8]。而一篇来自 Cochrane 的综述显示,尽管目前证据较少,但相较于生理盐水,次氯酸钠和氯己定（洗必泰）能够更有效地减少细菌培养物[49]。但是,这两种冲洗剂不可以同时使用,因为次氯酸钠和洗必泰组合会形成含对氯苯胺的沉淀物,这种沉淀不但难以清除,且有可能具有潜在的毒性和致癌性。

基于临床微生物学和体外微生物学数据,欧洲牙髓病学会（ESE）根管冲洗指南推荐使用既具有消毒作用,又具有组织溶解作用的根管冲洗剂[45]。

额外的消毒／药物

为了进一步改善感染根管的清洁和消毒效果,学者们研究了使用各种消毒剂的不同方案,包括含有抗生素或类固醇的物质（如 MTAD,Ledermix®）、2% 洗必泰或碘化钾、声波或超声波活化冲洗剂以及使用光或激光的光动力消毒等。研究发现,类固醇类的处理效果不如抗生素类[120]。一些消毒剂在体外和离体研究中展现出来有意义的结果[162]。

目前尚缺乏足够的证据确定额外的消毒程序、药物或其他方式是否对根管治疗的结果有影响[8, 162]。

单次就诊与多次就诊

随机对照试验证实,单次就诊和多次就诊的治疗结果没有差异。然而,目前尚缺乏关于单次就诊或多次就诊根管治疗术后疼痛的发生率及复发率差异的证据。

根管充填质量

根管治疗需要彻底地充填根管内的所有空间,因为如果存在空隙,残留或侵入的细菌引起的感染会导致治疗失败。

基于患者的队列研究和综述显示,根管充填的长度可能会影响根管治疗的结果。恰填（距离根尖 0~2mm）的疗效优于欠填或超填[12, 98, 118, 120, 147]。

此外,还有关于根管充填质量和感染／非感染根管之间相互作用的研究,结果显示,当术前不存在根尖周病变时,根管充填的长度就不那么重要[46, 57, 167]。若是术前存在根尖周病变,那么恰填将显著提高根管治疗的成功率[156-157, 164, 167]。

当发生超填时,超出根尖孔的材料可能对根尖周组织产生刺激,从而延迟愈合时间。因此,可能需要更长的观察时间才能对治疗结果进行可靠的评估[62, 120, 181]。超填往往伴随着之前的过度预备,此时,残髓或微生物可能已经被推出根尖孔,这同样会影响根管治疗的结果[12]。

根管充填的均匀性同样受到关注,相关研究结果显示,根管充填均匀,没有可见的空隙时预后更好[101, 118, 120, 169]。然而,此类研究大部分是基于患者的回顾性队列研究,因此对其结果的解读应当谨慎。SBU 于 2010 年的研究发现,尚缺乏证据来确定根管充填质量对治疗结果的影响[8]。

横断面研究指出,在进行了充分的根管治疗（长度／侧方密封）和充分的修复治疗的牙齿中,根尖周炎的发病率更低[59]。然而,在基于人群的队列研究中,当调整根尖周炎的基线信息时,根管充填质量对根尖周炎发病率的影响会降低,这表明根管充填质量不佳可能与根尖周炎的愈合有关,而不是与根尖周炎的发展有关[90-91]。

总之,根管充填质量欠佳会对根管治疗的结果产生负面影响,尤其是存在术前感染的牙齿。

5.5.3.3 术后危险因素

冠方修复

根管充填后的冠方修复可以防止根管系统再次感染,并恢复牙齿的功能。

大多数研究发现,根管充填和冠方修复的质

量都可能影响根尖周状况 [59, 90-91, 118, 120, 146, 173]。然而，Chugal 等人没有发现这种影响（2007），并认为缺乏对关键混杂因素的分层，导致高估了冠方修复对根管治疗成功的贡献 [28]。

研究发现，冠方修复的质量会影响根管治疗的疗效，冠方修复质量越差，疗效越差。

5.5.4 结语

即使支持我们诊断和临床程序选择的高质量研究很少，治疗也应以最佳可用证据为基础。目前，迫切需要更多高质量的研究，而在这样的研究被实施、分析、发表以前，临床操作必须依靠医生对现有研究结果的谨慎阐释。

许多不同的因素被认为会影响治疗结果，但是很难明确哪些因素对治疗的成功最重要。医生知道细菌会导致根尖周炎，因此，对于治疗前不存在根尖周炎的牙齿，以最高的临床标准进行治疗时，根管治疗的成功率高也就不足为奇了。

尽管如此，根尖周炎显然是大多数人群中的常见病。在普通人群中，30%~40% 的人至少有一颗牙患根尖周炎，而 25%~50% 的根管充填后的牙齿仍存在根尖周炎。这些结果可能表明，在非专科医院中进行的根管治疗并非总是遵循根管治疗的国际指南来开展的 [39, 45]。基于人群的队列研究发现，很少有患者在治疗后 3~5 年出现疼痛，且根管治疗后 10 年的牙齿保留率很高。

参考文献

[1] Adenubi J O, Rule D C. Success rate for root fillings in young patients. A retrospective analysis of treated cases. Br Dent J, 1976, 141: 237–241.

[2] Ahmad I A. Rubber dam usage for endodontic treatment: a review. Int Endod J, 2009, 42: 963–972.

[3] Al-Omari M A, Hazaa A, Haddad F. Frequency and distribution of root filled teeth and apical periodontitis in a Jordanian subpopulation. Oral Surg Oral Med Oral Pathol Oral Radiol Endod, 2011, 111, e59–65.

[4] Aleksejuniene J, et al. Apical periodontitis and related factors in an adult Lithuanian population. Oral Surg Oral Med Oral Pathol Oral Radiol Endod, 2000, 90: 95–101.

[5] Allard U. Palmqvist S. A radiographic survey of periapical conditions in elderly people in a Swedish county population. Endod Dent Traumatol, 1986, 2: 103–108.

[6] Aminoshariae A, et al. Association between Systemic Diseases and Endodontic Outcome: A Systematic Review. J Endod, 2017, 43: 514–519.

[7] Arya S, et al. Healing of apical periodontitis after nonsurgical treatment in patients with type 2 diabetes. J Endod, 2017, 43: 1623–1627.

[8] Assessment SCoHT. Rotfyllning-ensystematisk litteratur oversikt [Methods of Diagnosis and Treatment in Endodontics]. Report 203. Stockholm: Swedish Council on Health Technology Assessment, 2010.

[9] Balto K. Single-or multiple-visit endodontics: which technique results in fewest postoperative problems? Evid Based Dent, 2009, 10, 16.

[10] Barbakow F H, Cleaton-Jones P, Friedman D. An evaluation of 566 cases of root canal therapy in general dental practice. 2. Postoperative observations. J Endod, 1980, 6: 485–489.

[11] Barborka B J, et al. Long-term clinical outcome of teeth obturated with resilon. J Endod, 2017, 43: 556–560.

[12] Basmadjian-Charles C L, et al. Factors influencing the long-term results of endodontic treatment: a review of the literature. Int Dent J, 2002, 52: 81–86.

[13] Benenati F W. Khajotia S S. A radiographic recall evaluation of 894 endodontic cases treated in a dental school setting. J Endod, 2002, 28: 391–395.

[14] Bergenholtz G, et al. Influence of apical overinstrumentation and overfilling on re-treated root canals. J Endod, 1979, 5: 310–314.

[15] Bergenholtz G M E, Milthon R. Endodontisk behandling och periapikalstatus. II. Rötgenologisk bedömning av rotfyllningens kvalitet ställd i relation till förekomst av periapikala destruktioner. Tandläkartidningen, 1973, 5: 269–279.

[16] Bergström J, Eliasson S, Ahlberg K F. Periapical status in subjects with regular dental care habits. Community Dent Oral Epidemiol, 1987, 15: 236–239.

[17] Berlin-Broner Y, Febbraio M, Levin L. Association between apical periodontitis and cardiovascular diseases: a systematic review of the literature. Int Endod J, 2017, 50: 847–859.

[18] Berlinck T, et al. Epidemiological evaluation of apical periodontitis prevalence in an urban Brazilian population. Braz Oral Res, 2015, 29, 51.

[19] Bernstein S D, et al. Outcomes of endodontic therapy in general practice: a study by the practitioners engaged in Applied Research and Learning Network. J Am Dent Assoc, 2012, 143: 478–487.

[20] Boucher Y, et al. Radiographic evaluation of the prevalence and technical quality of root canal treatment in a French subpopulation. Int Endod J, 2002, 35: 229–238.

[21] Brynolf I. A histological and roentgenological study of the periapical region of human upper incisors Odontologisk Revy, 1967, 18.

[22] Buckley M. Spångberg L S. The prevalence and technical quality of endodontic treatment in an American subpopulation. Oral Surg Oral Med Oral Pathol Oral Radiol Endod, 1995, 79: 92–100.

[23] Burry J C, et al. Outcomes of primary endodontic therapy provided by endodontic specialists compared with other providers. J Endod, 2016, 42: 702–705.

[24] Byström A, et al. Healing of periapical lesions of pulpless teeth after endodontic treatment with controlled asepsis. Endod Dent Traumatol, 1987, 3: 58–63.

[25] Chen C Y, et al. Prevalence and quality of endodontic treatment in the Northern Manhattan elderly. J Endod, 2007, 33: 230–234.

[26] Cheung G S. Survival of first-time nonsurgical root canal treatment performed in a dental teaching hospital. Oral Surg Oral Med Oral Pathol Oral Radiol Endod, 2002, 93: 596–604.

[27] Chugal N M, Clive J M, Spångberg L S. A prognostic model for: ssessment of the outcome of endodontic treatment: Effect of biologic and diagnostic variables. Oral Surg Oral Med Oral Pathol Oral Radiol Endod, 2001, 91: 342–352.

[28] Chugal N M, Clive J M, Spångberg L S. Endodontic treatment outcome: effect of the permanent restoration. Oral Surg Oral Med Oral Pathol Oral Radiol Endod, 2007, 104: 576–582.

[29] Cvek M, Granath L, Lundberg M. Failures and healing in endodontically treated non-vital anterior teeth with posttraumatically reduced pulpal lumen. Acta Odontol Scand, 1982, 40: 223–228.

[30] Da Silva K, et al. Cross-sectional study of endodontic treatment in an Australian population. Aust Endod J, 2009, 35: 140–146.

[31] Dahlstrom L, Molander A, Reit C. Introducing nickel-titanium rotary instrumentation in a public dental service: the long-term effect on root filling quality. Oral Surg Oral Med Oral Pathol Oral Radiol Endod ,2011,112: 814–819.

[32] De Cleen M J, et al. Periapical status and prevalence of endodontic treatment in an adult Dutch population. Int Endod J ,1993, 26: 112–119.

[33] De Moor R J, et al. Periapical health related to the quality of root canal treatment in a Belgian population. Int Endod J, 2000, 33: 113–120.

[34] Doyle S L, et al. Retrospective cross sectional comparison of initial nonsurgical endodontic treatment and single-tooth implants. Compend Contin Educ Dent, 2007, 28: 296–301.

[35] Dugas N N, et al. Periapical health and treatment quality assessment of rootfilled teeth in two Canadian populations. Int Endod J, 2003, 36: 181–192.

[36] Eckerbom M, Andersson J E, Magnusson T. Frequency and technical standard of endodontic treatment in a Swedish population. Endod Dent Traumatol, 1987, 3: 245–248.

[37] Eckerbom M, Andersson J E, Magnusson T. A longitudinal study of changes in frequency and technical standard of endodontic treatment in a Swedish population. Endod Dent Traumatol, 1989, 5: 27–31.

[38] Eckerbom M, Flygare L, Magnusson T. A 20-year follow-up study of endodontic variables and apical status in a Swedish population. Int Endod J, 2007, 40: 940–948.

[39] Endodontists AAE. Guide to Clinical Endodontics. Sixth Edition. Chicago IL: AAE,2013.

[40] Engström B. Frostell G. Experiences of bacteriological root canal control. Acta Odontol Scand, 1964, 22: 43–69.

[41] Eriksen H M, et al. Changes in endodontic status 1973–1993 among 35-year-olds in Oslo, Norway. Int Endod J, 1995, 28: 129–132.

[42] Eriksen H M, Bjertness E. Prevalence of apical periodontitis and results of endodontic treatment in middleaged adults in Norway. Endod Dent Traumatol, 1991, 7: 1–4.

[43] Eriksen H M, Bjertness E, Ørstavik D. Prevalence and quality of endodontic treatment in an urban adult population in Norway. Endod Dent: raumatol, 1988, 4: 122–126.

[44] Eriksen H M, Ørstavik D, Kerekes K. Healing of apical periodontitis after endodontic treatment using three different root canal sealers. Endod Dent Traumatol, 1988, 4: 114–117.

[45] European Society of Endodontology. Quality guidelines for endodontic treatment: consensus report of the European Society of Endodontology. Int Endod J, 2006, 39: 921–930.

[46] Fabricius L, et al. Influence of residual bacteria on periapical tissue healing after chemomechanical treatment and root filling of experimentally infected monkey teeth. Eur J Oral Sci, 2006, 114: 278–285.

[47] Farzaneh M, Abitbol S, Friedman S. Treatment outcome in endodontics: the Toronto study. Phases II and II: Orthograde retreatment. J Endod, 2004, 30: 627–633.

[48] Farzaneh M, et al. Treatment outcome in endodontics-the Toronto Study. Phase II: initial treatment. J Endod, 2004, 30: 302–309.

[49] Fedorowicz Z, et al. Irrigants for non-surgical root canal treatment in mature permanent teeth. Cochrane nDatabase Syst Rev, 2012, CD008948.

[50] Figini L, et al. Single versus multiple visits for endodontic treatment of permanent teeth: a Cochrane systematic review. J Endod, 2008, 34: 1041–1047.

[51] Fletcher R H, Fletcher S W, Fletcher G S. Clinical epidemiology. The essentials. Baltimore: Williams & Wilkins, 2014.

[52] Fransson H, et al. Survival of root-filled teeth in the Swedish adult population. J Endod, 2016, 42: 216–220.

[53] Frisk F, Hakeberg M. A 24-year follow-up of root filled teeth and periapical health amongst middle aged and elderly women in Goteborg, Sweden. Int Endod J, 2005, 38: 246–254.

[54] Frisk F, Hakeberg M. Socioeconomic risk indicators for apical periodontitis. Acta Odontol Scand, 2006, 64: 123–128.

[55] Frisk F, Hugoson A, Hakeberg M. Technical quality of root fillings and periapical status in root filled teeth in Jonkoping, Sweden. Int Endod J, 2008, 41: 958–968.

[56] Georgopoulou M K, et al. Frequency and distribution of root filled teeth and apical periodontitis in a Greek population. Int Endod J, 2005, 38: 105–111.

[57] Gesi A, et al. Incidence of periapical lesions and clinical symptoms after pulpectomy-a clinical and radiographic evaluation of 1-versus 2-session treatment. Oral Surg Oral Med Oral Pathol Oral Radiol Endod, 2006, 101: 379–388.

[58] Gilbert G H, et al. Outcomes of root canal treatment in Dental Practice-Based Research Network practices. Gen Dent, 2010, 58: 28–36.

[59] Gillen B M, et al. Impact of the quality of coronal restoration versus the quality of root canal fillings on success of root canal treatment: a systematic review and meta-analysis. J Endod, 2011, 37: 895–902.

[60] Gulsahi K, et al. Frequency of root-filled teeth and prevalence of apical periodontitis in an adult Turkish population. Int Endod J, 2008, 41: 78–85.

[61] Gumru B, et al. Retrospective radiological assessment of root canal treatment in young permanent dentition in a Turkish subpopulation. Int Endod J, 2011, 44: 850–856.

[62] Halse A, Molven O. Overextended gutta-percha and Kloroperka N-O root canal fillings. Radiographic findings after 10–17 years. Acta Odontol Scand, 1987, 45: 171–177.

[63] Hamedy R, et al. Prevalence of root canal treatment and periapical radiolucency in elders: a systematic review. Gerodontology, 2016, 33: 116–127.

[64] Harrell F. Regression Modeling Strategies: With Applications to Linear Models, Logistic and Ordinal Regression, and Survival Analysis. Switzerland: Springer International Publishing AG, 2015.

[65] Harty F J, Parkins B J, Wengraf A M. Success rate in root canal therapy. A retrospective study of conventional cases. Br Dent J, 1970, 128: 65–70.

[66] He J, et al. Clinical and patientcentered outcomes of nonsurgical root canal retreatment in first molars using contemporary techniques. J Endod, 2017, 43: 231–237.

[67] Hebling E, et al. Periapical status and prevalence of endodontic treatment in institutionalized elderly. Braz Dent J, 2014, 25: 123–128.

[68] Hollanda A C, et al. Prevalence o endodontically treated teeth in a Brazilian adult population. Braz Dent J, 2008, 19: 313–317.

[69] Hoskinson S E, et al. A retrospective comparison of outcome of root canal treatment using two different protocols. Oral Surg Oral Med Oral Pathol Oral Radiol Endod, 2002, 93: 705–715.

[70] Huumonen S, et al. Healing of napical periodontitis after endodontic treatment: a comparison between a silicone-based and a zinc oxide-eugenolbased sealer. Int Endod J, 2003, 36: 296–301.

[71] Huumonen S, Ørstavik D. Radiographic follow-up of periapical status after endodontic treatment of teeth with and without apical periodontitis. Clinical Oral Investigations, 2013, 17: 2099–2104.

[72] Huumonen S, Suominen A L, Vehkalahti M M. Prevalence of apical periodontitis in root filled teeth: findings from a nationwide survey in Finland. Int Endod J, 2017, 50: 229–236.

[73] Huumonen S, Vehkalahti M M, Nordblad A. Radiographic assessments on prevalence and technical quality of endodontically-treated teeth in the Finnish population, aged 30 years and older. Acta Odontol Scand, 2012, 70: 234–240.

[74] Hülsmann M P, Peters O A, Dummer P M H. Mechanical preparation of root canals: shaping goals, techniques and means. Endodontic Topics, 2005, 10: 30–76.

[75] Imfeld T N. Prevalence and quality of endodontic treatment in an elderly urban population of Switzerland. J Endod, 1991, 17: 604–607.

[76] Imura N, et al. The outcome of endodontic treatment: a retrospective study of 2000 cases performed by a specialist. J Endod, 2007, 33: 1278–1282.

[77] Jersa I. Kundzina R. Periapical status and quality of root fillings in a selected adult Riga population. Stomatologija, 2013, 15: 73–77.

[78] Jiménez-Pinzón A, et al. Prevalence of apical periodontitis and frequency of root-filled teeth in an adult Spanish population. Int Endod J, 2004, 37: 167–173.

[79] Jokinen M A, et al. Clinical and radiographic study of pulpectomy and root canal therapy. Scand J Dent Res, 1978, 86: 366–373.

[80] Kabak Y. Abbott P V, Prevalence of apical periodontitis and the quality of endodontic treatment in an adult Belarusian population. Int Endod J, 2005, 38: 238–245.

[81] Kalender A, et al. Influence of the quality of endodontic treatment and coronal restorations on the prevalence of apical periodontitis in a Turkish Cypriot population. Med Princ Pract, 2013, 22: 173–177.

[82] Kerekes K, Tronstad L. Long-term results of endodontic treatment performed with a standardized technique. J Endod, 1979, 5: 83–90.

[83] Kerekes K B, Bervell S F A. En røntgenologisk vurdering av endodontisk behandlingsbehov. Den Norske Tannlægeforenings Tidende, 1976, 86: 248–254.

[84] Khalighinejad N, et al. The influence of periodontal status on endodontically treated teeth: 9-year survival analysis. J Endod, 2017, 43: 1781–1785.

[85] Kielbassa A M, Frank W, Madaus T. Radiologic assessment of quality of root canal fillings and periapical status in an

Austrian subpopulation-An observational study. PLoS One, 2017, 12, e0176724.

[86] Kirkevang L L, Hørsted-Bindslev P. Technical aspects of treatment in relation to treatment outcome. Endodontic Topics, 2002, 2: 89–102.

[87] Kirkevang L L, et al. A comparison of the quality of root canal treatment in two Danish subpopulations examined 1974–75 and 1997–98. Int Endod J, 2001, 34: 607–612.

[88] Kirkevang L L, et al. Frequency and distribution of endodontically treated teeth and apical periodontitis in an urban Danish population. Int Endod J, 2001, 34: 198–205.

[89] Kirkevang L L, et al. Prediction of periapical status and tooth extraction. Int Endod J, 2017, 50: 5–14.

[90] Kirkevang L L, et al. Prognostic value of the full-scale Periapical Index. Int Endod J, 2015, 48: 1051–1058.

[91] Kirkevang L L, et al. Risk factors for developing apical periodontitis in a general population. Int Endod J, 2007, 40: 290–299.

[92] Kirkevang L L, Vaeth M Wenzel A. Ten-year follow-up observations of periapical and endodontic status in a Danish population. Int Endod J, 2012, 45: 829–839.

[93] Kirkevang L L, Vaeth M, Wenzel A. Ten-year follow-up of root filled teeth: a radiographic study of a Danish population. Int Endod J, 2014, 47: 980–988.

[94] Kirkevang L L, Wenzel A. Risk indicators for apical periodontitis. Community Dent Oral Epidemiol, 2003, 31: 59–67.

[95] Kirkwood B R S, Sterne J A C. Essential medical statistics. Second Edition ed. Oxford UK: Blackwell Science Ltd, 2003.

[96] Koch M. On implementation of an endodontic program. Swedish Dental Journal, 2013, 230: 9–97.

[97] Koch M, et al. Effect of education intervention on the quality and long-term outcomes of root canal treatment in general practice. Int Endod J, 2015, 48: 680–689.

[98] Kojima K, et al. Success rate of endodontic treatment of teeth with vital and nonvital pulps. A meta-analysis. Oral Surg Oral Med Oral Pathol Oral Radiol Endod, 2004, 97: 95–99.

[99] Krupp C, et al. Treatment outcome after repair of root perforations with mineral trioxide aggregate: a retrospective evaluation of 90 teeth. J Endod, 2013, 39: 1364–1368.

[100] Landys Boren D, Jonasson P, Kvist T. Longterm survival of endodontically treated teeth at a public dental specialist clinic. J Endod, 2015, 41: 176–181.

[101] Lee A H, Cheung G S, Wong M C. Long-term outcome of primary non-surgical root canal treatment. Clin Oral Investig, 2012, 16: 1607–1617.

[102] Lin P Y, et al. The effect of rubber dam usage on the survival rate of teeth receiving initial root canal treatment: a nationwide population-based study. Journal of Endodontics, 2014, 40: 1733–1737.

[103] Loftus J J, Keating A P, McCartan B E. Periapical status and quality of endodontic treatment in an adult Irish population. Int Endod J, 2005, 38: 81–86.

[104] Lopez-Lopez J, et al. Frequency and distribution of root-filled teeth and apical periodontitis in an adult population of Barcelona, Spain. Int Dent J, 2012, 62: 40–46.

[105] Lupi-Pegurier L, et al. Periapical status, prevalence and quality of endodontic treatment in an adult French population. Int Endod J, 2002, 35: 690–697.

[106] Marending M, Peters O A, Zehnder M. Factors affecting the outcome of orthograde root canal therapy in a general dentistry hospital practice. Oral Surg Oral Med Oral Pathol Oral Radiol Endod, 2005, 99: 119–124.

[107] Marques M D, Moreira B, Eriksen H M. Prevalence of apical periodontitis and results of endodontic treatment in an adult, Portuguese population. Int Endod J, 1998, 31: 161–165.

[108] Marquis V L, et al. Treatment outcome in endodontics: the Toronto Study. Phase III: initial treatment. J Endod, 2006, 32: 299–306.

[109] Matijevic J, et al. Prevalence of apical periodontitis and quality of root canal fillings in population of Zagreb, Croatia: a cross-sectional study. Croat Med J, 2011, 52: 679–687.

[110] Mokkink L B, et al. Inter-rater agreement and reliability of the COSMIN (COnsensus-based Standards for the selection of health status Measurement Instruments, checklist. BMC Med Res Methodol, 2010, 10, 82.

[111] Mokkink L B, et al. The COSMIN checklist for evaluating the methodological quality of studies on measurement properties: a clarification of its content. BMC Med Res Methodol, 2010, 10, 22.

[112] Molander A, et al. Improved quality of root fillings provided by general dental practitioners educated in nickeltitanium rotary instrumentation. Int Endod J, 2007, 40: 254–260.

[113] Molven O, Halse A, Grung B. Observer strategy and the radiographic classification of healing after endodontic surgery. Int J Oral Maxillofac Surg, 1987, 16: 432–439.

[114] Montero J, et al. Patient-centered outcomes of root canal treatment: a cohort follow-up study. J Endod, 2015, 41: 1456–1461.

[115] Negishi J, Kawanami M, Ogami E. Risk analysis of failure of root canal treatment for teeth with inaccessible apical constriction. J Dent, 2005, 33: 399–404.

[116] Ng Y L, Mann V, Gulabivala K. Outcome of secondary root canal treatment: a systematic review of the literature. Int Endod J, 2008, 41: 1026–1046.

[117] Ng Y L, Mann V, Gulabivala K. Tooth survival following nonsurgical root canal treatment: a systematic review of the literature. Int Endod J, 2010, 43: 171–189.

[118] Ng Y L, Mann V, Gulabivala K. A prospective study of the factors affecting outcomes of non-surgical root canal treatment: part 2: tooth survival. Int Endod J, 2011, 44: 610–625.

[119] Ng Y L, et al. Outcome of primary root canal treatment: systematic review of the literature-part 1. Effects of study characteristics on probability of success. Int Endod J, 2007, 40: 921–939.

[120] Ng Y L, et al. Outcome of primary root canal treatment: systematic review of the literature-part 2. Influence of clinical factors. Int Endod J, 2008, 41: 6–31.

[121] Nixdorf D R, et al. Frequency, impact, and predictors of persistent pain after root canal treatment: a national dental PBRN study. Pain, 2016, 157: 159–165.

[122] Nixdorf D R, et al. Frequency of persistent tooth pain after root canal therapy: a systematic review and metaanalysis. J Endod, 2010, 36: 224–230.

[123] Odesjo B, et al. Prevalence of previous endodontic treatment, technical standard and occurrence of periapical lesions in a randomly selected adult, general population. Endod Dent Traumatol, 1990, 6: 265–272.

[124] Oginni A O, Adeleke A A, Chandler N P. Root canal treatment and prevalence of apical periodontitis in a Nigerian adult subpopulation: a radiographic study. Oral Health Prev Dent, 2015, 13: 85–90.

[125] Oliet S. Single-visit endodontics: a clinical study. J Endod, 1983, 9: 147–152.

[126] Ørstavik D. Time-course and risk analyses of the development and healing of chronic apical periodontitis in man. Int Endod J, 1996, 29: 150–155.

[127] Ørstavik D, Horsted-Bindslev P. A comparison of endodontic treatment results at two dental schools. Int Endod J, 1993, 26: 348–354.

[128] Ørstavik D, Kerekes K, Eriksen H M. The periapical index: a scoring system for radiographic assessment of apical periodontitis. Endod Dent Traumatol, 1986, 2: 20–34.

[129] Ørstavik D, Kerekes K, Eriksen H M, Clinical performance of three endodontic sealers. Endod Dent Traumatol, 1987, 3: 178–186.

[130] Ørstavik D, Qvist V, Stoltze K. A multivariate analysis of the outcome of endodontic treatment. Eur J Oral Sci, 2004, 112: 224–230.

[131] Pak J G, Fayazi S, White S N. Prevalence of periapical radiolucency and root canal treatment: a systematic review of cross-sectional studies. J Endod, 2012, 38: 170–6.

[132] Pak J G, White S N. Pain prevalence and severity before, during, and after root canal treatment: a systematic review. Journal of Endodontics, 2011, 37: 429–438.

[133] Peciuliene V, et al. Apical periodontitis in root filled teeth associated with the quality of root fillings. Stomatologija, 2006, 8: 122–126.

[134] Peters L B, et al. Prevalence of apical periodontitis relative to endodontic treatment in an adult Dutch population: a repeated crosssectional study. Oral Surg Oral Med Oral Pathol Oral Radiol Endod, 2011, 111: 523–528.

[135] Peters L B, Wesselink P R. Periapical healing of endodontically treated teeth in one and two visits obturated in the presence or absence of detectable microorganisms. Int Endod J, 2002, 35: 660–667.

[136] Peters O A, Barbakow F, Peters C I. An analysis of endodontic treatment with three nickel-titanium rotary root canal preparation techniques. Int Endod J, 2004, 37: 849–859.

[137] Petersson K. Endodontic status of mandibular premolars and molars in an adult Swedish population. A longitudinal study 1974–1985. Endod Dent Traumatol, 1993, 9: 13–18.

[138] Petersson K, et al. Twenty-year follow-up of root filled teeth in a Swedish population receiving high-cost dental care. Int Endod J, 2016, 49: 636–6345.

[139] Petersson K, et al. Follow-up study of endodontic status in an adult Swedish population. Endod Dent Traumatol, 1991, 7: 221–225.

[140] Petersson K, et al. Endodontic status and suggested treatment in a population requiring substantial dental care. Endod Dent Traumatol, 1989, 5: 153–158.

[141] Petersson K, et al. Technical quality of root fillings in an adult Swedish population. Endod Dent Traumatol, 1986, 2: 99–102.

[142] Pettiette M T, Delano E O, Trope M. Evaluation of success rate of endodontic treatment performed by students with stainless-steel K-files and nickel-titanium hand files. J Endod, 2001, 27: 124–127.

[143] Pirani C, et al. Survival and periapical health after root canal treatment with carrier-based root fillings: five-year retrospective assessment. Int Endod J, 2017,

[144] Pontius V, et al. Retrospective evaluation of perforation repairs in 6 private practices. J Endod, 2013, 39: 1346–1358.

[145] Pretzl B, et al. Endodontic status and retention of molars in periodontally treated patients: results after 10 or more years of supportive periodontal therapy. J Clin Periodontol, 2016, 43: 1116–1123.

[146] Ray H A, Trope M. Periapical status of endodontically treated teeth in relation to the technical quality of the root filling and the coronal restoration. Int Endod J, 1995, 28: 12–18.

[147] Ricucci D, et al. A prospective cohort study of endodontic treatments of 1,369 root canals: results after 5 years. Oral Surg Oral Med Oral Pathol Oral Radiol Endod, 2011, 112: 825–842.

[148] Ridell K, et al. Periapical status and technical quality of root-filled teeth in Swedish adolescents and young adults. A

retrospective study. Acta Odontol Scand, 2006, 64: 104–110.

[149] Rud J, Andreasen J O, Jensen J E. Radiographic criteria for the assessment of healing after endodontic surgery. Int J Oral Surg, 1972, 1: 195–214.

[150] Salehrabi R, Rotstein I. Endodontic treatment outcomes in a large patient population in the USA: an epidemiological study. J Endod, 2004, 30: 846–850.

[151] Salehrabi R, Rotstein I. Epidemiologic evaluation of the outcomes of orthograde endodontic retreatment. Journal of Endodontics, 2010, 36: 790–792.

[152] Sathorn C, Parashos P, Messer H. The prevalence of postoperative pain and flare-up in single-and multiplevisit endodontic treatment: a systematic review. International Endodontic Journal, 2008, 41: 91–99.

[153] Sathorn C, Parashos P, Messer H H. Effectiveness of single-versus multiple-visit endodontic treatment of teeth with apical periodontitis: a systematic review and meta-analysis. International Endodontic Journal, 2005, 38: 347–355.

[154] Saunders W P, et al. Technical standard of root canal treatment in an adult Scottish sub-population. British Dental Journal, 1997, 182: 382–386.

[155] Schäfer E, Burklein S. Impact of nickel-titanium instrumentation of the root canal on clinical outcomes: a focused review. Odontology, 2012, 100: 130–136.

[156] Seltzer S, et al. Endodontic failures-an analysis based on clinical, roentgenographic, and histologic findings. I. Oral Surg Oral Med Oral Pathol, 1967, 23: 500–516.

[157] Seltzer S, et al. Endodontic failures-an analysis based on clinical, roentgenographic, and histologic findings. II. Oral Surg Oral Med Oral Pathol, 1967, 23: 517–530.

[158] Seltzer S, Bender I B, Turkenkopf S. Factors Affecting Successful Repair after Root Canal Therapy. J Am Dent Assoc, 1963, 67: 651–662.

[159] Setzer F C, et al. Long-term prognosis of endodontically treated teeth: a retrospective analysis of preoperative factors in molars. J Endod, 2011, 37: 21–25.

[160] Shakiba B, et al. Influence of increased patient age on longitudinal outcomes of root canal treatment: a systematic review. Gerodontology, 2017, 34: 101–109.

[161] Sidaravicius B, Aleksejuniene J, Eriksen H M. Endodontic treatment and prevalence of apical periodontitis in an adult population of Vilnius, Lithuania. Endod Dent Traumatol, 1999, 15: 210–215.

[162] Siqueira J F Jr, Rôças I N. Optimising single-visit disinfection with supplementary approaches: a quest for predictability. Aust Endod J, 2011, 37: 92–98.

[163] Sjögren U, et al. Influence of infection at the time of root filling on the outcome of endodontic treatment of teeth with apical periodontitis. International Endodontic Journal, 1997, 30: 297–306.

[164] Sjögren U, et al. Factors affecting the long-term results of endodontic treatment. J Endod, 1990, 16: 498–504.

[165] Skudutyte-Rysstad R, Eriksen H M. Endodontic status amongst 35-year-old Oslo citizens and changes over a 30-year period. International Endodontic Journal, 2006, 39: 637–642.

[166] Skupien J A, et al. Survival of restored endodontically treated teeth in relation to periodontal status. Braz Dent J, 2016, 27: 37–40.

[167] Smith C S, Setchell D J, Harty F J. Factors influencing the success of conventional root canal therapy-a fiveyear retrospective study. Int Endod J, 1993, 26: 321–333.

[168] Soikkonen K T. Endodontically treated teeth and periapical findings in the elderly. Int Endod J, 1995,28: 200–203.

[169] Strindberg L Z. The dependence of the results of pulp therapy on certain factors. An analytic study based on radiographic and clinical follow-up examinations. Acta Odontologica Scandinavia, 1956, 14.

[170] Su Y Y, Wang C L, Ye L. Healing Rate and Post-obturation Pain of Single-versus Multiple-visit Endodontic Treatment for Infected Root Canals: A Systematic Review. Journal of Endodontics, 2011, 37: 125–132.

[171] Sunay H, et al. Cross-sectional evaluation of the periapical status and quality of root canal treatment in a selected population of urban Turkish adults. International Endodontic Journal, 2007, 40: 139–145.

[172] Swartz D B, Skidmore A E, Griffin J A Jr. Twenty years of endodontic success and failure. J Endod, 1983, 9: 198–202.

[173] Tolias D, et al. Apical periodontitis in association with the quality of root fillings and coronal restorations: a 14-year investigation in young Greek adults. Oral Health Prev Dent, 2012, 10: 297–303.

[174] Torabinejad M, et al. Outcomes of nonsurgical retreatment and endodontic surgery: a systematic review. J Endod, 2009, 35: 930–937.

[175] Touré B, et al. Prevalence and technical quality of root fillings in Dakar, Senegal. Int Endod J, 2008, 41: 41–49.

[176] Trope M, Delano E O, Ørstavik D. Endodontic treatment of teeth with apical periodontitis: single vs. multivisit treatment. J Endod, 1999, 25: 345–350.

[177] Tsuneish M, et al. Radiographic evaluation of periapical status and prevalence of endodontic treatment in an adult Japanese population. Oral Surg Oral Med Oral Pathol Oral Radiol Endod, 2005, 100: 631–635.

[178] Van Nieuwenhuysen J P, Aouar M, D'Hoore W. Retreatment or radiographic monitoring in endodontics. Int Endod J, 1994, 27: 75–81.

[179] Vena D A, et al. Prevalence of persistent pain 3 to 5 years post primary root canal therapy and its impact on oral health-related quality of life: PEARL Network findings. J

Endod, 2014, 40: 1917–1921.

[180] Walter C, et al. Association of tobacco use and periapical pathosis-a systematic review. International Endodontic Journal, 2012, 45: 1065–1073.

[181] Weiger R, Axmann-Krcmar D, Lost C. Prognosis of conventional root canal treatment reconsidered. Endod Dent Traumatol, 1998, 14: 1–9.

[182] Weiger R, et al. Periapical status, quality of root canal fillings and estimated endodontic treatment needs in an urban German population. Endod Dent Traumatol, 1997, 13: 69–74.

[183] Weiger R, Rosendahl R, Lost C. Influence of calcium hydroxide intracanal dressings on the prognosis of teeth with endodontically induced periapical lesions. Int Endod J, 2000, 33: 219–226.

[184] WHO. Epidemiology [2019-06-21]. https://www. who.int/topics/epidemiology/en/ (accessed 21 June 2019).

[185] Zhong Y, et al. Extension and density of root fillings and postoperative apical radiolucencies in the Veterans Affairs Dental Longitudinal Study. J Endod, 2008, 34: 798–803.

第 6 章　根尖周炎的影像学检查

Shanon Patel, Conor Durack

6.1　概述

根尖周炎是发生在牙根周围的炎症。来自根管系统的感染通常会引起根尖周骨组织的破坏[61, 73, 108]。

作为一种常见的口腔疾病，根尖周炎的发病率随着年龄的增长而增加。流行病学研究发现约70%的个体与7%的牙齿存在根尖周炎[39]。对于初步诊断为急性根尖周炎的患牙，可以通过它的临床表现进行确诊，而对于慢性根尖周炎的诊断通常依赖于影像学表现。

牙髓治疗的目的是预防，或在某些病例中治愈根尖周炎。无论患牙的牙髓状态如何，需要根管（再）治疗或根管外科手术治疗，牙髓治疗的诊断、治疗过程以及最终的疗效评价都依赖于影像学检查[40, 49, 125]。

根尖 X 线片和锥形束 CT（CBCT）是检查根尖周炎的主要影像学方法。

根尖 X 线片是目前评估根尖周组织影像的首选方法。它是一种快捷简单的检查技术，并且图像相对容易解读。此外，它还具有良好的特异性和较高的图像分辨率。根尖 X 线片的局限性主要是存在解剖结构的影像重叠；得到的是二维的图像；存在几何失真（图6.1）。这些因素导致检查的灵敏度欠理想[93]。

高分辨率小视野 CBCT 扫描所产生的辐射剂量高于传统的 X 线片。然而，随着对 CBCT 软件和硬件的不断改进，使得辐射暴露逐渐减少[7]。由于克服了根尖 X 线片的局限，CBCT 能够实现对牙槽骨解剖更为精确的解析，但是设备（和扫描）成本明显高于传统 X 线片。此外，对于扫描仪的使用以及对结果的判读需要经过特殊的培训[19]。

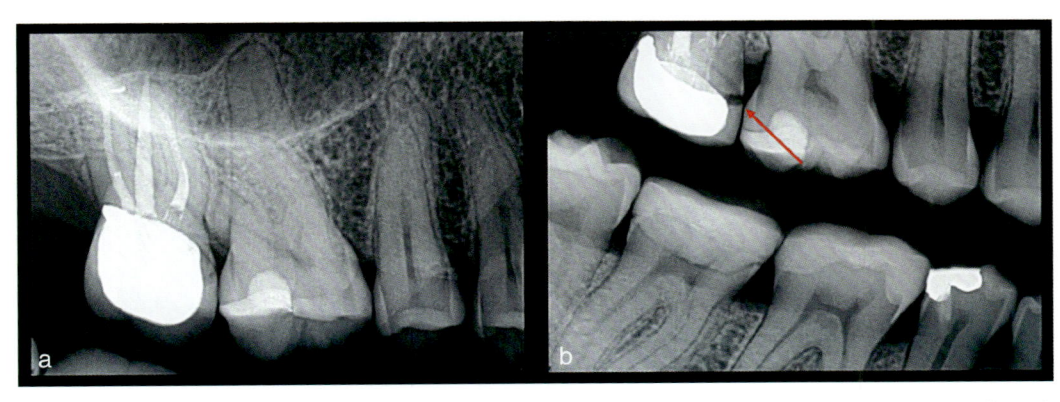

图 6.1　几何失真。a. 根管治疗后的右上磨牙根尖片未见明显异常。b. 咬合翼片显示牙冠边缘缺损表现（红色箭头）

牙髓病学基础：根尖周炎的预防和治疗

在不久的将来，CBCT 可能成为根尖周炎影像学评估和治疗过程中的重要组成部分。这已经体现在欧洲牙髓病学学会（ESE）近期发表的关于 CBCT 的立场声明 [91] 中，以及美国牙髓病学协会和美国颌面部放射学会（AAE/AAOMR）的联合声明中 [3]。考虑到这一点，本章节将同时对根尖周炎的根尖 X 线片和 CBCT 检查特征进行讲解。

随着 CBCT 在牙髓病学中的应用，关于根尖周炎影像学解读的研究和出版物的数量不断增加 [62, 88, 90, 116]。

本章节将对健康和病变的根尖周组织在诊断及后续治疗过程中的影像学表现进行解读。同时还会讨论鉴别诊断、导致错误的原因以及用于根尖周炎评估的其他影像学技术。

6.2 正常的根尖周组织

牙周组织由牙骨质、牙周膜以及牙槽骨组成。根尖周组织是特指这些结构在牙齿根尖处的相互关系。在根尖处一系列的影像学特征中，牙周膜和牙槽骨的硬骨板被认为是正常根尖周组织的典型特征。这些所谓的"典型"影像学特征被用作评估是否存在根尖周炎的参考标准。然而牙根的形态在不同牙齿间存在明显的变异，这些变异在同类牙齿之间虽然较小但同样存在。此外，由于观察区域重叠的解剖结构所产生的"干扰"，使得根尖周组织的影像解读变得更为复杂。这导致使用传统的 X 线片难以确定正常的根尖周组织影像学特征，从而使得对轻微病变的诊断较为困难。

在评估患牙是否存在根尖周炎时，需要对根尖周组织以及与其邻近的解剖结构加以识别，并评估是否存在异常的影像学变化（图 6.2）。

6.2.1 根尖及根尖孔

感染牙髓组织内的微生物毒素及炎症介质侵入到牙周膜间隙和牙槽骨处时，会发生典型的根尖周炎症状并出现影像学改变。根尖孔是这些毒素和炎症介质最主要的扩散途径，有时也可经根尖分歧扩散。因此在评估影像学图像是否存在疾病表现时，应首先了解根尖处的正常影像学表现。

根尖的顶点通常与牙根长轴存在一定角度的偏移 [72]。这种偏移可以发生在任何方向。在某种程度上，偏移方向取决于牙齿的类型。当根尖的顶点与牙长轴方向一致时，根尖孔通常位于影像学根尖的冠方。这些特征对于根尖孔位置的影像学分析有重要的影响。

常规 X 线片：由于根尖孔没有典型的影像学表现，因此为了尽可能准确评估它的位置，应当将根尖顶点作为典型标志 [127]。

通常，健康牙齿的根尖影像学表现为一个圆形，边界清楚的结构。然而正如上文所述的原因，影像学根尖很少与根尖孔重合，根尖孔的位置通

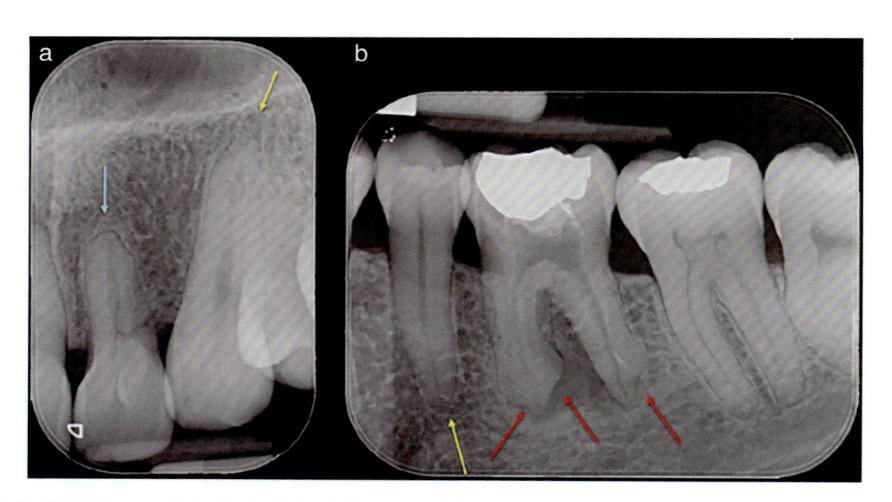

图 6.2 正常的根尖牙周膜。a. 固定矫治器治疗导致 22 牙根吸收，牙根缩短和牙根末端变钝（蓝色箭头）。相邻的 23 牙根末端（黄色箭头）呈边界清晰的圆形影像，即根尖未发生因疾病或压力导致吸收的典型影像。b. 感染坏死的根管和根尖周炎导致 36 根尖发生炎症性外吸收。与未受根尖周炎影响的 35 根尖（黄色箭头）相比，36 根尖变平且不均匀

常会偏向冠方[72]。由正畸治疗、创伤或慢性根尖周炎引起的根尖周吸收，会导致根尖形状的改变[112]。根尖变钝是正畸治疗中牙移动的典型特征，而慢性根尖周炎会导致根尖变平或出现参差不齐的不规则形态。这些形态变化在创伤后患牙的根尖均可能发生。由于牙根吸收而受损的根尖可以通过新的牙骨质沉积进行修复，但患牙损伤的特征往往会持续存在（图 6.3）。

CBCT：借助 CBCT 能够准确定位根尖顶点，观察牙根的走向，并追踪根尖 1/3 任何平面的偏移方向。根尖孔及其相对于根尖顶点的位置关系通常能够准确识别，特别是宽大的根管。对于牙髓钙化的患牙或根管狭窄的患牙，根尖孔可能无法识别（图 6.4）。此外，通过 CBCT 易于了解牙根吸收的过程及其对根尖形态的影响[8]。

6.2.2 牙骨质

牙骨质在根尖处的沉积过程可持续终生。咬合面的磨损和磨耗使得根尖处发生代偿性牙骨质沉积。有时，咬合压力或牙髓损伤可导致根尖处

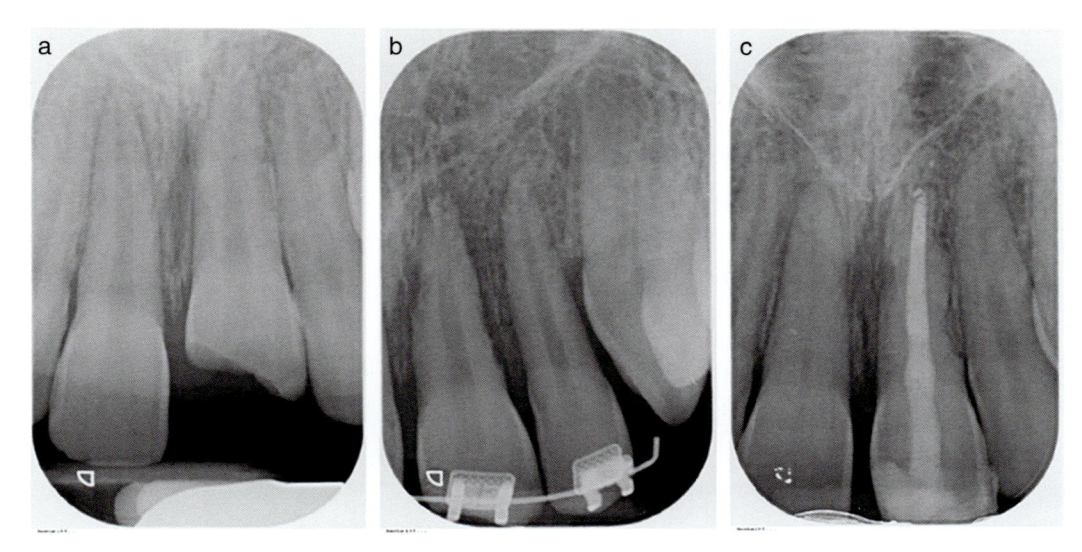

图 6.3 外伤伴炎症性外吸收。a. 牙外伤后上颌中切牙根尖片见 21 严重嵌入脱位。b. 1 周后 21 已发生炎症性外吸收，牙根表面出现陷凹，临近的牙槽骨可见透射影，累及整个根长，包括根尖 1/3。c. 外伤后 1 年，22 根尖片显示根尖周炎已消退，牙根吸收停止，牙根表面形态已发生永久性改变

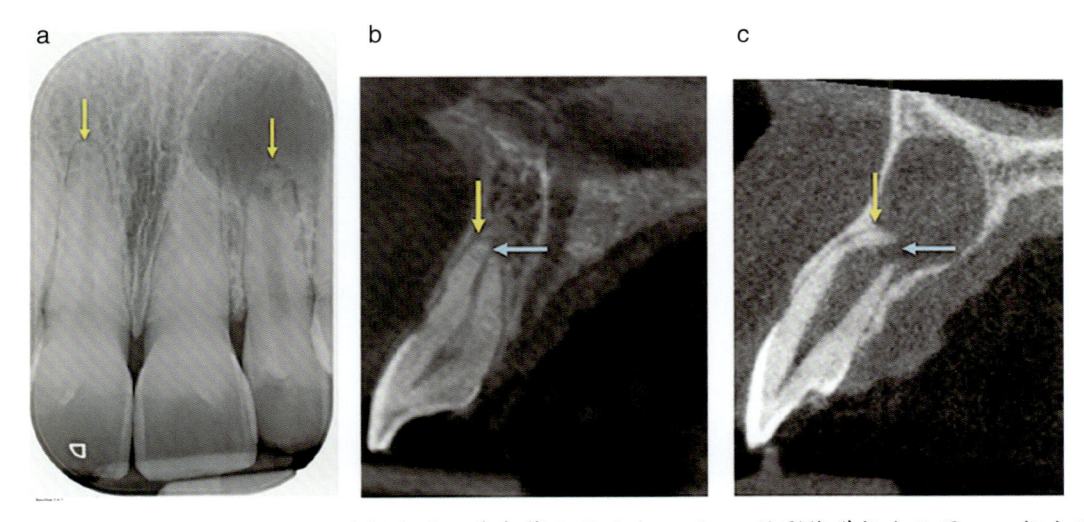

图 6.4 根尖牙周膜。a. 11、21 和 22 的根尖片。黄色箭头所示为 11 和 22 的影像学根尖位置，22 根尖周可见大面积透射影。b、c. 11（b）和 22（c）的 CBCT 矢状位。黄色箭头所示为根尖最顶端的位置，与传统根尖片上的影像学根尖相对应。根尖孔（蓝色箭头）位于稍向冠方的位置

牙骨质过度形成（牙骨质增生）。

常规X线片：牙骨质沉积增加的影像学特征较为多变，主要取决于沉积的部位。当牙骨质沉积在根尖顶点时，表现为牙根明显增长，而当其沉积在根尖1/3的部分时，则形成一个球状的根尖（牙骨质增生）。由于沉积的牙骨质通常比邻近的牙本质具有更高的阻射性，因此在常规X线片上能够对这两种组织进行区分。然而情况并非总是如此，两种组织之间也可能没有明显的分界。

CBCT：CBCT检查能够更准确地反映牙根部牙骨质沉积增加或牙骨质增生所处的位置和分布。

6.2.3　牙周膜间隙

常规X线片：牙周膜是连接牙骨质和周围牙槽骨硬骨板的软组织。由于牙周膜韧带具有透射性，而牙周膜间隙的边界结构矿化，具有相对较高的阻射性，因此牙周膜韧带的影像学表现为包绕着牙根的一条细窄的、边界清晰的透射影像。牙周膜韧带有效地将牙齿支撑在牙槽骨内，并使其具有一定的生理动度。当发生晚期边缘性牙周炎或存在创伤性咬合时，牙齿的活动度增加，牙周膜间隙的宽度可能增大（图6.5，图6.6）。

CBCT：牙周膜间隙在CBCT检查中的表现与常规X线片类似。然而借助CBCT能够在任意平面上观察牙周膜间隙，避免临近解剖结构的干扰（图6.7）。体外和体内研究证据显示，与传统X线片相比，CBCT能够更好地观察模拟的牙周膜韧带和天然的牙周膜间隙[58, 98]。

6.2.4　硬骨板

硬骨板是指紧邻牙周膜间隙处的骨组织，它是颌骨骨皮质的延续，表面有多个开孔供神经和血管通过。

常规X线片：通常，硬骨板比邻近的骨松质阻射性高，但也可能发生变化。在没有明显的解剖性干扰时，硬骨板可能表现为一个包绕牙根的、连续的阻射性边界影像。血管和神经的穿孔可能很大，以至于在X线片上能够识别。

CBCT：硬骨板在CBCT检查中的表现与常规X线片类似。但是由于CBCT具有3D系统特性，因此能够观察到更多的细节[98]。

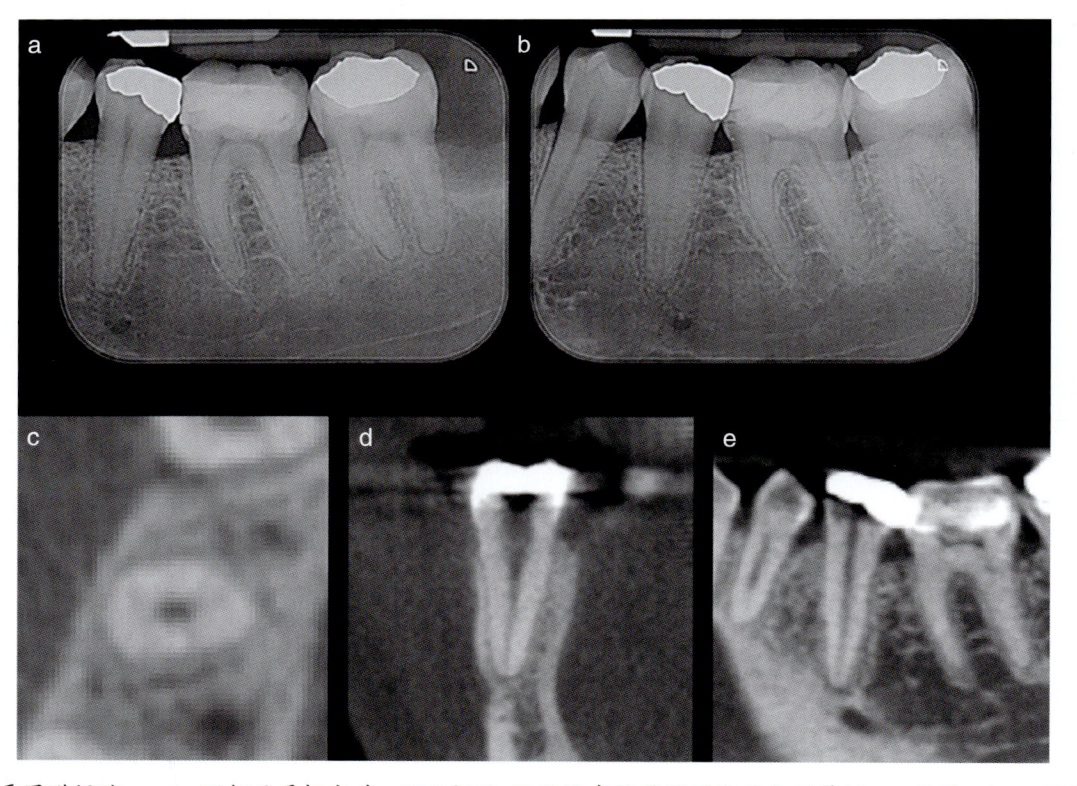

图6.5　牙周膜间隙。a、b. 下颌后牙根尖片。可以评估45近远中的牙周膜间隙和硬骨板。c. 轴面。d、e. 冠状面（d）和矢状面（e）能够更客观的了解牙齿的牙周膜间隙和硬骨板

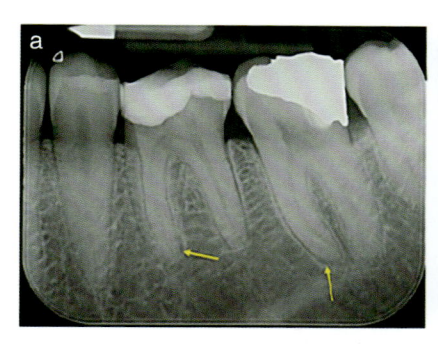

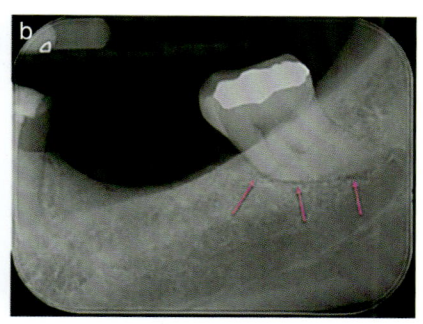

图 6.6　牙周膜间隙。a. 36 和 37 的根尖片显示近中根牙周膜间隙增宽（黄色箭头）。两颗牙均有不可复性牙髓炎症状。b. 37 根尖片，该牙孤立于牙弓末端，其近中侧牙周膜间隙增宽（粉色箭头）是由咬合创伤所致

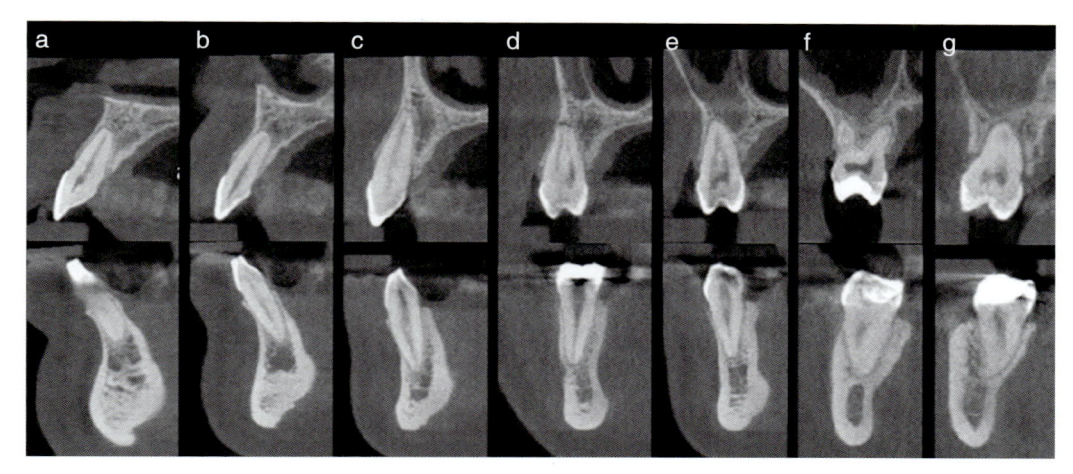

图 6.7　牙周膜间隙。a~e. 上颌（上排）和下颌（下排）前牙（a~c）和后牙（d~g）的 CBCT 矢状面和冠状面影像。这些影像准确地展示了牙根与皮质骨板的关系，以及牙齿在颌骨内的定位。同时易于了解颌骨局部的厚度和形状变化

6.2.5　皮质骨

上颌骨和下颌骨表面被一层致密骨所覆盖，称作皮质骨。上下颌骨的皮质骨厚度和完整性存在区域性差异。在上颌，唇颊侧皮质骨板较薄，自中线向后延伸至第一磨牙远中颊根时，骨皮质变宽变厚，包绕第一磨牙、第二磨牙颊侧。腭侧皮质骨通常比唇颊侧厚。但是在磨牙区，特别是第一磨牙处，腭侧皮质骨较薄，这是由于腭根向腭侧倾斜导致。

通常，上颌牙根的唇颊侧面与对应的皮质骨密切接触，但侧切牙例外，其牙根往往更向腭侧倾斜。事实上，除了侧切牙以外，上颌牙齿的根尖通常与唇颊侧皮质骨接触。此外，某些上颌牙根对应的唇颊侧皮质骨存在缺损，当患牙发生根尖病损时，可导致骨开裂。有时，这种开裂可以从根尖向牙周组织边缘延伸至任意位置。

下颌切牙区唇侧皮质骨较薄。然而，自尖牙向后延伸至第三磨牙时，唇颊侧皮质骨不断增厚。在第二磨牙、第三磨牙颊侧，皮质骨厚度最大，形成外斜嵴。

在下颌切牙区牙槽突非常窄。向后延伸过程中牙槽突不断增宽，尽管存在颌下腺窝（颌下腺所在的下颌骨凹陷处），磨牙区的牙槽突宽度仍明显增大。

在下颌前牙和前磨牙区，舌侧皮质骨通常比唇颊侧厚，而在磨牙区则相反。

下颌前牙区牙根的唇侧面通常与唇侧皮质骨紧密接触。当唇侧皮质骨非常薄时，下颌切牙的根尖有时会暴露在其缺损处。下颌前磨牙往往也较为接近颊侧皮质骨，但相对于下颌前牙略偏向舌侧。事实上，有时下颌前磨牙完全被髓质骨包绕，不与皮质骨接触。下颌磨牙的牙根通常向舌

侧倾斜，其牙根舌侧面和根尖往往与舌侧皮质骨接触。

常规X线片：在对常规X线片上的解剖结构影像进行解读时，需要首先深入了解面部骨骼的解剖学知识，这是由于在X线片上，邻近的解剖结构所造成的影像重叠和压缩往往会对了解真实的结构形态造成干扰。借助常规X线片无法了解皮质骨与牙根的关系以及覆盖在根尖处皮质骨的厚度。同时，也无法鉴别皮质骨是否存在骨开裂。

CBCT：合适的CBCT切面能够精确的测量皮质骨的厚度，还可以帮助医生观察皮质骨与邻近牙根的位置关系，检查皮质骨的完整性，确定是否存在骨开裂。

6.2.6 松质骨

致密的外层皮质骨构成了颌面部骨骼的保护层，包绕着内部的松质骨。松质骨是一种轻而多孔的骨组织，它是由皮质骨发出的骨突，即骨小梁相互交织形成的（图6.8）。骨小梁之间的间隙内有血管和骨髓。在X线片上，牙根周围包绕的牙槽突骨组织表现为颗粒状，这是由骨小梁的排列方式导致的。下颌骨的骨小梁较厚，呈水平状条纹排列，骨髓腔较宽。与之相比，上颌骨骨小梁较薄，排列更为致密，因此骨髓腔较小。然而，骨小梁的排列形态存在明显的个体差异，而且不同位点的骨小梁和骨髓腔的影像学表现与该处牙齿所承受的功能应力有关[15, 47, 50]。

常规X线片：在二维的根尖X线片上，松质骨中骨小梁和骨髓腔的界定会受到重叠的皮质骨以及邻近解剖结构的干扰。因此，由根尖周炎引起的松质骨排列的微小变化往往难以识别。有时，经验不足的临床医生会将根尖处边界清晰的、较大的骨髓腔误认为根尖周炎。

CBCT：通过选择合适的CBCT切面，能够排除解剖因素的干扰，真实观察检查区域的松质骨结构及其与牙根的关系。

6.2.7 邻近解剖结构

在对特定的牙齿进行X线片检查时，上颌骨和下颌骨正常的解剖结构可能被同时拍摄到。在使用常规X线片对根尖周炎进行评估时，与检查区域重叠的这些解剖结构可能会给影像的解读带来困难[55]。下文列举的颌骨的解剖结构在常规X线片上的表现可能被误解为根尖周炎。

切牙管和切牙孔　切牙管是位于上颌骨内的一个管道，其从鼻腔底部延伸至硬腭前部，开口位于上颌中切牙腭侧中线处。切牙孔内有上行的腭大动脉和下行的鼻腭神经穿过（图6.9）。在X线片上，切牙管和切牙孔表现为透射影像，形态可能为心形、卵圆形、圆形或楔形。在X线片上，当切牙管和（或）切牙孔与上颌中切牙根尖重叠时，可能表现出类似根尖周炎的透射影像。

鼻腔　鼻腔位于上颌骨腭突（硬腭）的正上方。鼻腔底部最前方正好位于上颌中切牙所在的牙槽突上方。鼻腔壁由皮质骨组成，在根尖X线

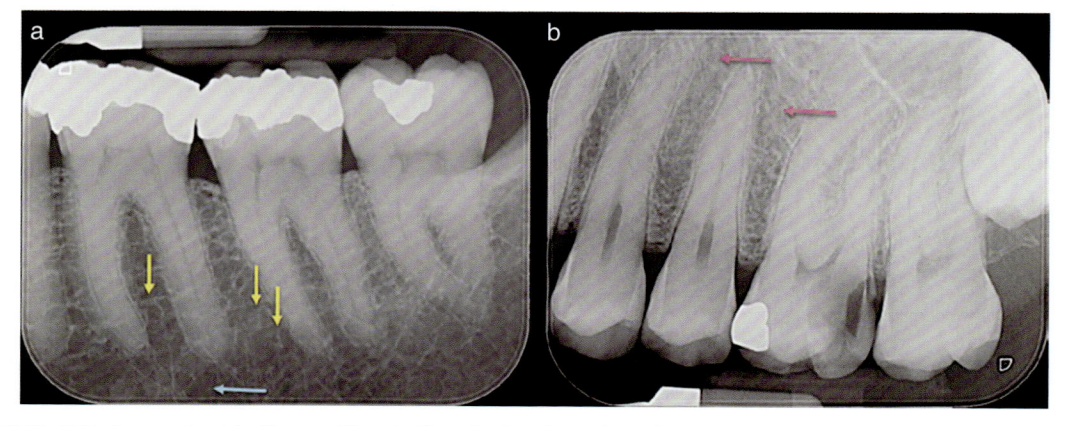

图6.8　牙周膜间隙。a. 右下颌第一、第二和第三磨牙的根尖片。多数为水平向分布的骨小梁（黄色箭头）。较宽的骨髓腔（蓝色箭头）可能被误认为根尖周透射影。b. 相较于下颌骨，上颌骨内的骨小梁（粉色箭头）较薄且更为紧密

片上，鼻腔底表现为阻射线。当其投射在上颌中切牙根尖处时，可能表现为有阻射边界的透射影像。

鼻尖 上颌前牙的根尖X线片可能包含鼻尖影像，表现为根尖处的弥散型密度增高影像。

尖牙窝 尖牙窝是位于上颌骨前部表面的一处凹陷，在尖牙隆凸的侧方。它可以表现为与上颌侧切牙根尖重叠的低密度透射影，类似根尖周炎表现。

上颌窦 上颌窦位于上颌骨体部内。作为一个充满空气的窦腔，上颌窦在X线片上表现为低密度透射影，其底部边界往往与磨牙和前磨牙牙根紧邻。然而，由于上颌窦被皮质骨包绕，其边界通常表现为一条或多条阻射线。从上颌窦边缘向腔内突出的皮质骨褶皱导致了多条阻射线的影像表现。

上颌窦的边缘可能表现为磨牙或前磨牙牙根上方的单房或双房透射影，其皮质骨构成的阻射边界可能被误解为邻近牙齿的硬骨板，窦腔可能被误认为根尖周炎病损。此外，由根尖周炎导致的真正的根尖周透射影则可能被上颌窦影像所掩盖（图6.10）。

上颌隆突 上颌隆突是由致密的皮质骨所组成的良性骨隆突，通常见于上颌骨牙槽突和腭突处。由于上颌隆突的高度矿化特性，其在常规X线片上表现为密度较高的阻射影像（图6.11）。因此，上颌隆突的影像学表现可能掩盖根尖区域正常的和病理性的影像学特征。

颏孔 颏神经穿过颏孔支配下唇和颏部的感觉神经。颏孔通常邻近下颌第二前磨牙根尖区，此外还多见于第一第二前磨牙之间的根尖下方处（图6.12）。颏孔的确切位置常常较为多变。由于颏孔的大小和形状多变，其影像学表现为多种形状的透射影。在X线片上，受其确切位置和投影角度影响，颏孔的影像可能与前磨牙牙根重叠（偶尔见于磨牙），类似根尖周炎影像。有时，由于颏孔位置过低，在根尖X线片上不可见。

下颌神经管 下牙槽神经和下牙槽动脉经下颌神经管穿过下颌骨体部。下颌神经管起自位于下颌升支内侧面的下颌孔，另一端延伸至颏孔，颏神经和血管分支经这里穿出。下颌神经管在X线片上表现为一个透射的管道影像，有时边缘放射密度较高。下颌神经管在下颌后牙根尖X线片上是否显影取决于管腔的垂直（上－下）位置。然而，当其在根尖X线片上显影时，位置接近

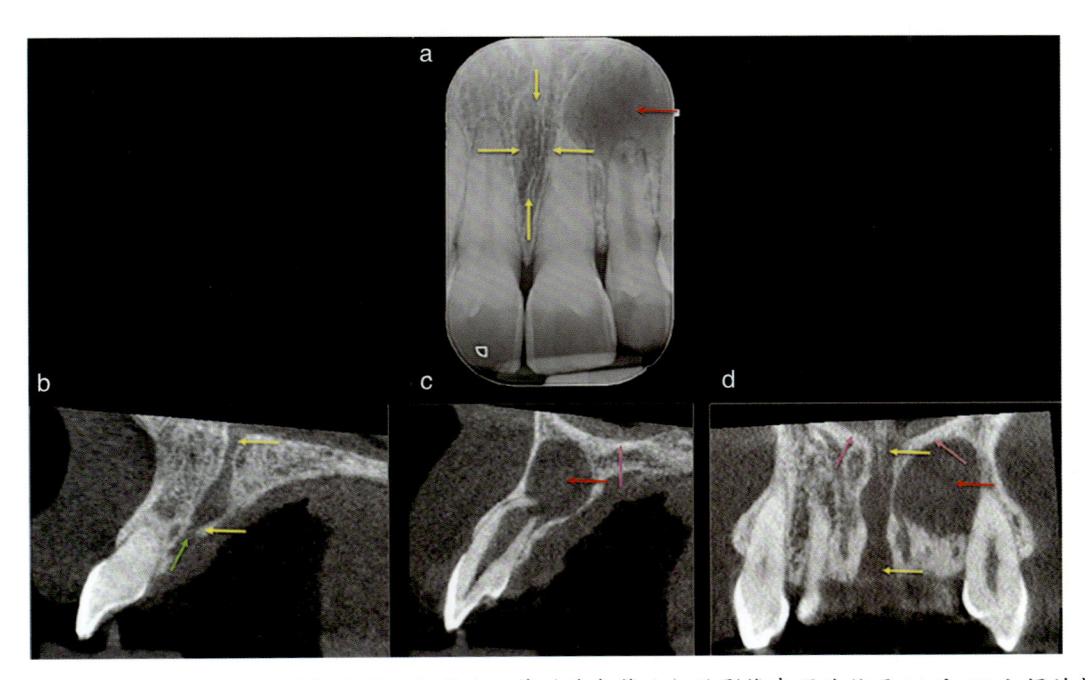

图6.9 切牙孔。a. 11、21和22的根尖片。切牙孔／管（黄色箭头）的影像表现为位于11和21之间的长形透射影。22根尖周可见大面积透射影（红色箭头）。b. CBCT矢状面上见切牙管（黄色箭头之间）和切牙孔（绿色箭头）。c. CBCT矢状面显示22根尖周透射影（红色箭头）及其与鼻腔（粉色箭头）的位置关系。d. CBCT冠状面显示切牙管（黄色箭头之间）与鼻腔（粉色箭头）和22根尖周透射影（红色箭头）的位置关系

牙齿的根尖处，可能掩盖根尖周组织的影像（图6.12）。

下颌隆突　下颌骨隆突在 X 线片上的表现与上颌隆突类似，因此对 X 线片的解读也有同样的影响（图 6.11）。

6.3　根尖周炎的影像学表现

6.3.1　常规 X 线片表现

通常，由根尖周炎引起的根尖周骨质破坏在常规 X 线片上很容易识别。然而，由于重叠的解

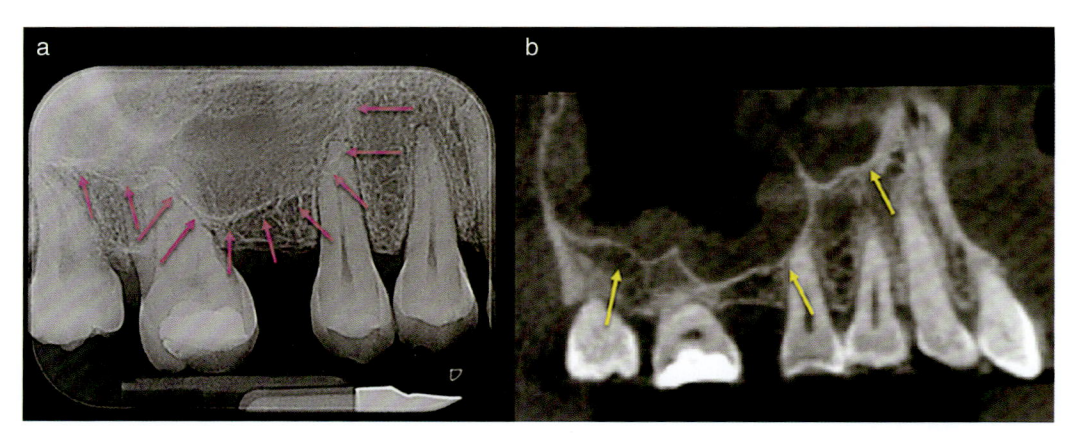

图 6.10　上颌窦。a. 右上颌后牙根尖片见右侧上颌窦下缘表现为一条细的，轮廓不清楚的阻射线（粉色箭头）。b. CBCT 矢状面准确显示了上颌窦的真实尺寸和多个分叶（黄色箭头）

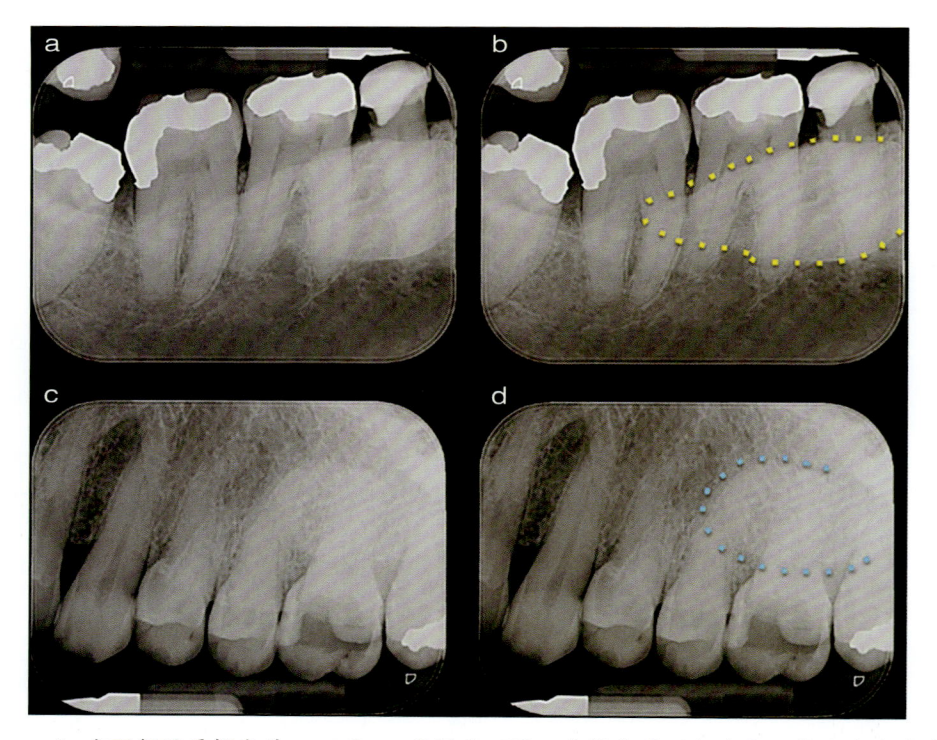

图 6.11　隆突。a、b. 右下颌后牙根尖片。45 和 46 牙根处可见一个较大的下颌隆突，表现为边界清楚的阻射影像（黄色虚线）。c、d. 左上颌后牙根尖片。25 和 26 牙根处可见一个较大的上颌隆突，表现为边界较为不清的阻射影像（蓝色虚线）

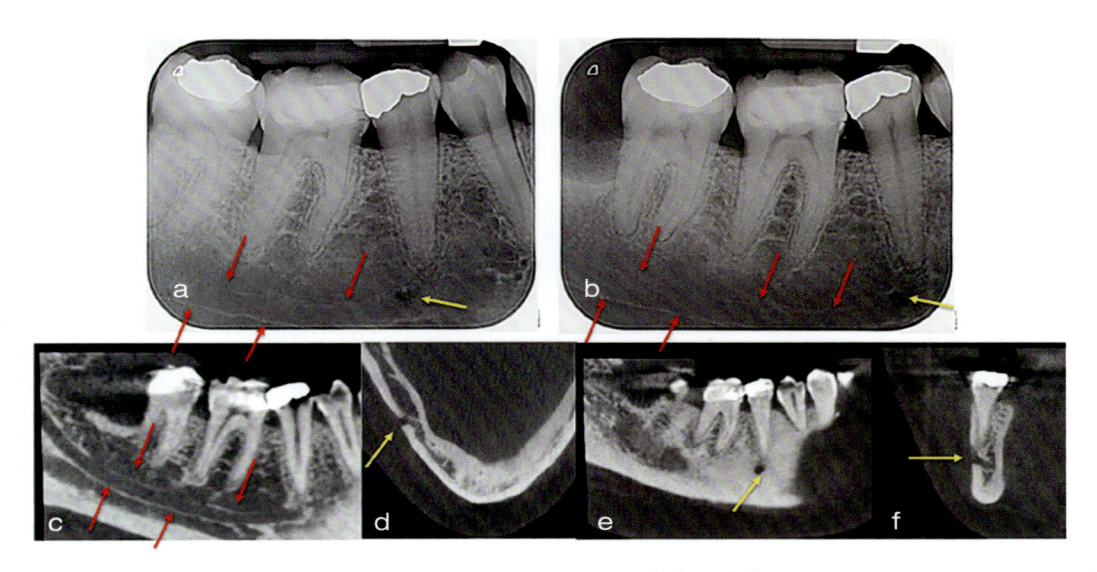

图 6.12 下颌骨解剖。a、b. 右下颌磨牙和前磨牙根尖片。下牙槽神经管表现为一组平行的、细的、阻射线（红色箭头），这些线沿近—远中方向走行，近中终止于颏孔，颏孔表现为边界清楚的椭圆形透射影（黄色箭头）。c. 下牙槽神经管的 CBCT 矢状面影像。显示神经管的真实走行及其与牙根尖的关系。d~f. CBCT 轴面（d）、矢状面（e）和冠状面（f）显示颏孔（黄色箭头）的位置

剖结构干扰，根尖周炎早期病损很难通过 X 线检测[11, 62]。根尖牙周组织结构和形态的改变，特别是牙周膜间隙、硬骨板和松质骨骨小梁的改变，往往是根尖周炎发展的早期表现[52]。因此，熟悉这些解剖结构的正常影像学表现对于疾病早期变化的识别至关重要。根尖孔仍然是根管系统内感染向牙周膜间隙和牙槽骨扩散的主要途径，侧支根管和根尖分歧往往也会成为感染扩散的通道。据文献报道，76% 的磨牙根分叉处存在副根管[22]。

6.3.2 早期根尖周炎的 X 线片表现

在常规 X 线片上，松质骨骨小梁正常结构发生细微改变是根尖周炎发展的早期指征之一。患牙根尖（或其他病菌出口处）周围的骨小梁开始出现结构破坏（正常功能改建除外）（图 6.13）。骨小梁破坏的区域可能是弥漫性的，难以与周围健康组织相区分，或者可能界限清晰，容易与邻近的骨组织区分[20]。

患牙的牙周膜间隙增宽通常是早期根尖周炎的特征之一。然而牙周膜间隙增宽并不仅仅与牙髓源性感染有关，其他原因包括咬合创伤、正畸创伤、边缘性牙周炎和神经源性炎症[23, 97]。即使是未受创伤的健康牙齿，在不使用平行投照技术的情况下，当垂直或水平方向投照角增大时，在常规 X 线片上也可看到牙周膜间隙变宽[13]。在

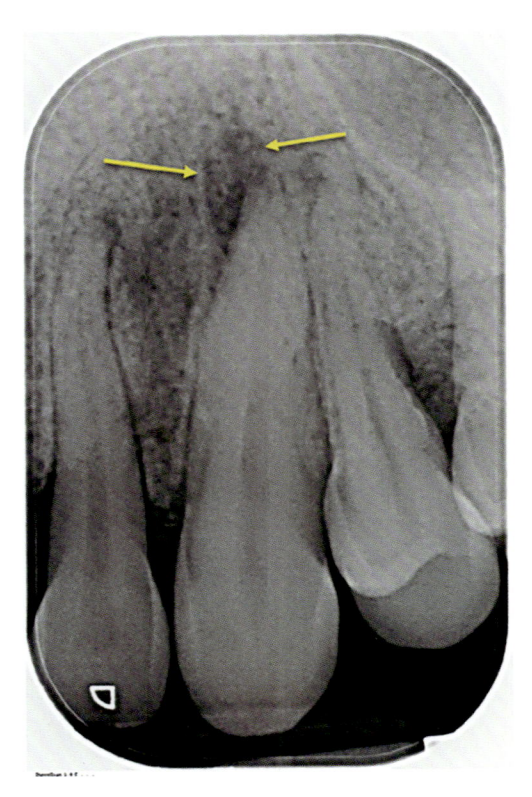

图 6.13 早期根尖周骨丧失。牙髓坏死的 23 的根尖片。23 根尖周骨质脱矿导致该区域呈现"霰弹枪"样影像（黄色箭头）

疾病的早期阶段，由牙髓感染导致的牙周膜间隙增宽会局限于感染扩散的主要通道周围的区域。邻近这些区域的牙周膜间隙不会受到影响，因此病变部位与正常部位之间会有明显的过渡。

早期根尖周炎的另一个指征是硬骨板的破坏。当疾病发生时，硬骨板的阻射密度可能降低，结构连续性可能会被破坏。这些变化会局限在微生物和毒性因子扩散的主要通道处。然而对于仅存在硬骨板连续性破坏的影像应当谨慎进行解读。硬骨板上存在的通道是松质骨和牙齿之间血管和神经供应的必经之路，这些通道可能在部分X线片上显影。此外，正常硬骨板的厚度和密度存在个体差异。而X线片的投照角度也会影响硬骨板这些特征的表现。

随着根尖周炎病程的发展，松质骨中骨小梁的矿物质逐渐耗尽，失去结构完整性。在常规X线片上表现为骨小梁变薄，放射密度降低，骨髓腔增大。这种明显的渗透性骨质破坏导致病变区域松质骨呈现出所谓的"霰弹枪"表现。虽然这一阶段并不总是能够被发现，但它代表了根尖周炎从硬骨板和牙周膜间隙的细微变化到形成明显透射影像的发展进程。

在根尖周炎的发展过程中，致密性骨炎的发生可能先于透射性影像表现的出现（图 6.14）。致密性骨炎是发生在感染患牙牙根周围牙槽骨内的一种炎症反应，可导致受累骨质发生局部硬化。至少在早期，硬化的骨质在X线片上表现为局限在患牙根尖周区域（或致病菌扩散周围的区域）的阻射影像。然而随着疾病的发展，致密性骨炎可能扩散到同一患牙或邻牙未发生感染的牙根周围的骨质。此外，骨内炎症区域还可向冠方扩展，累及远离根尖的牙槽骨。致密性骨炎病损的边缘可能呈现弥散性或界限分明。致密性骨炎的界限、形状和范围较为多变。硬化骨质的放射密度同样较为多变，在某些情况下，其密度可能过高，以至于掩盖了所包绕患牙的解剖表现。

6.3.3 晚期根尖周炎的 X 线片表现

当骨质破坏达到一定程度时，就会出现透射影像。根尖周透射影像的发展可能是上述根尖牙周组织结构变化的结果，也可能与其同时发生。当疾病进展迅速时，根尖周出现明显的透射影像可能是根尖周炎的第一个影像学表现。当疾病发展到这个阶段时，诊断就较为容易。然而，患牙所处的位置、X线片的投照角度，以及邻近解剖结构的影像可能仍然会与骨质破坏区域重叠，从而使透射影像难以识别。

为了在X线片上检测到根尖周炎，骨丧失的量需要达到一个阈值，以便与周围健康或未受影响的骨组织区分。早期的体外研究报道，当相关的骨质破坏局限在松质骨内，即皮质骨未受累时，无法检测出模拟的根尖周炎病损[11-12, 96, 103]。同时期的其他研究表明，当根尖周炎发生在上颌前部时，即使仅累及松质骨且皮质骨完整，也能通过X线检测到病损[105]。目前普遍认为根尖周炎的影像学检测与骨的矿化和脱矿比例（由疾病进展所致）、累及的颌骨、患牙在颌骨内的位置以及个体差异相关。而骨的矿化和脱矿比例本身就是反映疾病进展程度的因素。

根尖周炎导致的透射影像形态多变，其大小

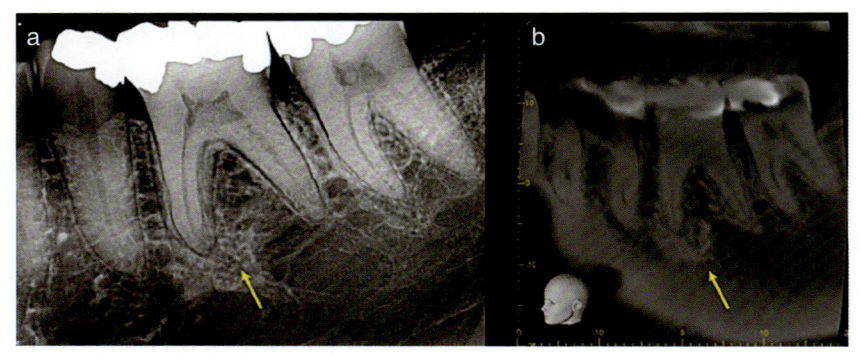

图 6.14 致密性骨炎。根尖片（a）和 CBCT 矢状面扫描（b）显示下颌磨牙近中根处阻射性增高，这是来自 46 的慢性刺激导致的反应性骨硬化（黄色箭头）的表现

与患牙牙髓感染的程度和组织对损伤产生的反应相关；其边界可以很清晰或是模糊（图 6.15、图 6.16）。有时，特别是在长期病损中，病损边界可能呈现类似皮质骨包围的外观。以往认为根尖周炎病损的影像学特征（如病损尺寸、阻射性边界的存在和性质）是预测病损组织学性质的因素[14]。这些关联后来受到了质疑，阻射性边界已不再被当作判定囊肿存在的证据[82-83, 100]。

由于根尖周炎影像学表现呈现多变性，并且对早期根尖周炎细微影像学变化的判定存在主观性，为了提高根尖周炎的客观评价，人们开发了带有参考量表的定量评分系统。根尖周指数（PAI）是通过可视的参考量表来评估牙根健康状态的评分系统[86]。

6.3.4 根尖周炎的 CBCT 表现

CBCT 扫描能够精确的表现根尖周炎的性质和尺寸。任何皮质骨的膨隆和（或）穿孔都可能被发现，并与临床表现相关联。

与传统 X 线片相比，CBCT 能够更为客观和定量地评价与疾病相关的骨质破坏的发生和进展程度，对致密性骨炎的显示也更为准确。

6.3.5 根管充填后患牙相关的根尖周炎

根尖周炎是骨质破坏和再矿化的动态过程，

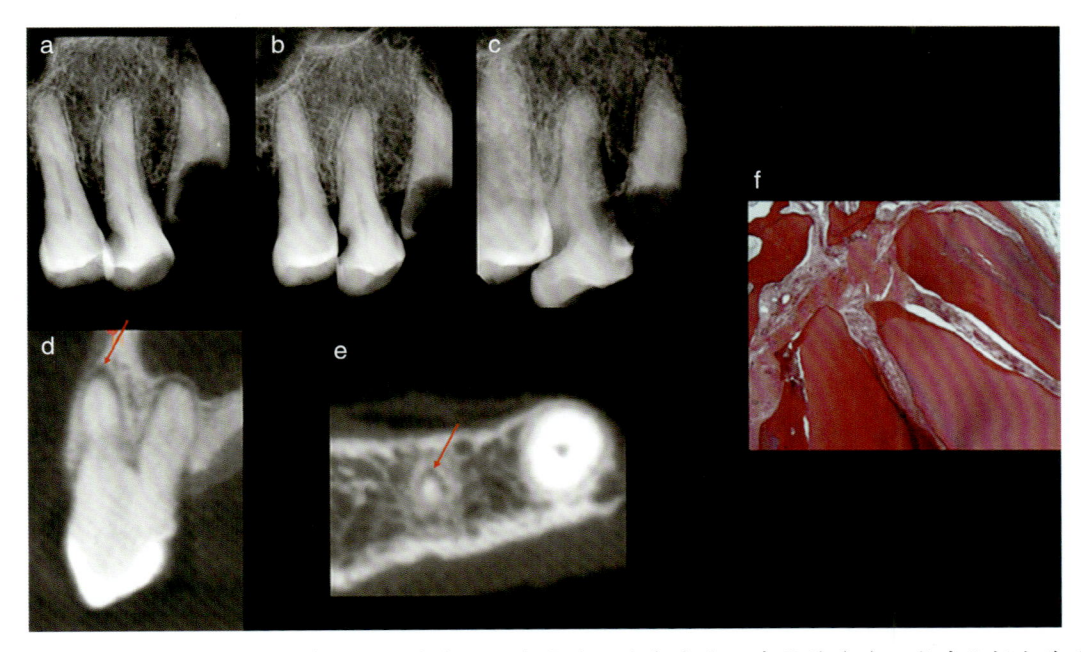

图 6.15 根尖周炎。胶片根尖片的中心视图（a）、近中偏移视图（b）和远中偏移（c）。数字化根尖片（d、e）。以上根尖片均未显示出 46 远中根根尖周病变。46 远中根组织学检查（f）显示存在根尖周炎：牙根脱矿，根尖牙髓组织坏死以及肉芽组织（放大 4 倍；HE 染色）。黄色箭头显示炎症区域伴随骨吸收（经许可转载自文献 92）

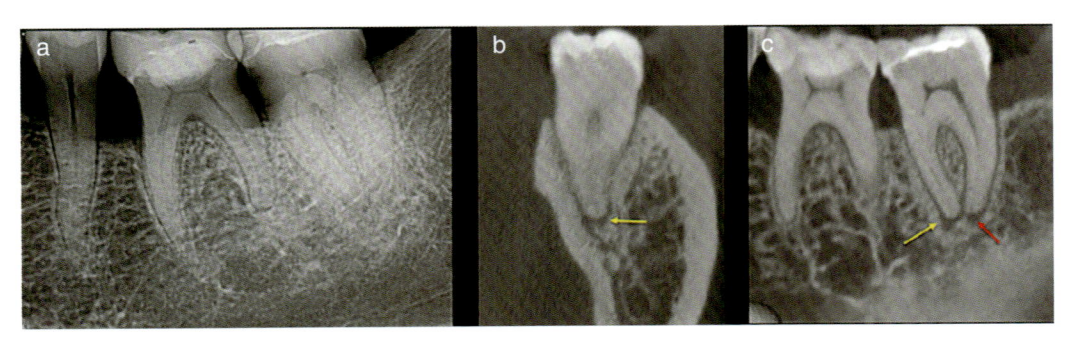

图 6.16 根尖周炎。a. 不可复性牙髓炎局部症状不明显患者的左下侧 X 线片。b、c. CBCT 冠状面和矢状面重建影像证实左下第二磨牙的近中（黄箭头）和远中（红箭头）牙根存在根尖周透射影

其变化无法通过常规 X 线片或三维影像学检查进行检测。在任何特定的时间点，对根管充填后患有根尖周炎的患牙拍摄 X 线片仅能说明透射影像当时的尺寸，对判定病变是否稳定，愈合或进展情况仅能提供很少的帮助。根管治疗后根尖周炎的愈合可能需要数年，甚至数十年的时间。虽然专家共识指南建议，治疗后 4 年仍持续存在的根尖周病损通常应考虑与治疗后疾病相关[40]，但是对于根管治疗后根尖周炎的愈合没有科学上公认的时间上限。一些长期疗效研究表明，根管治疗后根尖周炎的晚期愈合可长达 5~10 年[110]、10~17 年[76-77] 和 20~27 年[75]。Molven 等人[74] 研究报道大多数病例的延迟愈合与治疗过程中根管充填材料侵入根尖周组织有关。

6.4 愈合的特点

6.4.1 非手术根管治疗后根尖周炎的愈合

目前，对根尖周炎的愈合过程在 X 线片上的表现知之甚少；愈合所需的时间差异很大。有证据表明，骨密度的短暂增加可能发生在愈合过程的最初几周[84-85]。然而，如上文所述，根尖周炎相关的透射影像在治疗后可能部分消失，但最终可持续数年[76-77, 110]。在愈合过程中，根尖周病损的放射密度随着新骨的沉积而增加。目前尚不清楚新骨是从病损边缘向中心沉积，还是骨突凸向病损中心并扩增来填充病损区域。如果皮质骨板发生穿孔，那么愈合过程起自皮质骨完整性的重建和骨质沉积，并从穿孔处向病损中心延伸[17]。新形成的骨质尚不成熟，与邻近健康骨组织相比其排列尚不整齐。最终，在愈合的病例中，牙周膜间隙和硬骨板将完成重建。由材料超充引起牙周膜间隙持续性增宽和持续性的骨质稀疏是根管充填后患牙愈合过程的影像学特征。完全愈合可能随着时间的推移而发生[76, 110]。

6.4.2 根管外科手术后的愈合

根管外科手术后的愈合与非手术治疗不同，在手术过程中，清理掉骨缺损处的肉芽组织后，骨腔内即刻充满血液，随后形成血凝块，为新骨的形成提供了支架。手术治疗后的愈合通常比非手术治疗更快。在手术中，为了获得到达病损体部的通道，必须去除其表面覆盖的所有矿化组织。因此，与术前相比，术后即刻的 X 线片透射影像更为明显。此外，在愈合过程中，其影像学表现较根管治疗后病变的愈合过程也更为多变。

当唇/颊侧和舌/腭侧皮质骨破坏严重无法重建时，新骨的形成将从完整的侧壁处开始，皮质骨破坏的区域被纤维组织修复，导致根尖"瘢痕组织"形成。根尖瘢痕组织的形成在组织学被归类为"不完全愈合"，但在临床上被认为是完全愈合。根尖瘢痕组织形成的特点是以一定角度延伸至牙周膜间隙的，逐渐缩小的透射影像。根尖周围透射影像的分布可能不对称。透射影内有时可见到清晰的骨结构。在持续愈合过程中，可能看到根尖周围硬骨板形成，将透射影与牙根末端分隔开[78]。根尖周病损已经导致唇/颊侧和舌/腭侧皮质骨板广泛破坏的患牙在非手术根管治疗后，有时也会出现具有类似特征的瘢痕组织[78]。

6.5 X 线片在根尖周炎评价中的应用

X 线片的二维属性、解剖干扰和几何扭曲限制了其评价根尖周炎影像学特征的准确性。

平行投照技术克服了根尖 X 线片的一些局限性[40]。Kangasingam 等人[62] 以根尖组织切片和组织病理学分析为参考标准的研究发现，额外增加近中和远中水平角度投照的 X 线片，可提高根尖周炎诊断的准确性。然而，拍摄多张根尖周 X 线片可能并不能确保获得更多的信息来识别所有相关解剖结构和病损表现[10, 70]。

射线束瞄准装置的使用增大了获得几何精确性图像的可能性[46, 117]。Forsberg[43-45] 的一系列研究发现，与分角投照相比，平行投照技术在根尖解剖影像呈现的精确度和可重复性方面表现更佳。

X 线片投照角度过高或过低（分角或平行投照技术）可能增大或减小根尖周病损的尺寸，甚至无法显示病损影像[11, 13, 57]。

目前，根尖周 X 线片被认为是影像学初步评估的首选检查技术。后续部分将介绍一些被用来克服根尖周炎评估局限性的影像检查技术。

6.6 牙髓诊断的先进影像学技术

一些替代性的成像技术克服了根尖X线片的局限性[80, 90]。

调节孔径计算机断层扫描（TACT）的工作原理是基于体层成像合成[121]。它是使用一个可编程的影像套件，在不同的投照几何体内拍摄8~10张X线片，再通过专用软件重建能够分层查看的三维数据集。

TACT的总放射剂量不超过根尖X线片的1~2倍，并且检查部位因解剖干扰导致的影像重叠更少[81]。此外，该技术还能够避免金属修复体导致的放射伪影。据报道，其清晰度类似二维的X线片[80]。

磁共振成像（MRI）是一种不利用电离辐射的特殊成像技术，它是借助氢原子在磁场中的运动来生成MR图像。Tutton和Goddard[114]认为可以通过皮质骨的存在、破坏和（或）增厚来确定根尖周病损的性质。Goto等人[51]比较了离体下颌骨和半侧下颌骨使用三维重建MRI和计算机断层成像的测量结果，研究发现，MRI的准确性与计算机断层扫描相似。Cotti和Campisi[30]认为MRI可能有助于评估牙髓病变的性质和制定根尖周手术计划。

然而，MRI分辨率低、扫描时间长以及较高的硬件成本意味着只有在专业放射科才能进行这种影像检查。此外，硬件的使用以及图像的解读还需要专业的培训。

超声的原理是超声波在具有不同声学特性的组织之间的界面发生反射（回声）[53]。

一些课题组提出超声可以区分囊肿和肉芽肿[6, 30, 53]。然而，这些研究的根尖活检组织都没有包含完整的牙根根尖，因此无法确定囊性病变是真性囊肿还是袋状囊肿。此外，这些病损没有进行连续切片[99]，无法进行准确的组织学诊断。因此，超声评估根尖周病损真实性质和类型（如真性囊肿和袋状囊肿）的能力存在疑问。超声会受骨组织影响，因此仅适用于评估覆盖的皮质骨很少或没有覆盖皮质骨的根尖周病变的范围[6]。

计算机断层扫描（CT）通过拍摄一系列二维的断层X线图像来生成目标物的三维图像。

在过去的50年里，CT技术取得了显著的发展，实现了在低放射剂量下获得软硬组织的高分辨率。目前常用的CT扫描仪称为多层CT（MSCT），其具有多个探测器呈线性排列，机架内的X线射线源和探测器围绕着患者旋转，从而实现同时进行"多层"扫描。这使得扫描时间更快，从而减少了患者的辐射暴露[111, 124]。

与常规X线片相比，CT还具有以下优势。它消除了解剖干扰，并且具有高对比度的分辨率，从而能够对物理密度差小于1%的组织进行区分，而在使用常规X线片时需要物理密度差达到10%[124]。Velvart等人[118]发现，对于拟行根尖手术的下颌后牙，CT比常规X线片更容易发现根尖透射影和下牙槽神经的位置。

目前，在牙髓病学诊疗方面，CT技术已被锥形束计算机断层扫描（CBCT）所取代。

锥形束计算机断层扫描或数字化体层扫描（DVT）的发展始于20世纪90年代末，能够通过明显低于传统计算机断层扫描（CT）的放射剂量对颌面骨骼进行三维扫描[9, 79]。因此，CBCT在牙髓病学中的应用明显增长[92]。

CBCT通过口外X射线源和探测器围绕患者头部进行同步旋转实现180°~360°的单次扫描，从而获得三维的数据。CBCT所用的X射线束为锥形，所捕获的圆柱形或球形的数据集称作视场（FOV）。CBCT的优点是能够减少患者所受的放射剂量。在牙髓病诊疗中建议使用小剂量（有限的）高分辨率的CBCT。

通过软件将收集到的数据处理成类似于医用CT扫描仪产生的格式。重建的CBCT图像可以同时显示在三个正交位面上，从而使临床医生能够获得观察区域的真正的三维视图。

目前已有证据显示，将制造商默认设置的曝光参数进行修改，明显降低放射剂量，仍能够保持CBCT图像的诊断价值[37, 60, 67]。

CBCT也具有一些局限性，其中包括空间和对比度分辨率较差[102, 128]，以及在放射密度较高的材料（如牙釉质、牙胶尖、金属桩）周围会有伪影产生（如射线束增强和散射），这些因素均会导致CBCT的诊断价值降低[21, 41, 65]。

6.7 鉴别诊断

虽然根尖周炎是颌骨最常见的病损，但其他发生在颌骨内的病损也可能被误诊为根尖周炎。使用 CBCT 和超声[29]等先进的影像技术有助于进行鉴别诊断。下文将对颌骨内最常见的透射影像进行简要的介绍。

6.7.1 伴发的牙周疾病

在慢性边缘性牙周炎的晚期，病损可能进展到牙根根尖 1/3。影像学上通常可见根周的透射影像，有时可累及根分叉区域。因此，需要仔细评估确认是否存在牙髓来源的病变（根尖周病损），从而决定是否需要进行牙周和（或）牙髓治疗。根尖炎症也可以逆向扩散或沿着牙根向冠方引流，可能形成类似牙周袋状的窦道。

因此，可能需要进行 CBCT 扫描来确定牙槽骨受累的程度，从而有助于医生制定治疗计划。

6.7.2 牙根纵裂

根管治疗后的患牙牙根纵裂（VRF）的发生率高于活髓牙[25,28]。据报道，根管治疗后的牙齿有 20%~32% 因牙根纵裂而被拔除[24,27]。

早期（不完全）牙根纵裂在临床上和影像学上可能不容易发现。然而，随着牙根纵裂的进展和感染的发生，牙根一侧的牙周膜间隙会增宽，进一步发展时，会出现明显的根周骨丧失[26]。在常规 X 线片上，只有当 X 线束与不完全折裂纹平行时才能检测到牙根纵裂（图 6.17、图 6.18），然而这种情况较为少见[18]。

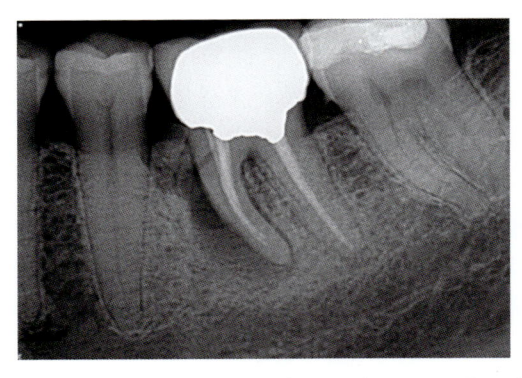

图 6.17 牙根纵裂；位于近中根近中侧的"J"形根周透射影提示近中根存在牙根纵裂

对于临床检查和常规 X 线检查难以确诊的病例，使用 CBCT 有助于检测疑似邻近牙根纵裂部位的根周骨组织的细微变化[91]。

6.7.3 骨髓炎

当感染扩散并破坏骨髓时，根尖周炎可能发展为骨髓炎[64]。这种情况更多见于下颌骨。受累的骨组织和骨膜的影像学表现多变，并与年龄相关[123]。邻近的骨膜处可能有新骨形成（骨膜反应）。骨髓炎的典型特征包括虫蚀样（模糊）的边界，致密的岛状死骨形成，坏死区域以外的骨膜下成骨，以及周围骨组织硬化。

6.7.4 咬合创伤

过大的咬合力引起的牙周组织损伤可导致牙周膜间隙增宽，硬骨板增厚或不连续[34]。与工作侧或非工作侧𬌗干扰相关的损伤可能是局限性的；但如果存在功能不良习惯、正畸治疗或牙周疾病时，影响可能更为广泛[59,119]。

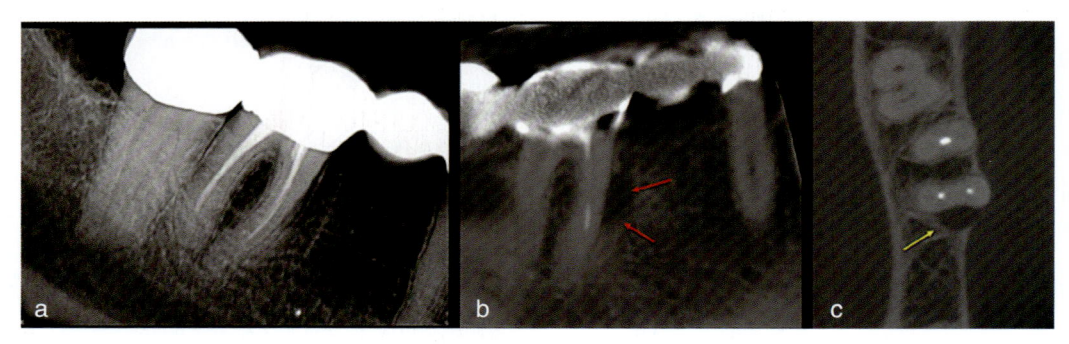

图 6.18 牙根纵裂。a. 右下磨牙根尖片未见异常，但 CBCT 矢状面（红色箭头）（b）和轴面（黄色箭头）（c）的影像显示近中根处存在明显的透射影

6.7.5 牙源性囊肿

根尖周囊肿 根尖周囊肿是颌骨内最为常见的囊肿，通常起源于 Malassez 上皮剩余细胞。这些囊肿多见于 30~50 岁的患者[122]，多发于死髓或根管治疗后的牙齿，其中最常见的是上颌侧切牙。这类囊肿表现为均匀的透射影像，为圆形、单房，边界光滑清晰，有密质骨围绕[123]。有时可见皮质骨板膨隆和邻近牙齿移位（图 6.19）。

牙源性角化囊性瘤 单房或多房的良性肿瘤，起源于牙板上皮，多见于颌骨后部和（或）下颌上颌尖牙区。表现为边界清晰，密度均匀的透射影，可在松质骨内明显扩张（图 6.20）。

含牙囊肿 含牙囊肿与未萌牙或阻生牙的牙冠相关，囊腔的衬里上皮细胞来自缩余釉上皮。含牙囊肿多见于 20~40 岁的患者，通常是在 X 线片检查时偶然发现，多见于下颌骨[36]。

该囊肿通常表现为边界清晰、单房、密度均匀的透射影，远离其所包绕的牙齿。有些病例的邻牙可能发生移位或出现相关的邻近牙根吸收。含牙囊肿可以在颊舌向和近远中向广泛扩张。

根侧囊肿 该囊肿的起源尚不清楚，可能来自 Malassez 上皮剩余细胞、牙板或缩余釉上皮。多见于下颌侧切牙或前磨牙区。囊肿累及的牙齿通常为活髓，这有助于进行鉴别诊断[104]。

影像学上，根侧囊肿表现为位于受累患牙侧方的，边界清晰的单房透射影像，也可能有牙周膜韧带和硬骨板的破坏[71]。

6.7.6 非牙源性囊肿和肿瘤

鼻腭（切牙）管囊肿 该囊肿的发病率约为 1%，多见于 40~60 岁男性。病变位于上颌中切牙后方中线处，表现为圆形或椭圆形透射影像，边界光滑清晰[123]。

该囊肿呈密度均匀的透射影像，当它发生扩张时，可能导致邻牙移位（图 6.21）。邻牙牙髓电活力测试通常有反应，可作为鉴别诊断的依据。

创伤性骨囊肿 该病损缺乏上皮衬里，不是真正的囊肿。创伤性骨囊肿多见于 10~20 岁的患者，好发于下颌骨，通常为检查时意外发现。这些病变通常位于牙根之间，为形态不规则的单房影像，边界光滑清晰。该病变对邻牙不会产生直接影响，也不会引起颌骨外形膨隆。

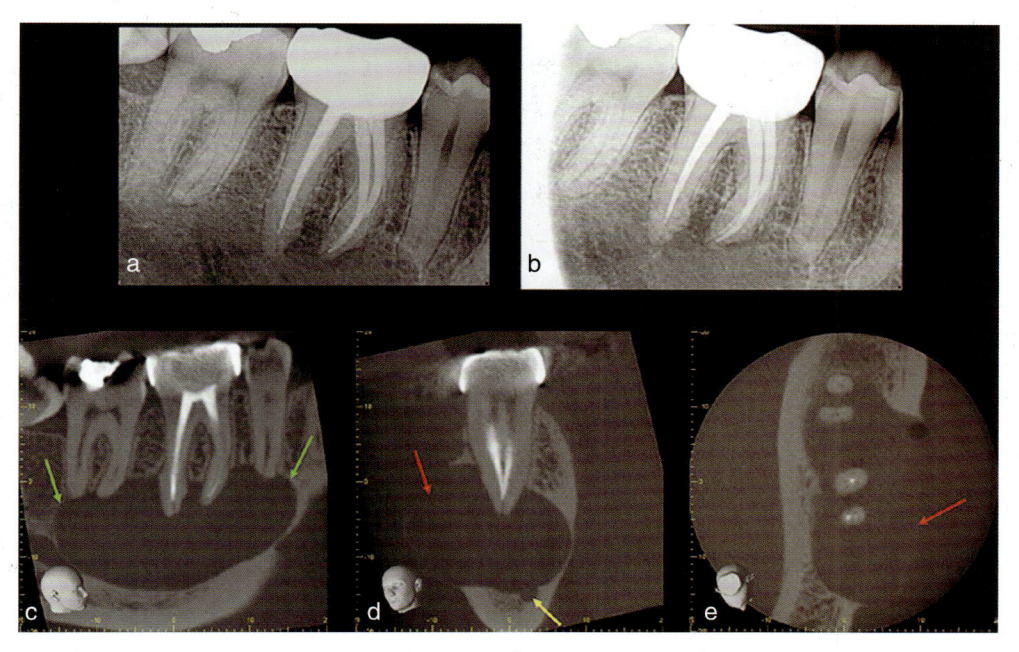

图 6.19 根尖周囊肿。a、b. 平行投照的根尖片显示根管治疗后的右下第一磨牙根尖周可见一个边界清楚的透射影相关。c. CBCT 矢状面重建影像显示一个边界清楚的透射影从右下第二前磨牙延伸到右下第二磨牙，且已经导致了根尖周吸收。CBCT 冠状面（d）和轴面（e）重建影像显示可见明显的颊侧扩张和颊侧皮质骨板穿孔（红色箭头）。下牙槽神经管（黄色箭头）已向下偏移

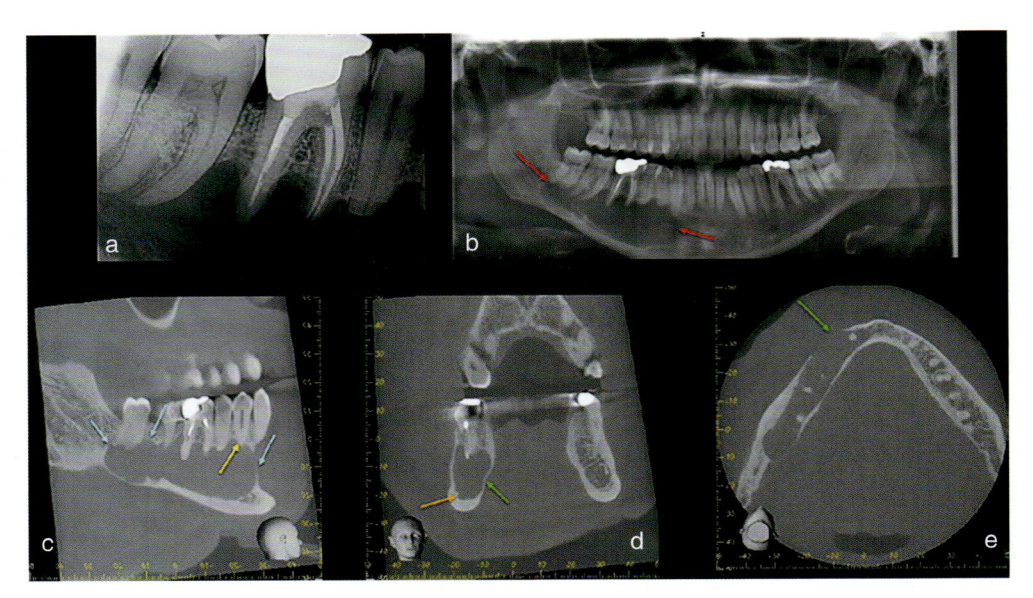

图6.20 牙源性角化囊肿。a. 根尖片显示右下前磨牙和根管治疗后的磨牙区可见大面积透射影。b. 曲面体层片显示病变累及的范围（红色箭头）。c~e. CBCT 矢状面、冠状面和轴面重建影像显示右侧下颌骨体内可见一较大的，边界清楚的假多房透射影，从右下切牙延伸至磨牙后区域，且在牙根之间向上延伸。右下前磨牙可见炎症性外吸收影像，但根管治疗后的右下第一磨牙未见吸收影像，提示这不是炎性病变。病变导致皮质骨板变薄并向颊侧扩张（绿色箭头），且临近下牙槽神经（橙色箭头）

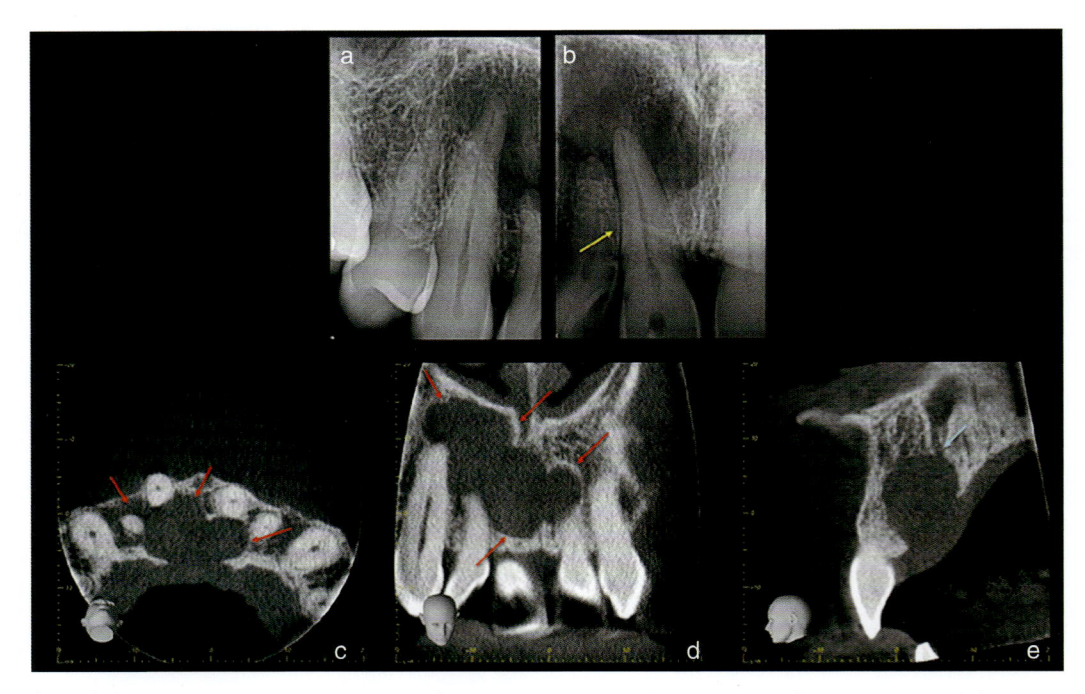

图6.21 鼻腭管囊肿。a、b. 根尖片显示右上中切牙可见开髓影像。13~21区域可见大面积透射影，边界清楚，部分区域见皮质骨影像。病变导致11牙（黄色箭头）移位，未见牙根吸收影像。CBCT 轴面（c）和冠状面（d）重建显示分叶状透射影像，皮质骨板未见明显扩张（红色箭头），矢状面（e）影像显示该透射影几乎与切牙孔融合（蓝色箭头）

6.7.7 骨相关的病损

巨细胞肉芽肿 巨细胞肉芽肿的病因包括刺激以及牙齿创伤。这些病损可以呈单房或多房，术后较易复发。病损边界光滑清晰，呈扇形。当较大的病损中存在薄的骨小梁时，可能呈现蜂窝样表现。邻牙可能移位和（或）吸收，邻近的颌骨可能出现膨隆。巨细胞肉芽肿的性质可以是非侵袭性的，也可以是侵袭性的。

根尖周牙骨质结构不良 牙骨质结构不良的病因尚不明确，经常被误诊为根尖周炎，特别是发生在中年人下颌切牙部位的病损，该病最常见于非洲裔的人群，女性发病率高于男性。患牙牙髓电活力测试结果通常有反应，除非存在其他因素的影响。

病损呈圆形，直径约为 5mm，通常累及多颗患牙。通常情况下，病损界限不清晰（图 6.22）。其影像学表现取决于所处的阶段，可能为透射影像（早期），出现阻射部分（中期），或呈现致密的阻射影像（晚期）。硬骨板可能消失。

6.7.8 肿瘤

成釉细胞瘤 一种侵袭性肿瘤，多见于 30~60 岁的患者，肿瘤可沿各个方向扩张，导致邻牙松动/移位。下颌骨成釉细胞瘤较上颌骨更为多见[123]。

影像学上，成釉细胞瘤通常表现为由骨小梁分隔的多房分叶状，有时可见蜂窝状表现。

恶性肿瘤 恶性肿瘤较为少见，其影像学表现取决于肿瘤的类型以及病程发展的时间。

影像学特征包括包绕一颗或多颗牙的边界不清，无皮质骨包围的透射影像，或是边界不清的"虫蚀样"（不规则）不均匀骨质破坏区。邻牙发生吸收可能是侵袭性的表现，提示为恶性肿瘤。生长缓慢，侵袭性较低的肿瘤可能导致牙齿移位，而不是吸收。

6.8 CBCT 在根尖周炎评估中的应用

6.8.1 诊断

临床研究表明，与根尖 X 线片相比，CBCT 将根尖周炎的检出率[5, 16, 32, 41, 69, 95]提高了 11% ~ 39%。此外，通过 CBCT 检查发现约 10% 的不可复性牙髓炎的牙齿存在根尖周炎[4]。

这些临床研究的结果已被体外实验所证实，在这些实验中，人为建立根尖周病损，即预先知道根尖周骨质的状态。对猪下颌骨上人为构建的不同尺寸根尖周病损的研究发现，CBCT 的诊断灵敏度约为数字化和常规 X 线片的两倍[109]。利用人类颌骨进行的体外研究同样发现，在评估根尖周病损是否存在方面，CBCT 比根尖 X 线片更为准确[87, 89, 107, 113]。CBCT 诊断的准确性已得到了体外实验系统评价和 meta 分析的证实[66]。

影像学表现和组织学特征的相关性对于区分病变组织和健康组织至关重要[48, 62-63]。根尖周炎

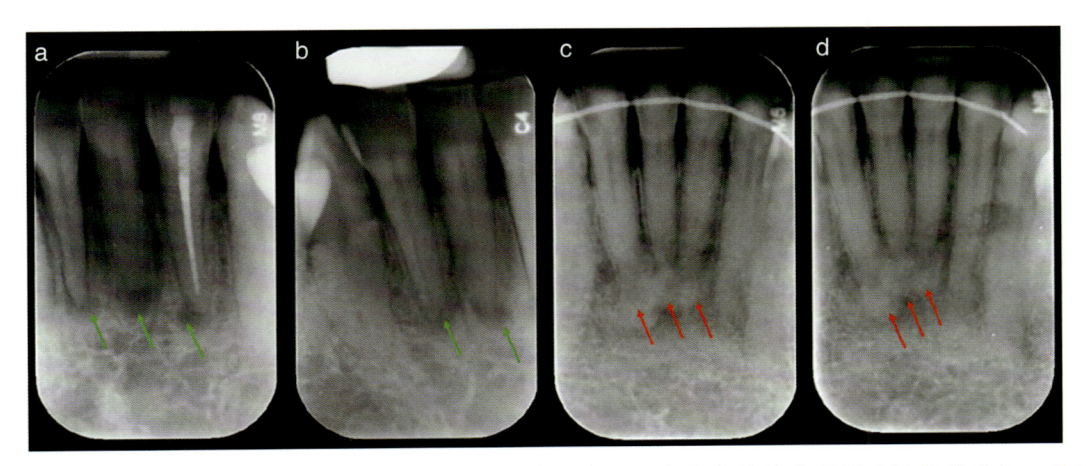

图 6.22 根尖周牙骨质结构不良。a、b. 早期：下颌切牙区均可见边界清楚的透射影（绿色箭头）。牙髓活力测试均为活髓，但 32 被误诊为根尖周炎进行了根管治疗。c、d. 中期：下颌切牙区根尖片可见边界不清的透射影，伴斑片状阻射影（红色箭头），所累及的患牙均为活髓

是一种炎症性疾病，其主要特征是细胞浸润和由炎症导致的继发性骨质破坏。由于健康组织中也可能存在类似病理改变骨质变化，因此将CBCT和根尖片的影像学特征与组织学相关联是至关重要的。一项在狗体内进行的对诱导性根尖周炎行根管治疗的研究以组织学作为参考标准，证实了CBCT的准确性[35]。X线片和CBCT的特异性和阳性预测值（positive predictive value，PPV）为1，即能够准确排除根尖周病变。然而，CBCT的灵敏度（0.91）明显高于根尖X线片（0.77）。CBCT和根尖X线片的阴性预测值（negative predictive value，NPV）分别为0.46和0.25。CBCT和X线片诊断根尖周炎的总体准确率分别为0.92和0.78[35]。

目前，来自人类研究的数据基本上确立了CBCT表现与其组织学反映的强相关性。Kanagasingam等人[62-63]采用与Brynolf[20]相似的方法，以组织学为金标准，在新鲜人体标本上评估了单一X线片、视差数字化X线片和CBCT在根尖周炎诊断中的准确性。研究共分析了67颗牙齿中的86个牙根。所有成像系统都表现出极好的特异性；也就是说当通过影像学技术诊断为根尖周炎时，其组织学表现也通常是一致的。然而，单视野X线片、视差图和CBCT的灵敏度（检测疾病的能力）分别为0.27、0.38和0.89。这些成像系统的总体准确率分别为0.63、0.69和0.94。因此，采用CBCT检测牙齿是否存在根尖周炎具有更高的可信度。

传统观点认为，由根尖周肉芽肿发展而来的根尖周囊肿可能需要手术切除。通过影像学表现区分囊肿和肉芽肿对治疗方案的选择是极为重要的[31]。有观点认为CBCT能够区分实性和囊性或腔性病变[106]，甚至区分肉芽肿和根尖周囊肿[54]。对于此类研究结果应当谨慎对待，因为鉴别根尖周病变类型的唯一可靠方法是将其完整切除后对样本行连续切片，但截至目前尚未完成。

CBCT在根尖周炎病变检测中的较高准确性已被证实有益于牙髓病诊断和治疗[33, 38, 101, 116]，以及根尖显微手术的术前评估。

对于根尖周病变的解读还取决于评估CBCT检查的临床医生或放射科医生所接受的培训，掌握的知识和积累的经验[88]。

即使CBCT在根尖周病变检测中具备较高的准确性，并不意味着应当将其常规用于牙髓病的诊断和治疗[66, 92]。它的使用应该限于可能对根尖周炎的诊断和（或）治疗带来潜在收益的特殊病例。根据欧洲牙髓病学学会对于CBCT的立场声明[91]建议，对于以下情况的根尖周炎应当考虑采用CBCT：①根尖周炎的影像学表现诊断与症状/体征相矛盾时；②确定非牙源性原因导致的症状/体征。

6.8.2 治疗结果

通过CBCT确定治疗的结果是其在牙髓病领域的一个令人兴奋的应用。治疗结果在很大程度上取决于缓解或消除慢性根尖周炎，或成功地防止其发展。因此，所有与CBCT在根尖周炎检测中的准确性相关的特性都将在关于牙髓治疗的后续研究中发挥作用。通过CBCT扫描应当能够更客观和准确地确定活髓治疗[56]和根管治疗[68, 94]的预后，并对牙根治疗后牙齿的进一步处理产生影响[33]。

CBCT在根尖周炎检测方面的灵敏度明显增高，因此对于同一颗因根尖周炎治疗后的患牙，在使用CBCT复查时其愈合率明显低于采用根尖X线片检测。Paula-Silva等人[48]以局部解剖的组织学评估为金标准，比较了根尖片和CBCT用于犬牙髓治疗结果的评估。根管治疗6个月后，通过根尖片评估可见79%的患牙治疗效果良好，然而在使用CBCT检查时仅为35%，即一半的在传统意义上"成功"的治疗被证明是失败的。当对术前已存在病变的患牙进行研究时，成功率甚至更低（25%）[48]。

Liang等人[68]采用根尖片和CBCT比较了根管治疗两年后的疗效。结果发现，采用根尖片评价时，87%的病例达到了良好的治疗效果，而采用CBCT评估时为74%；这一差距明显小于已有病变的患牙。

在对磨牙进行的随访研究中，CBCT的高灵敏度则更为明显[33, 94]。采用CBCT评估磨牙的治疗效果时失败率更高，这可能是由于其复杂的根管解剖导致初次治疗和再治疗过程中消毒的难度更大。

未来的研究可能会表明在常规 X 线片上表现为"愈合"的根尖周围组织，在使用 CBCT 成像时可能仍然有根尖周围疾病的表现（如牙周膜间隙变宽、根尖周透射影）。因此，在对已接受过根管治疗且影像学提示已经成功愈合的患牙行（再次）冠修复时，以上结果可能影响决策的制定和标准的选择[1]。在采用 CBCT 评估治疗结果时，可能会发现不同的疗效预测因素，这可能有助于医生理解根管治疗后患牙的愈合动态，并发现不同的疗效预测因素[126]。

应当制定符合临床情况的最小视场，以保证较低的辐射剂量[93]。

6.9 结语

影像学检查是成功诊断和治疗根尖周炎的基础之一。深入了解传统 X 线片的局限性和充分掌握牙槽骨解剖的相关知识对于准确解读 X 线片至关重要。

CBCT 的使用者必须熟悉该领域的相关立场声明，例如欧洲牙髓病学学会或美国牙髓病学协会/口腔颌面放射协会关于 CBCT 的立场声明[2,91]，并定期学习更新关于 CBCT 的核心知识[19]。当将患者暴露于电离辐射时，确保辐射剂量尽可能保持在合理可达的较低水平[42]。因此，每一次辐射暴露都必须是合理的，并对放射影像和患者的辐射剂量进行优化。

参考文献

[1] FGDP. The Royal College of Surgeons of England. Selection criteria for dental radiography. Good Practice Guidelines. London: FGDP, 2004,

[2] AAE. AAE and AAOMR Joint Position Statement: Use of Cone Beam Computed Tomography in Endodontics 2015 Update. Oral Surg Oral Med Oral Pathol Oral Radiol, 2015, 120: 508–512.

[3] AAE and AAOMR. AAE and AAOMR Joint Position Statement: Use of Cone Beam Computed Tomography in Endodontics 2015 Update. Oral Surg Oral Med Oral Pathol Oral Radiol, 2015, 120: 508–512.

[4] Abella F, et al. Evaluating the periapical status of teeth with irreversible pulpitis by using cone-beam computed tomography scanning and periapical radiographs. J Endod. 2012, 38: 1588–1591.

[5] Abella F, et al. An evaluation of the periapical status of teeth with necrotic pulps using periapical radiography and cone-beam computed tomography. Int Endod J, 2014, 47: 387–396.

[6] Aggarwal V, Singla M. Use of computed tomography scans and ultrasound in differential diagnosis and evaluation of nonsurgical management of periapical lesions. Oral Surg Oral Med Oral Pathol Oral Radiol Endod, 2010, 109: 917–923.

[7] Al-Nuaimi N, et al. The detection of simulated periapical lesions in human dry mandibles with cone-beam computed tomography: a dose reduction study. Int Endod J, 2016, 49: 1095–1104.

[8] Alqerban A, et al. Comparison of two cone beam computed tomographic systems versus panoramic imaging for localization of impacted maxillary canines and detection of root resorption. Eur J Orthod, 2011, 33: 93–102.

[9] Arai Y, et al. Practical model "3DX" of limited cone-beam X-ray CT for dental use. International Congress Series, 2001, 1230: 713–718.

[10] Barton D J, et al. Tuned-aperture computed tomography versus parallax analog and digital radiographic images in detecting second mesiobuccal canals in maxillary first molars. Oral Surg Oral Med Oral Pathol Oral Radiol Endod, 2003, 96: 223–228.

[11] Bender I B, Seltzer S. Roentgenographic and direct observation of experimental lesions in bone: I. 1961. J Endod, 2003, 29: 702–706, discussion 1.

[12] Bender I B, Seltzer S. Roentgenographic and direct observation of experimental lesions in bone: II. 1961. J Endod, 2003, 29: 707–712, discussion 1.

[13] Bender I B, Seltzer S, Soltanoff W. Endodontic success -a reappraisal of criteria. 1. Oral Surg Oral Med Oral Pathol, 1966, 22: 780–789.

[14] Bhaskar S N. Oral surgery-oral pathology conference No. 17, Walter Reed Army Medical Center. Periapical lesions-types, incidence, clinical features. Oral Surg Oral Med Oral Pathol, 1966, 21: 657–671.

[15] Biewener A A, et al. Adaptive changes in trabecular architecture in relation to functional strain patterns and disuse. Bone, 1996, 19: 1–8.

[16] Bornstein M M, et al. Comparison of periapical radiography and limited cone-beam computed tomography in mandibular molars for analysis of anatomical landmarks before apical surgery. J Endod, 2011, 37: 151–157.

[17] Boyne P J, Lyon H W, Miller C W. The effects of osseous implant materials on regeneration of alveolar cortex. Oral Surgery, Oral Medicine, Oral Pathology, 1961, 14: 369–378.

[18] Brady E, et al. A comparison of cone beam computed tomography and periapical radiography for the detection of vertical root fractures in nonendodontically treated teeth. Int

Endod J, 2014, 47: 735–746.
[19] Brown J, et al. Basic training requirements for the use of dental CBCT by dentists: a position paper prepared by the European Academy of DentoMaxilloFacial Radiology. Dentomaxillofac Radiol, 2014, 43: 20130291.
[20] Brynolf I. A histological and roentgenological study of the periapical region of human upper incisors. Odontologisk revy, Supplement, 1967, 11: 176s.
[21] Bueno M R, et al. Map-reading strategy to diagnose root perforations near metallic intracanal posts by using cone beam computed tomography. J Endod, 2011, 37: 85–90.
[22] Burch J G, Hulen S. A study of the presence of accessory foramina and the topography of molar furcations. Oral Surg Oral Med Oral Pathol, 1974, 38: 451–455.
[23] Caliskan M K. Pulpotomy of carious vital teeth with periapical involvement. Int Endod J, 1995, 28: 172–176.
[24] Caplan D J, Weintraub J A. Factors related to loss of root canal filled teeth. J Public Health Dent, 1997, 57: 31–39.
[25] Chan C P, et al. Vertical root fracture in endodontically versus nonendodontically treated teeth: a survey of 315 cases in Chinese patients. Oral Surgery, Oral Medicine, Oral Pathology, Oral Radiology Oral Radiol Endod, 1999, 87: 504–507.
[26] Chavda R, et al. Comparing the in vivo diagnostic accuracy of digital periapical radiography with cone-beam computed tomography for the detection of vertical root fracture. J Endod, 2014, 40: 1524–1529.
[27] Chen S C, et al. First untoward events and reasons for tooth extraction after nonsurgical endodontic treatment in Taiwan. J Endod, 2008, 34: 671–674.
[28] Cohen S, Blanco L, Berman L. Vertical root fractures: clinical and radiographic diagnosis. J Am Dent Assoc, 2003, 134: 434–441.
[29] Cotti E. Advanced techniques for detecting lesions in bone. Dent Clin North Am, 2010, 54: 215–235.
[30] Cotti E, Campisi G. Advanced radiographic techniques for the detection of lesions in bone. Endodontic Topics 7, 2004: 52–72.
[31] Cotti E, et al. A new technique for the study of periapical bone lesions: ultrasound real time imaging. Int Endod J, 2002, 35: 148–152.
[32] Davies A, et al. The detection of periapical pathoses in root filled teeth using single and parallax periapical radiographs versus cone beam computed tomography-a clinical study. Int Endod J, 2015, 48: 582–592.
[33] Davies A, et al. The detection of periapical pathoses using digital periapical radiography and cone beam computed tomography in endodontically re-treated teeth-part 2: a 1 year post-treatment follow-up. Int Endod J, 2016, 49: 623–635.
[34] Davies S J, et al. Occlusal considerations in periodontics. Br Dent J, 2001, 191: 597–604.
[35] De Paula-Silva F W, et al. Conebeam computerized tomographic, radiographic, histologic evaluation of periapical repair in dogs' post-endodontic treatment. Oral Surg Oral Med Oral Pathol Oral Radiol Endod, 2009, 108: 796–805. 206 6 Radiology of Apical Periodontitis
[36] Dunfee B L, et al. Radiologic and pathologic characteristics of benign and malignant lesions of the mandible. Radiographics, 2006, 26: 1751–1768.
[37] Durack C, et al. Diagnostic accuracy of small volume cone beam computed tomography and intraoral periapical radiography for the detection of simulated external inflammatory root resorption. Int Endod J, 2011, 44: 136–147.
[38] Ee J, Fayad M I, Johnson B R. Comparison of endodontic diagnosis and treatment planning decisions using conebeam volumetric tomography versus periapical radiography. J Endod, 2014, 40: 910–916.
[39] Eriksen H M. Epidemiology of apical Periodontitis// Østavik D P F, Pitt Ford T R. Essential Endodontology: Prevention and Treatment of Apical Periodontitis. Oxford: Wiley, 2008:262–274.
[40] ESE. Quality guidelines for endodontic treatment: consensus report of the European Society of Endodontology. Int Endod J, 2006, 39: 921–930.
[41] Estrela C, et al. Accuracy of cone beam computed tomography and panoramic and periapical radiography for detection of apical periodontitis. J Endod, 2008, 34: 273–279.
[42] Farman A G. ALARA still applies. Oral Surg Oral Med Oral Pathol Oral Radiol Endod, 2005, 100: 395–397.
[43] Forsberg J. A comparison of the paralleling and bisecting-angle radiographic techniques in endodontics. Int Endod J, 1987, 20: 177–182.
[44] Forsberg J. Estimation of the root filling length with the paralleling and bisecting-angle techniques performed by undergraduate students. Int Endod J, 1987, 20: 282–286.
[45] Forsberg J. Radiographic reproduction of endodontic "working length" comparing the paralleling and the bisecting-angle techniques. Oral Surg Oral Med Oral Pathol, 1987, 64: 353–360.
[46] Forsberg J, Halse A. Radiographic simulation of a periapical lesion comparing the paralleling and the bisecting-angle techniques. Int Endod J, 1994, 27: 133–138.
[47] Frost H M. Wolff's Law and bone's structural adaptations to mechanical usage: an overview for clinicians. Angle Orthod, 1994, 64: 175–188.
[48] Garcia de Paula-Silva F W, et al. Outcome of root canal treatment in dogs determined by periapical radiography and cone-beam computed tomography scans. J Endod, 2009, 35: 723–726.
[49] Glickman G W, Pettiette M T. Preparation for treatment//

Cohen S, Hargreaves K.M. Pathways of the Pulp. St Louis MO: Mosby Elsevier, 2006.

[50] Goldstein S A, et al. Trabecular bone remodeling: an experimental model. J Biomech ,1991, 24 Suppl 1: 135–150.

[51] Goto T K, et al. The accuracy of 3-dimensional magnetic resonance 3D vibe images of the mandible: an in vitro comparison of magnetic resonance imaging and computed tomography. Oral Surg Oral Med Oral Pathol Oral Radiol Endod, 2007, 103: 550–559.

[52] Grödahl H-G, Huumonen S. Radiographic manifestations of periapical inflammatory lesions. Endodontic Topics, 2004, 8: 55–67.

[53] Gundappa M, Ng S Y, Whaites E J. Comparison of ultrasound, digital and conventional radiography in differentiating periapical lesions. Dentomaxillofac Radiol, 2006, 35: 326–333.

[54] Guo J, et al. Evaluation of the reliability and accuracy of using cone-beam computed tomography for diagnosing periapical cysts from granulomas. J Endod, 2013, 39: 1485–1490.

[55] Halstead C L, Hoard B C. Dental radiology and oral pathology. Curr Probl Diagn Radiol, 1991, 20: 187–235.

[56] Hashem D, et al. Clinical and radiographic assessment of the efficacy of calcium silicate indirect pulp capping: a randomized controlled clinical trial. J Dent Res, 2015, 94: 562–568.

[57] Huumonen S, Østavik D. Radiological aspects of apical periodontitis. Endodontic Topics, 2002, 1: 3–25.

[58] Jervoe-Storm P M, et al. Comparison of cone-beam computerized tomography and intraoral radiographs for determination of the periodontal ligament in a variable phantom. Oral Surg Oral Med Oral Pathol Oral Radiol Endod, 2010, 109: e95–101.

[59] Jin L J, Cao C F. Clinical diagnosis of trauma from occlusion and its relation with severity of periodontitis. J Clin Periodontol, 1992, 19: 92–97.

[60] Jones D, et al. The effect of alteration of the exposure parameters of a cone-beam computed tomographic scan on the diagnosis of simulated horizontal root fractures. J Endod, 2015, 41: 520–525.

[61] Kakekashi S, Stanley H R, Fitzgerald R J. The effects of surgical exposures of dental pulps in germ-free and conventional laboratory rats. Oral Surg Oral Med Oral Pathol, 1965, 20: 340–349.

[62] Kanagasingam S, et al. Accuracy of single and parallax film and digital periapical radiographs in diagnosing apical periodontitis-a cadaver study. Int Endod J, 2017, 50: 427–436.

[63] Kanagasingam S, et al. Diagnostic accuracy of periapical radiography and cone beam computed tomography in detecting apical periodontitis using histopathological findings as a reference standard. Int Endod J, 2017, 50: 417–426.

[64] Kashima I, et al. Diagnostic imaging of diseases affecting the mandible with the use of computed panoramic radiography. Oral Surg Oral Med Oral Pathol, 1990, 70: 110–116.

[65] Krithikadatta J, et al. Mandibular first molar having an unusual mesial root canal morphology with contradictory cone-beam computed tomography findings: a case report. J Endod, 2010, 36: 1712–1716.

[66] Kruse C, et al. Cone beam computed tomography and periapical lesions: a systematic review analysing studies on diagnostic efficacy by a hierarchical model. Int Endod J, 2015, 48: 815–828.

[67] Lennon S, et al. Diagnostic accuracy of limited-volume cone-beam computed tomography in the detection of periapical bone loss: 360 degrees scans versus 180 degrees scans. Int Endod J, 2011, 44: 1118–1127.

[68] Liang Y H, et al. Endodontic outcome predictors identified with periapical radiographs and cone-beam computed tomography scans. J Endod, 2011, 37: 326–331.

[69] Lofthag-Hansen S, et al. Limited cone-beam CT and intraoral radiography for the diagnosis of periapical pathology. Oral Surg Oral Med Oral Pathol Oral Radiol Endod, 2007, 103: 114–119.

[70] Matherne R P, et al. Use of conebeam computed tomography to identify root canal systems in vitro. J Endod, 2008, 34: 87–89.

[71] Mendes R A, van der Waal I. An unusual clinicoradiographic presentation of a lateral periodontal cyst-report of two cases. Med Oral Patol Oral Cir Bucal, 2006, 11: E185–187.

[72] Mizutani T, Ohno N, Nakamura H. Anatomical study of the root apex in the maxillary anterior teeth. J Endod, 1992, 18: 344–347.

[73] Möler A J, et al. Influence on periapical tissues of indigenous oral bacteria and necrotic pulp tissue in monkeys. Scand J Dent Res, 1981, 89: 475–484.

[74] Molven O, Halse A, Fristad I. Long-term reliability and observer comparisons in the radiographic diagnosis of periapical disease. International Endodontic Journal, 2002, 35: 142–147.

[75] Molven O, et al. Periapical changes following root-canal treatment observed 20–27 years postoperatively. Int Endod J, 2002, 35: 784–790.

[76] Molven O, et al. Periapical changes following root-canal treatment observed 20–27 years postoperatively. International Endodontic Journal, 2002, 35: 784–790.

[77] Molven O, Halse A, Grung B. Observer strategy and the radiographic classification of healing after endodontic surgery. Int J Oral Maxillofac Surg, 1987, 16: 432–439.

[78] Molven O, Halse A, Grung B. Incomplete healing (scar

tissue, after periapical surgery-radiographic findings 8 to 12 years after treatment. J Endod, 1996, 22: 264–268.

[79] Mozzo P, et al. A new volumetric CT machine for dental imaging based on the cone-beam technique: preliminary results. Eur Radiol, 1998, 8: 1558–1564.

[80] Nair M K, Nair U P. Digital and advanced imaging in endodontics: a review. J Endod, 2007, 33: 1–6.

[81] Nair M K, et al. The effects of restorative material and location on the detection of simulated recurrent caries. A comparison of dental film, direct digital radiography and tuned aperture computed tomography. Dentomaxillofac Radiol, 1998, 27: 80–84.

[82] Nair P N. New perspectives on radicular cysts: do they heal? International Endodontic Journal, 1998, 31: 155–160.

[83] Nair P N, et al. Persistent periapical radiolucencies of root-filled human teeth, failed endodontic treatments, periapical scars. Oral Surg Oral Med Oral Pathol Oral Radiol Endod, 1999, 87: 617–627.

[84] Østavik D. Radiographic evaluation of apical periodontitis and endodontic treatment results: a computer approach. International Dental Journal, 1991, 41: 89–98.

[85] Østavik D, et al. Image analysis of endodontic radiographs: digital subtraction and quantitative densitometry. Endodontics and Dental Traumatology, 1990, 6: 6–11.

[86] Østavik D, Kerekes K, Eriksen H M. The periapical index: a scoring system for radiographic assessment of apical periodontitis. Endod Dent Traumatol, 1986, 2: 20–34.

[87] Ozen T, et al. Interpretation of chemically created periapical lesions using two different dental cone-beam computerized tomography units, an intraoral digital sensor, and conventional film. Oral Surg Oral Med Oral Pathol Oral Radiol Endod, 2009, 107: 426–432.

[88] Parker J M, et al. Cone-beam computed tomography uses in clinical endodontics: observer variability in detecting periapical lesions. J Endod, 2017, 43: 184–187.

[89] Patel S, et al. Detection of periapical bone defects in human jaws using cone beam computed tomography and intraoral radiography. Int Endod J, 2009, 42: 507–515.

[90] Patel S, et al. New dimensions in endodontic imaging: part 1. Conventional and alternative radiographic systems. Int Endod J, 2009, 42: 447–462.

[91] Patel S, et al. European Society of Endodontology position statement: the use of CBCT in endodontics. Int Endod J, 2019, doi: 10. 1111/iej.13187.

[92] Patel S, et al. Cone beam computed tomography in endodontics-a review. Int Endod J, 2015, 48: 3–15.

[93] Patel S, Horner K. The use of cone beam computed tomography in endodontics. Int Endod J, 2009, 42: 755–756.

[94] Patel S, et al. The detection of periapical pathosis using digital periapical radiography and cone beam computed tomography-part 2: a 1-year posttreatment follow-up. Int Endod J, 2012, 45: 711–723.

[95] Patel S, et al. The detection of periapical pathosis using periapical radiography and cone beam computed tomography-part 1: pre-operative status. International Endodontic Journal, 2012, 45: 702–710.

[96] Pauls V, Trott J R. A radiological study of experimentally produced lesions in bone. Dent Pract Dent Rec, 1966, 16: 254–258.

[97] Pope O, Sathorn C, Parashos P. A comparative investigation of cone-beam computed tomography and periapical radiography in the diagnosis of a healthy periapex. J Endod, 2014, 40: 360–365.

[98] Prakash N, et al. Visibility of lamina dura and periodontal space on periapical radiographs and its comparison with cone beam computed tomography. Contemp Clin Dent, 2015, 6: 21–25.

[99] Ramachandran Nair P N, Pajarola G, Schroeder H E. Types and incidence of human periapical lesions obtained with extracted teeth. Oral Surg Oral Med Oral Pathol Oral Radiol Endod, 1996, 81: 93–102.

[100] Ricucci D, Mannocci F, Ford T R. A study of periapical lesions correlating the presence of a radiopaque lamina with histological findings. Oral Surg Oral Med Oral Pathol Oral Radiol Endod, 2006, 101: 389–394.

[101] Rodriguez G, et al. Influence of Cone-beam Computed Tomography in Clinical Decision Making among Specialists. J Endod, 2017, 43: 194–199.

[102] Scarfe W C, et al. Use of cone beam computed tomography in endodontics. Int J Dent, 2009: 634567.

[103] Schwartz S F, Foster J K Jr. Roentgenographic interpretation of experimentally produced bony lesions. I. Oral Surg Oral Med Oral Pathol, 1971, 32: 606–612.

[104] Scuibba J J, Fantasia J E, Kahn L B. Tumours and cysts of the jaws// Rosai J, Sobin L. Atlas of Tumour Pathology. Washington DC: Armed Forces Institute of Pathology, 2001.

[105] Shoha R R, Dowson J, Richards A G. Radiographic interpretation of experimentally produced bony lesions. Oral Surg Oral Med Oral Pathol, 1974, 38: 294–303.

[106] Simon J H, et al. Differential diagnosis of large periapical lesions using cone-beam computed tomography measurements and biopsy. J Endod, 2006, 32: 833–837.

[107] Sogur E, et al. Detectability of chemically induced periapical lesions by limited cone beam computed tomography, intra-oral digital and conventional film radiography. Dentomaxillofac Radiol, 2009, 38: 458–464.

[108] Stashenko P, Yu S M. T helper and T suppressor cell reversal during the development of induced rat periapical lesions. J Dent Res, 1989, 68: 830–834.

[109] Stavropoulos A, Wenzel A. Accuracy of cone beam dental

[109] CT, intraoral digital and conventional film radiography for the detection of periapical lesions. An ex vivo study in pig jaws. Clin Oral Investig, 2007, 11: 101–106.

[110] Strindberg L. The dependence of the results of pulp therapy on certain factors. Acta Odontol Scand, 1956, 14 (Suppl) 21: 1–175.

[111] Sukovic P. Cone beam computed tomography in craniofacial imaging. Orthod Craniofac Res, 2003, 6 Suppl 1: 31–36; discussion 179–182.

[112] Tronstad L. Root resorption-etiology, terminology and clinical manifestations. Endod Dent Traumatol, 1988, 4: 241–252.

[113] Tsai P, et al. Accuracy of conebeam computed tomography and periapical radiography in detecting small periapical lesions. J Endod, 2012, 38: 965–970.

[114] Tutton L M, Goddard P R. MRI of the teeth. Br J Radiol, 2002, 75: 552–562.

[115] Tyndall D A, et al. TACT imaging of primary caries. Oral Surg Oral Med Oral Pathol Oral Radiol Endod, 1997, 84: 214–225.

[116] Uraba S, et al. Ability of conebeam computed tomography to detect periapical lesions that were not detected by periapical radiography: a retrospective assessment according to tooth group. J Endod, 2016, 42: 1186–1190.

[117] Vande Voorde H E, Bjorndahl A M. Estimating endodontic "working length" with paralleling radiographs. Oral Surg Oral Med Oral Pathol, 1969, 27: 106–110.

[118] Velvart P, Hecker H, Tillinger G. Detection of the apical lesion and the mandibular canal in conventional radiography and computed tomography. Oral Surg Oral Med Oral Pathol Oral Radiol Endod, 2001, 92: 682–688.

[119] Walton G, Heasman P. The role of occlusion in periodontal disease. Dent Update, 1998, 25: 209–210: 212–214, 216.

[120] Webber R L, et al. Comparison of film, direct digital, and tuned-aperture computed tomography images to identify the location of crestal defects around endosseous titanium implants. Oral Surg Oral Med Oral Pathol Oral Radiol Endod, 1996, 81: 480–90.

[121] Webber R L, Messura J K. An in vivo comparison of diagnostic information obtained from tunedaperture computed tomography and conventional dental radiographic imaging modalities. Oral Surg Oral Med Oral Pathol Oral Radiol Endod, 1999, 88: 239–247.

[122] Weber A L, Imaging of cysts and odontogenic tumors of the jaw. Definition and classification. Radiol Clin North Am, 1993, 31: 101–120.

[123] Whaites E. Differential diagnosis of radiolucent lesions of the jaws// Whaites E. Essentials of Dental Radiology and Radiography. Edinburgh: Churchill Livingston Elsevier, 2007: 329–354.

[124] White S, Pharoah M. Other imaging modalities// White S, Pharoah M. Oral Radiology: Principles and Interpretation. Louis MO: Mosby St, 2014:229–249.

[125] Wu M K, Shemesh H, Wesselink P R. Limitations of previously published systematic reviews evaluating the outcome of endodontic treatment. International Endodontic Journal, 2009, 42: 656–666.

[126] Wu M K, Wesselink P, Shemesh H. New terms for categorizing the outcome of root canal treatment. Int Endod J, 2011, 44: 1079–1080.

[127] Wu M K, Wesselink P R, Walton R E. Apical terminus location of root canal treatment procedures. Oral Surg Oral Med Oral Pathol Oral Radiol Endod, 2000, 89: 99–103.

[128] Yamamoto K, et al. Development of dento-maxillofacial cone beam X-ray computed tomography system. Orthod Craniofac Res 6 Suppl, 2003, 1: 160–162.

第7章 临床表现和诊断

Asgeir Sigurdsson

7.1 概述

正确的诊断是牙髓治疗的关键。在开髓或对牙齿进行任何其他治疗前，对牙髓和根尖周组织进行临床诊断至关重要。根据现病史、主诉、症状、诊断性测试和临床检查得出临床诊断。如果无法确诊或不能排除鉴别诊断，则应在完成进一步评估或会诊后再开始治疗。

据报道，临床症状与牙髓组织病理学之间的相关性较差[5, 31, 42, 107]。医生曾尝试仅根据临床表现和症状、牙髓电活力检测或热诊以及影像学检查对牙髓状况进行准确的诊断，但多数未能显示出任何相关性[25, 31, 83]。很多情况下，医生使用了各种不同的牙髓诊断术语，至少有部分术语是详细的，而几乎所有分类都有一个共同点，即对假定的牙髓组织学表现进行了详细描述[5, 105]。但显而易见的是，目前的技术无法对牙髓进行组织学评估，除非取出牙髓并在显微镜下进行观察。最近的趋势是不再使用这些复杂的分类，而是使用Morse等人在1977年提出的稍加修改的版本，后来美国牙髓病学学会又对其进行了简化[1, 82]。这种分类在一定程度上涉及牙髓的组织学状态，有助于临床医生确定治疗计划，因为不同的诊断所需的治疗方法之间没有交叉。近期的研究表明，使用更明确的标准对牙髓状态进行临床和组织学分类可以得到良好的一致性，尤其是对于牙髓正常或可复性牙髓炎的病例[101]。

症状或测试结果对牙髓和根尖周状态的预测作用有限，因此应尽可能多地收集有关主诉和病史的信息，并在明确最终诊断之前进行完善的检查[89]。只有全面了解临床体征和症状、诊断测试，以及牙髓组织对龋、手术操作、创伤和牙周病的反应，才能够让医生根据经验建立对牙髓病的诊断。

7.2 牙髓诊断术语

7.2.1 正常牙髓

根据定义，正常牙髓是有活力、无症状的，且没有任何炎症。此诊断术语仅在牙髓因修复等原因需要去髓和根管充填时使用，例如，需要预备桩道或对移位牙进行截冠时。此外，因外伤导致冠折露髓的患牙，在30~48h内进行治疗时，也可使用该术语[49]。

7.2.2 可复性牙髓炎

可复性牙髓炎是指牙髓为活髓，但在一定程度上存在感染；其症状常常被误解，可能完全无症状，也可能表现为热刺激引发尖锐疼痛。通过检查所收集的信息（见下文）可以被预测，刺激物（如深龋）一旦被去除，或暴露的牙本质得到封闭，炎症就会愈合并恢复正常。轻度创伤及继发炎症会引起小范围的神经源性炎症，足够的机械损伤也会导致神经芽生反应[20-21]，因此可能导致患者对活力测试的过度反应，提示存在更为严重的炎症，而事实并非如此。如前所述，临床症状、体征或诊断测试并不总是与牙髓的组织病理状态相对应。然而，将症状轻微的不可复性牙髓炎诊断为可复性炎症存在较高的风险（见下文）。因此，对所有诊断为可复性牙髓炎的患者，在治疗数周后复查评估其症状非常重要，包括所有可能的体征和症状变化，以及重新进行适当的牙髓活力测试。对这些病例仅进行电话随访是不够的，因为牙髓可能已经坏死，从而导致患者误以为问题已经得到了解决。诊断可复性牙髓炎时，其现病史主要表现为激发痛，即只有当患牙遇热和（或）冷或其他刺激时才会出现症状。

7.2.3 有症状的不可复性牙髓炎

这一诊断意味着牙髓仍有活力，但炎症严重，即使去除刺激物或引起症状的原因，牙髓也无法恢复正常。因此，需要去髓并进行根管治疗。对几乎所有的病例，如果不加以治疗，牙髓终将发生坏死，细菌将很容易侵入根尖和根尖周组织。这是基于主观和客观检查的临床诊断，患者除了抱怨与直接刺激相关的疼痛外，还会有热刺激延迟痛、自发痛和（或）牵涉痛[34]。

7.2.4 无症状的不可复性牙髓炎

这类患牙的症状可能具有极强的误导性。有充分的文献证明，在许多病例中不可复性牙髓炎是无症状的。研究报告表明，在 26%~60% 的病例中，牙髓可以在无痛的状态下发生坏死[4,79]。值得注意的是，性别和牙齿类型的差异似乎对无症状牙髓炎的发生没有影响[80]。

因此，该临床诊断是基于主观和客观检查，提示这种炎性牙髓虽然仍有活力，但无法恢复正常，因为龋坏或创伤的直接或间接作用，导致牙髓长期暴露于细菌及其产物中[12]。

7.2.5 牙髓坏死

当牙髓坏死时，最好的情况为髓腔内的坏死部分充满无菌碎屑，没有活髓[11]。对于年轻恒牙，区分部分坏死还是完全坏死非常重要，因为根尖区的健康牙髓组织可能会诱导牙根继续发育。此时，确认牙髓活性的唯一方法是开髓并去除坏死的碎屑，直至暴露活髓，这是因为对于年轻恒牙，即使牙髓正常时牙髓活力测试也并不准确[40]。

7.2.6 感染性牙髓/感染性髓腔

牙髓感染可能仅累及部分牙髓腔，例如发生在近期的外伤或龋齿导致的牙髓暴露，或者多根牙中只有一个或两个牙根受累。在外伤的病例中，牙髓完全坏死后留下的髓腔可以是无菌的，这是因为牙齿的血供被切断，但没有来自冠方的细菌侵入生长[11]。然而，在大多数病例中，由于龋齿或冠折/隐裂引起的细菌入侵会导致牙髓坏死，因此髓腔处于感染状态。研究表明，所有发生根尖周病变的患牙都存在髓腔感染[11]。众所周知，对于没有明确的根尖周病变的牙齿难以确定是否存在感染，因为只有存在明显骨缺损时才会出现影像学改变[9-10]。

7.3 牙髓病的症状

牙科培训的重点是通过视诊进行疾病诊断，如评估修复体、口腔健康或疾病的临床表现以及 X 线片。然而，当诊断疼痛的来源时，大多数诊断是通过收集病史信息来完成的，如医生所听到的，而不是看到的[91]。事实上，视觉的线索可能会使医生偏离正轨，导致错误的诊断。因此，在得出结论之前，仔细听取患者的倾诉并系统地回顾他/她目前的所有症状以及病史是很重要的。

7.3.1 主诉症状

根据定义，主诉症状是指在就诊时可识别的症状。主诉症状虽然具有提示性，但不能仅以此进行最终诊断。

无 痛

众所周知，牙髓炎可以是无痛的[7, 31, 49, 79]。因此，无痛不可作为判断牙髓炎存在与否、严重程度或可复性的指标。然而，牙髓炎疼痛症状多变的原因尚不清楚。至少在某些病例中，炎症的进展可能非常迅速，以至于没有疼痛；炎症进展非常缓慢时，参与疼痛过程的经典炎症介质未达到临界水平[79]。最可能的原因是局部和中央的调解系统能够产生有效的调节。在牙髓中有许多局部调节因子和系统，包括内源性阿片类物质、肾上腺素交感神经和一氧化氮系统[20, 55, 92]。有很好的研究表明：在特定条件下生长激素抑制素可能会抑制牙髓疼痛的激活[23, 113-114]。最近，一项对诊断为不可复性牙髓炎患者的牙髓进行的研究表明，几种已知的调节疼痛和炎症的基因在无症状和轻度疼痛患者中的表达与中度至重度疼痛患者中的表达存在差异；与痛感更强的患者相比，在无症状或轻度疼痛患者的牙髓样本中，具有疼痛调节作用的关键炎症反应因子表达水平相对较低，如 IL8、TNFA 和 ILIB [41]。

锐痛

如果疼痛是短暂的且仅与刺激有关，如冷的空气或饮品，则很可能仅由活跃在牙本质-牙髓复合体中的 Aδ 神经纤维介导 [7, 85]。因此，主诉为仅存在激发痛时表明可能仅有轻度（可复）炎症。这种情况可能仅需要活髓保存治疗，例如去除浅层龋损、更换存在渗漏的修复体，或覆盖暴露的牙根表面。

持续性剧痛

越来越多的证据表明，导致疼痛的经典炎症介质在牙髓中的释放与损伤成正比。5-羟色胺可使牙内 A 纤维变得更敏感，从而提高其反应性 [60, 92]，而有研究证明缓激肽在发生不可复性炎症的牙髓中的浓度显著提高 [67]。牙髓疼痛不仅仅与炎性介质有关。近来研究还发现，牙髓中疼痛性神经纤维来源的神经肽 [降钙素基因相关肽（CGRP）、神经激肽 A（NKA）和神经肽 P 物质] 在症状牙髓中的浓度明显高于无症状牙髓 [17, 48, 86]。最初，这些介质和肽主要影响更外围的 Aδ 纤维，但当炎症扩展至深部结构时，C 纤维也将受到影响。这将导致发作阈值降低，并使感受区域变大。因此，当询问患者延迟痛的情况时，不仅要询问去除刺激因素后疼痛持续的时间，还要询问疼痛的程度，这一点很重要。当延迟痛表现为钝痛、跳痛时，说明病变累及了更多的 C 纤维，意味着可能存在重度炎症。这可用于辅助预测牙髓炎症是否可复。

热痛冷缓解

人们普遍认为对于正常牙髓，主诉为冷刺激引发的敏感明显多于热刺激。然而，当牙髓出现重度炎症时，似乎对热刺激极为敏感，尤其是在疾病的后期。关于这方面的研究很少，但临床经验表明，当患者主诉为严重的热刺激敏感时，几乎可以肯定牙髓存在不可复性炎症。以往对此现象的理论解释为当患牙受热时，会导致髓腔内压力增加，从而导致神经活性增强 [14]。然而，相同程度的冷刺激却无法引起这种反应 [53]，因此推断这与压力升高有关。很明显，这不是一个理想的解释。临床中热刺激敏感更可能是由于热敏感的牙髓神经的反应。热敏性 C 纤维在正常情况下不易受到刺激，但随着炎症的扩散，它们变得更加活跃 [20]。当牙髓发炎时，炎症区域集聚的炎性介质以及神经肽的分泌可引起神经反应。这种反应将导致神经发生局部和中枢介导的变化，这可能是导致牙髓炎中牙髓敏感性变化的原因。例如：发生牙髓炎时跳痛的症状 [20] 可能是由压力敏感性纤维所引起。同样的情况也适用于热痛冷缓解的患牙。炎症介质可能会大大降低热敏纤维的激活阈值，在极端情况下，正常体温都会激活牙髓神经并引起疼痛；缓解疼痛的唯一方法是将牙齿冷却到环境温度以下 [62]。

活髓牙咬合痛

这表明牙髓和牙周组织可能存在严重炎症，同时必须与非牙髓来源的疾病进行仔细的鉴别诊断。如果牙髓受累，临床检查表现为至少部分牙髓坏死，其余活髓表现为不可复性牙髓炎 [10]。

牵涉痛

随着牙髓炎症的进展，疼痛会逐渐向远离患牙的部位转移。已有研究表明，一颗牙齿的疼痛可以牵涉到邻牙，对颌、甚至耳朵、锁骨和太阳穴等较远部位。在一项关于牙髓炎牵涉痛模式的经典研究中，Glick [44] 发现该模式存在一定规律。上牙的疼痛一般会牵涉至颧部或颞部。下颌磨牙疼痛更易牵涉至耳部甚至枕部。牙齿疼痛可能发生在牙弓之间，但不会跨越面部中线。牵涉痛产生的机制尚不清楚，但很明显，其与外周和中枢神经作用机制都有关系 [110]。有趣的是，软组织结构（如颞肌和咬肌）可以以类似的方式将软组织疼痛牵涉至牙齿 [115]。因此，对患者报告的发生在头颈部牙齿以外区域的任何疼痛进行触诊是非常重要的。如果对面部和（或）颈部肌肉的触诊加重了疼痛反应，则患者很可能是肌肉疼痛而不是牙痛（见下文 7.10）。

7.3.2 现病史

在患者的主诉病史中，存在许多对预测不可复性牙髓炎至关重要的相关因素。这些因素包括以下内容。

疼痛的特征，牙痛与牙髓疼痛

在牙本质疼痛中，外部刺激引起的剧烈而迅速的疼痛是由快速传导的 Aδ 纤维反应所导致的。Aδ 纤维延伸到牙本质内 150μm，通常在整个牙本质 - 牙髓复合体中都很活跃[47, 74, 76]。在正常牙髓中，位于更深层、慢传导且无髓鞘的 C 纤维在多数情况下对刺激无反应，非常强烈的刺激除外[20, 86]。当对健康牙髓施加长时间且足够强烈的刺激时，首先会出现由 Aδ 纤维介导的剧烈疼痛，随后是难以定位的钝痛感[58-59]。因此，主诉仅为存在刺激痛时，提示可能只有轻微（可复）的炎症，此时仅需活髓保存治疗，如去除浅层龋损、更换存在渗漏的修复体或遮盖暴露的牙根表面。但是，当细菌及其产物开始侵入牙髓，炎症介质会影响神经纤维，降低神经激活阈值，特别是 C 纤维的激活阈值[48, 67]。如果疼痛史最初表现为温度刺激敏感，伴间歇性剧烈的疼痛，随后转变为不断加重的更为迟钝的跳痛，则该病史具有很好的启示性。原因如下：首先，这表示疼痛的变化与 C 纤维的进一步激活有关，提示炎症加重；第二，研究表明，牙痛强度和性质的主诉是判断牙髓炎症是否可逆的有效预测指标[109]。

剧　痛

关于牙痛强度和性质的主诉似乎是预测牙髓炎症是否可逆的有效因素[46]。研究还表明，疼痛越严重，症状持续时间越长，越有可能出现不可复的炎症[7]。然而，由于感觉的主观性，关于疼痛严重程度的主诉可能具有误导性。例如，有研究证明患者对牙医的恐惧会增强其对疼痛的感知和对诊断性刺激的反应[63]。

自发性（非刺激性）牙髓疼痛

不可复性牙髓炎最明显的体征可能是自发性疼痛史，这种疼痛会在没有任何热刺激的情况下产生，甚至可能将患者从睡梦中唤醒[108]。病变区域的炎症可引起自发性疼痛，有时也可能延长对无害刺激的反应，这些刺激在没有炎症存在的情况下不会引起任何疼痛感（痛觉超敏）。这种自发痛被认为至少部分是由炎症介质对外周疼痛性神经末梢（主要是 C 纤维）产生的作用所引起[88]。这将激活和（或）导致神经末梢敏感，并导致局部和中枢释放 P 物质和降钙素基因相关肽（CGRP）[30, 48, 117]，这些神经肽可以进一步促进炎症介质的释放，产生正反馈回路或恶性循环。这种恶性循环有时被称为神经源性炎症。

7.4 临床检查

除了熟识牙髓对外界刺激物的反应，临床检查的结果对得到正确诊断也至关重要。牙髓炎通常是无痛的，而且症状、诊断性测试和牙髓组织病理状态之间缺乏相关性，因此临床检查至关重要。

7.4.1 龋源性露髓

科学证据表明，当龋病导致牙髓直接暴露时，细菌已经先于龋损侵犯牙髓并形成微脓肿[65,72,102]。因此，如果患牙存在龋源性露髓，则应考虑牙髓存在不可复性炎症。建议在牙根发育不完全的病例中，应尝试评估牙髓发炎或感染的程度，去除感染牙髓并尝试进行根尖诱导成形治疗。研究报道，硅酸钙材料作为盖髓剂应用于临床获得了成功，特别是在没有明显疼痛的不可复性牙髓炎病例中[19]。近来，对根尖发育完全伴龋源性露髓的患牙用这些新材料行盖髓术是研究的热点[68]。总的来说该方法成功率较为理想，特别是患者主诉无痛、牙髓活力测试的反应正常，并且牙髓没有直接暴露时[16]（见第 9 章）。

7.4.2 增龄性变化

随着年龄的增长，由于牙本质持续形成，牙髓的大小和体积不断减小。相对于胶原纤维的数量和厚度，细胞成分的含量会减少[29]。此外，血管和神经的数量也不断减少，而钙化和髓石的发生率增加[51]。虽然还没有实验证明，但相较于年轻牙髓，这些增龄性变化被认为会导致牙髓炎症无法逆转。此外，在发生广泛的退行性改变后，牙髓仍可能在不确定的时间内存在活性。

7.4.3 牙周病

据报道，中度至重度牙周病会导致牙髓过早衰老[13, 66, 103, 107]。因此，与牙髓健康的牙齿相比，牙周病患牙的牙髓对炎症的抵抗力也较低。然而，这一观点并未被普遍接受，因为 Mazur 和 Massler[75]发现牙周病并不影响牙齿的牙髓状态。

7.4.4 早期牙髓损伤

早期牙髓损伤，如龋齿、去龋和修复治疗都可能导致牙本质小管硬化、修复性牙本质形成和牙髓纤维化。据推测，牙髓的这种过早衰老可能导致其愈合能力低于未受应力的牙髓[84, 108]。当患牙存在较大的修复体或全冠时，如果没有注意车针冷却或在没有足够湿润的情况下进行预备，则会增大成牙本质细胞层受损的风险[52]。

7.5 诊断性测试

不幸的是，许多临床医生仅仅依靠诊断性测试进行诊断。需要注意的是，多数常用的检测方法实际上并不能评估牙髓的活力（血液循环），也不能明确指出牙髓是否存在炎症或炎症的严重程度。进行牙髓测试的主要原因是对症状进行重现和定位，并评估症状的严重程度。还需要注意的是，这些测试的反应都是主观的，一些患者会有夸大的倾向，而另一些患者则会低估其痛感[32, 64]。

7.5.1 敏感性测试

敏感性测试包括电活力测试（EPT）和温度测试。这些测试的主要功能是区分活髓和死髓[56, 116]。通过这些测试，牙髓中的神经纤维被激活，引起患者的反应。患者的反应是主观的，因此必须注意区分阳性反应是由恐惧引发还是真实反应[32, 64]。通常可以与对侧或邻牙的反应进行比较，并重新检查受试牙齿以确保检测结果一致性。同时，必须注意清洁和干燥患牙，以尽量减少刺激向牙周膜或邻近牙齿的传导。

在进行这些敏感性测试之前，还需要询问患者最近有无服用的止痛药。研究发现：对已诊断为牙髓源性疼痛的患者，在进行冷诊、叩诊、触诊和咬合力测试前 1 小时服用 800mg 布洛芬会显著影响诊断测试的结果[99]。

如上所述，除了主观性外，这些测试的主要缺点是必须假设牙髓内存在有血供的神经纤维。虽然多数情况下该假设是合理的，但在许多情况下，牙髓中的血供会在牙髓中的神经退化之前丧失，从而导致对牙髓活力的错误诊断[97]。相反，众所周知，在脱位性损伤后，有活力的牙髓有时在创伤后不久对敏感性测试没有反应，但在几周到几个月后的随访中，牙髓恢复正常反应[78, 111]。

7.5.1.1 电活力试验

牙髓电活力测试仪可激活牙髓中的神经束，可能主要是 Aδ 纤维。牙髓中的无髓鞘 C 纤维可能产生反应[83]或没有反应[87]。这类测试存在的主要问题是需要考虑许多变量，且其中一些变量无法控制。关键问题包括探测头在牙齿上的位置（尽可能远离牙龈），仪器与牙齿之间的传导性，刺激强度增加的速率，测试牙与邻牙的隔离，以及干燥牙冠防止电流转导至牙龈。此外，无法控制牙釉质和牙本质的厚度和电阻、修复体和龋齿的存在以及牙髓中神经复合体的功能。

步　骤

干燥患牙及邻近的牙齿。将探测头放置在切缘或与髓角对应的牙尖上[8, 39]（图 7.1）。使用传导介质（如牙膏或氟化物凝胶）加强探头和牙齿之间的接触。通过接触嘴唇或由患者握住牙髓电活力测试仪的手柄来形成电流回路。随着电流缓慢增大，告知患者在出现刺痛或其他感觉时及时示意（如举手）。

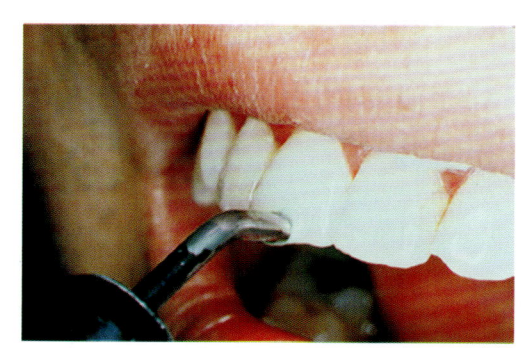

图 7.1　将牙髓电测仪（EPT）的探头放置于上颌前牙的切缘。测试牙需充分干燥，通过传导介质（如牙膏或氟化物凝胶）促进探头与牙冠表面的接触

诊断信息

在合理的强度范围内，对刺激有反应说明牙髓组织有活力。然而，反应水平并不能表明牙髓的健康状况或牙髓内可能存在的炎症是否可复，因为牙髓的电刺激痛阈与组织学状况之间没有相关性[69, 83]。对于大多数牙齿而言，没有反应即说明牙髓坏死[97, 108]。Seltzer 等人发现 72% 的牙髓完全坏死的患牙和 25.7% 的牙髓局部坏死的患牙对牙髓电活力测试没有反应。因此，如果认为恒牙即使是局部坏死也需要进行去髓治疗的话，那么当牙髓电活力测试无反应时，约 97% 的病例都将需要进行去髓治疗或牙髓坏死的清创术。最近的一项研究证实了 1963 年以来的研究结果，即牙髓电活力测试的总体准确率为 75%。然而，其阴性预测值为 90%，表明当仪器与牙齿接触良好时，没有反应表明牙髓坏死的可能性很高。反之则不然，因为阳性预测值只有 58%[56]。

此外，还需要意识到牙外伤后短期内[111]以及牙根发育不完全的牙齿[39-40]对牙髓电活力测试的反应是不准确的。这可能是由于拉施科夫神经丛在牙根发育的晚期才完全发育成熟。因此，不同于发育完全的牙齿达到正常咬合时的状态，此时牙髓神经无法到达成牙本质细胞、前期牙本质或牙本质区域。对于年轻患牙，冷测试，尤其是使用干冰进行测试比牙髓电活力测试更可靠[39]。

7.5.1.2 冷诊

牙科最常用的测验方法应该是不同形式的冷诊[98]。重要的是要认识到，这种测试方法也像牙髓电活力测试和热诊一样，只代表存在有功能的神经纤维，而不能反映牙髓活力状态（血流）。

冷刺激导致的最初反应是由于流体动力激活了冷刺激敏感的 Aδ 纤维[59]。温度变化导致牙本质小管中的液体快速移动，继而激活管内神经[17-18]。此外，在动物模型中，当牙齿温度快速降低时，冷敏感的 Aδ 纤维即产生反应[59]，而当温度变化率降低时，神经纤维最初的高频放电率也继而下降，在温度达到稳定水平时完全停止。这充分解释了当牙齿受到冷刺激时，最初的尖锐性疼痛是由 Aδ 纤维引起的，当管内液体停止运动时，神经纤维停止放电，感觉也随即消失。C 纤维同样表现出独特的不同的反应。C 纤维在短暂的延迟后开始放电，放电率较低[59]。在一项人体实验研究中[77]，受试者所报告的感觉与动物研究中 A 和 C 纤维的阶段性激活模式相类似。当牙齿被迅速冷却时，会感觉到明显的、尖锐的、潜伏期短（1.6s）的疼痛。随后表现为难以定位的钝痛、灼烧痛。这些研究结果证实了人类牙髓神经的反应行为与动物模型相似的假说：最初的剧烈疼痛是由牙内 Aδ 纤维引起的，随后，一旦牙内温度升高到一定程度，C 纤维就会被激活，并产生钝痛、跳痛。尽管研究方法稍有不同，其他研究小组的后期研究也得出了类似或相同的结论。然而，值得注意的是，这些研究数据是对相对正常、健康的牙髓进行实验所得到的[2]。

针对牙髓炎患者痛感的研究目前较少见。在临床诊断为牙髓炎的患者中，疼痛程度的估值与总的 Aδ 神经活性之间似乎仅有较弱的关联性[3]。然而，存在不同程度牙髓感染的患牙，其牙髓测试反应虽然通常表现为阳性，但有异常。因此，冷诊反应阳性仅表明牙髓有活力，但不能确定牙髓炎症是否可复；然而，没有反应即说明牙髓坏死。

过去，冷诊测试通常使用冰棒和氯乙烷喷雾。这两种方法的温度都不够低；氯乙烷的温度仅为 −4℃左右，冰的温度为 0℃或略高于 0℃。此外还存在一个问题，即材料一旦融化，冰水会滴落在相邻的牙齿上，导致假阳性反应。干冰笔的使用已有二十多年的历史，它们可以安全地用于活髓牙，不会损伤牙釉质或牙髓组织[54, 95-96]。使用干冰测试得到的阳性反应也比氯乙烷和冰棒更准确，此外，对于牙根未发育完全的年轻患牙，使用干冰测试似乎比牙髓电活力测试更可靠[40]。此外，对于正在接受正畸治疗患者的患牙，干冰也比牙髓电活力测试更可靠[24]。

近来，人们开始使用制冷剂喷雾——1, 1, 1, 2 四氟乙烷。它的优点是以喷雾罐形式储存；可以存放于椅旁；此外，与干冰相比成本更低。然而，它达不到干冰的低温（−26.2℃，−15.4°F）。无论牙齿的类型或修复情况如何，四氟乙烷和干冰在产生牙髓反应的方面似乎没有区别[57]。

牙髓病学基础：根尖周炎的预防和治疗

如果计划对一名患者进行几次活力测试，牙髓电活力测试和制冷剂喷雾冷诊之间的顺序和间隔并不会影响牙髓诊断测试的准确性[93]。

步 骤

与牙髓电活力测试一样，需要注意患牙和周围牙齿的干燥和隔湿。为了获得最佳效果，冷刺激物应放在切缘或靠近髓角的位置。冷诊应轻柔地进行，因为接触极冷的冰或物体可能会引起快速而剧烈的疼痛，尤其是前牙（图 7.2）。

诊断信息

异常的阳性反应在所有类型的牙髓炎中均可能发生[31,108]。因此，阳性反应表明至少部分牙髓有活性，但它不能表明炎症是否可逆。尽管冷刺激反应与牙髓组织学表现之间缺乏明显的相关性，但临床经验表明，当剧烈的疼痛迅速转变为钝痛，并伴有其他体征，如疼痛和自发痛史时，则提示很大可能为不可复性牙髓炎。

7.5.1.3 热诊

热诊是一种不太常用的温度测试，但可能会提供更多有用的临床信息。这种方法的主要问题是许多常用的测试方法会导致温度过高，损伤牙髓或邻近组织，而其他方法的应用较为繁杂。因此，热诊的临床应用存在一定的局限性。

正常牙髓对热刺激的反应和感觉与冷刺激相似。在多数情况下，反映呈现双相性，即 Aδ 纤维先被激活，如果刺激持续存在，随即出现钝痛、放散性疼痛[18, 86]。人的体内研究表明，热牙胶刺激诱导的神经反应模式比氯乙烷更为复杂。热牙胶会引发三个阶段的反应，其中第三阶段是在没有物理刺激的情况下出现缓慢的自发的神经活性，而受试者感觉不到这种反应，这表明更多的 C 纤维被激活[3]。

步 骤

目前存在多种热诊测试方法。一种是将牙胶置于火焰上加热，然后放置在涂有润滑剂的牙冠上靠近切缘处[83]。这种方法的问题在于难以控制温度，且牙胶容易粘在牙齿上，导致大块材料被去除后残留的牙胶依然持续对患牙进行加热。也有主张使用不加润滑剂的抛光杯或橡皮轮，但同样无法控制产热量。一种更好但烦琐的方法是将患者置于仰卧位，用橡皮障隔离单个牙齿，然后将暴露的牙齿浸在热水中。一旦患者有反应，将橡皮障移动至近中邻牙并重复该过程。从可疑患牙的远中邻牙开始检查，这样即使橡皮障封闭不

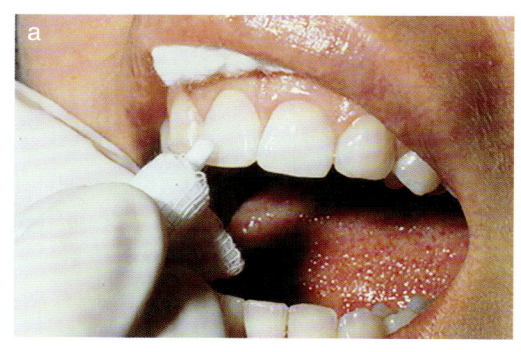

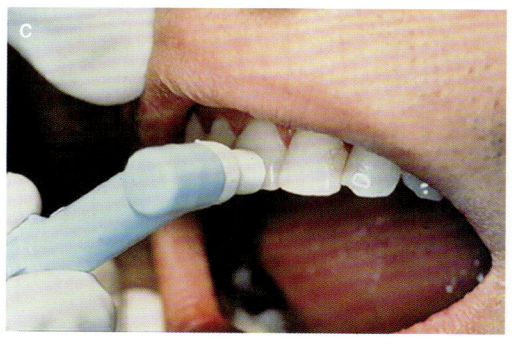

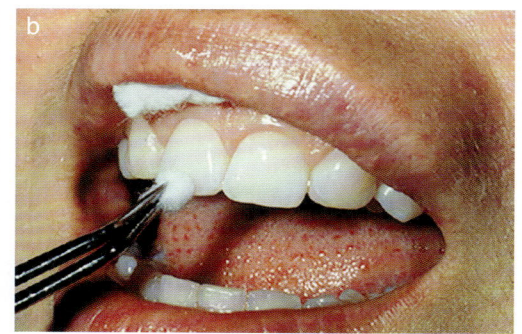

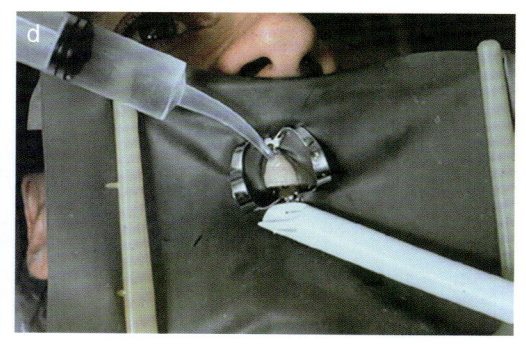

图 7.2 温度敏感性测试。a. 干冰棒（−70℃）。b. 喷有 1, 1, 1, 2− 四氟乙烷的棉球（−26℃）。c. 使用无润滑剂的橡皮杯加热牙齿表面。d. 橡皮障隔离单颗牙齿后使用热水冲洗

严，热水也不会滴落至可疑的患牙，从而产生假阳性反应。

诊断信息

目前，尚未发现热诊的异常反应和组织学诊断之间的相关性[31, 108]。然而，通常认为当牙髓存在严重炎症时，会对热反应较敏感。关于这方面的研究较少，但临床经验表明，当患者主诉存在严重的热刺激痛时，牙髓通常发生了不可逆的炎症。一些动物研究在某种程度上证实了以上问题，研究发现，对于有症状的牙髓炎，热刺激所激活的神经与疼痛反应标志物的分布区域相类似[26-27]。

7.5.2 机械性测试

叩诊和触诊测试不是活力测试，而是检测牙周和（或）根尖周组织炎症的方法。有研究指出，当牙髓出现部分或全部坏死时，叩诊更有可能引起疼痛[106]，从而间接对牙髓状态进行评估。显然，对于其他可能导致叩诊敏感的原因需要排除，比如最近的咬合创伤、充填体高点等。同样还包括根尖区扪诊不适但牙髓有活力的患牙。当活髓患牙对叩诊和（或）扪诊敏感并且对热刺激反应特别敏感时，提示牙髓很大可能存在不可逆的炎症[106]。若牙齿对叩诊和（或）扪诊不敏感，不能证明炎症不存在[10]。

叩 诊

正确的测试方法是使用口镜手柄。目的是确定根尖牙周组织是否存在炎症。

步 骤

使用口镜手柄轻叩咬合面、颊面和舌面。叩诊应按随机顺序进行，以避免患者会有所"预期"，而不是对真正的疼痛作出反应。

诊断信息

如前所述，叩诊阳性反应表明根尖周组织存在炎症。在分析叩诊结果时，必须注意排除牙周病或牙尖折裂导致的阳性反应。这对于牙髓活力测试为活髓的患牙尤其困难，需要结合其他诊断性测试的结果和症状来区分牙周源性或牙髓源性的感染。

扪 诊

该测试用于检测牙根周围黏骨膜的炎症。在出现广泛肿胀之前，可能检测到压痛、波动、质硬或捻发音。

步 骤

使用食指通过黏膜按压牙槽骨。当患者感觉到压力时晃动手指，如果存在炎症，则会出现不适感。与叩诊一样，应以随机方式进行测试，并将测试结果与对侧牙或邻牙进行比较。

诊断信息

与叩诊类似，根尖区扪诊的阳性反应是证实根尖周存在炎症的可靠依据。但是，如果反应为阴性，也并不能说明不存在炎症[10]。

7.5.3 影像学检查

影像学检查是常用的检查方法之一，其结果应与症状、临床检查以及其他检查结果相结合进行分析。所有 X 线片均应使用支架进行拍摄，以确保平行投照和标准化。如果随访时需要进行 X 线片对比，可制作一个橡胶咬合垫，以确保随访的 X 线片拍摄角度尽可能一致（图 7.3）。

诊断信息

X 线片不能直接检测牙髓炎症。然而，X 线片显示龋齿或不良修复体可提示牙髓存在炎症[73]。致密性根尖周炎的病变表现与牙髓炎类似（图 7.4）。当髓腔出现闭塞和钙化表现时（弥漫性或牙髓结石）可以考虑牙髓是否存在炎症，但两者之间没有直接关系。此外，若存在牙髓来源的根尖透射影，提示牙髓坏死或部分坏死。

7.5.4 试验性测试

方 法

牙髓活力测试需要有功能性神经对刺激作出反应。当牙髓存在有效的血液循环和有活力的细胞，但有神经被切断或受损时，可能会被误诊为牙髓坏死或无活力。因此，人们试图通过血液循环来判断牙髓的活力。目前已有几种试验性方法，如测量牙冠表面温度[36-37]、注射氙-133 放射性同位素[61]、脉冲血氧仪[104]、双波长分光光度法[90]和激光多普勒血流仪[43]。在这些方法中，激光多普勒血流仪和脉冲血氧仪似乎最有可能准确地评估牙髓活力[71]。然而，非常不幸的是，这些方法对于牙髓炎症水平的评估能力有限，尽管实验证

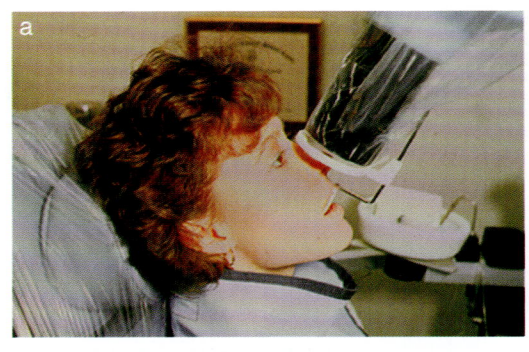

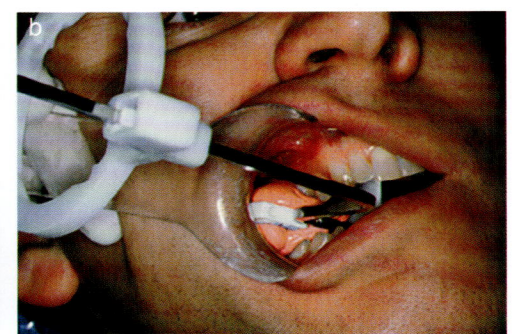

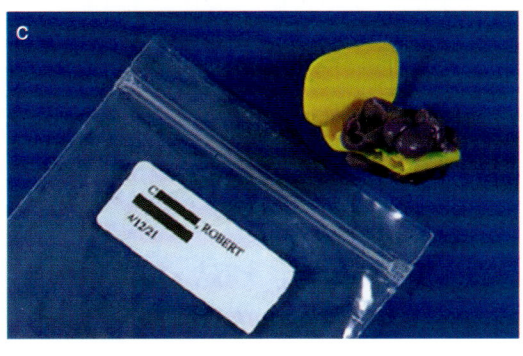

牙髓病学基础：根尖周炎的预防和治疗

图 7.3　a. 应使用胶片支架进行 X 线片拍摄以确保平行投照和标准化。b. 如果随访时需要 X 线片对比，可使用硅橡胶材料制作定制的橡胶咬合垫。c. 将咬合垫与胶片支架一起保存

明其中多数方法具有很高的准确性和可靠性，但从未出现商业化产品用于牙髓活力评估。

7.6　牙髓诊断

利用上述所得的信息进行诊断（表 7.1）。

7.6.1　关键因素

死髓与活髓

根据患者的主诉症状和尽可能多的诊断性测试结果，应该能够准确地确定牙髓是坏死的还是有活力的。如果牙髓坏死，则需要进行根管治疗来保存患牙。区分可复性牙髓炎和不可复性牙髓炎是一个更大的挑战，这需要结合症状、病史（主观的）和临床检查加以确定。

牙髓暴露

如前所述，如果在去龋时发现牙髓已暴露于细菌感染，则可以确诊为不可复性牙髓炎。治疗计划是去除全部牙髓并行预防性根管充填。然而，牙根未发育完成的非常年轻的牙齿除外。在这种情况下，可尝试行暂时（几个月到一年）的部分牙髓切断术，待根尖完全成形后再行完善的根管治疗。

7.6.2　相关因素

剧烈疼痛史、自发痛史、同一牙齿的既往疼痛史或牵涉痛都是不可复性牙髓炎的表现。必须考虑其他所有的相关因素，如年龄、牙周状态、既往牙髓治疗史，但这些因素的参考价值有限。

7.6.3　治疗计划

一直以来，人们都在不断强调，根据目前可用的诊断方法对不可复性牙髓炎进行的诊断最多

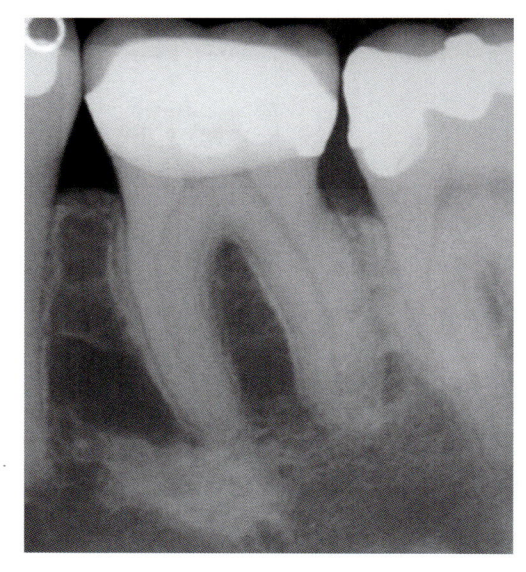

图 7.4　X 线片示下颌磨牙近中根处致密性根尖周炎。这颗患牙于几年前行修复治疗，似乎是进行了直接盖髓术。患者诉就诊前几周出现冷刺激敏感

表 7.1 牙髓诊断的制定

症状，测试，支持信息	牙髓坏死	活髓	
		不可复性牙髓炎	可复性牙髓炎
牙髓测试	阴性	阳性	阳性
重要因素			
髓腔暴露		存在	不存在
叩诊疼痛		存在	不存在
相关因素			
剧烈疼痛		存在	不存在
自发痛		存在	不存在
疼痛史		存在	不存在
延迟痛		存在	不存在
热痛冷缓解		存在	不存在
治疗计划相关因素			
年龄、牙周病史、牙髓治疗史		不确定（复杂治疗方案）	不确定（简单治疗方案）

是一种"有根据的猜测"，误诊是不可避免的。因此，患者的总体治疗计划应在去髓术或保守治疗中选择。

例如，如果患牙是牙弓中唯一需要治疗的牙齿，且仅需使用银汞合金或树脂修复（图 7.5），则即使一些因素表明牙髓存在中度炎症，也可以尝试保守方法治疗，而非去髓治疗。然而，当具有相同的症状和体征的患牙需要作为桥基牙时，若保守治疗可能失败则难以进行牙髓治疗，因此可能会优先选择去髓术，而非保守治疗。

7.7 根尖周的诊断

"根尖周炎"指由牙髓感染或牙髓坏死引起的牙周膜炎症。有害物质和细菌产物通过根尖孔进入牙周组织。如果髓腔和牙周组织之间通过根分叉或副根管形成交通，牙周炎症也可发生于这些部位。组织学上，病变主要为慢性炎症细胞浸润，总体表现为肉芽肿或囊肿[15]。

与牙髓炎症一样，根尖周炎可以是无症状的，仅在发展为慢性根尖周炎时才可通过 X 线片进行诊断。然而，如果在 X 线片上可以检测到根尖周

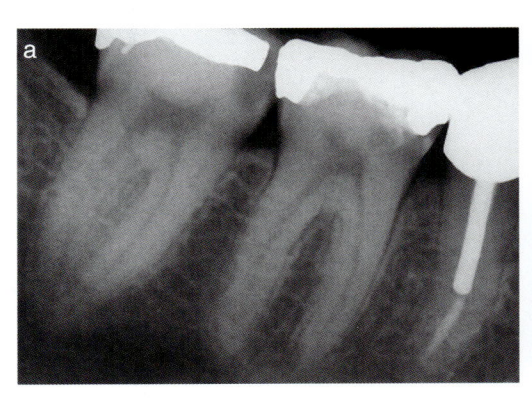

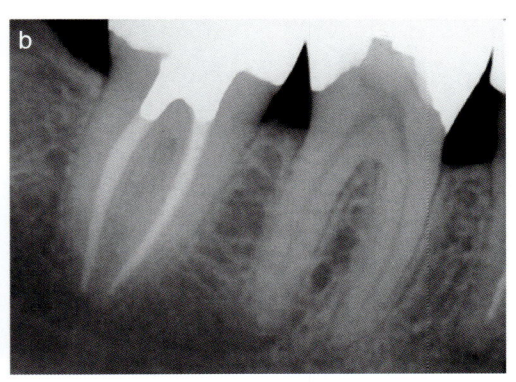

图 7.5 a. 两颗下颌磨牙均存在大面积深龋。患者主诉持续数天的剧烈疼痛，但无法确定疼痛是由哪颗牙引起。牙髓测试无法确定哪颗牙的牙髓炎症较重。去龋后发现第二磨牙有穿髓孔，而第一磨牙未穿髓。对第二磨牙进行根管治疗。对第一磨牙行活髓保存术及修复治疗。b. 1 年后随访，第一磨牙牙髓测试反应正常，两颗牙齿叩诊和扣诊反应均正常

病变，则几乎可以肯定是由根管系统感染引起的，不论牙齿是否有病史或有无症状[11]。通常，如果患者有症状，那么在治疗前明确病因是很重要的。治疗通常是去除引起症状或病变的刺激物。如果根尖周炎是由咬合创伤引起，则通过简单的咬合调整即可解决。根尖周炎的病因通常是根管系统中存在的细菌，因此唯一有效的治疗方法则是彻底消毒根管，然后进行根管充填和良好的冠方封闭。单独使用抗生素治疗是无效的[38]。

7.7.1 正常根尖组织

7.7.1.1 有症状的根尖周炎（SAP）

这一术语通常意味着根尖炎症始于急性期，导致了咬合及叩诊不适和（或）扪诊不适的临床症状。通常，有症状的根尖周炎仅有很少或几乎没有影像学改变。然而，这一诊断也可能存在根尖透射区。这种炎症可能有多种原因。最好的情况是咬合创伤，此时牙髓应该是有活力的，没有受损。然而，在细菌感染的情况下，牙髓可能存在严重的或不可逆的炎症，通常出现部分或全部坏死。急性根尖周炎也可由先前存在的慢性病变转变而来（见7.7.1.3）。

7.7.1.2 无症状的根尖周炎（AAP）

这一术语意味着根尖周炎在一定时间内没有症状。当牙髓坏死并伴有根尖周炎的影像学表现（透射影或阻射性降低）时，可以考虑为无症状的根尖周炎。

7.7.1.3 急性根尖周脓肿（AAA）

根尖周炎导致根尖周组织出现化脓性病损，伴随脓液在牙周组织、骨膜下、黏膜下和（或）皮下积聚，患者的症状有快速出现的疼痛、压痛和肿胀。通常，这种来源于之前存在的慢性根尖周炎的急性炎症被称为再发性根尖周脓肿。

7.7.1.4 慢性根尖周脓肿

慢性根尖周脓肿是由牙髓坏死及随后的感染导致的进展缓慢的炎症反应。通常情况下，慢性根尖周脓肿很少或没有不适感，并且存在可追踪的窦道，根尖周分泌物经此排放到体表（口内或口外），形成根尖周引流的窦道（图7.6，图7.7）。

7.7.1.5 致密性骨炎

这类疾病通常是无症状的，表现为根尖区弥

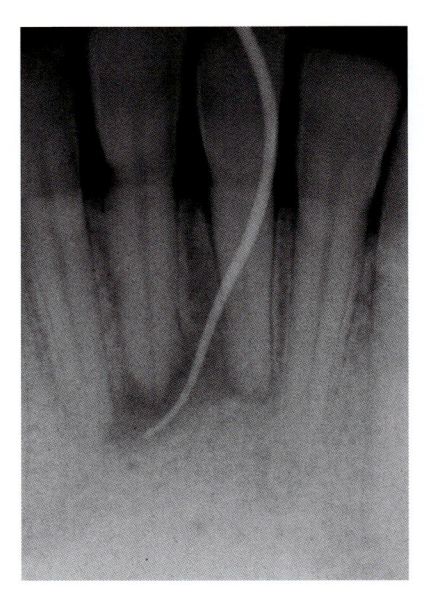

图7.6　X线片示使用#40牙胶尖进行窦道示踪。注意，窦道的开口位于左侧中切牙的远中，示踪其来源为右侧中切牙

漫性阻射影（图7.4）。该病被认为与牙髓轻度炎症刺激有关，对人类标本研究发现，这些炎症或无炎症区域被不同宽度的致密层状骨所包围，内部充满取代了松质骨和骨髓的结缔组织[45]。

7.8 根尖周病的症状

根尖周病变的诊断步骤应与上述牙髓病的诊断步骤相同。仔细评估患者的症状，进行诊断性测试，记录临床检查结果，汇总信息以做出初步诊断（表7.2）。

表7.2　牙髓源性窦道与牙周袋的鉴别诊断

测试	牙周袋	牙髓源性窦道
活力测试	正常	无反应
牙周探查	较宽的牙周袋	较窄的通道
患牙的临床表现	龋坏或修复体少见	明显的龋坏或修复体
全口牙周情况	差	正常
暗视野螺旋体计数	>30%	<10%

7.8.1 有症状的根尖周炎

咬合创伤

症状　患者主诉进食、咬物或"牙齿接触时"疼痛。

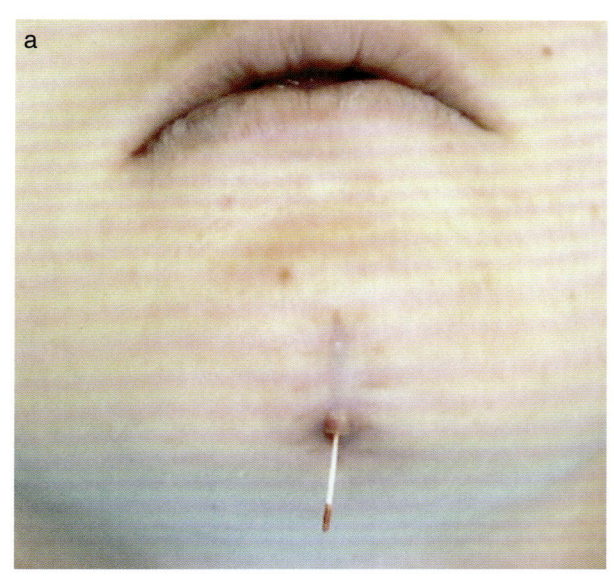

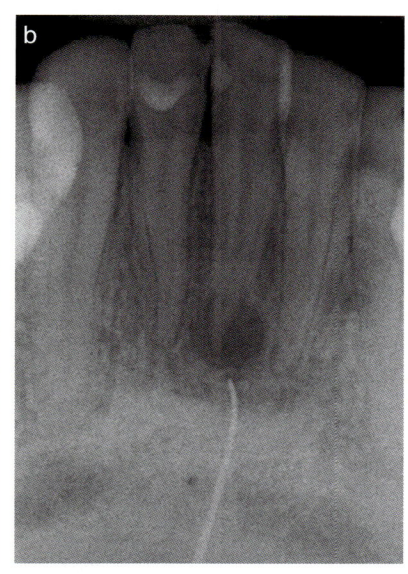

图 7.7 a. 患有癫痫大发作的患者曾因"颏部囊肿"接受多位医生的治疗,导致颏部瘢痕组织形成和局部感觉异常。最终,前往牙髓病专科医生处就诊,使用牙胶尖进行窦道的示踪。b. 示踪片显示病变来源于左下中切牙。牙髓敏感性测试无反应,X 线片示存在根尖周病变。在第一次就诊时进行了根管清理和氢氧化钙封药,窦道愈合,两年随访评估时未见复发(Buttke 博士提供)

病史 通常患者近期曾接受牙齿治疗,导致修复体咬合不均衡,存在咬合高点。

临床检查 患区经常可见新的修复体。

诊断性测试 牙髓热诊和电活力测试反应正常。叩诊疼痛,偶尔可见扪诊疼痛。影像学检查通常未见异常。

治疗 调整咬合以消除早接触,包括所有侧方接触的咬合干扰。随访患者以确保急性根尖炎症消退且牙髓活力正常。

有症状的根尖周炎伴急性牙髓炎

这种情况已经在牙髓诊断中讨论过。急性根尖周炎合并急性牙髓炎提示存在不可复性牙髓炎。

治疗 牙髓摘除术/根管治疗(见第 10 章)。根管充填后应尽快进行永久性修复,以防止冠方渗漏和由此引发的慢性根尖周炎[70]。

无症状根尖周炎的急性发作

症状 患者主诉咬物、进食或"牙齿接触时"疼痛。也可能出现自发性剧烈疼痛,以及肿胀和不适。

病史 这些案例的病史是多种多样的。有时,患者诉曾有疼痛史或近期修复治疗史。在其他情况下,患者可能曾有牙髓疼痛史,后来疼痛缓解。有时,患牙曾接受过根管治疗。

临床检查 与牙髓坏死或根管治疗后的患牙表现一致。如可见深龋、盖髓术后、大面积修复体或全冠。

诊断性测试 对热诊和电活力测试无反应。叩诊和(或)扪诊疼痛。影像学检查显示根尖透射影,提示慢性根尖周炎急性发作。

治疗 治疗包括完整的根管机械预备和消毒,使用抗菌剂进行根管冲洗以及根管内封药[22](见第 10 章)。由于脓肿尚未形成,无法引流。因此无须进行抗生素治疗。可根据需要开具止痛药。应在 1~4 周后再次评估以确认根管充填后根尖炎症已消退。为了防止冠方渗漏,应尽快进行永久性修复。

7.8.2 无症状根尖周炎

症状 根据定义,患者无症状或至少仅有轻度不适。这种情况可能通过常规的随访 X 线片,或者在牙齿进行修复治疗前,因牙髓活力测试无反应而被诊断出来。

病史和临床检查 与无症状根尖周炎急性发作类似,也可能完全没有疼痛史。

诊断测试 热诊和牙髓电活力测试无反应。

叩诊和（或）扣诊检查通常为阴性，可能存在轻度不适。

影像学检查 由于这些病例大部分无症状，因此慢性根尖周炎的诊断主要基于影像学表现，即存在透射影（或阻射性较低）（见第6章）（图7.8）。根尖周炎也可能没有影像学改变[9-10]，因此只有在进行牙髓治疗时才发现牙髓坏死和感染。需要修改诊断为无症状根尖周炎，并进行相应治疗（第11章）。

治疗 对根管系统进行有效的消毒可以消除慢性根尖周炎。

7.8.3 急性根尖周炎伴脓肿

在根尖周炎的急性期（原发性急性病变或慢性病变急性发作），感染可能发展并导致脓液积聚和脓肿形成。这样一来，病变可能会转变为慢性炎症，但有时会继续形成有症状的脓肿。随着组织压力增加，炎症介质导致骨吸收，脓液首先穿过骨和骨膜下层，穿透骨膜进入组织间隙。

脓液积聚的确切位置取决于根尖相对应面部肌肉的解剖位置[81]。最常见的是从颊侧引流至口腔前庭。罕见的并发症是经上颌和下颌第三磨牙及翼丛扩散，导致海绵窦血栓性静脉炎和脑血管引流障碍[50]（图7.9）。在下颌牙齿中，最严重的情况是从前磨牙或磨牙舌侧的下颌舌骨肌下扩散到咽后间隙。路德维希咽峡炎是由双侧咽后扩散所致，严重者可能会导致气道阻塞[112]。在大多数情况下，脓液会穿透口腔黏膜表面。有时脓肿会向口外引流到颏部、颏下或下颌下。

症状 症状会根据炎症过程的进展而有所不同。最初，可能为咬物、进食或咬合接触时的轻微疼痛。当脓液在骨膜下积聚时，疼痛加剧，患者有时会非常痛苦。当脓液穿透骨膜时，可能出现弥漫性肿胀（图7.9）。脓液穿透骨膜通常伴随着压力的释放，疼痛明显减轻。

病史和临床表现 与有症状的根尖周炎类似。

诊断性测试 热诊或电活力测试无反应。叩诊和（或）触诊疼痛，根据病程的不同阶段，疼痛有时会很剧烈。

影像学表现 脓肿的发展阶段决定了影像学表现。在脓肿形成的早期阶段，炎症的影像学表现可能不明显（如果有的话）。随着脓肿的扩散和更多的骨组织被破坏，根尖周炎的影像学表现将更加明显。对于慢性病变急性发作的病例，根尖周炎的影像学表现始终存在。

治疗 治疗原则与所有根尖周炎的患牙齿相同，即根管消毒（见第9章）。此外，在发生急性脓肿的情况下，治疗方案需要考虑感染在组织间隙内扩散（蜂窝组织炎）和疼痛控制的问题。急诊治疗的主要目的是消除脓肿的来源，即髓腔

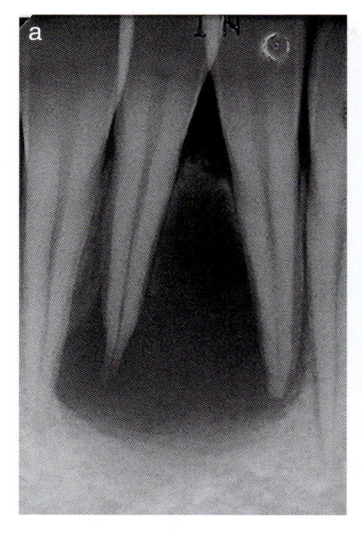

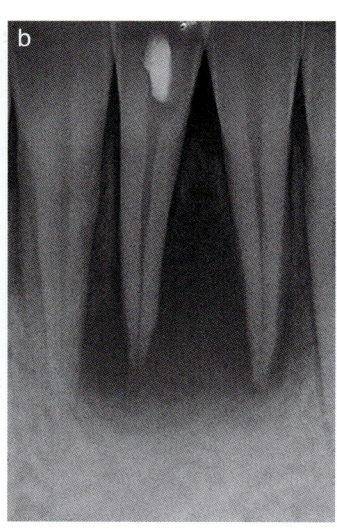

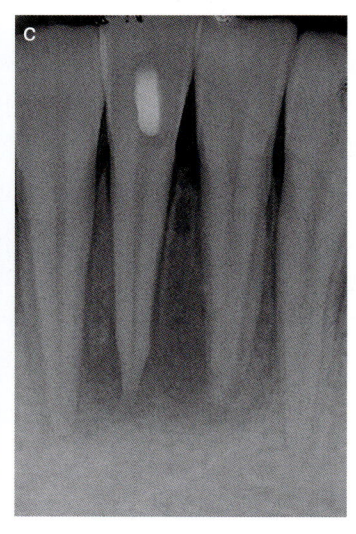

图7.8 a.13岁患者，下前牙唇侧出现无症状、质硬的肿胀。X线检查显示根尖周有较大的透射影像，且中切牙的牙根被推向了远中。冷诊示右侧中切牙无反应，但左侧中切牙有反应。诊断为牙髓坏死伴慢性根尖周炎。b.根管系统内封氢氧化钙6周后，根尖周病变明显改善。c.氢氧化钙封药3个月后，病变几乎完全消退

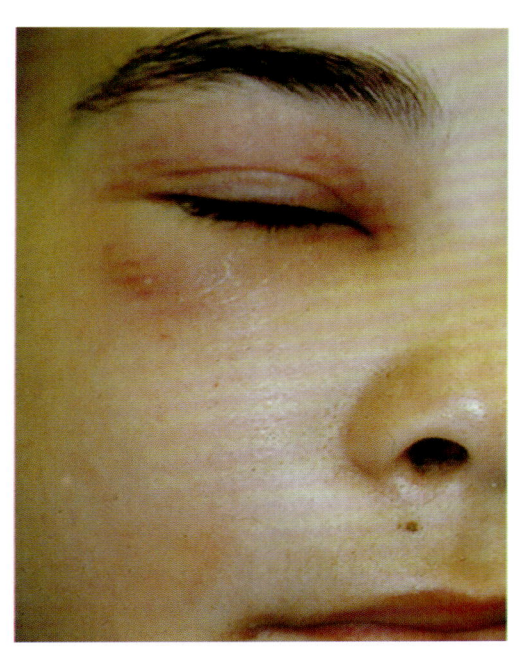

图 7.9 上颌第一前磨牙脓肿引起的严重肿胀。脓液突破了骨膜引起眶周严重的肿胀

内的感染，仅在患者出现系统性感染时使用抗生素作为补充治疗。在严重病例中，如怀疑感染向咽后间隙或眶部扩散时，建议请口腔外科医生或急诊医生急诊会诊。

7.8.4 慢性根尖周脓肿

发生慢性根尖周脓肿时，根尖炎性渗出液经口内或口外引流至体表。窦道的形成可能是机体控制感染的机制，也可能表明存在某些特殊的细菌混合感染——目前尚不清楚的。它可能是由上述脓肿引起的，也可能没有前期症状，因此，诊断甚至可能是在患者不知道其存在的情况下作出的。长期存在的窦道可完全上皮化[6]。随着根管的充分消毒和根尖周炎症的消退，上皮组织（如果存在）在大多数情况下会分解。通常窦道会在患牙附近的黏膜处引流。但窦道开口也可能与患牙有一定的距离（图 7.6），可通过牙周膜引流，形成类似的牙周袋，甚至引流至口外，导致误诊（图 7.7）。因此，必须进行彻底的检查来明确诊断，而不是依赖于窦道开口的位置来诊断。

症状　当根尖周炎伴窦道存在时，患者无疼痛感或痛感很轻微，无明显肿胀。这是由于骨膜或邻近组织下没有压力积聚所致。

病史和临床发现　与无症状根尖周炎和有症状根尖周炎类似。

诊断测试　热诊或电活力测试阴性。叩诊和（或）扪诊没有或仅有轻微疼痛。

影像学检查　慢性根尖周炎通常存在影像学改变，但窦道在黏膜上的位置并不总是与患牙相对应。因此，需要用 X 线阻射物（例如 #35 或 #40 的牙胶尖）追踪窦道，以确定窦道的来源。必须注意不要用力推牙胶尖，避免造成假的通道而导致误诊。

治疗方法　对根管系统进行消毒应该能够消除慢性根尖周炎，窦道可在几天到几周内消失。在极少数情况下，窦道无法愈合，这是由于感染主要位于牙根外，因此需抗生素治疗和（或）手术治疗。

7.8.5 致密性骨炎

如前所述，致密性骨炎通常表现为临近牙齿根尖区的弥漫性阻射影[118]。

症状　患者通常无明显症状，且大多数情况下患牙为活髓。患者可能对活力测试反应敏感。

病史和临床检查　理论上，牙髓受到了长期的慢性刺激，如较深的和（或）存在微渗漏的填充物导致牙髓发生轻度炎症，并伴有根尖周骨质改变，骨髓腔和松质骨被密质骨替代，脂肪性骨髓处发生纤维化[45]。

诊断性测试　牙髓通常对热诊或电活力测试有反应。叩诊和（或）触诊无痛。

影像学检查　可见围绕根尖呈同心排列的弥漫性阻射区域，有时可能存在炎性透射影，但根尖牙周膜间隙没有变化[35]。

治疗　评估牙齿修复体以排除牙髓的刺激源，无须其他治疗。

7.9　根尖周炎的诊断

只有在获得上述所有信息后才能进行诊断，见表 7.3 中的总结。

7.9.1　关键因素

与根管系统相关的根尖周病几乎总是由细菌和（或）细菌副产物引起。因此，应消除感染以确保疾病的消退和愈合。

表 7.3 根尖周炎的诊断

	临床表现		影像学表现	其他表现
	疼痛	肿胀		
急性根尖周炎	是	否	牙周膜间隙正常	
慢性根尖周炎	否	否	根尖周透射影	
根尖周炎伴脓肿	是/否	是	起初牙周膜间隙正常，后期可能增宽	
根尖周炎伴窦道	否	否	常见根尖周透射影	引流的窦道

7.9.2 相关因素

确定根尖周炎属于牙周源性还是牙髓源性，对于疾病的正确治疗至关重要（表 7.2）。

7.10 牙髓和根尖周病诊断的展望

最近，多种生物标记物，如基质金属蛋白酶，被认为可能是评估牙髓炎症水平的有效工具[119]。这是因为已有学者证明，至少在一般情况下，与健康牙髓相比，不可复性牙髓炎与多种生物标记物的不同表达相关，其中许多生物标记物甚至可以在龋损或其他修复治疗未露髓的情况下，通过无创的方法从龈沟液或牙本质/牙本质内组织液中收集[100]。这些生物标记物之间的相互作用不仅可用于评估牙髓炎症水平，还可提供足够的信息来区分根尖周囊肿和肉芽肿[28,33,94,100]。然而，我们还没有完全将其实现，因为在近期的一项对牙髓炎症生物标志物的系统评价中，作者提出生物标志物临床应用的主要挑战在于确定与牙髓炎症确实相关的生物标志物或生物标志物亚群、改进样本采集方法，以及应对生物标记物与非牙髓源性炎症的互相干扰[100]。

在进行任何侵入性牙髓治疗，甚至任何牙科治疗之前，明确牙髓病的诊断是至关重要的。很明显，医生进行临床诊断需要具备临床技能、对临床体征和症状有良好的理解以及认识到常用牙髓活力测试方法的局限性。这一后天技能的发展需要时间来培养，并且总是存在主观或偏见的风险。

参考文献

[1] AAE. AAE consensus conference recommended diagnostic terminology. J Endod, 2009, 35: 1634.

[2] Ahlquist M L, Franzen O G. Encoding of the subjective intensity of sharp dental pain. Endod Dent Traumatol, 1994, 10 (4): 153–166.

[3] Ahlquist M L, Franzen O G. Inflammation and dental pain in man. Endod Dent Traumatol, 1994, 10 (5): 201–209.

[4] Barbakow F H, Cleaton-Jones P E, Friedman D. Endodontic treatment of teeth with periapical radiolucent areas ina general dental practice. Oral Surg Oral Med Oral Pathol, 1981, 51 (5): 552–559.

[5] Baume L J. Diagnosis of diseases of the pulp. Oral Surg Oral Med Oral Pathol, 1970, 29 (1): 102–116.

[6] Baumgartner J C, Picket A B, Muller J T. Microscopic examination of oral sinus tracts and their associated periapical lesions. J Endod, 1984, 10 (4): 146–152.

[7] Bender I B. Reversible and irreversible painful pulpitides: diagnosis and treatment. Aust Endod J, 2000, 26 (1): 10–14.

[8] Bender I B, et al. The optimum placement-site of the electrode in electric pulp testing of the 12 anterior teeth. J Am Dent Assoc, 1989, 118 (3): 305–310.

[9] Bender I B, Seltzer S. Roentgenographic and direct observation of experimental lesions in bone: I JADA, 1961, 62 (2): 152–160.

[10] Bender I B, Seltzer S. Roentgenographic and direct observation of experimental lesions in bone: Ⅱ. JADA, 1961, 62 (6): 708–716.

[11] Bergenholtz G. Micro-organisms from necrotic pulp of traumatized teeth. Odontol Revy, 1974, 25 (4): 347–358.

[12] Bergenholtz G. Effect of bacterial products on inflammatory reactions in the dental pulp. Scand J Dent Res, 1977, 85 (2): 122–129.

[13] Bergenholtz G, Lindhe J. Effect of experimentally induced marginal periodontitis and periodontal scaling on the dental pulp. J Clin Periodontol, 1978, 5 (1): 59–73.

[14] Beveridge E E, Brown A C. The measurement of human dental intrapulpal pressure and its response to clinical variables. Oral Surg Oral Med Oral Pathol, 1965, 19: 655–668.

[15] Bhaskar S N. Oral surgery-oral pathology conference No. 17, Walter Reed Army Medical Center. Periapical lesions-

types, incidence, and clinical features. Oral Surg Oral Med Oral Pathol, 1966, 21 (5): 657–671.

[16] Bjørndal L, et al. Randomized clinical trials on deep carious lesions: 5-year follow-up. J Dent Res, 2017, 96 (7): 747–753.

[17] Bowles W R, et al. Tissue levels of immunoreactive substance P are increased in patients with irreversible pulpitis. J Endod, 2003, 29 (4): 265–267.

[18] Brannstrom M, Johnson G. Movements of the dentine and pulp liquids on application of thermal stimuli. An in vitro study. Acta Odontol Scand, 1970, 28 (1): 59–70.

[19] Brizuela C, et al. Direct pulp capping with calcium hydroxide, mineral trioxide aggregate, and biodentine in permanent young teeth with caries: a randomized clinical trial. J Endod, 2017, 43 (11): 1776–1780.

[20] Byers M R, Narhi M V. Dental injury models: experimental tools for understanding neuroinflammatory interactions and polymodal nociceptor functions. Crit Rev Oral Biol Med, 1999, 10 (1): 4–39.

[21] Byers M R, et al. Acute and chronic reactions of dental sensory nerve fibers to cavities and desiccation in rat molars. Anat Rec, 1988, 221 (4): 872–883.

[22] Byström A, Claesson R, Sundqvist G. The antibacterial effect of camphorated paramonochlorophenol, camphorated phenol and calcium hydroxide in the treatment of infected root canals. Endod Dent Traumatol, 1985, 1 (5): 170–175.

[23] Casasco A, et al, Peptidergicnerves in human dental pulp. An immunocytochemical study. Histochemistry, 1990, 95 (2): 115–121.

[24] Cave S G, Freer T J, Podlich H M. Pulp-test responses in orthodontic patients. Aust Orthod J, 2002, 18 (1): 27–34.

[25] Chambers I G. The role and methods of pulp testing in oral diagnosis: a review. Int Endod J, 1982, 15 (1): 1–15.

[26] Chattipakorn S C, et al. The effect of fentanyl on c-fos expression in the trigeminal brainstem complex produced by pulpal heat stimulation in the ferret. Pain, 1999, 82 (2): 207–215.

[27] Chattipakorn S C, et al. Trigeminal c-Fos expression and behavioral responses to pulpal inflammation in ferrets. Pain , 2002,99 (1–2): 61–69.

[28] de Paula-Silva F W, et al.High matrix metalloproteinase activity is a hallmark of periapical granulomas. J Endod, 2009, 35 (9): 1234–1242.

[29] Domine L, Holz J. The aging of the human pulp-dentin organ . Schweiz Monatsschr Zahnmed, 1991, 101 (6): 725–733.

[30] Dubner R, Ruda M A. Activitydependent neuronal plasticity following tissue injury and inflammation. Trends Neurosci, 1992, 15 (3): 96–103.

[31] Dummer P M, Hicks R, Huws D. Clinical signs and symptoms in pulp disease. Int Endod J, 1980, 13 (1): 27–35.

[32] Eli I. Dental anxiety: a cause for possible misdiagnosis of tooth vitality. Int Endod J, 1993, 26 (4): 251–253.

[33] Emilia E. Neelakantan P. Biomarkers in the dentin-pulp complex: role in health and disease. J Clin Pediatr Dent, 2015, 39 (2): 94–99.

[34] Estrela C, et al. Diagnostic and clinical factors associated with pulpal and periapical pain. Braz Dent J, 2011, 22 (4): 306–311.

[35] Eversole R, et al. Benign fibroosseous lesions of the craniofacial complex. A review. Head Neck Pathol, 2008, 2 (3): 177–202.

[36] Fanibunda K B. The feasibility of temperature measurement as a diagnostic procedure in human teeth. J Dent, 1986, 14 (3): 126–129.

[37] Fanibunda K B. A method of measuring the volume of human dental pulp cavities. Int Endod J, 1986, 19 (4): 194–197.

[38] Fouad A F, Rivera E M, Walton R E. Penicillin as a supplement in resolving the localized acute apical abscess. Oral Surg Oral Med Oral Pathol Oral Radiol Endod, 1996, 81 (5): 590–595.

[39] Fulling H J, Andreasen J O. Influence of maturation status and tooth type of permanent teeth upon electrometric and thermal pulp testing. Scand J Dent Res, 1976, 84 (5): 286–290.

[40] Fuss Z, et al. Assessment of reliability of electrical and thermal pulp testing agents. J Endod, 1986, 12 (7): 301–305.

[41] Galicia J C, et al.Gene expression profile of pulpitis. Genes Immun, 2016, 17 (4): 239–243.

[42] Garfunkel A, Sela J, Ulmansky M. Dental pulp pathosis. Clinicopathologic correlations based on 109 cases. Oral Surg Oral Med Oral Pathol, 1973, 35 (1): 110–117.

[43] Gazelius B, et al. Non-invasive recording of blood flow in human dental pulp. Endod Dent Traumatol, 1986, 2 (5): 219–221.

[44] Glick D H. Locating referred pulpal pains. Oral Surg Oral Med Oral Pathol, 1962, 15: 613–623.

[45] Green T L, et al. Histologic examination of condensing osteitis in cadaver specimens. J Endod, 2013, 39 (8): 977–979.

[46] Grushka M, Sessle B J. Applicability of the McGill Pain Questionnaire to the differentiation of "toothache" pain. Pain, 1984, 19 (1): 49–57.

[47] Haegerstam G. The origin of impulses recorded from dentinal cavities in the tooth of the cat. Acta Physiol Scand, 1976, 97 (1): 121–128.

[48] Heidari A, et al. Comparative study of substance P and neurokinin A in gingival crevicular fluid of healthy and painful carious permanent teeth. Dent Res J Isfahan, 2017, 14 (1): 57–61.

[49] Heide S, Mjör I A. Pulp reactions to experimental exposures in young permanent monkey teeth. Int Endod J, 1983, 16 (1): 11–19.

[50] Henig E F, et al. Brain abscess following dental infection. Oral Surg Oral Med Oral Pathol, 1978, 45 (6): 955–958.

[51] Hillmann G, Geurtsen W. Light-microscopical investigation of the distribution of extracellular matrix molecules and calcifications in human dental pulps of various ages. Cell Tissue Res, 1997, 289 (1): 145–154.

[52] Holt K G, Eleazer P D, Scheetz J P. Wet and dry deep cavity preparations compared by a novel odontoblast culture technique. J Endod, 2001, 27 (2): 103–106.

[53] Ingle J I, Beveridge E E, Olson C E. Rapid processing of endodontic "working" roentgenograms. Oral Surg Oral Med Oral Pathol, 1965, 19: 101–107.

[54] Ingram T A, Peters D D. Evaluation of the effects of carbon dioxide used as a pulpal test. Part 2. In vivo effect on canine enamel and pulpal tissues. J Endod, 1983, 9 (7): 296–303.

[55] Jaber L, Swaim W D, Dionne R A. Immunohistochemical localization of mu-opioid receptors in human dental pulp. J Endod, 2003, 29 (2): 108–110.

[56] Jespersen J J, et al. Evaluation of dental pulp sensibility tests in a clinical setting. J Endod, 2014, 40 (3): 351–354.

[57] Jones V R, Rivera E M, Walton R E. Comparison of carbon dioxide versus refrigerant spray to determine pulpal responsiveness. J Endod, 2002, 28 (7): 531–533.

[58] Jyvasjarvi E. Electrophysiological studies of afferent C-fiber innervation in the dental pulp. Proc Finn Dent Soc, 1987, 83 (4): 221–223.

[59] Jyvasjarvi E, Kniffki K D. Cold stimulation of teeth: a comparison between the responses of cat intradental A delta and C fibres and human sensation. J Physiol, 1987, 391: 193–207.

[60] Kaida K, et al. Suppressive effects of D-glucosamine on the 5-HT sensitive nociceptive units in the rat tooth pulpal nerve. Biomed Res Int, 2014 : 187989.

[61] Kim S, Schuessler G, Chien S. Measurement of blood flow in the dental pulp of dogs with the 133xenon washout method. Arch Oral Biol, 1983, 28 (6): 501–505.

[62] Klausen B, Helbo M, Dabelsteen E. differential diagnostic approach to the symptomatology of acute dental pain. Oral Surg Oral Med Oral Pathol, 1985, A 59 (3): 297–301.

[63] Klepac R K, et al. Reports of pain after dental treatment, electrical tooth pulp stimulation, and cutaneous shock. J Am Dent Assoc, 1980, 100 (5): 692–695.

[64] Klepac R K, et al. Reactions to pain among subjects high and low in dental fear. J Behav Med, 1980, 3 (4): 373–384.

[65] Langeland K. Management of the ninflamed pulp associated with deep carious lesion. J Endod, 1981, 7 (4): 169–181.

[66] Langeland K, Rodrigues H, Dowden W. Periodontal disease, bacteria, and pulpal histopathology. Oral Surg Oral Med Oral Pathol, 1974, 37 (2): 257–270.

[67] Lepinski A M, et al. Bradykinin levels in dental pulp by microdialysis. J Endod, 2000, 26 (12): 744–747.

[68] Lipski M, et al. Factors affecting the outcomes of direct pulp capping using Biodentine. Clin Oral Investig, 2017,

[69] Lundy T, Stanley H R. Correlation of pulpal histopathology and clinical symptoms in human teeth subjected to experimental irritation. Oral Surg Oral Med Oral Pathol, 1969, 27 (2): 187–201.

[70] Madison S, Wilcox L R. An evaluation of coronal microleakage in endodontically treated teeth. Part III. In vivo study. J Endod, 1988, 14 (9): 455–458.

[71] Mainkar A, Kim S G. Diagnostic Accuracy of 5 Dental Pulp Tests: A Systematic Review and Metaanalysis. J Endod, 2018

[72] Martin F E. Carious pulpitis: microbiological and histopathological considerations. Aust Endod J, 2003, 29 (3): 134–137.

[73] Massler M. Pulpal reactions to dental caries. Int Dent J 17, 1967, (2): 441–460.

[74] Matthews B, Searle B N. Electrical stimulation of teeth. Pain, 1976, 2 (3): 245–251.

[75] Mazur B, Massler M. Influence of periodontal disease of the dental pulp. Oral Surg Oral Med Oral Pathol, 1964, 17: 592–603.

[76] McGrath P A, et al. Non-pain and pain sensations evoked by tooth pulp stimulation. Pain, 1983, 15 (4): 377–388.

[77] Mengel M K, et al. Pain sensation during cold stimulation of the teeth: differential reflection of A delta and C fibre activity? Pain, 1993, 55 (2): 159–169.

[78] Mesaros S V, Trope M. Revascularization of traumatized teeth assessed by laser Doppler flowmetry: case report. Endod Dent Traumatol, 1997, 13 (1): 24–30.

[79] Michaelson P L, Holland G R. Is pulpitis painful? Int Endod J, 2002, 35 (10): 829–832.

[80] Michaelson R E, Seidberg B H, Guttuso J. An in vivo evaluation of interface media used with the electric pulp tester. J Am Dent Assoc, 1975, 91 (1): 118–121.

[81] Morse D R. Oral pathways of infection, with special reference to endodontics. J Br Endod Soc, 1972, 6 (1): 13–16.

[82] Morse D R, et al. Endodontic classification. J Am Dent Assoc, 1977, 94 (4): 685–689.

[83] Mumford J M. Thermal and electrical stimulation of teeth in the diagnosis of pulpal and periapical disease. Proc R Soc Med, 1967, 60 (2): 197–200.

[84] Murray P E, et al. Restorative pulpal and repair responses. J Am Dent Assoc, 2001, 132 (4): 482–491.

[85] Narhi M, Hirvonen T, Huopaniemi T. The function of intradental nerves in relation to the sensations induced by dental stimulation. Acupunct Electrother Res, 1984, 9 (2): 107–113.

[86] Narhi M, et al. Activation of heat-sensitive nerve fibres in

[87] Narhi M, et al. Electrical stimulation of teeth with a pulp tester in the cat. Scand J Dent Res, 1979, 87 (1): 32–38.

[88] Narhi M V O, et al. Role of intradental A and C type nerve fibers in dental pain mchanisms. Proceedings of the Finnish Dental Society, 1992, 88: 507–516.

[89] Newton C W, et al. Identify and determine the metrics, hierarchy, and predictive value of all the parameters and/ or methods used during endodontic diagnosis. J Endod, 2009, 35 (12): 1635–1644.

[90] Nissan R, et al. Dual wavelength spectrophotometry as a diagnostic test of the pulp chamber contents. Oral Surg Oral Med Oral Pathol, 1992, 74 (4): 508–514.

[91] Okeson J P, Falace D A. Nonodontogenic toothache. Dent Clin North Am, 1997, 41 (2): 367–383.

[92] Olgart L. Neural control of pulpal blood flow. Crit Rev Oral Biol Med, 1996, 7 (2): 159–171.

[93] Pantera E A Jr, Anderson R W, Pantera C T. Reliability of electric pulp testing after pulpal testing with dichlorodifluoromethane. J Endod, 1993, 19 (6): 312–314.

[94] Paula-Silva F W, da Silva L A, Kapila Y L. Matrix metalloproteinase expression in teeth with apical periodontitis is differentially modulated by the modality of root canal treatment. J Endod, 2010, 36 (2): 231–237.

[95] Peters D D, et al. Evaluation of the effects of carbon dioxide used as a pulpal test. 1. In vitro effect on human enamel. J Endod, 1983, 9 (6): 219–227.

[96] Peters D D, Mader C L, Donnelly J C. Evaluation of the effects of carbon dioxide used as a pulpal test. 3. In vivo effect on human enamel. J Endod, 1986, 12 (1): 13–20.

[97] Petersson K, et al. Evaluation of the ability of thermal and electrical tests to register pulp vitality. Endod Dent Traumatol, 1999, 15 (3): 127–131.

[98] Pigg M, et al. Validity of Preoperative Clinical Findings to Identify Dental Pulp Status: A National Dental Practice-Based Research Network Study. J Endod, 2016, 42 (6): 935–942.

[99] Read J K, et al. Effect of Ibuprofen on masking endodontic diagnosis. J Endod, 2014, 40 (8): 1058–1062.

[100] Rechenberg D K, Galicia J C, Peters O A. Biological Markers for Pulpal Inflammation: A Systematic Review. PLoS One, 2016, 11 (11): e0167289.

[101] Ricucci D, Loghin S, Siqueira J F Jr. Correlation between clinical and histologic pulp diagnoses. J Endod, 2014, 40 (12): 1932–1939.

[102] Rodd H D, Boissonade F M. Vascular status in human primary and permanent teeth in health and disease. Eur J Oral Sci, 2005, 113 (2): 128–134.

[103] Rubach W C, Mitchell D F. Periodontal Disease, Accessory Canals 236 7 Clinical Manifestations and Diagnosis and Pulp Pathosis. J Periodontol, 1965, 36: 34–38.

[104] Schnettler J M, Wallace J A. Pulse oximetry as a diagnostic tool of pulpal vitality. J Endod, 1991, 17 (10): 488–490.

[105] Seltzer S. Classification of pulpal pathosis. Oral Surg Oral Med Oral Pathol, 1972, 34 (2): 269–287.

[106] Seltzer S. Odontalgia (tooth pain) diagnosis and therapeutic considerations. Philadelphia, PG Temple University, 1990.

[107] Seltzer S, Bender I B, Ziontz M. The dynamics of pulp inflammation: correlations between diagnostic data and actual histologic findings in the pulp. Oral Surg Oral Med Oral Pathol, 1963, 16: 969–977.

[108] Seltzer S, Bender I B, Ziontz M. The interrelationship of pulp and periodontal disease. Oral Surg Oral Med Oral Pathol, 1963, 16: 1474–1490.

[109] Sessle B J. Neurophysiology of orofacial pain. Dent Clin North Am, 1987, 31 (4): 595–613.

[110] Sigurdsson A, Maixner W. Effects of experimental and clinical noxious counterirritants on pain perception. Pain, 1994, 57 (3): 265–275.

[111] Skieller V. The prognosis for young teeth loosened after mechanical injuries. Acta Odontologica Scand, 1960, 18: 171–177.

[112] Stone A, Straitigos G T. Mandibular odontogenic infection with serious complications. Oral Surg Oral Med Oral Pathol, 1979, 47 (5): 395–400.

[113] Taddese A, Nah S Y, McCleskey E W. Selective opioid inhibition of small nociceptive neurons. Science, 1995, 270 (5240): 1366–1369.

[114] Takahashi M, Takeda M, Matsumoto S. Somatostatin inhibits tooth-pulp-evoked rat cervical dorsal horn neuronal activity. Exp Brain Res, 2008, 184 (4): 617–622.

[115] Travell J, Rinzler S H. The myofascial genesis of pain. Postgrad Med, 1952, 11 (5): 425–434.

[116] Weisleder R, et al. The validity of pulp testing: a clinical study. J Am Dent Assoc, 2009, 140 (8): 1013–1017.

[117] Woolf C J, Costigan M. Transcriptional and posttranslational plasticity and the generation of inflammatory pain. Proc Natl Acad SciU S A,1999, 96 (14): 7723–7730.

[118] Yonetsu K, Yuasa K, Kanda S. Idiopathic osteosclerosis of the jaws: panoramic radiographic and computed tomographic findings. Oral Surg Oral Med Oral Pathol Oral Radiol Endod, 1997, 83 (4): 517–521.

[119] Zehnder M, Wegehaupt F J, Attin T. A first study on the usefulness of matrix metalloproteinase 9 from dentinal fluid to indicate pulp inflammation. J Endod, 2011, 37 (1): 17–20.

第8章 牙髓修复和再生的生物学基础

Kerstin M. Galler

8.1 再生和修复的原则

牙髓病和根尖周病的患者可通过根管治疗保留天然牙，但这不是一种具有生物学基础的方法。牙髓生物学和组织工程技术的发展对惰性合成材料替代脱落牙髓的传统概念提出了挑战。再生策略的目标是形成在形态、结构和功能上与原组织相似的新鲜有活力的组织。几十年前人们就知道牙髓组织具有再生能力，牙科医生一直致力于开拓再生方法，例如使用氢氧化钙等药物促进盖髓手术后的愈合[41]。这些治疗措施大多是经验性的，但随着我们了解生物学原理并开始理解再生和修复的机制，再生医学也为牙髓病学领域提供了广阔的发展空间。

名词解释

修复：用健康的新细胞替换组织或器官中死亡或受损细胞的总称。

再生修复：激活干细胞以实现结构的自然更新；牙髓中的第三期牙本质形成。

替代修复：瘢痕组织；在牙髓间隙中生长的纤维/类骨质组织，如当前的再生程序。

组织工程修复：用干细胞制造人体组织；组织工程牙髓组织再生。

"再生"一词指的是对特定组织类型的原始结构、形式和功能的再创造。"修复"指的是通过形成新的组织以修复原有组织已丧失的部分生物学功能。在临床中，区分修复和再生往往是很困难的。而且，作为生物学过程，两者在大多数情况下是重叠的。通常，长骨的复杂骨折通过骨骼本身几乎完全再生和愈合，但表面伤口可以通过纤维组织的形成和皮肤瘢痕而愈合。

8.1.1 牙髓和根尖周再生过程

根尖周围的骨组织在去掉炎症刺激后具有完全再生的能力。骨损伤的愈合是牙髓治疗的主要目标，如果临床医生成功地消除或充分减少根管系统内的细菌活动，就会发生骨愈合。因此，根尖周骨结构的结缔组织具有先天的再生能力以及充足的多能细胞供应，可在适当的情况下使牙周韧带和牙槽骨完全再生。

牙髓组织也能再生，但是，要确切阐明在什么情况下会再生仍然是一个挑战。确认可以被激活再生组织的细胞来源非常重要，剩余的活髓可以成为再生牙髓组织的起点[77]。年轻恒牙的根尖乳头干细胞是另一种可增殖、分化并形成成牙本质细胞和牙髓组织的细胞来源[44]。这些细胞可能通过血运重建使牙髓再生。对于牙根形成不完全和牙髓坏死的牙齿，牙髓血运重建可以作为根尖诱导成形术的替代治疗，在这种治疗中，含有根尖乳头上各个细胞的血液流入根管[54]。即使在牙根完全形成的牙齿中，牙根周围组织中也含有可被输送到根管中的间充质干细胞[14]；然而，目前尚不清楚，成熟牙齿在牙髓坏死后是否能形成牙髓样组织。再生手术后在根管内形成的组织中含有牙髓组织成分（成纤维细胞、结缔组织、血管、胶原蛋白），但其他细胞类型缺失，特别是成牙本质细胞，而非靶向的细胞类型或组织可能存在，如成骨细胞和牙骨质[56, 97]。因此，恢复过程可能不是通过再生，而是通过修复来实现的。

8.2 活髓保存治疗

间接或直接盖髓或牙髓摘除等治疗，旨在保存牙髓的活力，并维持其固有的再生和修复能力。无论是哪种治疗，牙髓都会形成第三期牙本质。第三期牙本质的形成是一种主动防御机制，可形成矿化屏障，将组织与损伤部位隔开；是一个可测量的愈合参数。第三期牙本质可以是反应性的，也可以是修复性的。在牙齿发育过程中，成牙本质细胞以每天 4~8μm 的速度分泌初级牙本质[49, 57]，在牙根形成完成后进入静止状态，分泌量减少到每天约 0.5μm [18, 79]。轻度刺激诱导成牙本质细胞活性上调，其中初级成牙本质细胞将其分泌活性上调至初始水平，导致反应性牙本质快速沉积，呈现管状结构[16, 81]。治疗干预后，牙髓组织内的可复炎症有望通过再生愈合。随着刺激强度的增加和干预的延迟，愈合将更有可能作为修复发生。如果原始的成牙本质细胞层丢失，如在强烈刺激或牙髓暴露后，干细胞可以分化成继发性成牙本质细胞将其替换[16, 22]。这些细胞沉积形成的修复性牙本质是一种矿化基质，可能不会表现出特征性的管状结构，而是类似于骨组织并常常显示细胞内包涵体[33]。目前尚不清楚骨样牙本质的形成是否与特定的细胞来源有关（非原始成牙本质细胞组成），或由于刺激强度的不同导致矿化组织迅速沉积但缺乏有序结构。此外，第三期牙本质还具有管周牙本质沉积增加的特征[81]，这是区分矿物晶体在管内钙化的一个关键过程[5]。因此，第三期牙本质的结构是高度可变的。

8.2.1 生物活性材料

长期以来，生物活性材料一直被用于诱导第三期牙本质形成并支持牙髓牙本质复合体的愈合。如果一种材料能够对活性组织产生积极影响并在界面处引起理想的生物反应，则称为生物活性材料[39]。反应可以通过抗菌活性间接，或直接与相邻细胞相互作用，例如：刺激增殖、分化和（或）生物矿化。约一百年前，氢氧化钙被引入到根管治疗中[40]，研究表明将这种材料与牙髓接触能使组织保持活力并形成矿化屏障[41]。氢氧化钙已被广泛用于牙髓病学和牙外伤学，几十年来一直是活髓保存治疗的首选材料。由于其强碱性，它不仅具有抗菌和抗真菌活性[80]，还会引起邻近细胞层的坏死和下层组织的炎症反应。促炎细胞因子和趋化因子会募集免疫细胞（通过清除损伤部位促进愈合）和干细胞（分化为继发性成牙本质细胞）。此外，氢氧化钙会释放结合在牙本质基质中的生长因子和分化因子[34, 94]，从而影响和调节细胞行为[94, 99]。使用氢氧化钙进行直接盖髓已被证明会形成矿化屏障[2, 29]，其厚度随着术后时间的延长而增加[29]。盖髓后的组织学分析显示，在氢氧化钙[29]和邻近的矿化屏障下面有一层浅层的组织碎片。该屏障可能显示出少量的与初级牙本质连续的管状结构和大量的弯曲小管[29, 67]，但更常见的表现为无定形和小管状钙化组织，并伴有细胞包涵体[33, 67, 71]。

氢氧化钙的应用具有多种能够通过再生进行愈合的效果；而其负面特性包括高溶解性和低机械稳定性，形成的矿化屏障可能是多孔的并表现出隧道样缺陷[19, 60]。与硅酸盐水门汀基质材料，如三氧化矿物聚合物（MTA）相比，氢氧化钙在新形成的矿化组织的厚度方面似乎较差。由于这些缺点，氢氧化钙逐渐被这种材料取代。这些材料统称为水硬性硅酸钙粘接剂，能形成稳定的水化硅酸钙基质，氢氧化钙和钙离子是这一反应的副产物，并产生生物活性效应[9-10]。与氢氧化钙相似，MTA 可溶解牙本质基质蛋白[91]，这可能有助于材料的生物活性。与氢氧化钙相比，水硬性硅酸钙粘接剂除了具有更高的稳定性之外，还具有密封性、消毒以及诱导牙本质或成骨矿化的能力，故而在牙髓学中得到了广泛的应用[21]。一些研究证据表明，与氢氧化钙相比，使用水硬性硅酸钙粘接剂可以减少坏死区、充血和炎症反应，第三期牙本质层更均匀和坚固，并且在失败率和牙髓活力方面有更好的临床表现[1, 42, 64, 89]。

8.3 参与牙髓修复的细胞类型

在构成牙髓组织的细胞中，首先受到外部刺激的是成牙本质细胞，因为它们位于牙髓组织的外围并延伸到牙本质中。成牙本质细胞是有丝分裂后的细胞，也就是说，在生理条件下，它们在生物体的生命过程中不会被替换。因此，它们与作为静态细胞群的神经元和心肌细胞具有某些共同特征[70, 92]。刺激源可以是热变化和生物力学力，也可以是微生物产生的分子产物。

8.3.1 第三期牙本质

牙髓防御的一个基本特征是第三期牙本质的形成。如上所述，必须将反应性牙本质与修复性牙本质区分开，由于它们来自两种不同的细胞群，它们的起源和性质是不同的。反应性牙本质是指有丝分裂后存活的成牙本质细胞在适当的刺激下分泌活性增加而分泌的第三期牙本质基质，将牙本质细胞外基质成分植入未露髓的牙洞中，可导致反应性牙本质的局部刺激[85]。这主要是由于转化生长因子β-1（TGFβ-1）的存在，它是牙本质基质中最丰富的生长因子，可显著上调成牙本质细胞的分泌活性[81]。此外，矿化前沿和沿着成牙本质细胞突分泌的基质会使管周牙本质厚度逐渐增加，磷酸钙晶体向心沉积导致牙本质小管逐渐闭塞、硬化，从而降低牙本质的通透性[91]。在龋病中，细菌产酸诱导的牙本质脱矿和随后生物活性分子的溶解释放，特别是TGFβ-1是负责启动对成牙本质细胞的刺激是反应性牙本质形成的主要原因。相比之下，修复性牙本质的生成是一个更为复杂的生物学过程，较强的刺激会导致成牙细胞死亡，但如果条件有利，新一代的成牙本质细胞样细胞可能会从牙髓内的干细胞或前体细胞分化出来。

8.3.2 干细胞：来源和激活

再生或修复的细胞来源主要是存在于牙髓、牙乳头和根尖周组织中的干细胞群。干细胞已经可从恒牙[35]和乳牙[59]的牙髓组织中分离出来，还可来源于年轻恒牙的根尖牙乳头[44,87]。最常见的是，基于细胞表面存在的特异性糖蛋白可将干细胞从体外培养的原代细胞群中分离出来。这样，通过识别间充质干细胞的特征并使用特异性抗体可对细胞进行分类。

根据定义，干细胞具有自我更新和分化为不同细胞类型的能力。干细胞一般通过取代老化的细胞来参与正常的组织更替、修复和再生过程。牙髓中的干细胞位于血管周围的壁龛中[78]，处于未分化阶段，在损伤发生之前处于静止状态。干细胞经历不对称分裂，这意味着一个细胞产生一个相同的细胞以保持干细胞库的恒定，而第二个子细胞则进入分化途径。趋化信号将干细胞募集到损伤部位，它们离开其细胞龛，迁移并分化为次级成牙本质细胞[22]，这些细胞可以在软组织和矿化组织的界面上产生矿化屏障。因此，干细胞在牙本质-牙髓复合体的再生和修复过程中发挥着重要作用，见图8.1和图8.2。

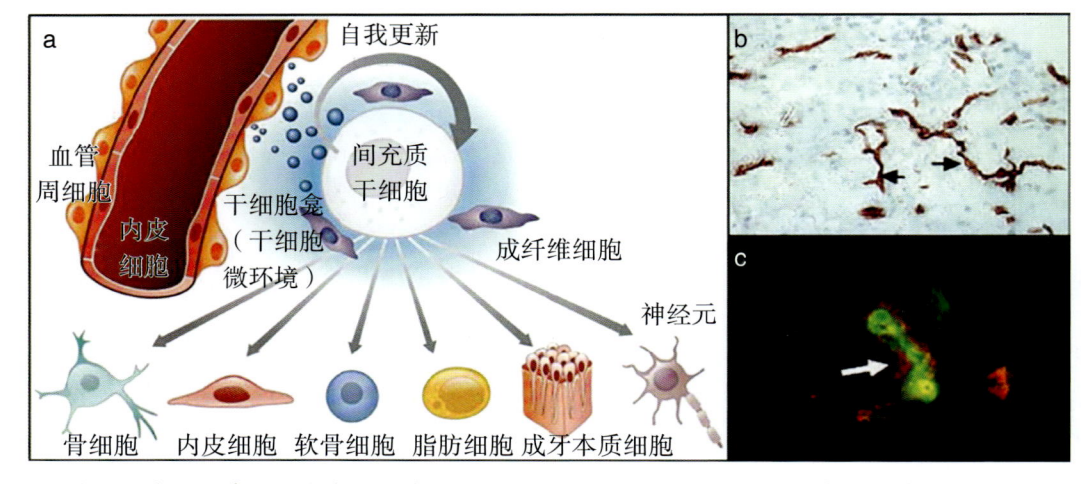

图8.1 间充质干细胞的血管周围生态位和多能性。a.间充质干细胞（MSC）存在于血管周围的壁龛中，可进行自我更新并维持周围的细胞或组织。在特定的信号转导条件下，MSC可以分化为不同的谱系[65]。b. CD146抗原（一种内皮细胞表面标志物）在人牙髓组织血管壁的免疫定位。c.牙髓中血管和间充质干细胞的共定位。双免疫荧光染色显示：用得克萨斯红标记的针对间充质干细胞标志物STRO-1的抗体与用异硫氰酸荧光素标记的针对血管内皮标志物CD146的血管发生反应[78]

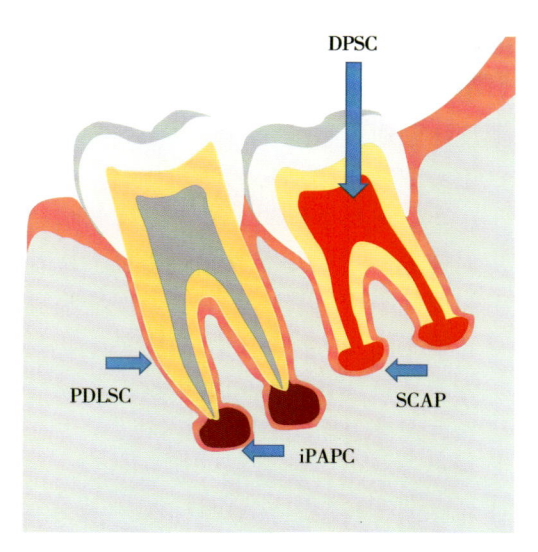

图 8.2 与牙髓和根尖组织再生相关的干细胞类型。
PDLSC：牙周膜干细胞。iPAPC：炎性根尖祖细胞。
DPSC：牙髓干细胞。SHED：人脱落乳牙干细胞。
SCAP：根尖牙乳头干细胞[38]

8.3.3 再生过程中的神经血管成分

牙髓炎症和随后的愈合也受到复杂的神经血管关系以及炎症过程与感觉神经纤维之间相互作用的影响。正常组织和损伤组织中的神经纤维除了具有感受深部痛觉作用外，还具有血管扩张和神经源性炎症等功能。伤害性刺激会触发神经肽的释放，特别是P物质（SP），它能引起血管舒张，增加牙髓血流量和血管通透性，并激活免疫细胞。龋齿牙髓中SP的表达显著上调[74]。神经肽可能通过增加成牙本质细胞样细胞的骨形态发生蛋白2（BMP-2）的表达，从而对成牙本质细胞产生刺激作用，诱导第三期牙本质的形成[12]。牙齿感觉纤维通过将它们的末端分支发芽到受伤部位下方的存活牙髓中来对损伤和炎症做出反应[51]。发芽纤维中升高的神经肽水平可通过募集免疫细胞和增加血管通透性来增强炎症[7,37]。与有神经支配的牙髓相比，失去神经支配的牙齿的血管牙髓存活较少、牙髓组织丢失加速[7]。因此，如果感觉神经在损伤前被切除，牙髓的自我防御能力就会降低，从而引发神经源性炎症并在牙髓暴露后愈合。

牙髓成纤维细胞在防御和再生过程中的作用已被广泛研究。牙髓成纤维细胞产生补体系统的所有成分，并能形成膜攻击复合物（MAC），对致龋细菌有效[48]。此外，细菌毒素刺激使牙髓成纤维细胞能够在牙髓再生过程中通过激活补体系统和产生神经营养因子来引导神经发芽[8,13]。

下文将详细讨论免疫细胞参与牙髓组织的再生和修复。

8.4 炎症的作用

随着龋病的进展，细菌毒素和细菌本身最终通过牙本质小管进入牙髓腔[53]。成牙本质细胞通过Toll样（TLR）和nod样（NLR）家族的受体感知细菌毒素（如细菌的细胞壁成分）[88]，并对牙髓免疫反应作出重大贡献。

牙髓对感染产生的炎症反应是最初的保护-宿主反应的一部分。龋病是微生物侵入牙髓最常见的原因。牙本质为管状结构，是一种可穿透的屏障，越靠近牙髓，牙本质小管密度和直径越大，其渗透性也随之增加。细菌毒素或成分以及完整的细菌通过牙本质小管到达牙髓，随着深度的增加，渗透也加速。微生物成分和毒素首先会激活先天免疫，一般来说，先天免疫不是抗原特异性的，而是识别细菌特有的分子模式，并通过吞噬细胞的杀伤力对细菌进行攻击和消除。由于细菌在龋损中的独特解剖位置，只有在龋坏前端到达牙髓时才会发生吞噬作用。牙本质-牙髓复合物的先天反应会调动多种保护措施，包括成牙本质细胞的反应、神经肽的产生、免疫细胞的激活以及趋化因子和细胞因子的产生[36]。

通常情况下，由于牙髓内的正压作用，牙本质液向外流动可防止口腔细菌从暴露的牙本质表面散发到牙髓中。因此，与死髓牙相比，活髓牙的细菌侵袭率明显较低[61]。作为预防龋齿发展的初始保护机制，牙髓内的感觉传入神经释放神经肽后可扩张血管，进而增加牙本质液向外流动的速度[55,58]。

8.4.1 牙髓对细菌侵入的反应

成牙本质细胞在解剖学上位于牙髓的外围，其细胞突起延伸至牙本质小管，因此它们是最先遇到细菌抗原的细胞。为了感知潜在的威胁，成牙本质细胞持续表达模式识别受体（PRRs），这些受体可识别并结合各种细菌成分。细菌成分与受体结合将导致细胞内信号转导的激活和白细胞介素、促炎细胞因子和趋化因子的分泌。这些信使物质会刺激白细胞的渗出，并招募不成熟的树突状细胞[25,43]加工和呈递抗原，从而充当先天免疫系统和适应性免疫系统之间的信使。

在急性期，成牙本质细胞产生的脂多糖结合蛋白（LBP）参与了防御机制。LBP中和细菌细胞壁成分，并通过抑制促炎细胞因子的产生来减弱免疫反应[26]。在细菌毒素的攻击下，成牙本质细胞会产生血管内皮生长因子（VEGF）。VEGF是一种血管通透性和血管生成的有效诱导因子[90]，还会分泌称为防御素的抗菌肽[23]。抑菌肽可在微生物的细胞膜中产生通道或微孔，从而发挥广谱抗菌活性。此外，成牙本质细胞分泌的TGF-β1可刺激牙本质基质分泌，同时可作为抗炎介质；TGF-β1在不可逆牙髓炎中表达增加[68]。牙髓细胞也可能产生抗炎信号分子，减弱免疫反应以限制组织损伤，同时刺激成牙本质细胞分化和新牙本质的形成[26]。

剩余的牙本质厚度很关键。评估龋病牙髓组织免疫反应的研究显示，如果牙本质层低于0.5mm，会引起全面的细胞宿主反应[15]。显然，龋病进展速度也很重要，与快速进展的龋病相比，缓慢进展的龋病具有不同的菌群、颜色和软硬程度[6]。发展缓慢的龋齿可以通过上述防御措施以及管周矿物质沉积导致牙本质硬化，从而关闭微生物入侵的大门。

8.4.2 炎症和再生之间的联系

先天免疫反应提供了一系列旨在恢复牙髓内稳态的保护机制，对龋病和其他感染源进行治疗干预和清除，可以缓解炎症并促进愈合。最初的炎症反应会促进再生。人们在动物实验中观察到皮质类固醇会抑制心肌梗死后的愈合过程，这证实了炎症反应与组织再生之间紧密联系的重要性[52]。治愈的先决条件是消除细菌病因以及宿主产生促炎介质。免疫系统产生促炎和抗炎信号分子。促炎介质启动免疫反应，而抗炎分子抑制过度反应并维持组织内稳态。去除病原体会导致反应减弱，残留的毒素最终会被中和[26]。当然，如果牙本质-牙髓复合体的损伤太严重，就不能通过愈合来解决。越来越多的免疫细胞迁移引起广泛的附带组织损伤。免疫细胞产生蛋白酶，一方面使免疫细胞通过组织，另一方面又会导致组织溶解。免疫细胞还会分泌活性氧和酶，不仅破坏细菌，还会损害局部细胞。来自坏死细胞的信号进一步促进炎症过程并导致病情恶化。长时间的刺激引起慢性炎症，表现为中度免疫细胞浸润、胶原纤维化和组织过早老化，宿主反应降低和（或）可能导致坏死组织和微生物扩散到根管系统，最终进入根尖周区域。

与龋齿时微生物缓慢侵入牙髓不同，牙髓在牙外伤和牙冠骨折后会迅速受到微生物污染和感染。在这种情况下，具有完全功能性免疫应答的健康组织将直接面对微生物。在猴子身上进行的一项经典研究发现，磨除或切断暴露的牙髓一周后，炎症区域的深度不会超过约2mm[20]，48h后的炎症穿透深度与之相比没有显著差异，说明健康的牙髓对细菌入侵具有显著的抵抗力。

8.5 牙本质中的信号分子

在牙齿发育过程中，牙乳头的神经嵴源性细胞最终分化为形成牙本质的成牙本质细胞。细胞分化完成后，成牙本质细胞开始进入分泌阶段，产生胶原和非胶原蛋白质的有机模板，随后与羟基磷灰石晶体一起矿化形成钙化牙本质。在这一合成过程中，成牙本质细胞不仅分泌前期牙本质，而且还表达多种生物活性分子，并将其分泌到细胞外基质中[28,73,100]。在矿化过程中，这些生物活性因子嵌入并固定在牙本质基质中。虽然活性蛋白质和生长因子的半衰期很短，但与细胞外基质成分结合可以使其免受蛋白水解降解从而延长其生命，并维持生物活性。生长因子结合化合物主要包括蛋白聚糖[72,96]，也包括特异性结合蛋白[3]、糖蛋白如纤连蛋白[69]和不同类型的胶原蛋白[66,86]。

由于牙本质的细胞外基质没有转换，生物活性调节分子从其结合中释放出来后可在后期重新激活。在龋病进展过程中，乳酸等细菌酸会暴露牙本质的有机成分并释放生物活性因子，这些生物活性因子可能会改变免疫反应、细胞募集和分化（图8.3）（表8.1）[24]。在牙本质上应用的牙科材料，例如氢氧化钙或水硬性硅酸钙粘接剂，以及

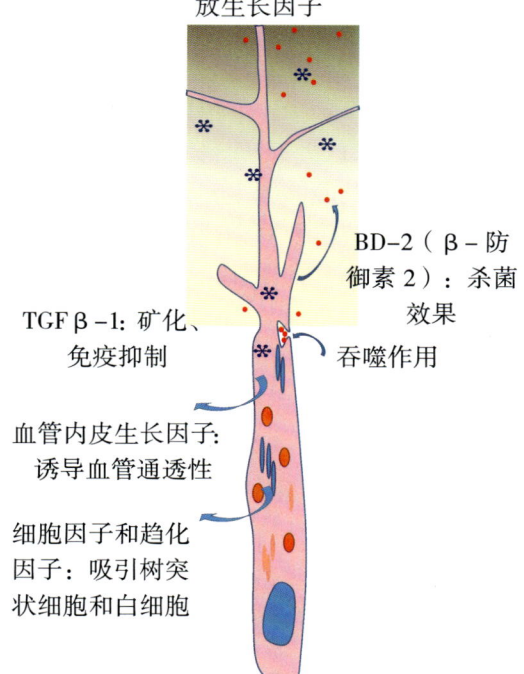

图 8.3 成牙本质细胞对龋损反应的简化示意图。成牙本质细胞表达 TLR（Toll 样受体）以识别各种细菌产物（红色）。受体结合激活细胞内信号通路。成牙本质细胞产生抗菌肽（如 β-防御素 2、细胞因子）和趋化因子以吸引免疫细胞、生长因子（如血管内皮生长因子），从而增加血管通透性和转化生长因子 β-1 来诱导矿化。成牙本质细胞具有吞噬活性。这种反应很可能受到细菌酸脱矿而引起的牙本质基质释放的生长因子的调节[36]

表 8.1 生物活性牙本质基质成分及其可能的功能，非详尽综述

生长因子和细胞因子	功能
转化生长因子 beta1（TGFβ1）（异构型 1、2、3）	抗炎药，诱导成牙本质细胞分化和基质分泌，趋化性
碱性成纤维细胞生长因子 (bFGF)	诱导细胞增殖，趋化性，血管生成
血管内皮生长因子 (VEGF)	血管生成
骨形态发生蛋白 (BMPs)（BMP2、BMP4 和 BMP7）	分化，矿化
肾上腺髓质素 (ADM)	抗炎药，成牙本质细胞分化
胰岛素样生长因子（IGF1 和 IGF2）	增殖，分化
血小板衍生生长因子（PDGF）	调节细胞生长和分裂，血管生成
胎盘生长因子 (PGF)	血管生成，趋化性，成牙本质细胞分化的调节
肝细胞生长因子 (HGF)	增殖，迁移，细胞存活
表皮生长因子 (EGF)	细胞生长和神经源性分化
白细胞介素（IL-8、IL-10）	抗炎药
生长因子和细胞因子	功能
降钙素 (CT)	钙的新陈代谢
降钙素基因相关肽	血管舒张，痛觉
神经肽 Y(NPY)	神经递质
P 物质 (SP)	神经递质，神经调节器

请注意，生物活性分子通常是多功能的（引自文献 82 和 84）

自酸蚀牙科粘接剂会释放生物活性因子[27, 34, 93]。有机酸或螯合剂，例如在牙髓治疗中常用的乙二胺四乙酸（EDTA）也适用于牙本质脱矿。在牙本质细胞外基质中已鉴定出多种生物活性分子（相关综述见文献84），其中包括调节矿化的非胶原蛋白、生长和分化因子、细胞因子、趋化因子和神经营养因子。存在于人牙本质细胞外基质中的生长因子包括转化生长因子β1（TGF-β1）、碱性成纤维细胞生长因子（bFGF）、骨形态发生蛋白2（BMP-2）、血小板衍生生长因子（PDGF）、胎盘生长因子（PIGF）和表皮生长因子（EGF），以及血管生成因子（如血管内皮生长因子）[11, 28, 73]。这些分子可在非常低的浓度下发挥作用，即使在皮克水平也能引起细胞反应。它们改变免疫反应，刺激血管生成，发挥趋化作用将细胞募集到损伤部位，并促进增殖、分化和矿化[4, 83, 98]。牙本质基质蛋白及其在愈合和再生中的作用正在不断研究中，并且学者们也在探索其生物活性，为组织工程的研究提供新思路。

8.6 牙髓再生的组织工程方法

组织工程是一个跨学科的研究领域，它涉及材料和细胞的使用，目的是了解组织的功能并最终使特定的组织能够新生。根据经典的组织工程例子，干细胞被接种到合适的载有生长因子的支架中，这些支架在移植到宿主后会诱导干细胞分化和组织形成（图8.4）。牙髓干细胞的分离为牙科组织工程的研究开辟了新的途径。恒牙[35]和乳牙[59]以及牙根未发育完全的根尖牙乳头中均可分离干细胞[44]。

牙髓组织也可以通过将牙髓干细胞移植到合适的载体系统中进行再生。将载有支架和牙齿干细胞的牙齿切片、牙本质段和整个牙根移植到小鼠背部皮下，几周后在原位形成类似于牙髓的血管化组织，与牙本质相邻的细胞分化为沉积管状

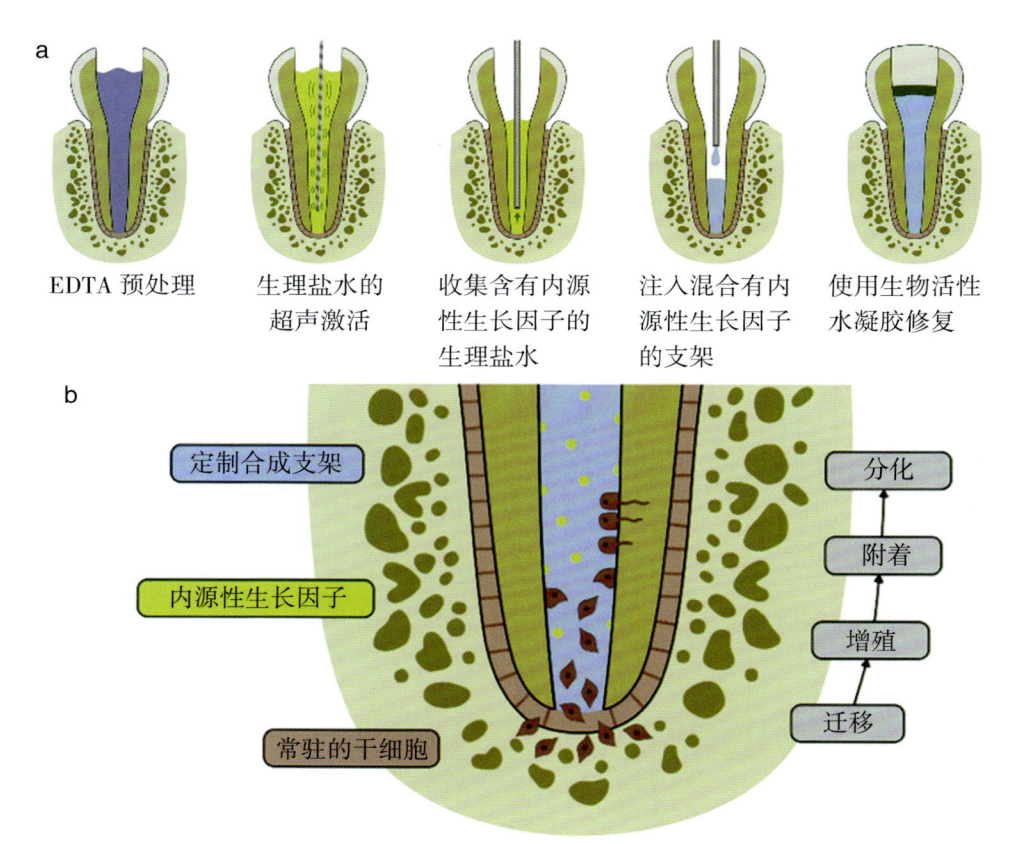

图8.4 牙髓组织工程的细胞归巢方法步骤的示意图。a. 经EDTA调节后，内源性生长因子被超声波激活并释放到生理盐水中。支架上装有分离的生长因子并注入根管内；用生物活性水凝胶和紧密的冠状密封修复牙齿。b. 示意图说明在成熟牙齿的细胞归巢方法中暴露或补充内源性生长因子引发的潜在作用。生物活性分子可诱导残留干细胞（如果存在残余的牙髓组织，则为DPSC、PDLSC或iPAPC）的趋化、增殖和黏附以及向成牙本质细胞样分化[32]。

牙本质[17, 31, 45, 76]。其他动物模型可以更接近地模拟临床再生牙髓治疗过程：将犬牙牙髓摘除后，用含有干细胞和重组生长因子的支架材料填充空隙，将会形成活的牙髓样组织[46-47, 62]。还有证据表明，自体牙髓干细胞移植到人类根管后，有恢复牙髓组织的功能的可能[63]。这些基于细胞的实验遵循了上述组织工程概念，即在载体材料中输送干细胞和重组生长因子。然而，干细胞移植存在几个问题，包括细胞来源有限、细胞收获和扩增的技术问题、运输、高成本以及审批和临床转化的监管障碍。

已有学者提出无细胞的牙髓组织工程方法[30, 50, 75]。遵循细胞归巢原则，可以通过重组或内源性牙本质衍生生长因子，将残余牙髓或根尖周组织中的常驻干细胞募集到专门设计的生物材料中。越来越多的证据表明，遵循细胞归巢原则的再生性牙髓手术可能是细胞移植的可行且经济的替代方法[32,50,75]。

表 8.2 列出了牙髓炎或牙髓坏死治疗方式中再生机制和组织工程方法的一般原则。

表 8.2 牙髓炎或牙髓坏死的治疗方式

目前的治疗方式					
侵入类型	牙齿类型	治疗	被激活/招募的细胞类型	愈合	可能的机制
感染-轻度刺激（可复性牙髓炎）	恒牙	间接盖髓修复	初级成牙本质细胞	再生或修复	成牙本质细胞分泌活性的上调
感染-强烈刺激（不可复性牙髓炎）	恒牙	直接盖髓或牙髓摘除术修复	牙髓干细胞	修复	干细胞分化为成牙本质细胞样或矿化细胞
牙髓坏死、根尖周炎	年轻恒牙	再生	根尖牙乳头干细胞或异位性细胞（骨，PDL）	再生，更多为修复	干细胞向成牙本质细胞分化，完成牙根形成或牙骨质形成，骨长入
	年轻恒牙	根尖诱导形成术	骨细胞、牙周膜细胞	与合成材料接触的骨修复再生	生物活性材料对矿化屏障的诱导作用
	恒牙	根管治疗	–	与合成材料接触的骨修复再生	与生物相容性材料接触的愈合
基于组织工程的治疗方式					
侵入类型	牙齿类型	治疗	被激活/招募的细胞类型	愈合	可能的机制
不可复性牙髓炎、牙髓坏死、根尖周炎	恒牙和未发育完成的恒牙	细胞移植组织工程	移植的细胞（如牙髓干细胞）	再生	移植干细胞的分化，血管系统的向内生长
	未发育完成的恒牙	细胞归巢组织工程	牙髓干细胞或根尖牙乳头干细胞	再生	常驻、募集干细胞的分化
	恒牙	细胞归巢组织工程	牙髓干细胞或根尖周间充质干细胞	再生	常驻、募集干细胞的分化

参考文献

[1] Aeinehchi M, et al. Mineral trioxide aggregate (MTA)and calcium hydroxide as pulp-capping agents in human teeth: a preliminary report. Int Endod J, 2003, 36: 225–231.

[2] Al-Hezaimi K, et al. Histomorphometric and micro-computed tomography analysis of pulpal response to three different pulp capping materials. J Endod, 2011, 37: 507–512.

[3] Arai T, Busby W Jr, Clemmons D R. Binding of insulin-like growth factor (IGF) I or II to IGF-binding protein-2 enables it to bind to heparin and extracellular matrix. Endocrinology, 1996, 137: 4571–4575.

[4] Barrientos S, et al. Growth factors and cytokines in wound healing. Wound Repair Regen, 2008, 16: 585–601.

[5] Baume L J. The biology of pulp and dentine. A historic, terminologictaxonomic, histologic-biochemical, embryonic and clinical survey. Monogr Oral Sci, 1980, 8: 1–220.

[6] Bjørndal L, Demant S, Dabelsteen S. Depth and activity of carious lesions as indicators for the regenerative potential of dental pulp after intervention. J Endod, 2014, 40, S76–81.

[7] Byers M R, Taylor P E. Effect of sensory denervation on the response of rat molar pulp to exposure injury. J Dent Res, 1993, 72: 613–618.

[8] Byers M R, Wheeler E F, Bothwell M. Altered expression of NGF and P75 NGF-receptor by fibroblasts of injured teeth precedes sensory nerve sprouting. Growth Factors, 1992, 6: 41–52.

[9] Camilleri J. Hydration characteristics of calcium silicate cements with: lternative radiopacifiers used as root-end filling materials. J Endod, 2010, 36: 502–508.

[10] Camilleri J. Tricalcium silicate cements with resins and alternative radiopacifiers. J Endod, 2014, 40: 2030–2035.

[11] Cassidy N, et al. Comparative analysis of transforming growth factor-beta isoforms 1–3 in human and rabbit dentine matrices. Arch Oral Biol, 1997, 42: 219–223.

[12] Caviedes-Bucheli J, et al. Neuropeptides in dental pulp: the silent protagonists. J Endod, 2008, 34: 773–788.

[13] Chmilewsky F, About I, Chung S H. Pulp fibroblasts control nerve regeneration through complement activation. J Dent Res, 2016, 95: 913–922.

[14] Chrepa V, et al. Delivery of apical mesenchymal stem cells into root canals of mature teeth. J Dent Res, 2015, 94: 1653–1659.

[15] Cooper P R, et al. Mediators of inflammation and regeneration. Adv Dent Re, 2011, 23: 290–295.

[16] Cooper P R, et al. Inflammationregeneration interplay in the dentine-pulp complex. J Dent, 2010, 38: 687–697.

[17] Cordeiro M M, et al. Dental pulp tissue engineering with stem cells from exfoliated deciduous teeth. J Endod, 2008, 34: 962–969.

[18] Couve E. Ultrastructural changes during the life cycle of human odontoblasts. Arch Oral Biol, 1986, 31: 643–651.

[19] Cox C F, et al. Tunnel defects in dentin bridges: their formation following direct pulp capping. Oper Dent, 1996, 21: 4–11.

[20] Cvek M, et al. Pulp reactions to exposure after experimental crown fractures or grinding in adult monkeys. J Endod, 1982, 8: 391–397.

[21] Darvell B W, Wu R C. "MTA"-an hydraulic silicate cement: review update and setting reaction. Dent Mater, 2011, 27: 407–422.

[22] Dimitrova-Nakov S, et al. Pulp stem cells: implication in reparative dentin formation. J Endod, 2014, 40: S13–18.

[23] Dommisch H, et al. Human beta-defensin (hBD-1)-2, expression in dental pulp. Oral Microbiol Immunol, 2005, 20: 163–166.

[24] Dung S Z, et al. Effect of lactic acid and proteolytic enzymes on the release of organic matrix components from human root dentin. Caries Res, 1995, 29: 483–489.

[25] Durand S H, et al. Lipoteichoic acid increases TLR and functional chemokine expression while reducing dentin formation in in vitro differentiated human odontoblasts. J Immunol, 2006, 176: 2880–2887.

[26] Farges J C, et al. Odontoblast control of dental pulp inflammation triggered by cariogenic bacteria. Front Physiol, 2013, 4, 326.

[27] Ferracane J L, Cooper P R, Smith A J. Dentin matrix component solubilization by solutions of pH relevant to self-etching dental adhesives. J Adhes: ent, 2013, 15: 407–412.

[28] Finkelman R D, et al. Quantitation of growth factors IGF-I, SGF/IGF-II, and TGF-beta in human dentin. J Bone Miner Res, 1990, 5: 717–723.

[29] Franz F E, Holz J, Baume L J. Ultrastructure (SEM) of dentine bridging in the human dental pulp. J Biol Buccale, 1984, 12: 239–246.

[30] Galler K M, Eidt A, Schmalz G. Cell-free approaches for dental pulp tissue engineering. J Endod, 2014, 40, S41–5.

[31] Galler K M, et al. A customized self-assembling peptide hydrogel for dental pulp tissue engineering. Tissue Eng Part A, 2012, 18: 176–184.

[32] Galler K M, Widbiller M. Perspectives for cell-homing approaches to engineer dental pulp. J Endod, 2017, 43, S40–s5.

[33] Goldberg M, et al. Application of bioactive molecules in pulp-capping situations. Adv Dent Res, 2001, 15: 91–95.

[34] Graham L, et al. The effect of calcium hydroxide on solubilisation of bio-active dentine matrix components. Biomaterials, 2006, 27: 2865–2873.

[35] Gronthos S, et al. Postnatal human dental pulp stem cells (DPSCs)in vitro and in vivo. Proc Natl Acad Sci U S A, 2000, 97: 13625–13630.

[36] Hahn C L, Liewehr F R. Innate immune responses of the

dental pulp to caries. J Endod, 2007, 33: 643–651.
[37] Hanoun M, et al. Neural regulation of hematopoiesis, inflammation, and cancer. Neuron, 2015, 86: 360–373.
[38] Hargreaves K M, Diogenes A, Teixeira F B. Treatment options: biological basis of regenerative endodontic procedures. Pediatr Dent, 2013, 35: 129–140.
[39] Hench L L, West J K. Biological application of bioactive glasses. Life Chemistry Reports, 1996, 13: 187–241.
[40] Herrmann B. Kalziumhydroxid als Mittel zum Behandeln und Füllen von Zahnwurzelkanälen. Dissertation, Würzburg, 1920.
[41] Herrmann B. Ein weiterer Beitrag zur Frage der Pulpenbehandlung. Zahnärztliche Rundschau, 1928, 37: 1327–1376.
[42] Hilton T J, Ferracane J L, Mancl L. Comparison of CaOH with MTA for direct pulp capping: a PBRN randomized clinical trial. J Dent Res, 2013, 92, 16S–22S.
[43] Huang G T, et al. Increased interleukin-8 expression in inflamed human dental pulps. Oral Surg Oral Med Oral Pathol Oral Radiol Endod, 1999, 88: 214–220.
[44] Huang G T, et al. The hidden treasure in apical papilla: the potential role in pulp/dentin regeneration and bioroot engineering. J Endod, 2008, 34: 645–651.
[45] Huang G T, et al. Stem/progenitor cell-mediated de novo regeneration of dental pulp with newly deposited continuous layer of dentin in an in vivo model. Tissue Eng Part A, 2010, 16: 605–615.
[46] Iohara K, et al. A novel combinatorial therapy with pulp stem cells and granulocyte colony-stimulating factor for total pulp regeneration. Stem Cells Transl Med, 2013, 2: 521–533.
[47] Iohara K, et al. Regeneration of dental pulp after pulpotomy by transplantation of CD31(-)/CD146(-) side population cells from a canine tooth. Regen Med, 2009, 4: 377–385.
[48] Jeanneau C, et al. Can pulp fibroblasts kill cariogenic bacteria? Role of complement activation. J Dent Res, 2015, 94: 1765–1772.
[49] Kawasaki K, Tanaka S, Ishikawa T. On the daily incremental lines in human dentine. Arch Oral Biol, 1979, 24: 939–943.
[50] Kim J Y, et al. Regeneration of dental-pulp-like tissue by chemotaxisinduced cell homing. Tissue Eng Part A, 2010, 16: 3023–3031.
[51] Kimberly C L, Byers M R. Inflammation of rat molar pulp and periodontium causes increased calcitonin gene-related peptide and axonal sprouting. Anat Rec, 1988, 222: 289–300.
[52] Kloner R A, et al. Mummification of the infarcted myocardium by high dose corticosteroids. Circulation, 1978, 57: 56–63.
[53] Love R M, Jenkinson H F. Invasion of dentinal tubules by oral bacteria. Crit Rev Oral Biol Med, 2002, 13: 171–183.
[54] Lovelace T W, et al. Evaluation of the delivery of mesenchymal stem cells into the root canal space of necrotic immature teeth after clinical regenerative endodontic procedure. J Endod, 2011, 37: 133–138.
[55] Maita E, et al. Fluid and protein flux across the pulpodentine complex of the dog in vivo. Arch Oral Biol, 1991, 36: 103–110.
[56] Martin G, et al. Histological findings of revascularized/revitalized immature permanent molar with apical periodontitis using platelet-rich plasma. J Endod, 2013, 39: 138–144.
[57] Massler M, Schour I. The appositional life span of the enamel and dentin-forming cells; human deciduous teeth and first permanent molars; introduction. J Dent Res, 1946, 25: 145–150.
[58] Matthews B, Vongsavan N. Interactions between neural and hydrodynamic mechanisms in dentine and pulp. Arch Oral Biol, 1994, 39 Suppl: 87s–95s.
[59] Miura M, et al. SHED: stem cells from human exfoliated deciduous teeth. Proc Natl Acad Sci U S A, 2003, 100: 5807–5812.
[60] Murray P E, Garcia-Godoy F. The incidence of pulp healing defects with direct capping materials. Am J Dent, 2006, 19: 171–177.
[61] Nagaoka S, et al. Bacterial invasion into dentinal tubules of human vital and nonvital teeth. J Endod, 1995, 21: 70–73.
[62] Nakashima M, Iohara K. Regeneration of dental pulp by stem cells. Adv Dent Res, 2011, 23: 313–319.
[63] Nakashima M, Iohara K. Recent progress in translation from bench to a pilot clinical study on total pulp regeneration. J Endod, 2017, 43: S82–86.
[64] Nowicka A, et al. Response of human dental pulp capped with biodentine and mineral trioxide aggregate. J Endod, 2013, 39: 743–747.
[65] Oh M, Nor J E. The perivascular niche and self-renewal of stem cells. Front Physiol, 2015, 6: 367.
[66] Paralkar V M, Vukicevic S, Reddi A H. Transforming growth factor beta type 1 binds to collagen IV of basement membrane matrix: implications for development. Dev Biol, 1991, 143: 303–308.
[67] Pavlica Z, Juntes P, Pogacnik M. Defence reaction in dental pulp after pulp capping and partial pulpectomy in dogs. Acta Vet Hung, 2000, 48: 23–34.
[68] Piattelli A, et al. Transforming growth factor-beta 1 (TGF-beta 1, expression in normal healthy pulps and in those with irreversible pulpitis. Int Endod J, 2004, 37: 114–119.
[69] Rahman S, et al. Novel hepatocyte growth factor (HGF, binding domains on fibronectin and vitronectin coordinate a distinct and amplified Met-integrin induced signalling pathway in endothelial cells. BMC Cell Biol, 2005, 6, 8.
[70] Rezzani R, Stacchiotti A, Rodella L F. Morphological and

[71] Ricucci D, et al. Is hard tissue formation in the dental pulp after the death of the primary odontoblasts a regenerative or a reparative process? J Dent, 2014, 42: 1156–1170.

[72] Rider C C, Mulloy B. Heparin, heparan sulphate and the TGF-beta cytokine superfamily. Molecules, 2017, 22.

[73] Robert-Clark D J, Smith A J. Angiogenic growth factors in human dentine matrix. Arch Oral Biol, 2000, 45: 1013–1016.

[74] Rodd H D, Boissonade F M. Substance P expression in human tooth pulp in relation to caries and pain experience. Eur J Oral Sci, 2000, 108: 467–474.

[75] Ruangsawasdi N, Zehnder M, Weber F E. Fibrin gel improves tissue ingrowth and cell differentiation in human immature premolars implanted in rats. J Endod, 2014, 40: 246–250.

[76] Sakai V T, et al. SHED differentiate into functional odontoblasts and endothelium. J Dent Res, 2010, 89: 791–796.

[77] Saoud T M, et al. Histological observations of pulpal replacement tissue in immature dog teeth after revascularization of infected pulps. Dent Traumatol, 2015, 31: 243–249.

[78] Shi S, Gronthos S. Perivascular niche of postnatal mesenchymal stem cells in human bone marrow and dental pulp. J Bone Miner Res, 2003, 18: 696–704.

[79] Simon S, et al. Molecular characterization of young and mature odontoblasts. Bone, 2009, 45: 693–703.

[80] Siqueira J F Jr, Lopes H P. Mechanisms of antimicrobial activity of calcium hydroxide: a critical review. Int Endod J, 1999, 32: 361–369.

[81] Smith A J, et al. Reactionary dentinogenesis. Int J Dev Biol, 1995, 39: 273–280.

[82] Smith A J, et al. Exploiting the bioactive properties of the dentin-pulp complex in regenerative endodontics. J Endod, 2016, 42: 47–56.

[83] Smith A J, et al. Trans-dentinal stimulation of tertiary dentinogenesis. Adv Dent Res, 2001, 15: 51–54.

[84] Smith A J, et al. Dentine as a bioactive extracellular matrix. Arch Oral Biol, 2012, 57: 109–121.

[85] Smith A J, et al. Odontoblast stimulation in ferrets by dentine matrix components. Arch Oral Biol, 1994, 39: 13–22.

[86] Somasundaram R, et al. Collagens serve as an extracellular store of bioactive interleukin 2. J Biol Chem, 2000, 275: 38170–38175.

[87] Sonoyama W, et al. Characterization of the apical papilla and its residing stem cells from human immature permanent teeth: a pilot study. J Endod, 2008, 34: 166–171.

[88] Staquet M J, et al. Patternrecognition receptors in pulp defense. Adv Dent Res, 2011, 23: 296–301.

[89] Tabarsi B, et al. A comparative study of dental pulp response to several pulpotomy agents. Int Endod J, 2010, 43: 565–571.

[90] Telles P D, et al. Lipoteichoic acid up-regulates VEGF expression in macrophages and pulp cells. J Dent Res, 2003, 82: 466–470.

[91] Ten Cate A A. Oral Histology: Development, Structure and Function. St. Louis MI: Mosby, 1994

[92] Terman A, et al. Mitochondrial turnover and aging of long-lived postmitotic cells: the mitochondriallysosomal axis theory of aging. Antioxid Redox Signal, 2010, 12: 503–535.

[93] Tomson P L, et al. Dissolution of bioactive dentine matrix components by mineral trioxide aggregate. J Dent, 2007, 35: 636–642.

[94] Tomson P L, et al. Growth factor release from dentine matrix by pulpcapping agents promotes pulp tissue repairassociated events. Int Endod J, 2017, 50: 281–292.

[95] Torabinejad M, et al. Bacterial leakage of mineral trioxide aggregate as a root-end filling material. J Endod, 1995, 21: 109–112.

[96] Vlodavsky I, et al. Extracellular sequestration and release of fibroblast growth factor: a regulatory mechanism? Trends Biochem Sci, 1991, 16: 268–271.

[97] Wang X, et al. Histologic characterization of regenerated tissues in canal space after the revitalization/ revascularization procedure of immature dog teeth with apical periodontitis. J Endod, 2010, 36: 56–63.

[98] Widbiller M, et al. Dentine matrix proteins: isolation and effects on human pulp cells. Int Endod J, 2017.

[99] Widbiller M, et al. Threedimensional culture of dental pulp stem cells in direct contact to tricalcium silicate cements. Clin Oral Investig, 2016, 20: 237–246.

[100] Zhao S, et al. Ultrastructural localisation of TGF-beta exposure in dentine by chemical treatment. Histochem J, 2000, 32: 489–494.

第 9 章 牙髓-牙本质复合体暴露的预防和治疗

Lars Bjørndal

9.1 深龋和外伤性露髓的诊断挑战

根尖周炎的预防首先要评估牙髓是否能被保留。然而，目前尚缺乏严格的牙髓诊断方法，评估真实的牙髓感染状态和炎症发展阶段仍是一项重大难点[61]。以下几点尤为重要的是：①为必然导致牙髓坏死的炎症情况确定准确的阈值；②评估能否避免牙髓-牙本质复合体的暴露；③在已暴露的情况下，确认是否可能进行盖髓术或活髓切断术，或者是否需要进行去髓术。

牙髓的炎症和感染状态的评估是诊断深龋的关键，将决定不同的治疗方案。治疗可以从严格的保守治疗，即保留部分感染性牙本质及修复性牙本质下方的牙髓，到彻底去除牙髓后行根管充填。基于对深龋 X 线片解读的问卷调查结果显示，在特定情况下，不同牙科医生在治疗方案的选择上存在较大差异[64, 76, 85-86]。在临床实践中，即使经过充分的主观判断和客观检查，是否保存牙髓的决定也会有所不同。大多数牙科医生倾向于采用侵入性手段，建议进行活髓切断术[64, 86]。不同治疗方案的选择也可能是因为医生对深龋定义的不明确，以及缺乏明确的临床体征和症状来判定牙髓状态。临床研究应努力为诊断程序以及与不同临床情况相关的治疗选择提供更坚实的证据基础。在实践中，这意味着医生需要在充分的临床证据的基础上对深部病变作出更准确的定义，同时也需要用先进的技术来评估炎症状态。虽然相关领域的临床研究众多，但目前仍有许多问题没有得到解答。

9.1.1 作为牙髓病学难题的深龋

牙髓病学作为一门学科掌握着提供最佳"牙髓护理"的关键。牙髓病学主要聚焦于无菌策略，这是成功保存牙髓活力的基础和必要措施，包括使用橡皮障隔离的无菌操作空间和消毒剂的应用。在治疗深龋的过程中，缺乏无菌操作、使用污染器械及龋坏牙本质碎屑进入暴露的髓腔可能是导致保守治疗失败的主要原因。目前看来，在使用橡皮障的无菌环境下操作的治疗结果通常是最好的。绝大多数从业人员治疗深龋及其引起的牙髓暴露并没有考虑无菌操作[15, 44, 70, 82]，这使盖髓术从一开始就是一种易于失败的治疗方案。我们需要明确：确保深龋的治疗及盖髓术的步骤是严格无菌操作的，才能达到预期效果的，而不是将治疗当成避免去髓的简易方法[49]。

这一章讨论了正确判断深龋牙髓状态的难点，也从生物学基础上强调了牙髓-牙本质复合体能够形成硬组织屏障的原因。此外，对牙髓炎症性疾病的各种治疗方案进行了回顾，包括避免牙髓暴露的方法。

9.2 牙髓病鉴别诊断

龋病是引起牙髓暴露及后续牙髓治疗的最常见原因[14]。深龋是诊断的难点。经典的牙髓病学观点认为，应当立即考虑牙髓的实际炎症状况。一般认为，客观检查时患者的体征和症状并不能让医生对牙髓的组织学状态做出准确诊断，因此很难评估牙髓炎症是否可逆[26, 78-79]（见第10章）。从组织病理学和细菌生物学的观点来看，定义不可复性牙髓炎的关键点在于微生物是否已通过第三期牙本质或直接进入牙髓组织而侵入髓腔[66, 69]。在临床上这种感染的临界阈值很难被检测出来。有牙髓暴露风险的深龋在治疗时，医生应通过病变进展阶段、细菌侵入深度、病变活动性及进展时间（患者年龄）等信息来更好地定义龋病。以上这些定义龋病的各要素将在下文进一步详细说明。

9.2.1 龋损穿透深度

临床上通常是基于牙科医生在去除龋坏后可能引起牙髓暴露的预期来定义龋坏的深度[18]。影像学上，深龋被定义为龋坏已进展到牙本质的髓方，但仍有清晰的放射状不透明的牙本质将病变与牙髓分隔开[7]。随着龋损的进一步发展，当脱矿的牙本质可能会影响到整个牙本质层的厚度时被定义为极深龋[17]。图 9.1 所示为深龋和极深龋。

根据龋的组织病理学知识，感染牙本质最初局限于脱矿牙本质的外层，该区域胶原降解，不可再矿化[31]，其内层是龋损进展的前沿，包括实际阻止微生物直接进入牙髓的非透射区和再矿化区。当再矿化区被破坏时，微生物将侵入第三期牙本质和牙髓的临界区[66]。这个阶段可能会出现与不可复性牙髓炎诊断相关的临床症状，牙髓内也会存在相应的细菌[69]。

因此，在咬合翼片上仔细检查病变深度成为评估细菌侵入牙髓风险的替代方法。在盖髓术相关的文献中，很少描述龋病的确切进展程度[10]。这意味着牙本质和牙髓感染的程度在不同的病例中可能存在较大的差异，这也可能是对照研究和预测直接盖髓术预后的困难之一。盖髓术是在深龋或极深龋情况下进行，还是在医源性牙髓暴露后进行，这一点非常重要。在后一种情况下，盖髓术是在窝洞制备或进行牙冠预备时，发生牙髓意外暴露（如髓角），而局部牙髓组织未受到龋的影响。以上这些信息在临床报告中鲜有说明[10, 28]，但它可能代表了结果的主要差异。去除龋坏组织过程中牙髓暴露后细菌感染的风险较高，而医源性暴露很有可能不发生细菌感染。

9.2.2 牙髓炎症：一把双刃剑

龋病是进行根管治疗的常见原因，也是引起牙髓炎症的主要原因，特别是在一些重要病例中[14]。龋损下方的牙髓炎症是无法停止的、不可逆的过程的观点已经站不稳。牙髓炎症和龋病病理学的最新研究认为：如果龋坏牙本质被人为保留，则对其下方的牙髓组织来说意味着一个强大且持续的挑战，终将导致持续的牙髓炎症。即使清除龋坏组织并对炎性牙髓行盖髓术，预期炎症会自行发展，最终导致坏死和治疗失败[63]。然而，牙髓炎症并不一定会导致牙髓坏死和感染；相反，较轻的炎症为修复和再生提供了平台[23]。当病源被移除后，牙髓仍然有能力和潜力上调硬组织形成细胞，包括成牙本质细胞[81]。此外，牙髓对龋的反应在本质上是动态的，龋病进展缓慢与迅速的反应不同。牙髓-牙本质复合体位于初级成牙

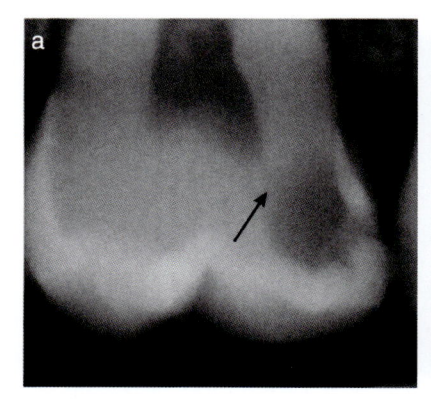

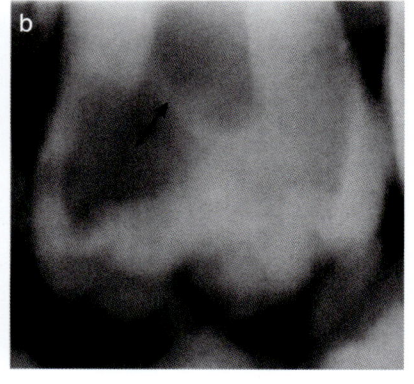

图 9.1　a. 深龋病变穿透到牙本质的髓方，放射状不透明的牙本质区将病灶与髓腔分离（箭头所示）。b. 极深龋病变贯穿整个牙本质厚度，未见没有牙本质辐射的不透明区，但在髓腔内可能有较薄的放射状不透明线（箭头）

本质细胞在低级别或缓慢进展的病变环境（通常是成人/老年患者，病变穿透一半牙本质）下形成的反应性及第三期牙本质下方[8]。在快速发展的病变（年轻患者，牙本质内四分之一的病变）下方，如果存在第三期牙本质，其特征是牙本质小管数量的减少，最终完全是非管状的，这一过程称为纤维牙本质生成[6]。这种情况下，初级成牙本质细胞已经凋亡，此反应被视为修复而不是再生[68]。

9.2.3 理解修复性牙本质的模型：未治疗的龋病

图9.2展示了磨牙咬合面龋病的不同进展阶段情况。龋坏牙本质由于大量地脱矿而萎缩，沿着釉-牙本质界的侧面形成一个沟或缝隙，这将为进一步扩大感染提供途径。已形成生物膜[12]的缝隙正在破坏健康牙釉质。在临床上，感染[9]向侧方进展，牙本质看上去呈乳白色、半透明状，围绕在龋洞周围（图9.2b箭头）。在咀嚼过程中，破坏的牙釉质崩解，较大的牙本质表面暴露在口腔中（图9.2c）。这反过来又改变了致龋生物膜的生长条件。尽管病变较深，但其较大的、暴露的表面使其转变为进展较慢的病变，在这些开放的深部病变的下方经常会发现大量的修复性牙本质形成。组织学上，在非管状牙本质[8]的下方有一层新形成的管状牙本质。不幸的是，即使有时牙髓炎症是可复性的，但当深部病变进展导致牙釉质被严重破坏时，这类牙齿也可能无法保留。

龋病"自然进展史"的关键是，当外部病变环境发生改变，龋源性负荷减少时，牙髓能反应形成修复性牙本质。原则上，这一观点能使医生通过保守治疗方法来改变深部龋损的病变活动。如果医生能够改变活跃的病变环境，那么将能产生有效的修复性牙本质。要注意的是：修复性牙本质的形成并不是生物学上或临床上成功的永久标志。新的细菌感染总会考验任何一种新形成的第三期牙本质屏障。因此，虽然牙本质屏障的形成是迈向成功的必要一步，但为了永久保存活髓，彻底控制并消除牙本质感染才至关重要。

表9.1列出了一些描述龋病临床特征的变量。结合主观、客观和椅旁临床信息，将牙髓状态分为正常牙髓、可复性牙髓炎及不可复性牙髓炎。

表9.1 可复性牙髓炎和不可复性牙髓炎的临床及影像学特征

鉴别要点	可复性牙髓炎	不可复性牙髓炎
自发性牙痛	无	有
冷诊及电活力测试结果	有	有
冷诊延迟痛	无	可能有
热诊延迟痛	无	可能有
冷刺激疼痛减轻	无	可能有
肿胀	无	无
牙齿松动度升高	无	可能有
咬诊或叩诊敏感	可能有	有
根尖周骨质破坏的影像学表现	可能有	可能有

9.3 盖髓术相关的牙髓生物学

9.3.1 硬组织形成

大量动物实验研究表明，在牙髓本身没有发生感染的前提下，牙髓-牙本质复合体具有形成

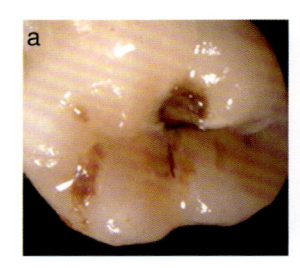

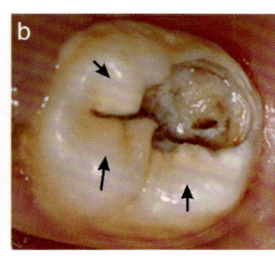

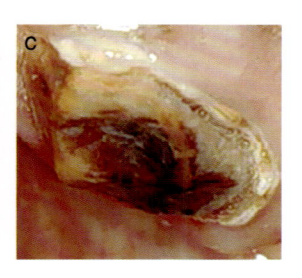

图9.2 未治疗龋齿的"自然进展史"。深部病变的三个阶段，牙釉质受损（a），因咀嚼导致釉质崩解（b中箭头所示）；病变环境从"封闭"转变为开放环境（c），病变中心部分转变为缓慢进展。在龋损进展过程中改变外部环境会使活跃、快速的病变转变为缓慢的、甚至停滞的状态（图由 Lars Bjørndal 医生提供）

第三期牙本质来封闭暴露牙髓的生物学潜能。经典的Kakehashi研究因证实了[45]根管感染在根尖周炎形成中的基本作用而闻名。该研究同时发现：在没有细菌的情况下，即使无菌鼠的牙髓发生暴露，仍能形成第三期牙本质愈合。若进一步详细说明其发生的生物学相互作用将超出本章范畴。因此，下文将简要讨论这些内容：形成修复性牙本质的细胞来源、盖髓材料的止血作用、生物学性能以及封闭性。

9.3.2 第三期牙本质形成的刺激因素和修复牙本质的细胞起源

第三期牙本质是与外部损伤[6]相关的新形成的牙本质。第三期牙本质分为反应性牙本质（由原代成牙本质细胞形成的牙本质）和修复性牙本质（由原代成牙本质细胞以外的其他细胞形成的硬组织），这反映了上文所述的与龋病相关的第三期牙本质形成的外部刺激因素类型[8,68]。完全非管状牙本质是龋损进展非常迅速的典型表现，也可以在急性医源性创伤后的牙髓组织中看到，例如，在车针快速旋转的窝洞预备过程中由于水冷却不足造成的创伤。非管状牙本质或纤维牙本质也可作为一种生理现象出现在没有外伤迹象的牙齿中[6]（例如，在髓角尖端或髓室底部[19]）。非管状牙本质或纤维牙本质不仅是成牙本质细胞，也反映了牙髓干细胞的矿化潜能。

事实上，第三期牙本质可以由非原始的成牙本质细胞形成，因此牙髓暴露后在直接盖髓术成功后可见到牙本质桥的重建（图9.3）。直接盖髓术后形成的牙本质桥中含有大量非矿化部分或所谓的"管道缺陷"，这些部位将很容易被微生物入侵[24]。因此，术后必须放置防止细菌微渗漏的冠方封闭材料，以确保长期疗效。

9.3.3 止血

任何成功的盖髓术（或活髓切断术）都必须进行止血以避免盖髓材料与牙髓组织之间形成血凝块。充分止血后将盖髓材料正确放置在干燥窝洞底部非常重要。此外，血凝块的存在可能与较高的感染风险有关[71-72]。止血的方法并不十分重要，对健康牙髓而言更是如此。一项在氢氧化钙盖髓前分别使用生理盐水、次氯酸钠或氯己定止血的研究发现，不同的液体与牙髓修复[4]相关的特异性葡萄糖-蛋白表达没有差异。此外，一项随机临床试验表明，如果在止血方案中使用消毒剂后再放置盖髓材料，那么最终疗效将会有所改

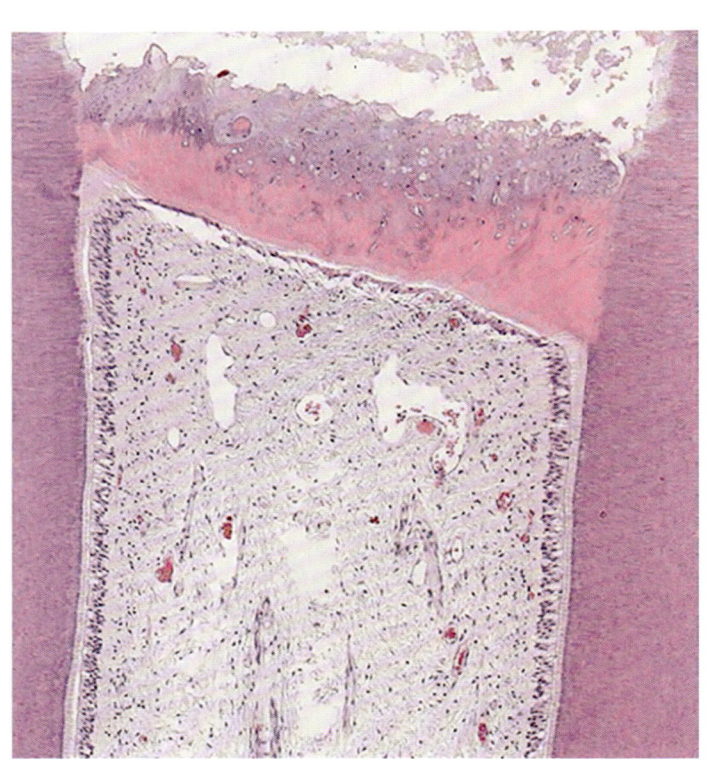

图9.3 人类牙齿直接盖髓术后，修复性牙本质的组织病理学表现

善[88]。令人矛盾的是血凝块虽然应当被清除掉，但它却含有大量的潜在生物活性分子，可以促进并有利于修复过程。因此，在牙髓血运重建术中要主动诱导出血[32-33]。总体来说，目前的盖髓术很可能尚未充分发挥牙髓的修复潜力。

9.3.4 盖髓材料

大多数证据来源于动物和人体研究中各种各样的氢氧化钙制剂。然而，许多体内研究仍缺乏足够的证据。大多数研究中都缺乏对照组[28]。大量盖髓术的研究是在无污染的环境中测试材料，即牙髓未发炎且没有龋齿的牙齿。这对于各种外伤和（或）医源性情况导致的牙髓暴露是适用的，在这种情况下，牙髓是相对健康的。然而，临床上最常见的是龋源性露髓，盖髓术应该在这些更接近现实的条件下进行测试。因此，尽管生物工程的抗炎盖髓材料已经存在了相当长的一段时间[49]，但目前仍缺乏实际的临床试验，这是其得到临床认可的阻碍。新型盖髓材料的市场营销往往先于强有力的临床证据。然而，最新的综述证明水凝性硅酸钙基材料，特别是各种形式的三氧化物矿合物（MTA）具有更好的效果[52,91]。但是，由于缺乏高质量的随机临床试验来比较和检测这些盖髓材料，不同盖髓剂的性能在很大程度上是未知的（见下文）。

9.4 活髓保存治疗成功的评价标准

综合各项症状和体征才能得出治疗成功的准确定义。因此，记录患者有无自发的或诱发的疼痛或不适等临床症状是评估治疗成功或失败的一个重要部分。牙髓坏死可能是治疗或感染的后果，但不一定会引起症状，这样一来，通过温度测试或电活力测试评估牙髓的敏感性是十分必要的。随着牙髓感染的扩散，病变最终将演变为根尖周炎，这可通过根尖片的对比反映出来。值得注意的是，在一些外伤性病例中，炎性牙髓可引起根尖周放射学改变，称为暂时性根尖碎裂[3]，这种牙髓是可以保留的。X 线片有时也被用于检查牙本质桥和第三期牙本质的形成。CBCT 可作为检测牙髓组织在盖髓术后反应变化的精细手段，它能更容易地检测到受龋源性影响的活髓牙在根尖处的影像学变化，CBCT 可作为一个灵敏的技术观察不同材料盖髓术后机体的反应差异[37]。

9.5 间接盖髓术和逐步去龋

传统观点认为一次性去净龋坏组织适用于任何龋损。然而，临床和实验证据已经逐渐建立了一个更为微妙的概念来处理深龋和极深龋损[39,47,67,74]。在部分病例中，完全去除龋坏组织直至健康牙本质（非选择性的去除龋坏组织）显然是不可取的[44,75]。临床随访研究表明，本章所定义的逐步去除深龋病变的方法比一次性完全去除龋坏组织的方法更好：牙髓暴露风险降低，术后 5 年牙髓仍有活力，疼痛较少且无根尖周炎。去除部分龋坏组织后同期行永久充填的方案是可行的[21,29]；霍尔技术将这一概念在乳牙龋病治疗中发挥到了极致，直接将不锈钢金属冠粘在有龋损的牙齿上，最终也显示出类似的高成功率[40,42]。然而，从临床牙髓病学的观点来看，医生很难对病变的深度做出明确的判断，而且成年人中定义明确的深龋的证据也很有限。因此，经典的间接盖髓术[47]在同期去除龋坏的基础上也永久留下了部分龋坏牙本质，目前尚不能推荐用于成人深龋的治疗，因为医生不清楚保留的龋坏牙本质将会收缩到什么程度，是否会影响冠方牙体组织的修复以及是否增加了牙髓并发症的风险。在侵袭性较低的龋病治疗中，暂时性或永久性的冠方封闭不足可能导致牙髓病变和根尖病变治疗失败[18,56]。

如上所述，当病变外部环境转变为不利于龋病进展时将能解释为何可采用低侵袭性的逐步去除龋坏组织的理念。因此，逐步法去除龋坏的第一阶段目的在于改变致龋性外环境（图9.4a~b）。

临床上普遍认为牙本质在进展性龋中呈质软、着色浅且湿润的状态（图 9.4c），当龋损静止后其质地更硬、颜色更深以及更加干燥（图9.4d）。首次去除龋坏组织后，活动性龋坏牙本质被保留在氢氧化钙基盖髓材料下方，随后使用玻璃离子进行临时修复（图 9.4c）。8~12 周后非选择性地去尽剩余龋坏组织，直到牙本质硬度与未被波及的牙本质相当。虽然影像学上很难判断

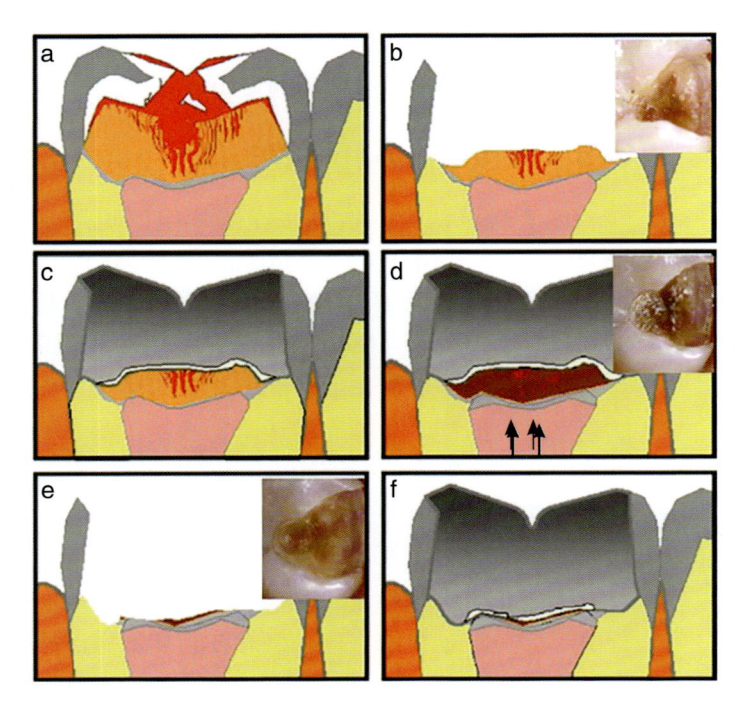

图 9.4 逐步去龋过程中的主要变化。a. 深龋中崩解破坏的釉质和未受干扰的致龋微生物，进展性龋的牙本质呈棕黄色、较湿润、质软。b. 第一次去龋后留下近髓的少量软龋（插图为一个临床样本）。c. 放置氢氧化钙基的盖髓材料后暂封。d. 复诊（2~9 个月后），龋坏牙本质的颜色更深、更干燥、质地更硬（插图为一个临床样本）。e. 第二次非选择性去除龋坏组织，窝洞底部留下硬化的第三期牙本质（插图为一个临床样本）。f. 组织不会进一步收缩后进行永久修复

两次就诊期间形成的第三期牙本质的质量及范围（图 9.4d 箭头）[54]，但这与临床操作步骤无关。

与直接、彻底地去净龋坏组织相比，逐步去除显著降低了牙髓暴露的风险。初诊后留下的龋坏牙本质最终转变为慢性或停滞性龋[13,55]。初次治疗后龋坏牙本质的停滞与感染程度的降低有关[13,65]。龋的进程停滞能刺激硬组织生成，因此，与一次法完全去净龋坏组织相比，经逐步法治疗的牙齿牙髓暴露的发生率更低。此外，有证据表明即使在第二次治疗过程中发生了牙髓暴露，经盖髓术治疗后的效果仍要好于第一次就诊时就发生暴露[51]；这可能与逐步法中第一次和第二次就诊时的感染程度不同有关。在牙本质龋坏停滞后，保留的牙本质皱缩导致其与临时修复体间产生间隙。因此，复诊时进一步去除龋坏可使窝洞的永久修复达到最佳状态。

9.6 非感染牙髓的盖髓术（Ⅰ类）

非感染牙髓的盖髓术是指在复杂牙外伤或意外穿髓导致牙髓表面暴露后进行的盖髓术。治疗前应确认牙髓完整且无炎症、无临床症状、穿孔要小（直径最好小于 1mm）且位于髓腔的冠三分之一（如髓角）。除此之外，必须用永久修复体恢复牙冠。深龋去除后发生的穿孔不能用这一治疗方法。一项随机研究记录了深龋穿髓后行盖髓术的不良后果；5 年后只有 5% 左右的牙髓存活[11]，这证实了早期的回顾性研究[5]。

9.7 龋相关的盖髓术（Ⅱ类）

此种方法适用于特别需要保存活髓的一类龋齿，如牙根发育不全的患牙。当龋坏已引起牙髓上方四分之一或更多牙本质脱矿时，只有活髓牙才能使盖髓术成为可能。牙髓是活的，且没有不可复性牙髓炎的疼痛指征，盖髓术是更为精良的治疗方案。该方案能应对严重的微生物挑战。基于目前的数据观察[20, 53, 57]该方法结果良好，但尚缺乏随机研究。此外，这类盖髓术的数据主要来源于儿童，即使龋损非常深，只要没有自发性、持续性疼痛则均诊断为"可复性牙髓炎"。

9.8 部分牙髓切断术

部分牙髓切断术即众所周知的"Cvek"牙髓切断术。最先应用于年轻恒牙外伤性露髓。在无菌条件下将已发生感染和可能感染的冠方浅表牙髓部分切除后将氢氧化钙或其他盖髓材料放置在牙髓表面[25, 30]。部分牙髓切断术也被应用于深龋的治疗[58-60, 92]，但只有少数病例有长期随访数据[1]。应用这项技术，盖髓材料的保留率可能会

得到改善，例如单根牙[25]中出现的复杂冠折，该技术的基本原理是要去净暴露部位表面的坏死物质和感染牙髓组织。对于牙根发育不完全的年轻恒牙，该技术有两方面的优势：①牙根可以继续发育完成；②牙颈部形成继发性和第三期牙本质，强化了牙颈部，降低了牙颈部折裂的风险。为去除潜在的感染组织而扩大的穿孔应尽可能小，因为在儿童治疗中穿孔越大[22]失败率越高。临床试验结果显示成人因龋露髓时，行直接盖髓术和部分牙髓切断术没有差异[11]。

9.9 活髓切断术

活髓切断术是乳牙活髓保存治疗的标准方法，其基本原理是完全切除冠部牙髓组织，提高感染牙髓的清除率。乳牙髓腔的特点使盖髓术操作困难。在未患龋病的牙齿中活髓切断术的适应证通常为复杂冠折和牙根尚未发育完全的牙齿。参见图9.5。

不可复性牙髓炎是活髓切断术的绝对禁忌证，例如牙髓温度测试后出现延迟痛或持续性疼痛（在儿童中难以评估）。影像学上，应注意区分与根尖敞开相关的囊腔样低密度影与慢性根尖周炎导致的透射影[89]。

系列病例报告发现，对于可复性牙髓炎的成年患者，活髓切断术可能成为一种永久性的治疗[80]。也有证据表明，不可复性牙髓炎可以通过活髓切断术成功治疗[27, 90]。根尖发育已完成的因龋露髓的恒牙由于某些原因无法进行根管治疗时，活髓切断术[2]可作为一种替代拔牙的治疗方案。需进一步开展比较活髓切断术和传统去髓术的临床试验，以全面评估其适应证。

9.10 活髓保存术的治疗细节

一般情况 治疗深龋和（或）已发生牙髓暴露患牙时必须使用橡皮障隔离、去净边缘龋坏并化学消毒操作界面。表面消毒后，用无菌器械进行龋坏组织清除和窝洞预备。当没有厚的血凝块时才能进行止血，通常用无菌生理盐水或次氯酸钠冲洗5min即可，如果出血不能止住，应改行去髓术。氢氧化钙或硅酸钙基水门汀可用于盖髓术和活髓切断术，其最小厚度为1.5mm。最终，在无菌条件下进行临时或永久充填，并进行临床和影像学随访。

分步去龋 经橡皮障隔离和表面消毒后，选择性地去除表层变色和湿软的龋坏组织（图9.4c），将氢氧化钙垫底材料放置在剩余的少量软化牙本质上方，最后用玻璃离子充填窝洞（图9.4c）。8~12周后再次打开窝洞，用无菌挖器非选择性地去除接近牙髓的颜色更深、质地更硬、更为干燥的牙本质，只留下硬度与正常牙本质相当的硬化牙本质（图9.4d）。在牙本质龋停滞后，作为第二阶段窝洞基底部的牙本质不会进一步缩小。这一系列步骤也消除了与牙本质皱缩相关的潜在问题，优化了永久修复体与窝洞间的操作界面。

意外性或外伤性穿髓（Ⅰ类） 用橡皮障隔离和表面消毒后，用无菌生理盐水轻轻冲洗窝洞和穿髓孔，清除碎屑，使创口干净无出血。冲洗和用棉球加压穿孔部位可能引起进一步出血，如果5min后仍未能止住，则放弃盖髓术，改行去髓术。最好在盖髓材料放置好后立即进行永久修复，或至少在近几天内进行，这样做可以显著改善愈后[5]。

龋相关盖髓术（Ⅱ类） 经橡皮障隔离和表面消毒后，使用放大镜或显微镜加强照明，在龋指示剂的指导下去除龋坏组织，直到在暴露的牙本质边缘看不到染料。不要试图扩大穿髓部位。盖髓材料上方用玻璃离子水门汀垫底后进行冠部的粘接修复。如果需要等盖髓材料完全凝固，那么建议分两步操作。图9.6所示为一个符合Ⅱ类盖髓术的案例。

部分牙髓切断术 在橡皮障隔离和表面消毒后，使用高速金刚砂车针切除约2mm的冠部牙髓组织并大量冲洗。当浅层牙髓切除完成并成功止血后，其余操作步骤与龋源性露髓的盖髓术步骤相同（图9.5）。

活髓切断术 在橡皮障隔离和表面消毒后，使用高速无菌金刚砂车针在喷水下去除整个冠部牙髓组织，断面应位于根管口下方1~2mm处。对于单根牙，断面应位于颈缘下2~3mm。纸尖（钝端朝向盖髓材料）是放置和压紧盖髓材料的简单工具。盖髓材料的厚度最好达到4~5mm。如果需要等盖髓材料硬化，建议分两步操作，但这不是必需的[48]。图9.7展示了一例活髓切断术。

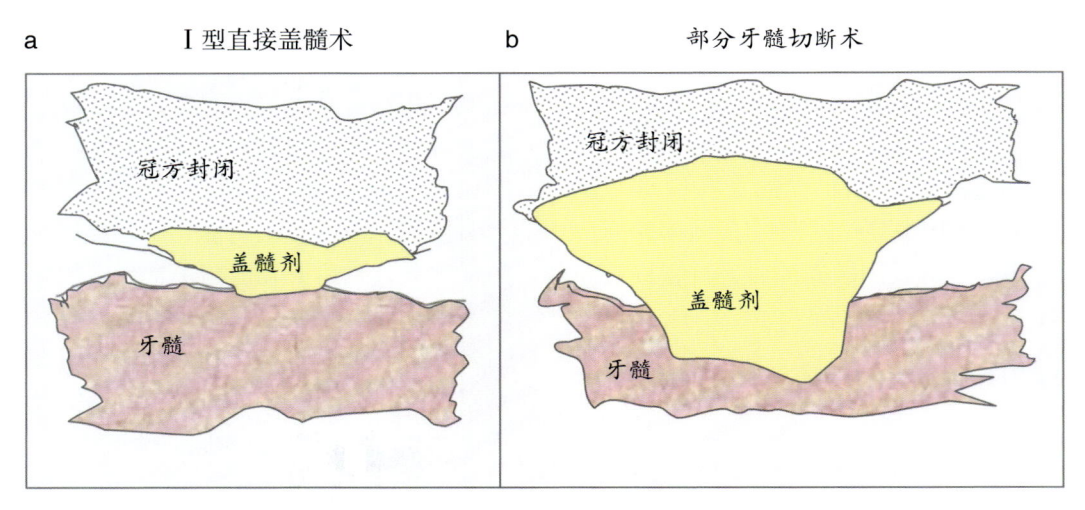

图 9.5 直接盖髓（a）和部分活髓切断术（b）间的差异。部分活髓切断术去除了感染或炎症的表面牙髓组织，增加了盖髓剂的放置

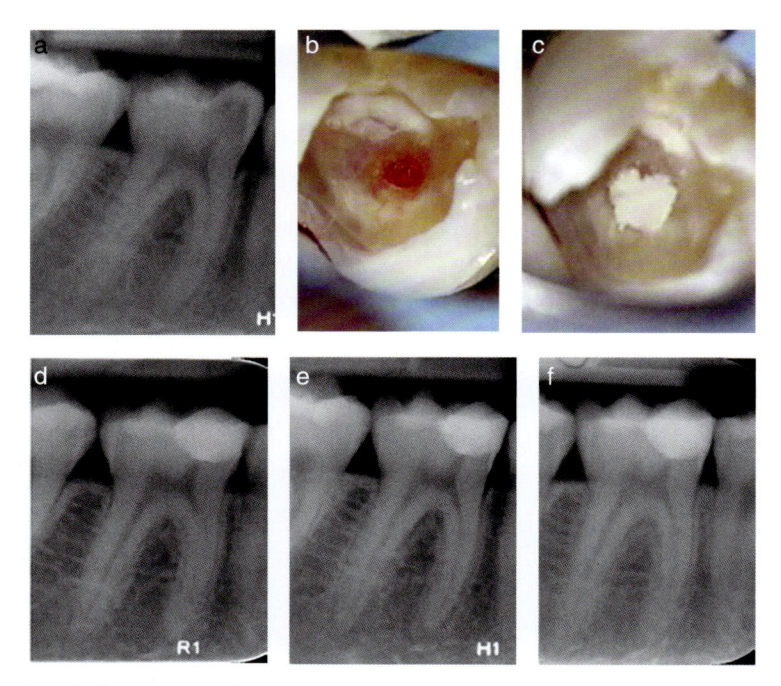

图 9.6 Ⅱ类直接盖髓术临床案例。a. 术前影像示病变较深，无根尖周病变。b. 使用手术显微镜非选择性去除龋坏后，无龋坏牙本质残留，出血停止。c. 将盖髓剂（MTA）分批放入。d. 术后影像示永久修复体就位。e.1 年随访。f.2 年后随访。感谢 Phu Le 医生提供病例

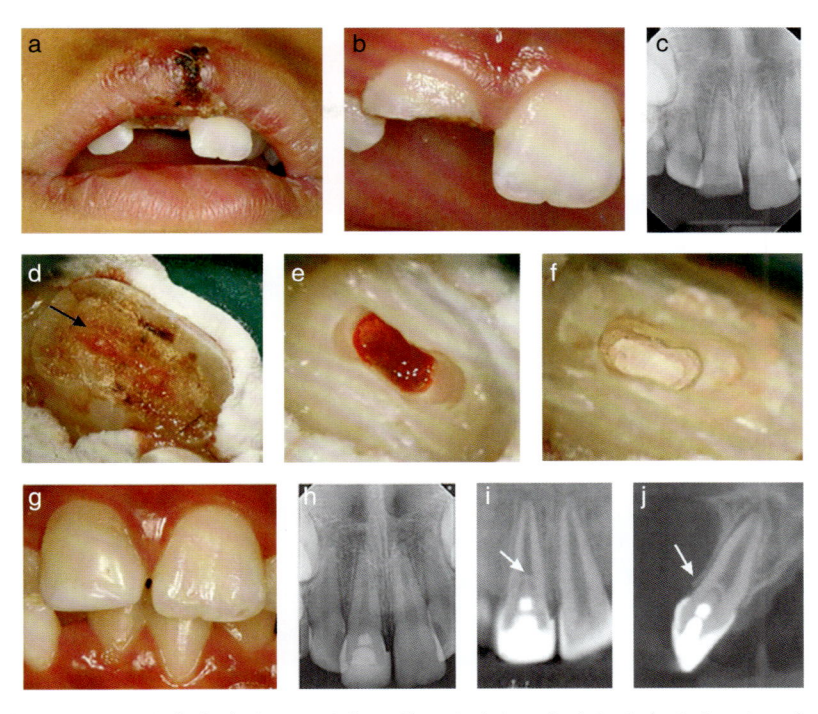

图 9.7　a. 一个 10 岁女孩，4 天前在急诊进行了唇部撕裂伤的缝合，未进行牙齿治疗，今日来牙体牙髓科进行治疗。临床（b）和影像学（c）显示为复杂冠折髓角暴露（d）（黑色箭头所示）。患牙对冷诊有剧烈的非持续反应，电活力测试有反应，诊断为可复性牙髓炎。e. 橡皮障充分隔湿，金刚砂车针伴大量水冲洗，去除冠部约 3mm 牙髓。f. 立即用硅酸钙基水门汀盖髓，玻璃离子垫底，复合树脂修复。g. 1 年后随访，患牙无症状，对电活力测试有反应，无变色等症状和体征。h. 影像学无根尖病变。i、j. 小视野 CBCT 显示出密集的矿化区（病例由 Anibal Diogenes 医生提供）

9.11　有关活髓保存优点的现有证据

9.11.1　多种结果和后续治疗的设想

根据已发表数据，可建立各种活髓保存治疗的成本－效果分析模拟场景[77]，这虽然不会改良现有数据，但可以扩展医生对结果的解读。在一个关于活髓保存治疗结果的病例中[77]，根据以下假设创建模拟场景：有敏感无疼痛症状的深龋磨牙，在去龋过程中发生牙髓暴露可行氢氧化钙或 MTA 直接盖髓后直接修复，也可行根管治疗（去髓术）后铸造冠修复。深龋可以是邻面龋或牙合面龋。使用状态转换图来模拟这类牙齿各种可能的寿命（图 9.8）。基于 2014 年之前收集的数据模型显示，直接盖髓术的最佳适应证是年轻患者（< 40 岁）的后牙咬合面露髓，而年龄较大的患者（> 40 岁）前牙露髓则愈后最差。其中许多病例在出现并发症后需要尽快接受牙髓治疗。

图 9.9 显示了Ⅱ类近中邻牙合面深龋牙髓暴露后直接盖髓术失败的情况。在这一案例中，邻面牙髓暴露后的盖髓操作在技术层面上执行得很好，但最终还是导致了牙髓坏死、感染以及根尖周炎。与牙髓摘除术相比，已确诊的根尖周炎的治疗预后更差。在这种情况下，对发炎的牙髓进行盖髓处理增加了治疗成本，而且很可能缩短了患牙的使用寿命。

9.11.2　获得最佳临床证据的策略

深龋患牙治疗方案有分次去龋或直接盖髓术，部分或全部牙髓切断术，以及去髓术。对于极深龋，建议只进行牙髓侵入治疗。目前的证据指出了一种更保守的方法，从这个意义上来说，牙髓在采用侵入性较小的技术治疗时，其存活情况比以往认为的要好。选择合适技术的进一步证据必须依赖精心开展的临床研究中的数据，最好是采用随机设计的临床研究数据。在设计这类试验时要有明确定义的纳入标准。例如，对龋损的大小和龋损活动性有更明确的定义，可能会得到更准确的数据分析（表 9.2）（图 9.10）；对样本量估计进行功效计算；采用中心随机化；以及进行无偏倚的，也就是盲法记录结果。

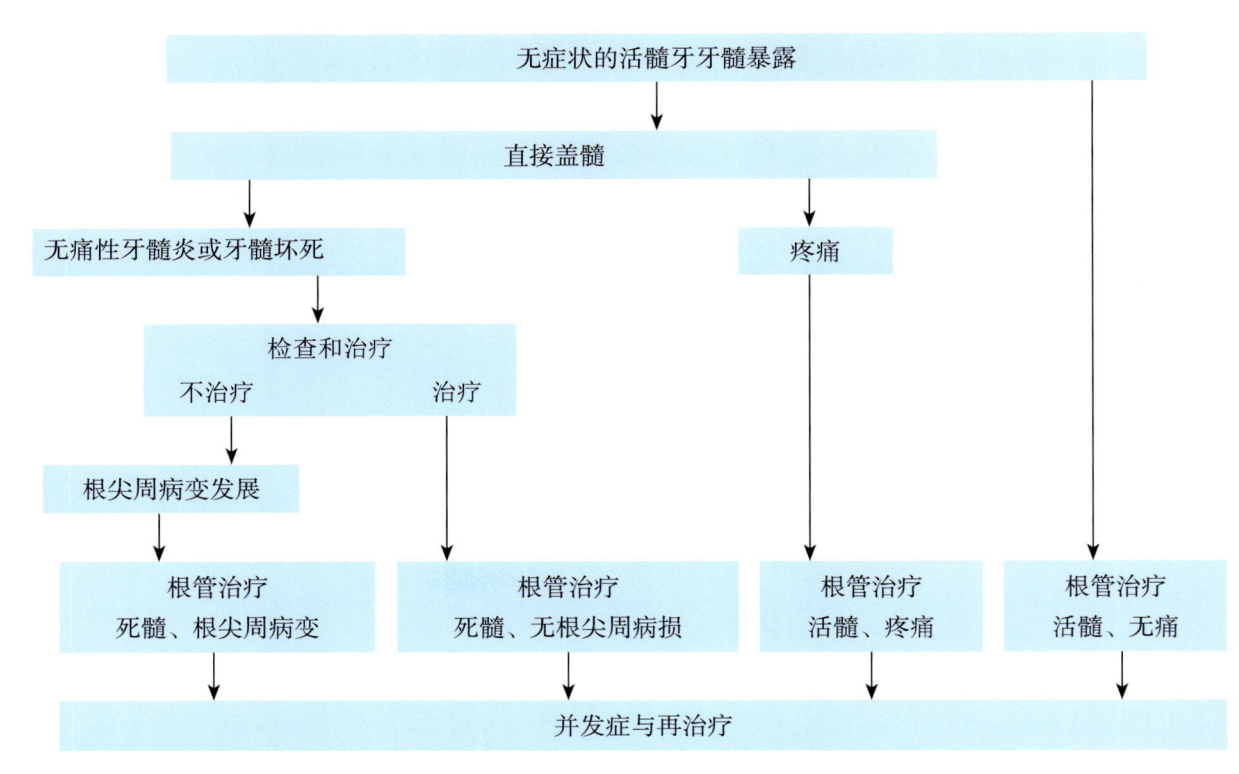

牙髓病学基础：根尖周炎的预防和治疗

图9.8 敏感无症状患牙在牙髓暴露后，多种治疗方案的状态转换图

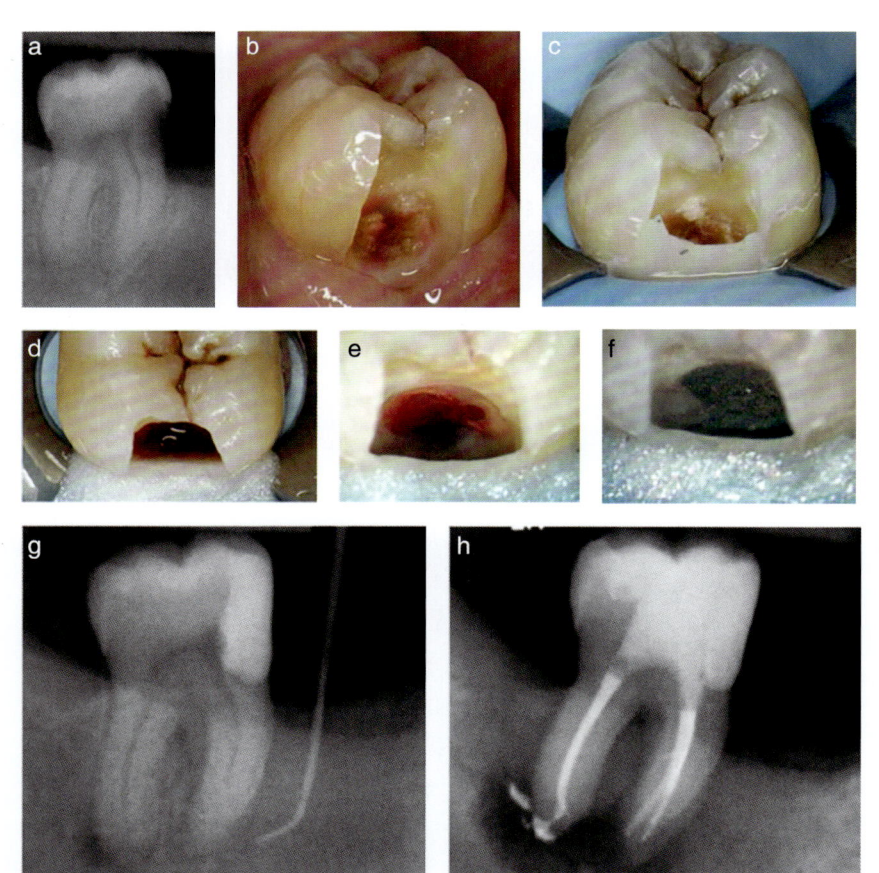

图9.9 Ⅱ类直接盖髓术的临床实例（男性，48岁）。a.术前X线片显示存在一个深龋，且无根尖病变。b.去除龋坏组织后，龋损位于邻面的较深部位。c.在边缘处放置了一个小的垫底充填物，以便于实现无菌操作。d.可见有出血的牙髓暴露情况。e.即将实现止血。f.应用硅酸钙基水门汀。g.3个月后，患者出现了窦道和根尖周炎。h.完成根管治疗后的即刻术后X线片（Pim Buurman医生提供病例）

9.11.3 临床试验缺乏标准化

表 9.3 列出了最新的随机临床试验结果，涵盖了本章提出的各个主题。虽然这些研究并不是为了进行比较，但它们都有相同的纳入标准：深龋和可复性牙髓炎的症状。然而，治疗方法包括了从活髓切断术到间接盖髓术以及逐步去龋，反映出目前在活髓保存治疗方案的选择上还没有全球共识。此外，即使治疗方法相同，技术细节也有很大的差异，这表明需要对临床试验的操作细节进行更多的标准化。

表 9.2 龋坏牙本质的状态和活髓保存治疗的预后

暴露牙髓周围牙本质的临床表现	各种龋活动状态下行Ⅱ类直接盖髓术的预后
牙本质质软、湿润、淡黄色	差（深龋或极深龋）
牙本质质硬、干燥、黑色	中等（二次去龋后）
牙本质质硬、干燥、灰色	好（中龋、医源性髓角暴露）

表 9.3 盖髓剂和保髓干预措施的随机临床试验结果

	Jang 等人 2015[43]	Kang 等人 2015[46]	Hashem 等人 2015[37]	Bjørndal 等人 2017[11]
研究材料				
牙齿	恒牙	乳牙	恒牙	恒牙
龋齿	乳牙和恒牙	乳牙	乳牙	乳牙
牙髓状态	可复性牙髓炎	?	可复性牙髓炎	可复性牙髓炎
年龄	>19 岁	3~10 岁	平均年龄 28 岁	平均年龄 29 岁
试验				
干预	15%	?	20%	20%
权重	80%	?	80%	90%
样本大小	23	47~48	36	156~158
材料	ProRoot MTA 和 Endocem	ProRoot MTA 和 OrthoMTA 和 RetroMTA	玻璃离子和 Biodentine	Dycal/Ketac cem
变量	年龄、𬌗面龋、邻面龋	–	窝洞大小、CBCT	操作步骤
方案				
间接盖髓			√	
分次去龋				√
直接盖髓	√			
活髓切断		√		
结果评估				
观察时间	1 年	1 年	1 年	5 年
牙髓活力测试	x	x	x	x
影像学检查	适中	适中	x	x
临床牙髓诊断	适中	适中	x	适中
结果变量				
材料	无显著差异	无显著差异	无显著差异	
方法			CBCT 更敏感	
治疗方案				分次比直接好
其他	邻面洞更差			

9.11.4 盖髓材料的选择

尽管一些研究表明，与氢氧化钙相比，MTA 在组织学上有更好的反应（即更同质的牙本质桥，无炎症或少量）[87]，临床队列研究也支持此观点[62]，但氢氧化钙仍然被认为适合活髓保存治疗。几项研究显示出两种类型的盖髓剂之间无显著差异，这表明穿髓孔的大小比盖髓材料的选择更为重要[22]。尽管 MTA 可能会提供更好的预后，但一项旨在真实反映临床情况的多中心随机实验未发现两种材料的治疗结果有显著差异[38]。

规范操作步骤及保证窝洞和牙髓创面无菌至关重要[20,24]，将这一基本原则转化为临床实践可能将面临重大挑战。

9.11.5 当前临床证据的现状

数据可以从证据金字塔的各个层次收集，从简单的病例到不同质量的队列和比较研究。然而，在比较不同盖髓材料的随机对照临床试验（表9.3）中，有些可能证据不足，这使得对临床实践的推断存在问题[43, 46, 84]。这些研究并不是都能充分随机化，但对于充分解释干预效果至关重要[34]。即使是设计良好的随机试验，也会出现病例特征（病损深度）在各组之间分布不均匀的风险[50]。因此，基于目前的研究，很难对盖髓材料的选择给出高质量的科学建议[73]。

表9.4是将每个干预因素与其当前证据水平相关联的交叉列表。

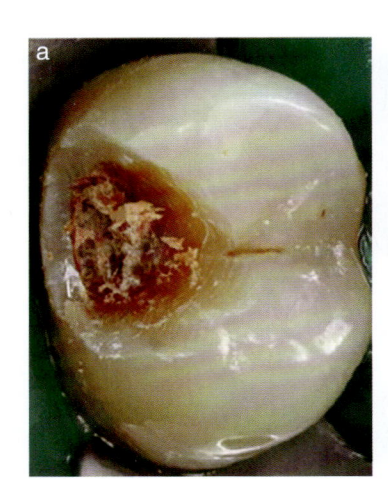

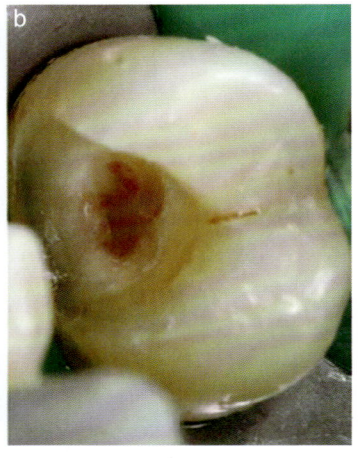

图9.10 纳入试验的临床标准。对于将行盖髓术的病变环境，精确数据将为纳入试验的标准提供更好的平台，从而更好地解释数据。a.病变中有病变活动停止迹象的龋齿组织被切除，牙本质颜色更深、质地更硬。b.据报道，牙髓暴露时的预后优于活跃病变环境下的暴露，其感染水平远低于活跃病变环境[51]（病例由Miguel Marqeus 医生提供）

表9.4 治疗和诊断因素交叉列表

治疗	诊断性因素					
	健康牙本质（创伤）	年轻人	年长者	影像学深龋（髓方1/4）	影像学极深龋（髓方4/4）	可复性牙髓炎	不可复性牙髓炎
Ⅰ类直接盖髓术	是（+）	是	是	否（++）	否	是	否
Ⅱ类直接盖髓术	否	是	是	是（+）	是（+）	是	否
部分活髓切断术	是	是	否	否	否	是	否
活髓切断术	是	是	是	？（+）	？	是	是
分次去龋	–	是	是	是（++）	否	是	否
间接盖髓术	–	是	是	是（+）	否	是	否
选择性去龋	–	是	？	？	？	是	否

++：采用RCT方式。+：采用基于观测的方式对比

9.12 未来展望：更先进的生物学方法

修复牙本质的细胞通常被描述为次级成牙本质细胞样细胞，它们来源于干细胞/祖细胞。这些细胞可在牙髓的不同部位表达，通常与血管[36]相关。修复活动并不局限于靠近原始牙本质的区域，这些细胞的普遍存在解释了为什么在成功形成牙本质桥的情况下，可以进行浅层的盖髓术和更深层的活髓切断术。然而，目前还不清楚究竟是哪些干细胞/祖细胞参与了牙本质修复[35]。这些细胞表达大量间充质和胚胎干细胞标记物，反映了牙髓内干细胞/祖细胞的变异[83]。简而言之，在更大规模的临床实践真正受益之前，还需要进行更多的研究。

增加有关牙本质和牙髓修复细胞来源的知识将指导未来的修复和再生性牙髓治疗，包括盖髓术和活髓切断术的技术和材料（见第10章）。

参考文献

[1] Aguilar P, Linsuwanont P. Vital pulp therapy in vital permanent teeth with cariously exposed pulp: a systematic review. J Endod, 2011, 37, (5): 581–587.

[2] Alqaderi H, et al. Coronal pulpotomy for cariously exposed permanent posterior teeth with closed apices: A systematic review and meta-analysis. J. Dent, 2016, 44: 1–7.

[3] Andreasen F M. Transient root resorption after dental trauma: the clinician's dilemma. J Esthet Restor Dent, 2003, 15（2）: 80–92.

[4] Baldissera E Z, et al. Tenascin and fibronectin expression after pulp capping with different hemostatic agents: a preliminary study. Braz. Dent J, 2013, 24 (3): 188–193.

[5] Barthel C R, et al. Pulp capping of carious exposures: treatment outcome after 5 and 10 years: a retrospective study. J Endod, 2000, 26 (9): 525–528.

[6] Baume L J. The Biology of Pulp and Dentine. A Historic, Terminologic-Taxonomic, Histologic-Biochemical, Embryonic and Clinical Survey. Karger: Basel, 1980：67–182.

[7] Bjørndal L. Vital pulp therapy for permanent molars// Peters O A. The Guidebook to Molar Endodontics. Berlin/Heidelberg: Springer, 2016: 125–139.

[8] Bjørndal L, Darvann T. A light microscopic study of odontoblastic and non-odontoblastic cells involved in tertiary dentinogenesis in well-defined cavitated carious lesions. Caries Res, 1999, 33（1）: 50–60.

[9] Bjørndal L, Darvann T, Lussi A. A computerized analysis of the relation between the occlusal enamel caries lesion and the demineralized dentin. Eur J Oral Sci, 1999, 107 (3): 176–82.

[10] Bjørndal L, Demant S, Dabelsteen S. Depth and activity of carious lesions as indicators for the regenerative potential of dental pulp after intervention. J Endod, 2014, 40 (4 Suppl): S76–81.

[11] Bjørndal L, et al. Randomized clinical trials on deep carious lesions: 5-year follow-up. J Dent Res, 2017, 96 (7): 747–753.

[12] Bjørndal L, Kidd E A. The treatment of deep dentine caries lesions. Dent Update, 2005, 32 (7): 402–404, 407–410, 413.

[13] Bjørndal L, Larsen T, Thylstrup A. A clinical and microbiological study of deep carious lesions during stepwise excavation using long treatment intervals. Caries Res, 1997, 31 (6): 411–417.

[14] Bjørndal L, Laustsen M H, Reit C. Root canal treatment in Denmark is most often carried out in carious vital molar teeth and retreatments are rare. Int Endod J, 2006, 39, 10, : 785–790.

[15] Bjørndal L, Reit C. The adoption of new endodontic technology amongst Danish general dental practitioners. Int Endod J, 2005, 38（1）: 52–58.

[16] Bjørndal L, et al. Treatment of deep caries lesions in adults: randomized clinical trials comparing stepwise vs. direct complete excavation, and direct pulp capping vs. partial pulpotomy. Eur J Oral Sci, 2010, 118 (3): 290–297.

[17] Bjørndal L, Ricucci D. Pulp inflammation: from the reversible pulpitis to pulp necrosis during caries progression// Goldberg M. The Dental Pulp: Biology, Pathology and Regenerative Therapies. Heidelberg: Springer, 2016: 125–139.

[18] Bjørndal L, Thylstrup A. A practice-based study on stepwise excavation of deep carious lesions in permanent teeth: a 1-year follow-up study. Community Dent Oral Epidemiol, 1998, 26（2）: 122–128.

[19] Bjørndal L, Thylstrup A, Ekstrand K R. A method for light microscopy examination of cellular and structural interrelations in undermineralized tooth specimens. Acta Odontol Scand, 1994, 52 (3): 182–190.

[20] Bogen G, Kim J S, Bakland L K. Direct pulp capping with mineral trioxide aggregate: an observational study. J Am Dent Assoc, 2008, 139 (3): 305–315; quiz 305–315.

[21] Casagrande L, et al. Indirect pulp treatment in primary teeth: 4-year results. Am J Dent, 2010, 23(1): 34–38.

[22] Chailertvanitkul P, et al. Randomized control trial comparing calcium hydroxide and mineral trioxide aggregate for partial pulpotomies in cariously exposed pulps of permanent molars. Int Endod J, 2014, 47 (9): 835–842.

[23] Cooper P R, et al. Inflammationregeneration interplay in the dentine-pulp complex. J Dent, 2010, 38 (9): 687–697.

[24] Cox C F, et al. Pulp capping of dental pulp mechanically

[25] Cvek M. A clinical report on partial pulpotomy and capping with calcium hydroxide in permanent incisors with complicated crown fracture. J Endod, 1978, 4 (8): 232–237.

[26] Dummer P M, Hicks R, Huws D. Clinical signs and symptoms in pulp disease. Int Endod J, 1980, 13 (1): 27–35.

[27] Eghbal M J, et al. MTA pulpotomy of human permanent molars with irreversible pulpitis. Aust Endod J, 2009, 35 (1): 4–8.

[28] Fransson H, Wolf E, Petersson K. Formation of a hard tissue barrier after experimental pulp capping or partial pulpotomy in humans: an updated systematic review. Int Endod J, 2016, 49 (6): 533–542.

[29] Franzon R, et al. Outcomes of one-step incomplete and complete excavation in primary teeth: a 24-month randomized controlled trial. Caries Res, 2014, 48 (5): 376–383.

[30] Fuks A B, Gavra S, Chosack A. Long-term follow-up of traumatized incisors treated by partial pulpotomy. Pediatr Dent, 1993, 15 (5): 334–336.

[31] Fusayama T. Two layers of carious dentin; diagnosis and treatment. Oper Dent, 1979, 4 (2): 63–70.

[32] Galler K M. Clinical procedures for revitalization: current knowledge and considerations. Int Endod J, 2016, 49, 10: 926–936.

[33] Galler K M, et al. European Society of Endodontology position statement: Revitalization procedures. Int Endod J, 2016, 49 (8): 717–723.

[34] Gluud L L. Bias in clinical intervention research. Am J Epidemiol, 2006, 163 (6): 493–501.

[35] Gronthos S, et al. Stem cell properties of human dental pulp stem cells. J Dent Res, 2002, 81 (8): 531–535.

[36] Gronthos S, et al. Postnatal human dental pulp stem cells (DPSCs) in vitro and in vivo. Proc Natl Acad Sci USA, 2000, 97, 25: 13625–13630.

[37] Hashem D, et al. Clinical and radiographic assessment of the efficacy of calcium silicate indirect pulp capping: a randomized controlled clinical trial. J Dent Res, 2015, 94 (4): 562–568.

[38] Hilton T J, Ferracane J L, Mancl L. Comparison of CaOH with MTA for direct pulp capping: a PBRN randomized clinical trial. J Dent Res, 2013, 92 (7)Suppl: 16S–22S.

[39] Hoefler V, Nagaoka H, Miller C S. Long-term survival and vitality outcomes of permanent teeth following deep caries treatment with step-wise and partial-caries-removal: A Systematic Review. J Dent, 2016, 54: 25–32.

[40] Innes N P, et al. The Hall Technique 10 years on: Questions and answers. Br Dent J, 2017, 222 (6): 478–483.

[41] Innes N P, et al. Managing Carious Lesions: Consensus Recommendations on Terminology. Adv Dent Res, 2016, 28（2）：49–57.

[42] Innes N P, et al. Preformed crowns for decayed primary molar teeth. Cochrane. Database. Syst Rev, 2015 (12): CD005512.

[43] Jang Y, et al. A randomized controlled study of the use of ProRoot mineral trioxide aggregate and Endocem as direct pulp capping materials: 3-month versus 1-year Outcomes. J Endod, 2015, 41 (8): 1201–1206.

[44] Jenkins S M, Hayes S J, Dummer P M. A study of endodontic treatment carried out in dental practice within the UK. Int Endod J, 2001, 34 (1): 16–22.

[45] Kakekashi S, Stanley H R, Fitzgerald R J. The effects of surgical exposures of dental pulps in germ-free and conventional laboratory rats. Oral Surg. Oral Med Oral Pathol, 1965, 20: 340–349.

[46] Kang C M, et al. A randomized controlled trial of ProRoot MTA, OrthoMTA and RetroMTA for pulpotomy in primary molars. Oral Dis, 2015, 21 (6): 785–791.

[47] Kerkhove B C Jr, et al. A clinical and television densitometric evaluation of the indirect pulp capping technique. J Dent Child, 1967, 34 (3): 192–201.

[48] Khalilak Z, et al. The effect of one-step or two-step MTA plug and tooth apical width on coronal leakage in open apex teeth. Iran Endod J, 2012, 7 (1): 10–14.

[49] Komabayashi T, Zhu Q. Innovative endodontic therapy for antiinflammatory direct pulp capping of permanent teeth with a mature apex. Oral Surg. Oral Med. Oral Pathol. Oral Radiol Endod, 2010, 109 (5): e75–e81.

[50] Kundzina R, et al. Capping carious exposures in adults: a randomized controlled trial investigating mineral trioxide aggregate versus calcium hydroxide. Int Endod J, 2017, 50 (10): 924–932.

[51] Leksell E, et al. Pulp exposure after stepwise versus direct complete excavation of deep carious lesions in young posterior permanent teeth. Endod Dent Traumatol, 1996, 12 (4): 192–196.

[52] Li Z, et al. Direct pulp capping with calcium hydroxide or mineral trioxide aggregate: a meta-analysis. J Endod, 2015, 41 (9): 1412–1417.

[53] Linu S, et al. Treatment outcome following direct pulp capping using bioceramic materials in mature permanent teeth with carious exposure: a pilot retrospective Study. J Endod, 2017, 43 (10): 1635–1639.

[54] Magnusson B O, Sundell S O. Stepwise excavation of deep carious lesions in primary molars. J Int Assoc Dent Child,1977, 8 (2): 36–40.

[55] Maltz M, et al. A clinical, microbiologic, and radiographic study of deep caries lesions after incomplete caries removal. Quintessence Int, 2002, 33 (2): 151–159.

[56] Maltz M, et al. Randomized trial of partial vs. stepwise caries removal: 3-year follow-up. J Dent Res, 2012, 91, 11: 1026–1031.

[57] Marques M S, Wesselink P R, Shemesh H. Outcome of direct pulp capping with mineral trioxide aggregate: a prospective study. J Endod, 2015, 41 (7):1026–1031.

[58] Mass E, Zilberman U. Clinical and radiographic evaluation of partial pulpotomy in carious exposure of permanent molars. Pediatr Dent, 1993, 15 (4): 257–259.

[59] Mass E, Zilberman U, Fuks A B. Partial pulpotomy: another treatment option for cariously exposed permanent molars. ASDC J Dent Child, 1995, 62 (5): 342–345.

[60] Mejare I, Cvek M. Partial pulpotomy in young permanent teeth with deep carious lesions. Endod Dent Traumatol, 1993, 9 (6): 238–242.

[61] Mejare I A, et al. Diagnosis of the condition of the dental pulp: a systematic review. Int Endod J, 2012, 45 (7): 597–613.

[62] Mente J, et al. Treatment outcome of mineral trioxide aggregate or calcium hydroxide direct pulp capping: long-term results. J Endod, 2014, 40(11) : 1746–1751.

[63] Nyborg H. Healing processes in the pulp on capping; a morphologic study; experiments on surgical lesions of the pulp in dog and man. Acta Odontol Scand, 1955, 13 (suppl) 16: 1–130.

[64] Oen K T, et al. Attitudes and expectations of treating deep caries: a PEARL Network survey. Gen Dent, 2007, 55 (3): 197–203.

[65] Paddick J S, et al. Phenotypic and genotypic selection of microbiota surviving under dental restorations. Appl Environ Microbiol, 2005, 71 (5): 2467–2472.

[66] Reeves R, Stanley H R. The relationship of bacterial penetration and pulpal pathosis in carious teeth. Oral Surg. Oral Med. Oral Pathol, 1966, 22 (1): 59–65.

[67] Ricketts D N, et al. Complete or ultraconservative removal of decayed tissue in unfilled teeth. Cochrane. Database. Syst Rev, 2006 (3): CD003808.

[68] Ricucci D, et al. Is hard tissue formation in the dental pulp after the death of the primary odontoblasts a regenerative or a reparative process? J Dent, 2014, 42 (9): 1156–1170.

[69] Ricucci D, Loghin S, Siqueira J F Jr. Correlation between clinical and histologic pulp diagnoses. J Endod, 2014, 40, 12: 1932–1939.

[70] Saunders W P, Chestnutt I G, Saunders E M. Factors influencing the diagnosis and management of teeth with pulpal and periradicular disease by general dental practitioners. Part 2. Br Dent J, 1999, 187(10): 548–554.

[71] Schroder U. Effects of calcium hydroxide-containing pulp-capping agents on pulp cell migration, proliferation, and differentiation. J Dent Res, 1985, 64 (4): 541–548.

[72] Schroder U, Granath L E. Scanning electron microscopy of hard tissue barrier following experimental pulpotomy of intact human teeth and capping with calcium hydroxide. Odontol Revy, 1972, 23 (2): 211–220.

[73] Schwendicke F, et al. Different materials for direct pulp capping: systematic review and meta-analysis and trial sequential analysis. Clin Oral Investig, 2016, 20 (6): 1121–1132.

[74] Schwendicke F, Dorfer C E, Paris S. Incomplete caries removal: a systematic review and meta-analysis. J Dent Res, 2013, 92 (4): 306–314.

[75] Schwendicke F, et al. Managing carious lesions: consensus recommendations on carious tissue removal. Adv Dent Res, 2016, 28 (2): 58–67.

[76] Schwendicke F, et al. Dentists' attitudes and behaviour regarding deep carious lesion management: a multinational survey. Clin Oral Investig, 2017, 21 (1): 191–198.

[77] Schwendicke F, Stolpe M. Direct pulp capping after a carious exposure versus root canal treatment: a cost-effectiveness analysis. J Endod, 2014, 40 (11): 1764–1770.

[78] Seltzer S, Bender I B, Ziontz M. The dynamics of pulp inflammation: correlations between diagnostic data and actual histologic findings in the pulp. Oral Surgery. Oral Medicine, Oral Pathology, Oral Radiology, 1963, 16: 846–871.

[79] Seltzer S, Bender I B, Ziontz M. The dynamics of pulp inflammation: correlations between diagnostic data and actual histologic findings in the pulp. Oral Surgery. Oral Medicine, Oral Pathology, Oral Radiology, 1963, 16: 969–977.

[80] Simon S, et al. Should pulp chamber pulpotomy be seen as a permanent treatment? Some preliminary thoughts. Int Endod J, 2013, 46 (1): 79–87.

[81] Simon S, et al. The MAP kinase pathway is involved in odontoblast stimulation via p38 phosphorylation. J Endod, 2010, 36 (2): 256–259.

[82] Slaus G, Bottenberg P. A survey of endodontic practice amongst Flemish dentists. Int Endod J, 2002, 35 (9): 759–67.

[83] Sloan A J, Waddington R J. Dental pulp stem cells: what, where, how? Int J Paediatr Dent, 2009, 19 (1): 61–70.

[84] Song M, et al. A randomized controlled study of the use of ProRoot mineral trioxide aggregate and Endocem as direct pulp capping materials. J Endod, 2015, 41 (1): 11–15.

[85] Stangvaltaite L, et al. Treatment preferences of deep carious lesions in mature teeth: Questionnaire study among dentists in Northern Norway. Acta Odontol Scand, 2013, 71 (6): 1532–1537.

[86] Stangvaltaite L, et al. Management of pulps exposed during carious tissue removal in adults: a multi-national questionnaire-based survey. Clin Oral Investig, 2016, 21 (7):

2303–2309

[87] Torabinejad M, Pitt Ford T R. Root end filling materials: a review. Endod Dent Traumatol, 1996, 12 (4): 161–178.

[88] Tuzuner T, et al. Clinical and radiographic outcomes of direct pulp capping therapy in primary molar teeth following haemostasis with various antiseptics: a randomised controlled trial. Eur J Paediatr Dent, 2012, 13 (4): 289–292.

[89] Webber R T. Apexogenesis versus apexification. Dent Clin North Am, 1984, 28 (4): 669–697.

[90] Witherspoon D E, Small J C, Harris G Z. Mineral trioxide aggregate pulpotomies: a case series outcomes assessment. J Am Dent Assoc, 2006, 137 (5): 610–8.

[91] Zhu C, Ju B, Ni R. Clinical outcome of direct pulp capping with MTA or calcium hydroxide: a systematic review and meta-analysis. Int J Clin Exp Med, 2015, 8 (10): 17055–17060.

[92] Zilberman U, Mass E, Sarnat H. Partial pulpotomy in carious permanent molars. Am J Dent, 1989, 2 (4): 147–150.

第 10 章 牙髓摘除术

John Whitworth

10.1 概述

健康牙齿中的牙髓组织在热敏和电敏试验测试时，大多数情况下都有反应。龋病牙髓炎的病理发展过程包括从拥有完全健康牙髓的原始牙齿，到严重龋坏，发展为有广泛的、不可复性牙髓炎的牙齿。重要的推论是，有牙髓活力的牙齿至少在根尖区域有轻微的或没有微生物感染[95]。因此，这类牙的临床治疗不同于那些牙髓组织完全坏死、感染和已确诊根尖周炎的牙。

假设根管治疗的理想结果是预防或治愈根尖周炎，术前未感染或影像学检查未发现根尖周病变的牙齿比有坏死/感染的牙髓和根尖周炎症的牙齿有更高治愈率[76]。在这种背景下，牙医可能会把活髓牙齿的治疗作为一种简单的技术性工作，即一种快速和可预测的机械任务，而且可达到立即缓解疼痛，术后X线片令人满意，并保证长期根尖周健康的效果。但医生在工作中往往忽视细节，包括在无菌条件下处理活髓牙髓腔，在治疗过程中预防临床获得性（医院）感染，以及防止微生物定植。为了促进根管治疗后牙齿的长期保存，牙医还应将结构重要的牙髓腔过度机械预备和化学治疗的风险降到最低，并在治疗后对其进行适当修复[74]。

虽然这类报告必须讨论一些器械、材料和技术，但重点应放在受损活髓牙的感染控制和活髓保存治疗的生物学原理上。

10.2 牙髓摘除术的定义和基本原理

牙髓摘除术即摘除牙齿中的牙髓组织以及切断靠近可能无菌的根尖孔的软组织，然后封闭的根管空间，并进行冠修复，以保护牙髓系统免受口腔环境的影响和防止牙齿折裂。

牙髓摘除术最显著的适应证是有症状的不可复性牙髓炎，摘除活髓以缓解疼痛，并防止牙髓最终完全坏死、牙髓腔感染和根尖周炎的发生。

许多人认为无症状因龋露髓的患牙是不可复性牙髓炎情况之一，不适合保守的盖髓或牙髓摘除术。在这种情况下，与活髓保存治疗相比，牙髓摘除术在保护根尖周健康方面有更强的证据基础，特别是在长期随访时[10]。未成熟的恒牙是例外，医生需要更加努力保存根髓，至少到牙根发育完成和根管壁获得足够的厚度和强度。在这种情况下，通常会进行深部牙髓摘除术，在无菌的水平上切断牙髓组织，然后进行盖髓和封闭冠修复体，以排除新的感染并保留活髓的功能（图 10.1）。

从上述情况和创伤牙髓暴露后成功切髓的证据推断[21]，直接盖髓术[14]和牙髓摘除术[59,94,106,119]作为龋齿受损恒牙可预测的治疗方法又重新引起大众兴趣。许多人将这些手术显著的成功归因于硅酸钙基水门汀的特性[65]；但也有报告指出，如果要获得良好的疗效，在临床治疗的所有阶段都需要关注细节。虽然这些方法看起来很有吸引力，

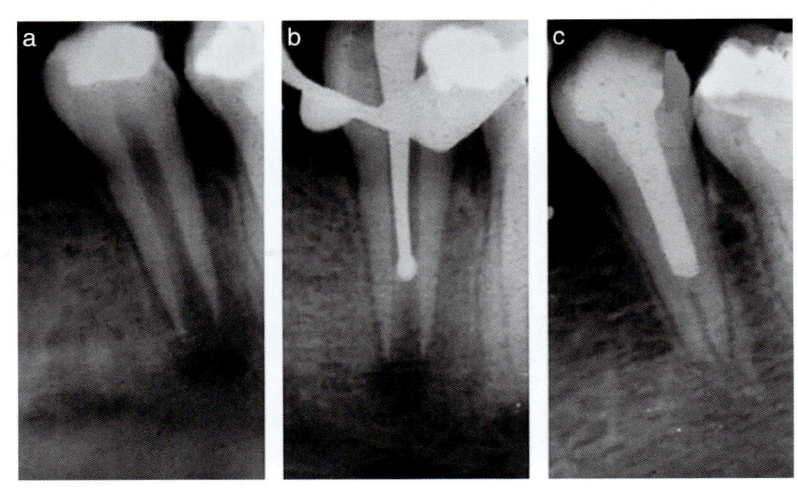

图 10.1 对部分牙髓坏死的未成熟牙进行深部牙髓摘除术。a. 患有复发性龋齿和牙髓根尖周炎的牙齿。牙根形成不完全。b. 在隔离牙齿、去龋和充填后，用长柄圆钻在距根端 5mm 处找到出血的牙髓组织。伤口经过长时间包扎，多次更换非凝固性 Ca(OH)$_2$。c. 治疗 1 年后，根尖完全形成，根管壁增厚，矿化桥将牙髓与上覆的修复材料隔开

但它们并不是快速简单的解决方法，而且目前还缺乏长期的数据结果。向患者提供这样的治疗选择的前提是：公开讨论潜在的益处和风险。只有这样，患者才可以获得这种治疗方案。在这个阶段，它们是实验性的干预措施，其结果不像牙髓摘除术那么确定。

无症状的不可复性牙髓炎的另一种形式是炎症性牙根内吸收，牙髓摘除术是阻止牙根内吸收过程唯一可靠的方法。

牙髓摘除术也适用于正常、健康的牙髓在修复过程中有严重损害风险的牙齿。例如，覆盖义齿基牙的牙齿附件，以及为弥补牙齿错位或扭转而进行的冠预备。

对于创伤后有进行性根管闭塞迹象的牙齿，也建议行选择性牙髓摘除术。临床数据表明，其中 10%~20% 的牙髓可能在 20 年内感染和坏死[41,99]。一些人认为这是干预的理由，应在根管变得无法进入之前将牙髓摘除。与此相关的是，硬组织沉积并不总是代表成牙本质细胞向中心移动而缩小髓腔，这不可避免地为根管治疗器械留下一个中央缩小的髓腔空间（图 10.2）。此外，沉积的硬组织结构相当混乱，有时甚至是骨质，没有根管腔让根管治疗器械进入（图 10.3）。

也有数据表明[22]，这种情况牙髓损坏的风险相对较低，不需要预防性治疗。显微镜前时代的报告表明[137]，如果病变随后发展为根尖周炎，80% 的牙齿可以成功治疗，并且情况很可能会得

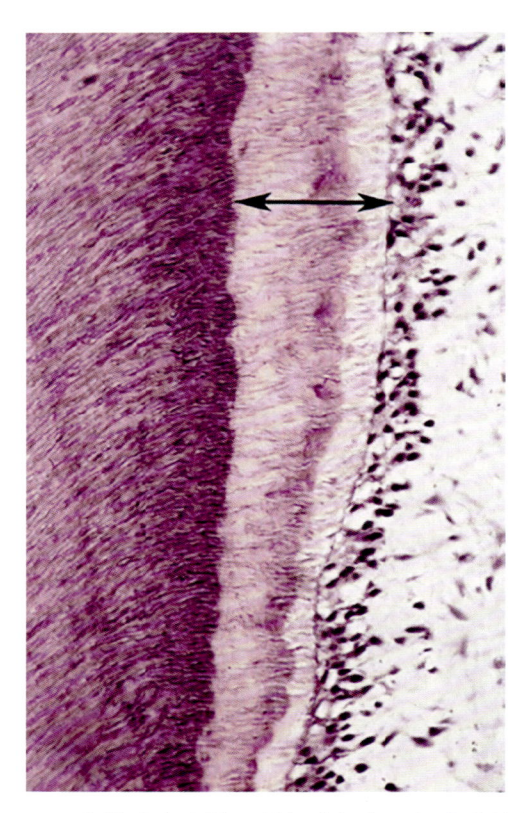

图 10.2 显微照片示龋洞预备过程中三级反应性牙本质基质在局部加速沉积。只要刺激存在，这种对轻微创伤的生理反应就会持续。它不会导致牙髓坏死或牙髓腔隙完全矿化

牙髓摘除术 | 第 10 章

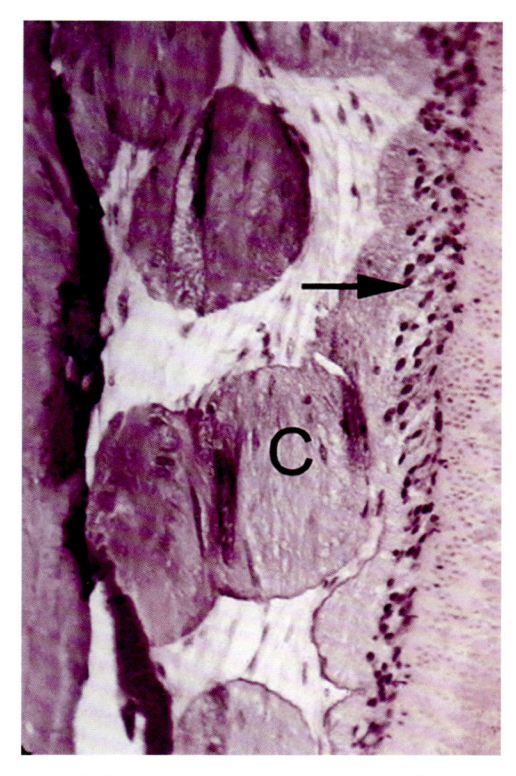

图 10.3 显微照片显示牙髓间隙矿化阻塞。矿化沉积物（C）与成牙本质细胞功能无关，而是牙髓健康不良的标志。请注意，矿化组织中包括成牙本质层（箭头所指）。矿化的进展是不可预测的，可能与牙髓坏死有关，也可能留下牙髓间隙，难以或无法用根管器械进行操作

到改善。3D 扫描和导板技术可用于控制钻的直线通路，为安全、保守和有效地进入髓腔狭窄的空间开辟了更多的机会，并进一步削弱了常规预防性干预的必要性。

10.3 有效局部麻醉面临的挑战

有效局部麻醉是急性牙髓炎的公认挑战。大多数临床医生会遇到下牙槽神经阻滞注射后嘴唇深度麻木的患者，但牙齿对操作干预仍非常敏感——即所谓的"热髓"[81]。虽然牙髓感觉神经兴奋性和中枢神经系统中央感受性的增强在疼痛的变化过程中起着重要的作用，但解释是复杂的，而且不完全被理解。增强麻醉的方法包括给予额外增加注射剂量以及将更长的感觉神经末支暴露于麻醉溶液中，如在下颌采用高位的 Gow-Gates[35] 和 Akinosi[3] 神经阻滞。阿替卡因的补充浸润对下颌骨[56]也有相当大的作用，一些最有

效的辅助技术包括局部骨内注射麻醉药，这包含牙周膜内注射、骨壁内注射和通过颊皮质板的穿孔直接向骨内输送[81]。急性牙髓炎时，不鼓励使用"失活剂"诱导牙髓坏死，因为有病例报告这些高毒性物质的局部作用会造成广泛的组织损伤[112]。麻醉药物仍然有必要直接注射到发炎的牙髓组织，以确保有效麻醉，这一过程伴随着麻药进入牙髓腔导致神经震荡而引起短暂的疼痛。

研究人员还探索了使用各种甾体和非甾体抗炎药物作为术前用药以提高麻醉成功率的潜能[103]。目前还没有术前用药方案被广泛接受。有时患者可能需要镇静剂来补充局部麻醉，以便舒适地摘除牙髓组织。

10.4 牙髓摘除术的核心原则

活髓保存治疗的核心原则是排除微生物感染，主要是口腔微生物群，也包括来自患者、牙科人员、临床材料和设备的共生和环境致病菌[78]。以下各段概述了标准措施。

10.4.1 无菌工作环境

10.4.1.1 术前准备

牙髓摘除术一般限于在治疗过程中与口腔环境隔离并在治疗完成后能够修复的牙齿。理想情况下，在根管治疗前应将所有修复体从牙齿上移除，并评估剩余的牙齿组织是否有龋齿、裂纹、剩余牙体组织的体积和分布[1]。通过这种方法，早期识别不可修复的牙齿、需要矫正带和（或）术前修复的牙齿可以得到适当的治疗。在新的、无菌器械进入髓腔之前，必须去除有缺陷的修复体，并去除龋损组织，避免穿髓，以降低髓腔感染的风险。在器械进入牙髓腔之前用橡皮障隔离患牙，同时清除牙龈上的牙结石和牙菌斑也是一个很好的做法。

10.4.1.2 橡皮障隔离

使用橡皮障将患牙与口腔环境隔离是公认的安全有效的根管治疗的先决条件。这一标准措施得到了专业团体的支持[27-28]，但橡皮障在全科医生中的使用可能有所差异[5, 73, 132]。橡皮障是防止术区感染[20]的重要组成部分，它还可以保护患者口腔部位免受如 NaClO 等刺激性和腐蚀性冲洗

203

溶液的伤害。已发表的报告显示，采用橡皮障隔离治疗后，根尖周病变的愈合得到改善，但效果并不强[58,128]。常规的橡皮障隔离也可以保护口咽不受器械错位的影响。虽然可能很少有根管治疗器械被吞咽或吸入[118]，但即使避免了一次这样的事故，也足以为常规应用这种简单而廉价的方法提供充分的理由。使用橡皮障的好处，包括改善医生的视野、患者的舒适度和医生的工作环境。鉴于感染与根尖周炎症之间明确的因果关系[70]，使用和不使用橡皮障的根管治疗结果的随机对照研究不太可能进行，而且进行这样的研究在伦理上是不合适的，橡皮障隔离的时间应根据临床情况而定。基于感染控制的理由上，在进入髓腔前隔离患牙是明智的，如果橡皮障阻碍了钻头直线通路和深度判断，应尽量平衡好过度去除组织和牙齿意外穿孔的风险。

10.4.1.3 术区消毒

去除龋坏组织和残缺修复体以及应用橡皮障是治疗过程中防止牙髓腔感染的机械手段。作为一项额外的防护措施，必须对患牙和橡皮障进行表面或术区消毒。必须在进入髓腔前使用双氧水、碘酊或洗必泰这些制剂进行消毒。术区消毒在多数外科治疗中都很常见，研究人员发现根管治疗过程中从根管内取出的是有菌样本，因此术区消毒在牙髓治疗中也得到了推广[71]。不同方法的相对有效性仍不确定[77]。

这些术前措施仅代表很小一部分感染控制步骤。通过这些步骤建立与最佳感染控制相兼容的环境，有利于提高临床成功率。采取这些措施的医生应尽可能将重点放在感染控制上，将术区消毒作为手术成功与否的决定因素，并将这种方法贯穿于其所有决策和治疗中。

10.4.1.4 无菌器械

手术器械在患者身上使用前必须进行消毒处理。在许多情况下，根管治疗器械是由制造商预先消毒的，并且通常标明只能一次性使用。对于在非无菌状态下供应的仪器，现代的洗涤剂/消毒剂和高压灭菌方案在使用前能完全清除环境污染物。使用过的根管治疗器械去污问题更大。在治疗过程中，使用热盐浸润、玻璃珠甚至熔化的锡来"消毒"根管治疗器械的做法已经有很长一段历史[29]。即使在现在严格控制的消毒过程中，众所周知，根管成形工具是难以清洁和有效消毒的。朊病毒为基础的疾病带来了特殊的挑战，由于无法彻底从根管治疗器械中消除这些病菌，在2007年，有学者建议所有的根管治疗器械的钻和锉都应被视为一次性器械[131]。尽管存在这些潜在的担忧，但目前还没有与牙科干预有关的基于朊病毒的病例报告。

根管治疗器械的刀刃和充填材料牙胶尖必须消毒灭菌，以减少来自皮肤和临床环境微生物的医院感染风险[78]。两项基于CBCT的根管治疗研究结果强调了医院感染的可能性，其中约20%的无根尖周炎患牙在牙髓摘除术后1~5年内发生病变[31, 87]。医院感染的真正影响仍然是研究的热点，3D成像在评估根管治疗疗效中的应用也是如此。

10.4.2 组织保存通路

为了消除整个髓腔的牙髓组织，必须打开所有的髓腔入口，使得成形、清洗和填充过程得到优化。同时，牙髓治疗的目的是为长期有效的修复提供可靠的基础，这使得微创原则和保存尽可能多的牙本质更有意义。在患牙牙颈区，这一点尤为重要，因为在颈区扩大洞口和大量的冠方预敞可能会不经意地削弱牙齿，增加牙齿折裂的风险[34]。

10.4.3 牙髓组织摘除及清除

"牙髓摘除术"一词可能让人联想到干净的外科切除术，但手术过程很少如此精确。尽管早在90多年前[23]学者们就讨论过这一概念，并提出了用于这一目的的改良器械[67]，但目前还不能使用微型手术刀来整齐地分割具有丰富神经管束网络的根尖牙髓组织。在去除髓室顶后，用带倒钩的拔髓针旋转半圈，将完整的牙髓从根管内拔出，有时可将年轻恒牙中的活髓组织完整取出（图10.4）；也将根管锉旋转或切削，以获取所需的工作长度，切断牙髓，同时修整周围的硬组织。这种切除不可避免地涉及根尖软组织的压迫、扭曲、拉伸和撕裂（图10.5）[82]，包括三叉神经传入纤维，这些纤维将保留在根尖创面内。很少有患者在活髓摘除后出现明显的持续症状[80]，尽管偶尔也会遇到与根管传导阻滞损伤相关的持续症状[79]。

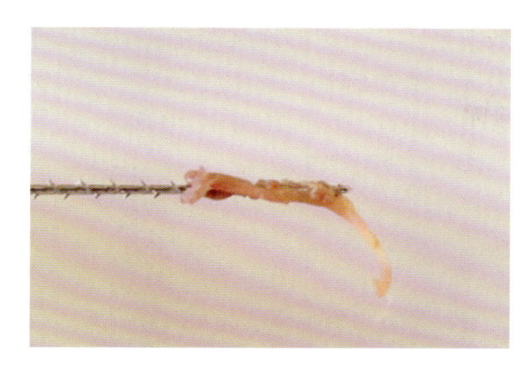

图 10.4 使用拔髓针拔除年轻恒牙的牙髓

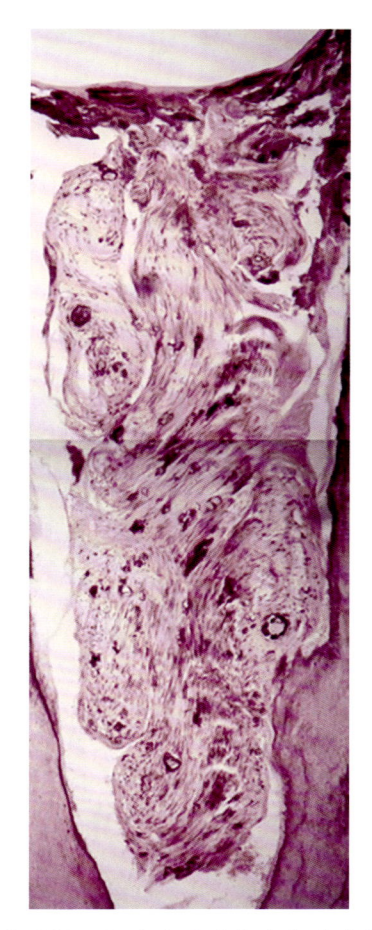

图 10.5 使用扩口锉清除牙髓摘除术后残留的牙髓组织。牙髓组织扭曲到根尖孔（感谢 H. Nyborg 博士供图）

在牙髓坏死、感染的病例中，为了从无血管和无防御的环境中去除微生物生物膜、受感染的牙本质及分解的牙髓组织，应将治疗器械应尽可能延长至根管末端[111]。在这种情况下，保持根尖开放的做法也被提倡，以确保在整个器械植入和消毒过程中能到达根管系统最深处[75]。对于有活髓的牙齿，情况有些不同，由于根髓和牙本质壁未受感染，建议将创面合理放置在 X 线片中离根尖 1~2mm 的位置[48, 51]，严格的无菌操作可使根尖残髓存活。在切除创伤后，较短根尖残髓可能比较长的残髓更容易重新形成血管，而超过 2mm 的根尖残髓可能无法恢复[110]。20 世纪 70 年代的实验研究提供了证据，如果以无菌方式去除牙髓，随后在离工作长度 2~4mm 的地方填充牙髓，可能会通过重组无菌血凝块来实现愈合[40, 83]。现代电子根尖定位仪提供了良好的长度控制，有助于医生将内固定装置控制在距离最大狭窄点 0.5~1.0mm 的位置[72]。此时，切断的髓部伤口可能在横切面上尽可能小，且不受管壁扩大程度的影响（图 10.6a）。器械放置超过最大收缩点可能会使根尖创面扩大到更大的横截面，并促进根管内出血，从而破坏根尖封闭。根尖止点预备方式（破坏根尖止点）有可能会导致根充材料的超填（图 10.6b）。虽然有必要用一个小号锉到达根尖周的韧带确保电子根尖定位仪"零"的读数，但保持根尖开放可能是不明智的，这会导致一个已经破坏了的根尖孔反复被穿刺。牙髓根尖部位和周围牙周组织在非感染性组织损伤后恢复能力较强，通常表现为根尖牙本质和牙骨质的根尖周炎初始吸收（图 10.7），这为根尖周结缔组织提供通往在牙髓摘除术中严重损坏的狭窄封闭的根尖牙髓的通道[82]。可能存活的牙髓将形成一层牙髓质壁，从而将重要的牙髓组织与随后的根管充填隔开。在大多数情况下，受损的牙髓组织被重新血管化，纤维结缔组织取代牙髓。当根尖吸收停止时，牙骨质将形成，以取代丢失的牙本质，并进一步封闭牙髓间隙（图 10.8）[30, 83]。如果牙髓摘除术后对根管进行充分且无菌的填充，过度器械切削引起的损伤将通过根尖修复而愈合[8, 40]。保持无菌是治疗成功的关键。

即使牙髓被完整地移除，也不能预期它已经完全从复杂的网状分支、侧支、根尖、峡部和侧管中被移除，也不能判断所有成牙本质的突起会随着牙髓组织的主体被整齐地从它们的小管中移除。新除去的牙髓根管壁和分支含有不同数量的细胞质、血液和微生物（图 10.9）。成功处理这种情况的关键是保持根尖残髓健康和未受感染的状态，尽可能多地从管壁和分支中去除细胞碎片与无血管的牙髓组织。这些材料可能会破坏根管充填的密封，并为微生物提供底物，这些微生物可能会进入根管系统。

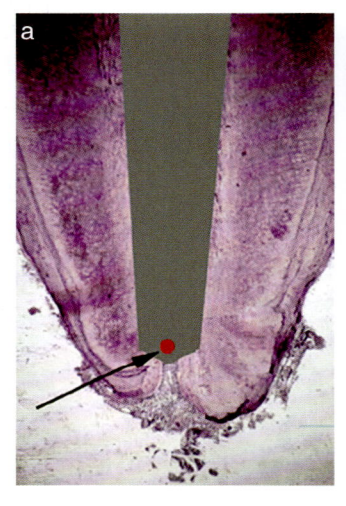

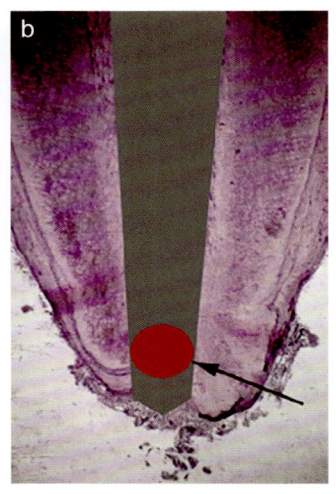

图10.6　a.在尽量减小伤口横截面积的前提下进行根尖牙髓摘除。无论器械在多大范围内切除根管壁，软组织伤口的表面积不会增加。b.同一的器械过度拉伸会大大增加伤口面积，并促使出血进入根管。如果使用锥度较小的器械，可能会失去根尖阻力形态，造成超充的风险

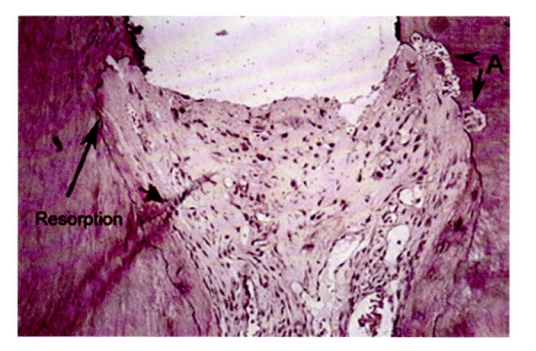

图10.7　牙髓摘除术后距根管顶端2~3 mm处的组织。根管侧壁发生了大面积吸收（箭头所指）和局部区域吸收（A）；未见炎性细胞浸润。Resorption：组织吸收

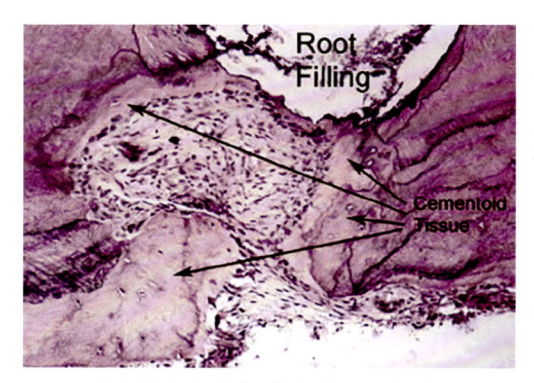

图10.8　牙髓摘除术和根管充填后距根尖2~3 mm处组织。牙髓摘除术后发生吸收的牙本质和牙骨质（图10.7）已经修复。在牙髓间隙周围可以看到牙骨质样组织附着（箭头所指）。Root Filling：根充物。Cementoid Tissue：牙骨质样组织

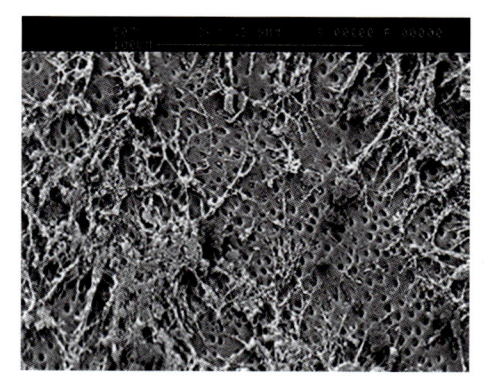

图10.9　用拔髓针拔除牙髓后根管壁被碎屑覆盖的SEM影像

10.5 根管预备

如果要对根管进行充分清洁和充填，大多数根管需要机械扩大。预备的根管应便于放置根管充填物，同时限制充填物对根尖周的挤压。最理想的根管形状是光滑的锥形，根尖最窄，冠方最宽。目前讨论的问题包括以下内容。

锥度 在不牺牲牙体组织的情况下，怎样才能达到有效的清理和充填效果？

根尖形态 在牙髓摘除术时的清理和牙根充填的封闭时是否有最佳的根尖形状？

根管壁接触 在牙髓摘除过程中，器械是否有必要甚至是预备所有的根管壁？

锥度（图 10.10a） 标准根管器械的锥度为 0.02mm/mm 或 2%。一些最流行的成形技术涉及用这样的器械进行后退或向下预备。从根尖开始以 1mm 的增量依次顺序施加，形成标准锥度为 0.05mm/mm 或 5%。这些技术的成功使用表明，这样锥度的根管已经进行了有效的清理和充填，其他技术已经在更小的锥度（如 Lightspeed[93]）和更大的锥度（GT rotary[17]）方面也取得了成功。

根尖形态 在根管充填过程中，对根充材料向根尖位移的阻力可以通过预备根尖止点、或锥度阻力形式来实现（图 10.10b）。传统上，主张活髓患牙采用的是止点准备[48]，而有些人可能主张预备达到或略超过根尖止点最大限度（图 10.10b）。虽然每一种方法的支持者可能都能够用成功治疗的病例来支持他们的观点，但几乎没有高水平的临床证据支持一种方法优于另一种方法。在牙髓摘除术中，根管扩大至必须足以切除牙髓组织，但与感染、坏死病例相比，根尖尺寸可能不需要太大，因为根管壁不太可能被微生物定植。

管壁接触 机械器械无疑在牙髓摘除术中起着清理根管壁的作用，同时也是锥度和根尖止点形成的必要条件。

然而，荒谬的想法是认为根管钻和锉会接触所有根管壁，特别是宽的、椭圆形的、带状的或不规则断面的根管壁[91, 133]。即使努力引导器材进入不规则根管，器材也无法控制，因为许多根管壁和根管弯曲的周围区域是预备不到的。根管器械同样不会进入复杂的二级解剖，包括侧支、网状分支、根尖、峡部和内吸收区域。这可能会限制器械在牙髓摘除术中清除细胞碎片，以及在活髓病例中清除坏死物质、微生物生物膜和被感染的牙本质的能力。因此，具有抗菌和软组织溶解特性的冲洗溶液是必要的，以弥补根管预备器械的局限性。

10.5.1 根管治疗器械运动方式

根管预备器械应以最佳切割效率的方式进入根管，同时将牙齿或器械折损的风险降至最低。具体的根管器械运作方式通常是由制造商根据仪器设计推荐的（见 10.5.2 节）。在初始根管通路预备过程中，小的手用器械通常在食指和拇指之间进行轻柔的往复运动（图 10.11）。这可能配合短时间的低幅度上下提拉、锉、切削等，从而打开根管的冠部，使器械更自由地前进。通过继续顺时针旋转手用器械和向外提拉根管壁进一步扩大根管。平衡力法[98]是捻转法方法上的发展，这种方法中仪器首先通过顺时针的轻柔旋转，轻轻地进入管中；然后将仪器以足够的轴向压力逆时针旋转，以试图平衡器械反向出根管的力。当器械的尖端接触到牙本质时，应力在柄内积聚，

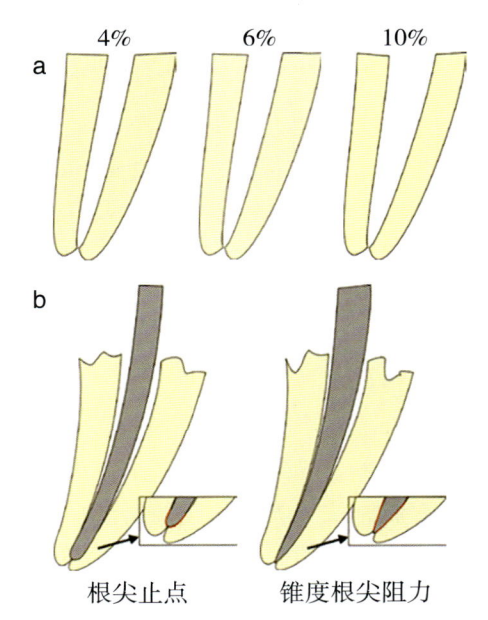

图 10.10 a. 不同的根管锥度，但多少才足够？ b. 根尖止点和锥度阻力形式

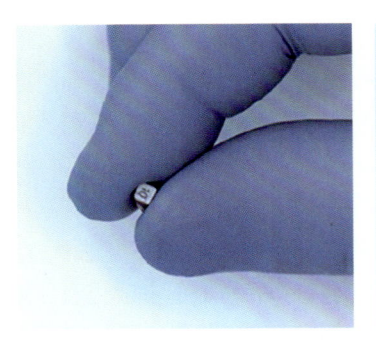

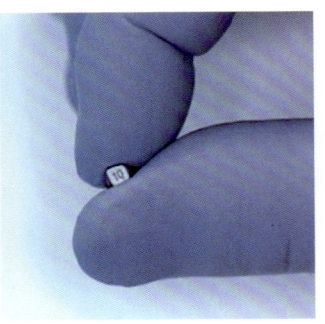

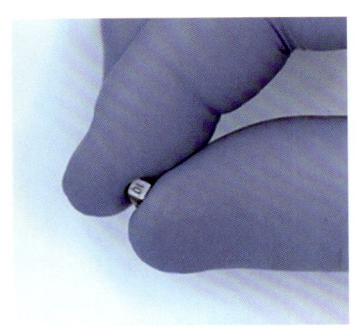

图 10.11　使用小型预弯不锈钢锉沿初始根管测量时的路径手动进行往复或旋转运动

直到管壁被阻止，牙本质被切削，通常着可听到咔嗒声。再顺时针方向轻轻推进器械，取出牙本质碎屑，然后将器械从根管中取出进行清洁和检查。平衡力法已被证明是安全有效的[19]，尽管它不是最容易概念化或掌握的方法。重点是医生要借助触觉来测量旋转的程度和轴向力，对于不同尺寸的器械以及由不锈钢和镍钛制造的器械而言，安全使用的情况差别很大。

Giromatic、牙髓光标仪（Endocursor）、牙髓提升器（Endolift）和 M4 等手用器械[38, 60-61]能使锉产生类似于捻转动作的往复运动，且顺时针和逆时针旋转角度相等（以牙髓光标仪为例，顺时针和逆时针旋转都为 60°）。多数器械都是连续顺时针旋转运动。顺时针旋转的器械有钻入根管壁和旋入根管内的倾向，同时也有损坏器械和牙齿的危险。机用器械在根管中的应用是由工程术语转速和扭矩定义的。转速是指器械旋转的速度，镍钛系统中，ProTaper Universal 转速为 300 转/分，BioRaCe 转速为 600 转/分；XPEndo Shaper 的转速为 800 转/分，扭矩是指器械进入根管内的方式。对于许多系统来说，镍钛器械预备时采用轻啄的方式，即通过施加瞬时、轻的轴向力以推动器械切割根管壁。通常需要 3/4 次扣动运动就要取出器械进行清洁和检查以及冲洗根管。另一种方法是刷法，将旋转器械插入根管中，并向外拖拽或刷擦根管壁。通过这种方式扩大根管腔，为器械在下一次更深的插入时进入创造了空间。这种扭转方法不太可能接触到管壁，也不太可能允许器械进入，但可能会牺牲更多的牙体组织。笔者感兴趣的是采用往复式运动的单支锉的出现，机用器械提供不等的顺时针/逆时针运动。最终结果是器械完全旋转，但被短时间的反转打断，这降低了旋入的风险。与连续旋转器械相比，单支锉更不容易折断[88]，可以通过啄食或刷擦动作将器械送入根管中。

10.5.2　成形器械

通常用不锈钢或镍钛合金器械来扩大根管，而其他区域则通过冲洗剂和药物的机械和化学作用进行清洁。

不锈钢锉

不锈钢锉和 ISO（国际标准化组织）标准手动锉并不是最理想的根管成形和清理工具，特别是那些具有任意曲度的根管（图 10.12）。

机械驱动的扩孔钻和 Peezo 锉通常用于根管冠方较直部分的扩大。但它们具有侵袭性和不可弯曲性，如果弯曲或进入根管弯曲部，可能会迅速硬化和折断。

即使是最专业的人使用，随着直径的增大，不锈钢器械的柔韧性变差，其刚度也可能导致偏差。使用不锈钢器械进行上下锉磨运动易造成根管偏移，而捻转法和平衡力法被认为更安全[98]（图 10.5.1）。据报道，25 或更大尺寸的不锈钢锉可疏通弯曲的根管。在磨牙弯曲根管中，通常将不锈钢器械的根尖预备限制在 25 或 30 左右[75]。矛盾的是，关于根管[47]根尖尺寸的经典形态学研究表明，这可能会导致许多活髓未被完全切除，并且许多根管未被扩大至最佳的清洁尺寸，特别是在根尖未预备的情况下。在一定程度上可以通过延长不锈钢器械预备时间，以及将根管长时间浸泡在能溶解组织的次氯酸钠（NaOCl）溶液中进行弥补。

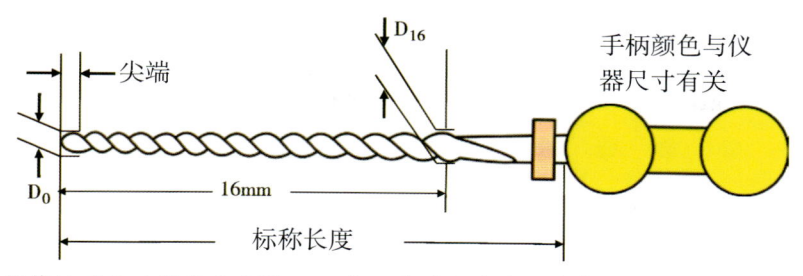

图 10.12 ISO 根管治疗手动器械示意图。D_0 表示靠近尖端的器械直径。器械的标称尺寸：10 号，D_0=0.01mm；30 号，D_0=0.03mm。所有仪器都有一个 16mm 的带刃区域，从 D_0 到 D_{16} 的锥度为 0.02 mm/mm 或 2%。因此，20 号仪器的 D16 直径为 0.52mm。标称长度表示仪器的总长度，通常为 21mm、25mm 或 31mm。手柄颜色与仪器尺寸有关。黄色：20 或 50；红色：25 或 55。

镍钛器械

大多数牙医现在都很熟悉镍钛器械的优点。镍钛预备器械和机用驱动系统的快速发展是临床需求和制造商的商业利益共同推动的结果。所有利益相关方，无论是患者、牙医还是商业公司，都对能够快速、安全预备根管而不存在器械折断或牙齿损坏风险的高效系统感兴趣。锉包装系统通常有与锉的尺寸匹配的纸尖用于干燥，匹配的牙胶用于填充。这一领域的变化速度使医生有必要从文献和领先的制造商网站寻找最新的信息。

以下是镍钛合金、器械设计以及它们发展过程中重要节点的简要总结。这将使医生能够在一定的背景下了解镍钛器械未来的发展方向。

10.5.3　镍钛合金的基本原理

20 世纪 60 年代，Beuhler 在美国海军实验室观察到等原子镍钛合金的独特性能[18]。直到 1988 年，Walia 描述了第一个镍钛根管锉[130]，这些合金在加工和制造方面的挑战限制了它们在牙髓病学中的应用。与不锈钢合金相比，镍钛合金具有更高的强度（抗压和抗拉强度更高），更低的硬度（更大的柔韧性，更低的弹性模量）[139]。这意味着与同等尺寸的不锈钢器械相比，镍钛器械可以用于弯曲根管的预备和扩大，发生器械分离的风险更低。室温中，该合金一般是奥氏体或"母"晶结构（图 10.13a）[125]。根管治疗器械通常制造成这种较直的奥氏体形态。通过弯曲或扭转镍钛器械施加应力来改变由刚性诱导相变过程的金属结构（图 10.13b）。在这种状态下，它们能够吸收相当大的能量而不产生永久变形，并在应力释放时恢复到原始的直奥氏体形态（图 10.13b → a）。在根管预备之后，当镍钛器械从弯曲的根管中取出时，可以观察到这种超弹性行为。因此，在使用前很难对镍钛器械预弯曲，在进行初步的探查和绕过台阶时预弯曲不锈钢器械是必需的。与镍钛器械不同，不锈钢器械的弯曲会导致金属晶粒结构的永久滑移，任何试图矫直弯曲的不锈钢仪器的尝试都会增加其机械硬化和断裂的风险。

镍钛器械并非坚不可摧。过大的应力可能导致金属结构的永久变形，当应力被消除时，金属结构不能完全回弹。临床表现为根管中出现弯曲或不规则切割的螺旋槽。在反转过程中，加热镍钛器械，使其高于阈值温度（图 10.13c），也可以恢复部分形态（不是全部）。这是形状记忆的一个例子，扭曲的器械会"记住"并返回母奥氏体状态（图 10.13a）。制造商可能会宣称，这样的修复处理能够让镍钛器械得以更安全地再次使用。使用者不知道在金属的晶体框架内是否发生了裂纹或其他不可修复的变化，以及器械是否会在下次使用时断裂。如果在经济允许的情况下，根管预备器械应视为一次性使用[46]，并在出现第一个变形迹象时丢弃它们可能是明智之举。

形状记忆现象最近被用来制造设计和性能完全不同的器械。已经生产出成形工具，在冷水或牙髓冷测试剂中冷却时变为直的，但在加热至体温时就会回复到其创新的螺旋形或其他形态，或最初形态（见 10.5.5）。

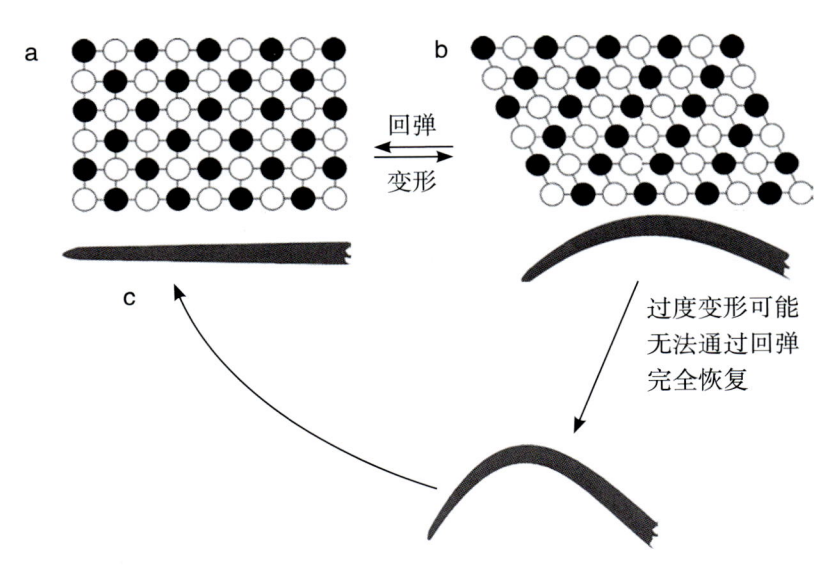

图 10.13 镍钛合金中应力和温度引起的相变示意图。a. 母体奥氏体形态的非变形镍钛锉。b. 仪器的弯曲导致应力诱导的马氏体转变为脱孪变形的马氏体。只要仪器变形不过度，应力释放后就会回弹到母体奥氏体形态；这是超弹性行为的一种表现。过度变形可能无法通过回弹完全恢复。c. 在阈值温度以上加热，可使合金通过反向转变部分或完全恢复到母体奥氏体形态；这是形状记忆的一种表现（改编自 Thomoson，2000）

随着人们对这些极其复杂的合金的了解不断加深，专门的热机械处理技术已经被开发出来，可以将合金加工成更加有用的形式。R 相镍钛合金代表奥氏体和马氏体之间的中间阶段，在这种形式下，仪器可能会比传统奥氏体形式表现出更大的灵活性和更强的循环抗疲劳性。M-Wire 是另一种热力学衍生的变体，在室温和体温下同时含有奥氏体和马氏体，同时增加了柔韧性和抗疲劳能力。奥氏体/马氏体混合合金也具有可控记忆，因此能够在临床使用前进行预弯曲，而在加热后再次恢复到正常状态[139]。这是一个快速发展的领域，最新技术的详细说明将很快公布。

从临床角度来看，镍钛合金的独特性能使得生产的器械具有以下优势。

（1）柔韧性增加 镍钛合金器械几乎消除了传统器械预备穿孔的风险，即使是使用直径较大的器械也没有穿孔风险。器械柔韧性的增加将允许根尖得到更大的扩大，潜在地改善活髓切除、根管清创和深层冲洗，而不存在根尖破坏的风险。

（2）断裂风险降低 与不锈钢锉相比，镍钛器械在断裂前能够吸收更多的能量。它们也远比不锈钢合金具有更强的抗循环疲劳断裂性能。

尽管有了这些改进，但器械断裂的风险仍然令人担忧。遵循制造商的使用说明，接受适当的培训，耐心而轻柔地使用器械，并学会感知器械无法前进时的手感，医生可将风险降到最低。任何推动的本能行为都应该被抵制。许多镍钛器械都有旋入根管的倾向，并达到与牙本质紧密锁定的程度。当器械继续转动时，它们可能会达到无法进一步旋转和前进的锁定位置，从而面临扭转过载和断裂的风险。这是锥度锁住的现象，可以通过温和的、渐进的工作和使用扭矩控制器械来避免，当器械不能自由旋转时，应停止转动甚至反转。工作硬化或循环疲劳是由于当器械围绕曲线旋转时，金属晶界的拉伸和压缩的重复循环引起的，伴随着微裂纹的形成，这些微裂纹通过器械传播并导致折断。控制这一情况的措施包括以正确的速度旋转，避免在急性弯曲根管中使用机械驱动的镍钛器械，因为重复压缩和拉伸的程度过大，保持器械在根管内上下移动，以避免弯曲循环集中在器械的一个水平上，并使器械在根管内旋转的时间尽可能短。此外，器械使用一次后丢弃也是有帮助的。

结论：在根管治疗（包括牙髓摘除术）中，目前的镍钛合金为弯曲根管的成形提供了前所未有的安全、快速和可预测的手动和机动机会。

10.5.4 仪器设计的基本原则

现代镍钛仪器是由各种复杂的研磨和扭曲技术制造的，在尺寸、锥度和切割槽设计上几乎无限制。为了追求更快、更锋利、更安全、更高效的镍钛器械系统，大量的工具相继问世，每一种工具都以比竞争对手以更优越的方式实现了自己的目标。图 10.14 展示了不同配置的镍钛根管治疗器械的选择，这些器械的设计目的都是执行类似的成形和清洁任务。

以下是创新重点的特性。

（1）尖端形状　几乎所有的镍钛根管锉都使用非切削尖端。不仅器械的引导点是圆形的，而且光滑的头部和刀片区域之间的过渡区域也是轻柔混合的（图 10.15）。这些特点降低了在预备过程中根管壁破坏、穿孔和器械分离的风险。

（2）锥度　由于柔韧性增加，镍钛器械增加了 6%、8%、10% 甚至 12% 的锥度，而且没有显著的器械分离风险。有时，锥度增大的器械

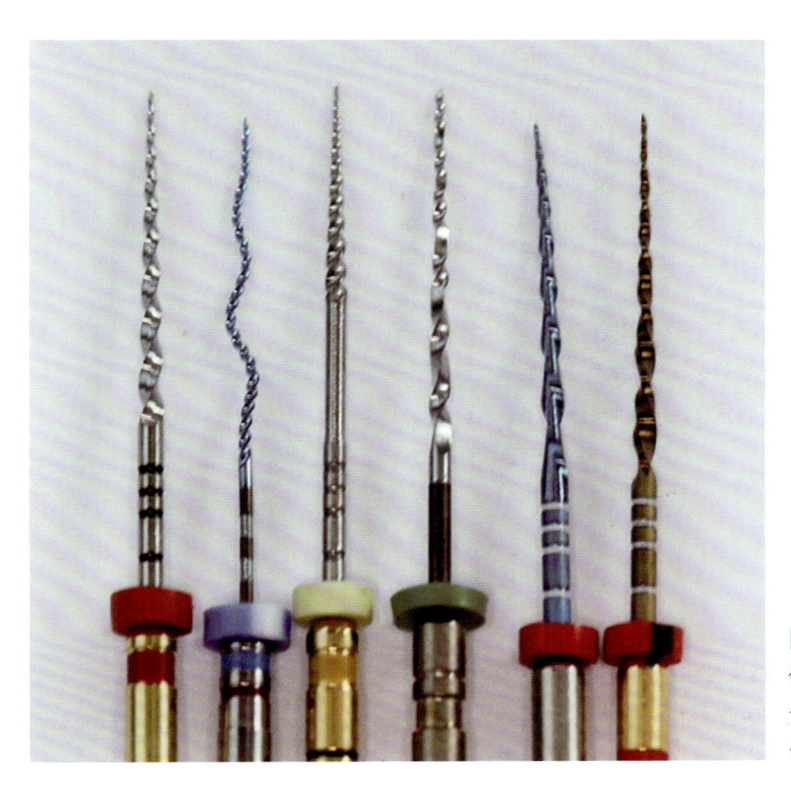

图 10.14　不同的镍钛根管成形器械。与不锈钢器械相比，它们都有许多优点。至于它们的哪些特点对安全和性能影响最大，目前仍不确定

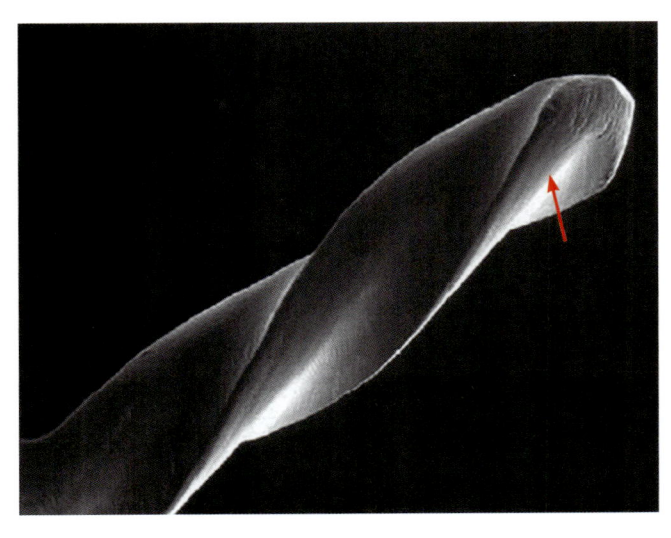

图 10.15　具有非切割尖端且尖端与刀刃区域（箭头）有平滑过渡角的器械，可最大限度地降低根管穿孔和根管壁损坏的风险（图片由 Paul Dummer 提供）

有相对较短的切割区域，以避免过度去除根管颈部三分之一的牙本质。同样，一些制造商设计了短切削头和无锥度的仪器，而另一些制造商则认为在整个器械长度中使用锥度可变是有益的，能尽可能限制器械旋入根管牙本质的风险。

（3）切削角　这是器械在根管内旋转时，前缘和横截面半径形成的角度（图10.16a）。许多早期的器械具有负的或中性的切削角，以平缓地修整根管壁，而其他的一些器械在去除牙本质时更积极，具有明显的自攻性，或许会有人认为这样效率更高。

（4）螺旋角　这是工作刃与器械长轴之间形成的角度（图10.16 b）。当这个角度较大时，器械的刀刃靠得很近，创造出更密集的工作刃，但它们之间的空间较小，无法容纳被切割的牙本质和其他碎屑的聚集。器械工作刃之间碎片可能聚集的空间称为切削空间。人们可能会争论刀刃数量和切削空间的相对优势。贯穿器械全长的恒定螺旋角可能会促使器械更多的旋入根管，这使得一些制造商在器械全长或其刀刃区域的某些点上改变螺旋角。

（5）核心直径和凹槽深度　与核心直径较大的器械相比，核心直径较小的金属器械柔韧性更佳（图10.16c）。薄的中央核心还可以使工作刃更深，使得它们在切割时更高效(具有自攻性)，并且被切割碎屑堵塞的可能性较低，前提是要经常清洁工作刃。

（6）横断面切削空间　许多设计都强调了器械的横断面形状，不仅涉及金属质量和柔韧性，而且再次强调了可收集切削碎屑的空间（图10.16d）。提供较小碎屑空间的器械开始可能会高效地切割，然而一旦它们的空间被碎屑堵塞，切割效率就会受到影响。这可能会阻碍器械的工作，甚至会因应力集中导致器械折断。所有器械每次使用几秒钟后都应立即从根管中取出，清洁工作刃，并检查是否有变形。在此期间，应彻底冲洗根管，清除切割碎屑，恢复冲洗剂的组织溶解性和抗菌活性。

（7）表面处理　大多数镍钛器械在制造时会将金属丝段铣削成不同的形状，这会在器械表面留下缺陷。这些瑕疵可能成为应力集中点，导致裂纹扩展和过早断裂。改善根管治疗器械表面质量的策略包括电抛光和氮离子表面处理技术。在一种完全不同的方法中，至少有一种器械的制造商通过喷砂粗化器械表面，以便在上下轻微振动时促进根管壁的清理。

器械的设计特点具有复杂的相互作用，不能只考虑单一因素。例如，具有锋利的正切角的器械可能切割效率较高，但如果横截面切屑空间较小，并且螺旋角度不佳，则可能影响其性能。这仍然是一个非常好的研究方向。

10.5.5　NiTi 系统的发展

镍钛成形器械的发展重点已经发生了转变，以应对新出现的挑战。以下简单总结了2013年以前的几代器械。[37]

第一代：大锥度和径向平面的设计

John McSpadden 博士和 Ben Johnson 博士分别于 1992 年和 1994 年将机械驱动的 NiTi 器械引入牙科。最初的工具锥度为 2%，较容易折断。随后便迅速生产了 4% 和 6% 锥度的 Profiles 器械并配有更大锥度的开口锉。与此同时，Steve Buchanan 博士正在开发 6%、8%、10% 和 12% 锥度的 Greater Taper 锉，Wildey 和 Senia 则采用了不同的方法——他们推出的无锥度的 Lightspeed 系列锉包含了 22 种锉，具有类似于 GG 钻的小切割头，尺寸从 20~140[33]。

第一代器械的一个共同特征是三重 U 形横截面设计，创建了三个切削空间，中性或略负的前角，可以轻柔地扩锉根管使其管壁平滑，其径向平面的设计可以使器械维持在根管的中央位置。所有锥形器械的全长锥度不变，螺旋角也是恒定的。

第二代：正向前角，变锥和螺旋角设计

关键的发展包括：正向前角可以更积极高效地(激进地)去除牙本质，同时还能避免根管交通，更小的螺旋角可以使切割刃部间距更大，并减少器械嵌入根管的倾向。ProTaper 系统成形器械设计为全长变锥，以促进不同器械对根管不同部分的扩大，并减少器械沿全长切削的风险(锥度锁)。ProTaper Finisher 器械为固定锥度，对根尖区进行最终的预备。包括 K3 和 Quantec 在内的其他

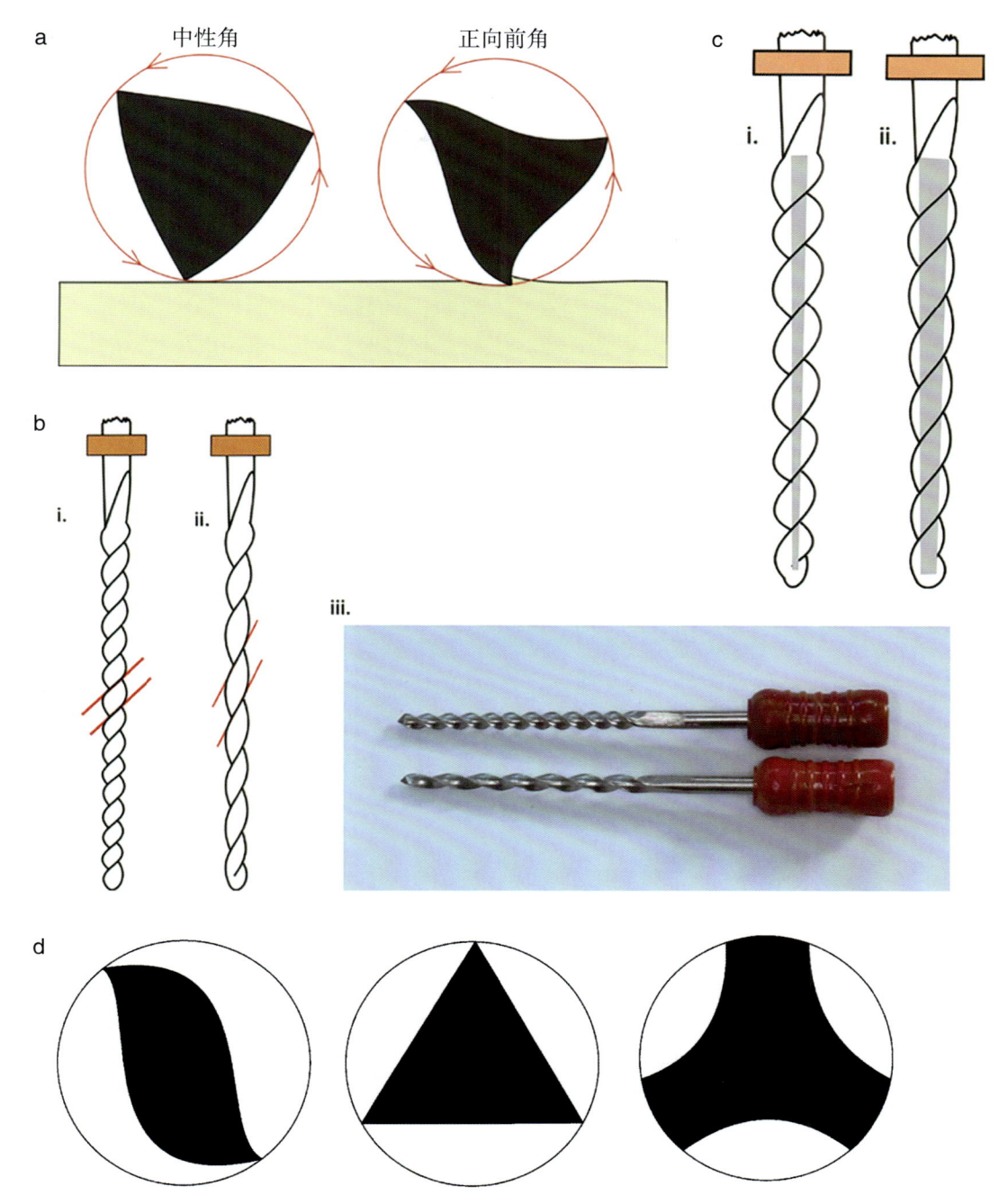

图 10.16 镍钛成形器械的设计特点。a. 切削角影响器械与牙本质接触的角度。中性角度可修整根管表面。正向的角度切割时更具自攻性。b. 螺旋角；(i)较浅的角度导致刀刃间距更紧密。(ii)较陡的角度导致刀刃间距更大。(iii)传统手锉（上）和镍钛器械（下）的螺旋角不同。c. 核心直径：中央核心较窄的器械（i）比核心较厚的器械（ii）更具柔韧性，它们的凹槽较深，切屑空间更大，因此可以更有效地切割牙本质。d. 切屑空间。器械的横截面形状可能影响切割碎屑积聚的空间大小

器械都在径向平面和切削空间上进行了调整，以优化根管成形的效率和安全性。BioRaCe 器械被设计为不连续的螺旋角度，以减少螺旋效应。这些器械还进行了电抛光处理，以平滑器械制造过程中产生的缺陷。BioRaCe 器械之所以被标记为 bio 是因为它的标准根尖完成锉（35# 和 40#，4% 锥度）具备相对较大的根尖直径和适中的锥度，这与牙齿的天然解剖形态是比较接近的，避免了

预备锥度过大以及冠方牙体组织的过度预备。

第三代：冶金技术的改进

从2007年开始，NiTi合金经热机械处理后，根管治疗器械具有更大的柔韧性和抗断裂性。第一种是M相器械，由508镍钛合金组成，经过特定的拉伸应力和温度处理[43]，早期的产品包括登士柏的ProFile GT第十代，ProFile Vortex和Vortex Blue（蓝色是制造过程中产生的氧化物）。2008年，SybronEndo开发了R相器械，它是通过扭转镍钛丝制造而成，而非切削，相关产品是K3XF和Twisted File。CM相（控制记忆型）器械出现于2010年，以HyFlex和Typhoon为代表。这些器械在进入根管之前可以预先弯曲，具有很大的柔韧性，并且可以通过高压灭菌恢复到原来的形状——这有利于再加工和重复使用。

第四代：往复式，单支锉和一次性器械

直到2011年，大多数机械驱动的NiTi器械都以恒定的方向旋转驱动。2008年，实验表明，单个ProTaper F2（25#，8%）即可安全有效地成形大多数根管，无须进一步使用其他器械[134]。由此产生了往复器械系统WaveOne和Reciproc，两者都是由M相金属丝制造的，也都是使用单支器械来预备根管，并均以顺时针+逆时针方向旋转驱动，即WaveOne顺时针旋转50°再逆时针旋转170°；Reciproc顺时针旋转30°再逆时针旋转150°。该过程主要为逆时针旋转，较短的反转是为了减少器械嵌入根管的倾向。这两种器械的刃部与大多数根管治疗器械的切削方向均相反，较大的逆时针运动是为了深入并切削根管。还有其他的一些创新，包括在器械顶端3mm处使用不连续的锥度，越靠近器械柄的方向锥度越小，以尽量减少冠三分之一牙体组织的损失。随后推出了热改良版本，如WaveOne Gold和Reciproc Blue，两者都有更大的柔韧性，提高了抗断裂性和预弯能力。

第五代：偏心轴

这一代器械的特点是旋转轴偏离中心，导致器械在进入根管时成蛇形运动或摆动，减少了器械与根管壁的接触，还有可能减少根管壁上的应力，为排除碎屑创造了更多的空间，并减少器械旋入和锁紧的可能性。主要产品包括ProTaper Next和Revo-S。

2013年后的创新：利用形状记忆创造更温和的器械。

2016年推出了利用热诱导形状记忆效应的仪器。例如XPEndo锉，它在冷态下锥度只有1%，但在加热时有至少锥度4%的螺旋。该器械以相对较高的转速（800转/分）运行，可以轻柔地接触根管壁，与传统的沿着根管钻孔的工具相比，它可能会在根管内牙本质中产生更小的应力。该器械质量相对较小，理论上也有利于冲洗液更好地运动并清除牙本质碎屑和其他根管内容物。

其他设计及使用范围

其他创新领域也仍在不断开发新的产品，包括自适应锉，它是通过激光切割镍钛管制成细密的网格结构，经喷砂处理其粗糙表面。在不断用次氯酸钠冲洗根管的条件下，低幅度上下振动自适应锉以完成根管预备。它们具有的类似于扩大狭窄冠状动脉的支架的设计使其能扩展到不规则的空间，并轻柔地从根管壁去除碎屑和牙本质，比传统的旋转器械切削范围更大。

随着根管预备系统的进步，锥度适当、发动机驱动的镍钛器械已成为安全有效的顺滑通路的工具[13]，并可以减少后续成形器械[12]的阻力。

镍钛系统似乎解决了许多不锈钢成形器械面临的难题、风险和低效率问题。然而，创新总是会引发更多的问题，而单支锉成形系统的出现也带来了新的问题和焦点。可以想象，许多经过单支锉的治疗会在根管壁上产生过多的应力，从而增加产生微裂纹的风险[89]，随着时间的推移，微裂纹可能会逐渐发展成纵向的根折。目前尚不清楚这种风险是否真实存在，以及会在多大程度上影响治疗结果。

也有人认为，旋转系统中的单支系统，特别是往复式系统可能会增加过量切削碎屑推出根尖孔的风险[126]。

这些问题的答案仍然没有解决，但突出了持续研究和提高临床警惕的必要性。

在结束这一相当具有技术性的讨论时，重新以生物学的视角审视是很重要的。镍钛器械的优点是使临床医生能够安全快速地成形弯曲的根管，而这些根管在不久以前都是很难或不可能治疗的。目前虽然已经克服了器械拉直根管带来的许多挑战，但器械断裂、牙齿抗力性降低、应力以及碎屑推出等问题仍有待进一步研究。它们对根管治疗后长期疗效的影响尚不完全清楚。目前还不确定根管扩大到何种程度（包括根尖宽度和锥度）疗效较好，器械成形的局限性只能通过有效的冲洗来处理。本章的重点是牙髓摘除术，目前尚不清楚哪种器械系统能够更好、更完整、创伤更小地去除根髓，或者形成更清洁、形状更好的根管。由于不同的器械系统相关的操作方法存在差异，临床医生必须在使用任何既定系统前经过培训并获得经验，至少需要了解所用器械在临床处理牙髓问题时工作的局限性。

10.5.6　根管成形的原则

在年轻的活髓牙病例中，最好在成形根管前用拔髓针去除牙髓组织。对于年长且纤维化牙髓，在 EDTA 凝胶润滑剂的辅助下，器械可以顺利穿过牙髓组织，而不是向根方压实并造成麻烦的根尖阻塞。典型的阻塞感表现为"有弹性""橡胶状"或"海绵状"，可阻碍小号器械通过，这需要反复扩锉，次氯酸钠冲洗和超声荡洗来处理并绕过阻塞物。

大多数制造商会向医生提供详细的操作指南，指导医者在简单的情况下如何有效地使用他们的仪器。通常遵循以下模式。

（1）用小号不锈钢手用器械或机用镍钛器械探查根管冠三分之一的部分。

（2）扩大根管冠部 1/2~2/3 区域。

（3）用电子测长仪和（或）放射学手段确定工作长度。

（4）扩大根尖 1/3~1/2 区域。

（5）测量根尖直径，根据需要完成根尖区预备。

机械预备还应伴随频繁、深入的冲洗，以清理切割的碎屑、辅助润滑锉、杀死微生物、并溶解有机物。

如果根管本身比较宽大，可能无须进行太多的机械扩大；如果需要扩大，器械可能仅限于扩大根尖部分以预备出一个合适的根尖抗力形态，防止根充物的超充。在这种情况下，主要是通过冲洗剂的机械和化学作用来清理根管而不是用器械预备了。

10.6　根管冲洗和药物治疗

10.6.1　冲洗液和置换

器械预备会产生大量的切割碎屑，如牙本质碎屑、残余牙髓组织和常见的微生物。至少需要冲洗掉碎屑，否则会导致根管阻塞和工作长度丧失。作为器械预备的辅助手段，冲洗可以润滑和防止根管堵塞，从而保持根管成形的效率并降低器械折断的风险。冲洗效率受冲洗剂输送深度和根管内流体动力学的影响。通常使用带有 Luer Lock 的细长针头的一个小注射器（3~10mL）进行冲洗。针头尽量靠近根尖，不要紧贴管道壁或伸入管内过长。30 号针头（直径 0.25mL；ISO 尺寸 25）通常被认为是最佳选择，有许多人仍然选择更宽的 27 号针头（直径 0.36mm；ISO 尺寸约 35）或更大号的针头，可能是为了避免使用次氯酸钠溶液时针头伸入根管内过长[36]。冲洗剂采用何种流动模式，取决于针头的设计和开口的位置、形状和方向[104]。一般来说，尖端封闭、侧向开口的针头可在有效冲洗和安全性之间取得平衡，被认为是最佳选择。一个一致的观察结果是，即使使用开口式针头，冲洗剂也不会在超过针尖[2]以外的 2~3mm 的区域流动，而且仅仅使用针头和注射器冲洗不能有效地冲洗整个根管中的碎屑。特别是当根管弯曲或狭窄时[15]。人们还认识到，冲洗剂的化学作用可通过对根管壁的频繁冲刷而实现优化。

由于这些原因，人们对"活化"冲洗产生了兴趣，机械能量可使冲洗剂实现深层次、高容量的交流，但不会增加侵入根尖周组织的风险[4]。方法包括手动活化、机械刷洗、声波和超声波振动，以及激光照射和负压吸引。

手动活化

"手动活化"是指在灌满冲洗剂的根管中，以低振幅上下移动牙胶尖，频率通常为 2Hz（大约每分钟 100 次）。在接近工作长度的地方，牙胶尖可使冲洗剂到达注射器可能无法到达的根尖三分之一处。随着牙胶尖的反复提拉，这种有节奏的运动使冲洗剂沿着根管壁快速运动，冲洗剂形成的膜的厚度在不断缩小和扩大[42]；也可以通过小幅度来回提拉成形器械达到同样的效果。

机械刷

根管刷是一种锥形的塑料工具，通过慢速手动器械将其推进到根管工作长度刷洗根管壁，不仅有利于冲洗剂的交流，还可产生湍流作用[45]。同样，用于控制牙菌斑的小间隙刷也可以应用于特别宽大的根管。

热诱导的形状记忆作用（参见 10.5.4）允许无锥度的镍钛器械（如：XPEndo Finisher）在口腔温度下采用螺旋式运动，其转速为每分钟600~1000转，这不仅能使冲洗剂产生湍流作用，还能在上下提拉时，与不规则的根管壁反复轻触。体外研究表明，这种方法在清理根尖区和控制牙内吸收方面具有一定的潜力[7,50]。

声波和超声波振动

声波振动方法包括会在冲洗根管时产生湍流的振动注射器系统[100]以及一些设备，例如"Endo Activator"[63]，使用非损伤型的塑料工作尖，在声波频率下（＜10 000 Hz）搅动冲洗剂（图10.17）。

超声波活化（20 000~45 000 Hz）已被广泛应用于临床[66]，可在冲洗剂中传递能量以产生复杂的声学微流动模式，使得冲洗剂流速增加并促进漩涡效应，以此达到深度清洁。除此之外还能加热冲洗剂，促进组织溶解和抗菌作用，也有学者指出超声可产生空穴效应[62]——当溶液中的气泡爆破时，可能会从根管壁分离沉积物。一段时间内，这被称为被动超声冲洗（PUI），通常建议在预备完成后用超声激活的15号器械活化冲洗剂20s，然后更新冲洗剂并重复两次[127]。该过程被描述为被动，因为超声激活的锉可以持续停留在冲洗剂中，并不与管壁接触。然而被激活的器械经常会与管壁接触，有时会造成损伤[16]。人们也认识到，管壁接触会抑制振动，并减弱活化效果。这个过程现在被简单地描述为超声活化冲洗。由于担忧超声波激活的金属器械可能对管壁造成损害，促使人们对塑料替代品产生了兴趣。

激光活化

光子诱导光声流（PIPS）是活化冲洗剂[53]的另一种方法。首先将根管系统被灌满冲洗剂，然后使用 E：YAG 激光将专门设计的尖端置于髓腔，激活激光后会产生光声冲击波。据说这种冲击波会传递至整个牙髓系统中，破坏碎屑、玷污层和生物膜。这个原理看起来非常可观，但硬件成本相当高。

负压冲洗

负压冲洗包含一个窄的吸引导管，先放置在根管冠 2/3 处，然后再置于根尖 1/3 处，同时不断将冲洗剂注入髓腔（图 10.18）。在这种情况下，溶液在被吸入根管时移动迅速，产生剪切力，有望提高管壁的清洁度[108]，并可以穿过解剖较为复杂的部位，而不会出现正压方法常发生的冲洗剂溢出根尖孔的风险[68]。该方法的一个变体是 Gentle Wave，它结合了负压技术和多频率声波活化[69]。早期的报告显示了相当大的潜力，6个月

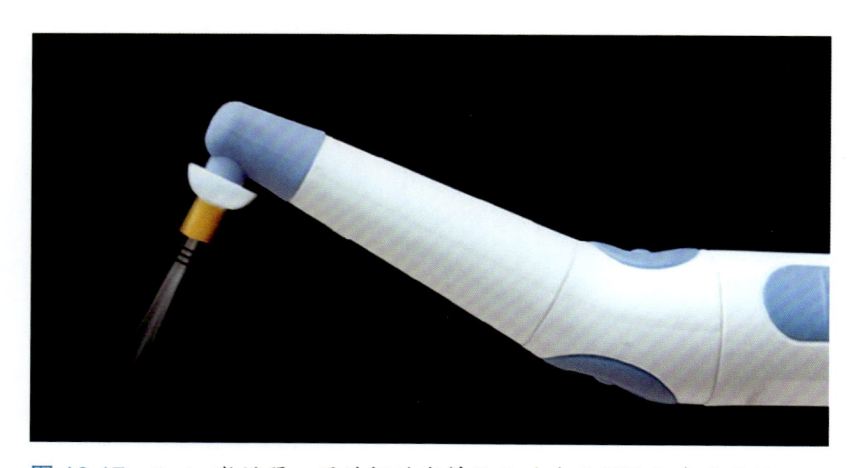

图 10.17　Endo 激活器，通过振动塑料针头对冲洗剂进行声波激活

的临床成功率很高[105]。

目前对冲洗活化及其传递的新兴技术的关注，从生物学和疗效的角度来看似乎是合理的。许多实验室研究可以证明，活化冲洗可促进清除碎屑、溶解组织并增强抗菌作用，但目前还没观察到活化冲洗对临床疗效的明显改善，无论是对坏死/感染病例还是在牙髓摘除术后[55]。能够控制单一变量（如活化冲洗剂）的临床试验可能不会很快出现，临床医生还是应该尽可能地应用他们认为能够优化清理的方法，无论根管的感染是否严重。

在整个机械预备过程中都应该用冲洗剂不断冲洗根管，但只有在完成根管成形后，才能最有效地冲洗管道的深层成分和复杂的侧支系统。牙髓摘除术的病例中，由于根管不太可能被严重感染，人们可能会忽略机械成形后的冲洗需求。然而，根管内尚未被机械预备区域的切割碎屑和牙髓残留物表明，在准备填充之前进行大量的活化冲洗可能是最佳选择。为了强调这一系列的步骤，以及机械预备后根管清理的优点，术语"成形和清理"对于感染和非感染的病例来说都会更有帮助，而不是"清理和成形"。

10.6.2 碎屑和软组织清除方案

在牙髓摘除术中，操作重点是无菌、保持根尖区残髓的活性和溶解根管分支内的有机物。对坏死/感染的病例，操作重点是破坏和消除已形成的生物膜和大块坏死组织。幸运的是，许多冲洗剂的特性都能适用于这两种情况。

次氯酸钠

追溯到100年前的证据表明，稀释的（0.5%）NaOCl溶液可以有效地清洁伤口和保护重要组织的健康[57]。这一结果在牙髓摘除术和盖髓术中也得到了印证，至少在短期内，用高浓度（5%）NaOCl溶液可以有效地处理这些创口[14]。

NaOCl在冲洗剂中是比较特殊的，它具有止血/溶解组织的作用，同时具有抗菌性，这些作用基于细胞破坏和生物膜基质内聚合物的溶解[121]。除溶解牙髓组织外，NaOCl还能从其接触的表面去除不同数量的低矿化前期牙本质（图10.19）。在牙髓摘除术中使用的最佳浓度尚未确定，NaOCl作用的有效性不仅受浓度的影响，还受温度、体积、交流深度、活化方法和时间的影响[107]。有些人可能会理性地认为，浓度较低（0.5%~2%）溶液在良好的活化和作用时间的情

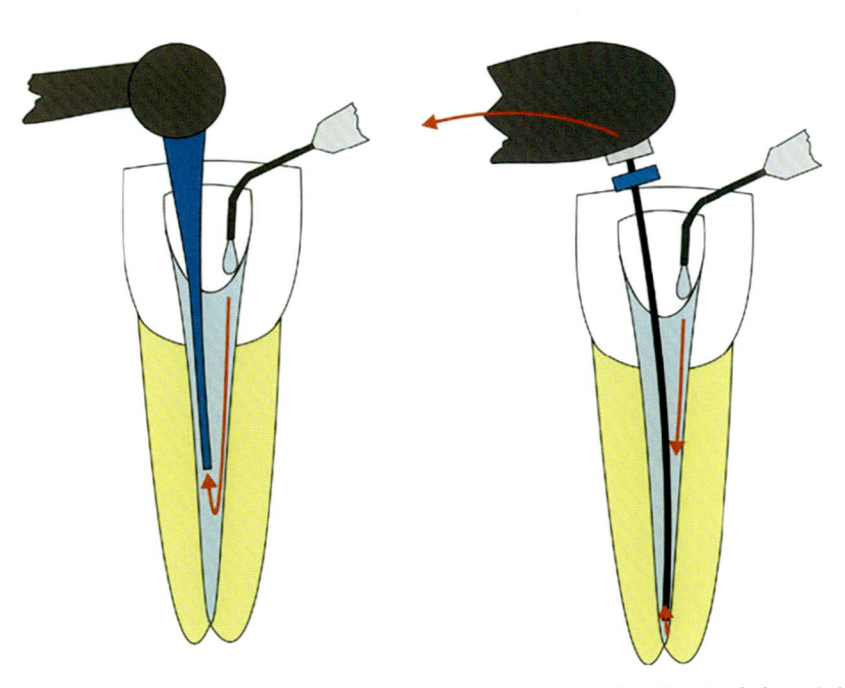

图10.18 EndoVac负压灌洗示意图。a. 根中部灌洗，溶液流入髓室，通过延伸至根中部的塑料套管负压抽吸。b. 将金属微型套管延伸至根管末端进行根尖液体交换

况下可能会达到清理目标，而另一些人则更喜欢浓度较高的溶液（3%~5%），无论病例是否感染。高浓度溶液，特别是加热的溶液，会造成脱蛋白，从而可能会增加牙本质损伤的风险[120,138]。

浓度为 0.5%~3% 的 NaOCl 是牙髓摘除术冲洗剂的金标准剂。

氯己定

氯己定（0.5%~2%）表现出广谱抗菌活性，可以被尖端的残髓所耐受，但它不具有组织溶解和止血作用，而这两种特性在牙髓摘除术中是非常重要的。氯己定可能是 NaOCl 的合理替代品，但通常被认为是 NaOCl 以外的第二选择。NaOCl 和氯己定混合后会立即产生氯苯胺，这是一种黏稠状的沉淀，不仅会引起阻塞，还对重要组织[11]有毒性。

其他冲洗剂，如碘化钾和苯扎氯铵对根管消毒有一定作用，但在牙髓摘除术中较少使用。

10.6.3 玷污层去除剂

机械成形后会在接触到的表面留下玷污层。一些人认为应该将其去除，特别是在感染病例中，因为 NaOCl 对残存在牙本质小管中的微生物的作用不大，而且人们可能担心生物膜和玷污层会影响根充糊剂的封闭性能。其他人则认为，玷污层对临床疗效的影响尚不确定[129]。常见的去除玷污层的冲洗剂包括 EDTA（通常为 17%）和柠檬酸（通常为 5%），它们在这一作用中的有效性得到了认可。如果使用加热或浓度较高的溶液，可能会导致脱矿和腐蚀牙本质。当 EDTA 或柠檬酸与高浓度 NaOCl 溶液交替使用时尤其会令人担忧，因为会产生脱矿和去蛋白化的反复循环，可能对牙本质造成化学损伤。NaOCl 与 EDTA 的结合也降低了 NaOCl 的抗菌活性。最近有报道提出了一种替代方案，将螯合作用较为温和的乙二胺四乙酸[86]或 1-羟乙基二膦酸（HEDP）与 NaOCl 混合，这样不会破坏其性质，形成"双重冲洗"溶液。

含抗生素的 MTAD（四环素异构体、酸和洗涤剂的混合物）和相关的 Tetraclean 等组合产品不仅有抗菌活性，还可以温和地去除玷污层。然而，使用广谱抗生素作为治疗局部生物膜感染的药物并不明智，因为抗生素耐药性的正在成为一场全球危机。在轻度感染或未感染的牙髓摘除术病例中，很难确定这些制剂的作用。QMix 是一种替代产品，将 EDTA、氯己定和一种去污剂相结合，以增强管壁润湿性和小管渗透性。它的大部分评价都集中在抗菌活性上，而 QMix 在牙髓摘除术中的具体优势尚不清楚[114]。

牙髓摘除术中的最佳冲洗溶液是什么，至今尚无确凿的科学依据。到目前为止，NaOCl 溶液应该是已被证明的最好的冲洗剂。

10.6.4 根管内封药

大家讨论单次或多次根管治疗的优点通常是针对坏死/感染病例[64]，即使如此，多次就诊的病例依旧缺乏强有力的证据支持。对于活髓牙病例，一般的共识是，治疗应尽可能在一次就诊中完成，主要是为了确保无菌[32]。

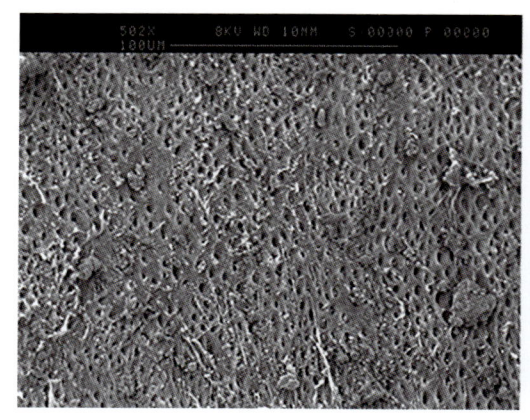

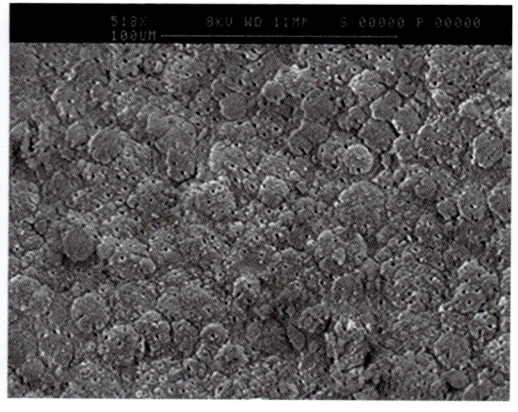

图 10.19 a. 被前期牙本质和少量组织碎屑覆盖的根管壁。b. 在 5% 的 NaOCl 溶液中暴露 10 min，去除细胞碎屑和前期牙本质，暴露根管壁上完全矿化的牙本质钙质小球

如果患者无法忍受一直躺在椅位上，或者医生没有足够的时间按标准流程完成治疗，抑或者根管内充满血液且无法干燥，可能需要对活髓病例进行分次治疗。

标准的根管内封药是在水溶液或次氯酸钠溶液中的氢氧化钙软浆[136]，这将有助于进一步清除根管中的有机物，并促进止血，同时对残髓作用温和。氢氧化钙还可能起到消毒作用，并有助于保持根管的无菌状态，直到完成根管充填。

当患牙有根管内吸收时，使用不固化的氢氧化钙可能会更有效，因为药物可能会在清除组织残留物时发挥重要作用，而器械无法触及这些残留组织。

在一些国家，很流行使用类固醇/抗生素软膏，据说有抗炎和抗菌活性等优点。在根管治疗中使用这类材料对于术后疼痛的控制还是伤口愈合的效果从文献中均无法得到有力的证明，而且局部应用广谱抗生素并不明智，因为抗生素耐药性日渐增加。

在这种情况下，重点是提供一个严密的冠方封闭，用轻柔切容易去除的材料，比如灰色的暂封膏（Cavit Grey），或先用一小块的无菌药棉、泡沫海绵或将聚四氟乙烯（PTFE）胶带搓成小球置于髓室内保护根管口，然后用至少 3mm 厚的水门汀暂封[102]。

10.7　保持无菌环境：根管充填和冠方修复

Kakehashi 的研究表明，机械性损伤和暴露的牙髓组织能够自我重组并保持健康，前提是它们处于是无菌环境[44]。类似的结果也出现在外伤性露髓和牙髓摘除术后，以及在关于牙科材料对牙髓影响的许多研究中[9]。经典文献中也观察到，根管治疗后无菌环境对根尖周健康的积极影响[109]。由此推断，根管充填和冠状修复应该提供无菌环境，以促进根尖区牙髓创面和根尖周组织的健康。与根尖软组织直接接触的根管充填材料是否必须具有任何特殊的"生物活性"尚不确定。由此推断氢氧化钙、特别是水硬性硅酸钙基水门汀可能在促进根尖残髓健康方面具有一定特性似乎是合乎逻辑的，因为它们在其他部位无菌处理的牙髓创面中也具有类似作用。根管充填时使用牙胶和一系列化学成分多样的根管糊剂进行根管治疗，可观察到良好的疗效，这表明临床治疗的成功可能更多地依赖于排除感染，而不是主动诱导生物学愈合过程。根据无菌原则，所有用于根管充填的材料和器械必须在无菌或有效消毒的条件下使用。

应采取非接触原则，将牙胶插入根管之前，最好将其浸泡在 2% 的氯己定中至少 1min[115]。其他物品，包括搅拌垫、搅拌刀和用于器械储存的泡沫海绵也可能是污染源。大多数新鲜混合的根管封闭在这种低水平的污染中还具有多少抗菌特性尚不清楚[101]，尽管再次强调，保持无菌性的一些小细节可能有利于治疗成功。

10.7.1　充填准备

根管成形和清理后，应确认没有来自根尖牙髓创面的明显渗出，并且根管可以干燥。根管充填时有血液或炎性液体不符合最佳封闭的要求，在此期间应进一步的根管冲洗和药物治疗后，改日进行根管充填。通常用吸水纸尖干燥根管，注意不要穿透根尖区的残髓，以免引起不必要的出血。

10.7.2　主尖的选择和试配

大多数根管充填技术中，选择合适的主尖是至关重要的第一步。牙胶尖仍然是最常见的充填材料，如今还有一些变体，如含有"生物陶瓷"颗粒的牙胶，常与硅酸钙类封闭剂结合使用。基于聚己酸酯的替代材料（如：Real Seal, Sybron）已经广泛应用，声称具有更好的封闭性并可以强固牙根、粘接根管充填物。然而理论可能比实际情况更简单，因为实际操作中还需要良好的酸蚀、预处理和粘接根管系统深处的牙本质壁[122]。这种类型的产品也可能通过污染的微生物被酶分解或碱性水解[122,124]。在根管这样深而窄的空腔中，结合面和非结合面的不良比例（特殊结构，或"c"因子）也会促使材料在聚合收缩过程中与管壁分离[135]。

另一项创新是 Cpoint，这是一种由类似于软性隐形眼镜的材料制成的产品，当它在水基根管封闭剂中时会横向膨胀以封闭根管[25]。

许多锥形镍钛器械系统都配备了匹配的主

尖。在许多情况下，根管可以用单尖和封闭剂填充；但在复杂的带状根管中，这可能就不太现实（图10.20）。ISO主尖也适用于那些使用ISO器械完成根尖准备的患者，这些锥度适中的主尖在填充剩余的根管空间之前起到根尖封闭，通常还要使用合适的根管封闭剂进行冷侧方加压充填。

主尖可以用锋利的手术刀进行修剪，保证顶端有回拉阻力，这样一来，在完整的工作长度或短0.5mm的情况下，尺寸合适并能被压实。

10.7.3 根充糊剂的选择

若没有根充糊剂，牙胶是不能单独用于根管充填的，目前应用于临床的所有核心充填材料也是如此。尽管根管封闭剂起着关键作用，但传统观念认为它们是根管充填中较薄弱的部分，特别是在大量使用根管封闭剂时，容易出现气泡和空隙的困扰，凝固过程还会出现收缩，并且性质不稳定、易溶解。不仅如此，在再治疗或桩道预备的病例中，还需要关注根管长度的控制和根管的可恢复性，所以并不提倡仅使用水门汀和大量使用水门汀充填根管。

如何选择封闭剂水门汀可能受到一系列因素的影响，其中一些因素可以从科学文献中找到合理的证据，另一些因素则可能与操作的便捷性和实际应用有关。

过去30年，对根管糊剂的研究主要集中在染料渗漏法和液体过滤法上，研究目的是确定根充材料和方法的封闭性。然而这些研究与临床结果缺乏相关性[84,117]，随后受到主流根管研究密集期刊的限制[24,26]，近些年这种评估和比较方法的应用已经减少了。目前根管充填研究的重点仍主要以实验室为基础，评估与培养组织接触的材料的生物相容性、抗菌性、与牙本质的结合强度、湿润牙本质的能力以及对牙本质小管的穿透能力。这些都可以反映出根充糊剂的潜在临床表现，几乎没有足够规模的体内研究来控制单个封闭剂对根管治疗临床结果的影响。还应认识到，粘接强度等参数不一定与封闭效果相关。

根管封闭剂的理想特性有以下几点。

（1）抗菌特性 封闭剂能杀灭或禁锢残留微生物[116]，并长期预防根管感染。

（2）封闭能力 能够阻止微生物和营养液进入根管系统，防止微生物内毒素等具有生物学意义的物质进入根尖周组织。水门汀在根管系统内应该是惰性的，且不会溶解的。它们的封闭性不应受到根管核心充填材料和冠方修复材料间不良的相互作用的影响。

（3）与宿主组织的相互作用 能充分地流入复杂的解剖结构内，能够湿润并适应根管壁、与根尖软组织接触时的体现出生物相容性，不会使硬组织和软组织产生不良染色。

（4）操作性能 确保易于混合和方便应用，有适当的工作和凝固时间，并且有足够的阻射度，以判断充填的程度和质量。

经济学也是材料选择的重要考虑因素，除非某一种材料的特性明显优于其他产品。

对每种类型的根管封闭剂的各项参数进行详细的评估，并试图在根管治疗中衡量它们的相对重要性是不现实的。当结合使用已非常成熟的牙胶加压技术时，无论是氧化锌丁香油酚、环氧树脂、氢氧化钙、聚乙烯基硅氧烷、玻璃离子、甲

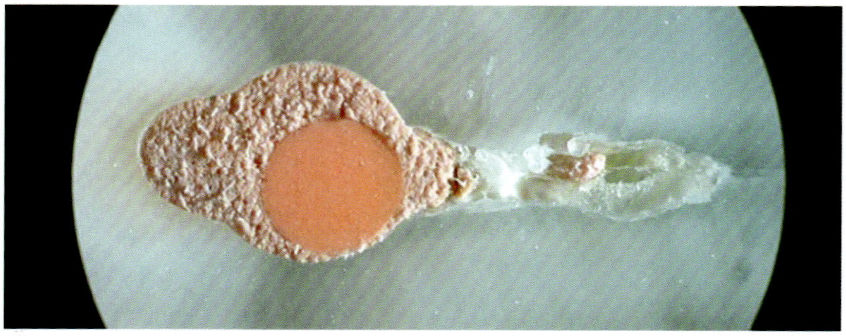

图10.20 形状不规则的根管系统，未彻底完成机械预备，未彻底完成清理，用单一的牙胶尖和封闭剂进行欠填

基丙烯酸酯树脂还是硅酸钙封闭剂，目前都没有临床依据可以证明它们能取得更好的根管治疗效果。封闭剂可能对临床预后产生系统性影响，但这种影响都不会太大，并且很快就会被其他生物和技术因素以及复杂的干预因素所掩盖，例如根管治疗[85]。关键在于保留无菌的根尖牙髓创面，避免大量的根充糊剂被挤压到根尖周组织。因此，在牙髓摘除术中，容易将大量牙胶或封闭剂挤入根尖残髓或超出根尖孔的技术似乎不太可取[54, 96]，如热塑性和载体基方法[90]。然而，有证据表明，与坏死/感染的炎症相比，活髓牙的根尖残髓可以提供更大的抵抗材料挤压能力，在牙髓摘除术后，不太可能出现精细的复杂解剖结构[97]。应始终注意避免根管治疗材料过度超充至邻近的结构，如下牙槽神经[92]和上颌窦[39]。

10.7.4　加压

尽管人们对系统的牙髓病学，以及使用合适的封闭剂进行单尖法充填的潜力越来越感兴趣，但考虑到对整个根管空间的填充，依然鼓励医生使用加压技术来优化牙胶的密度，并将封闭剂推向尽可能多的分支。

冷牙胶侧向加压充填术仍然很受医生的欢迎并被广泛传授，该技术不需要昂贵的设备，且临床效果良好[52]。冷侧压是一个通用术语，包括使用 ISO 或有锥度的主尖，ISO 或有锥度的侧方加压器以及副牙胶尖，不锈钢或镍钛加压器，不同型号的加压器控制插入深度和加载程度，以及冠方切除和垂直加压法。如果主尖是锥形的，用加压器和辅尖可能很难深入到根管中，加压可能会受到影响。需要特别注意的是，侧向加压时施加在根管内部的楔力可能会导致牙本质的隐裂或裂纹，或加剧在预备过程中出现的缺陷。这种操作过程相对较慢的技术需要一个凝固速度较慢的封闭剂，而大规模超出根尖孔的风险相对较低，这意味着根管内可以使用大量的封闭剂，随着根充物的压实和堆积，过量的封闭剂会逐渐向冠状方向推移。

冷压胶侧向加压往往是热充以及本文介绍的许多技术的基础。在热熔加压过程中，将一个旋转的器械应用于冷凝材料，并扫至根管中部，通过摩擦产生的热量将材料热塑化，从而将熔化的材料移至器械凹槽尖端。一个小号的超声活化用的锉也可以在冷加压的牙胶中推进，当被活化的锉升温时可以软化材料，并在撤出后为之后插入冷加压器和辅尖提供通路[6]。此外，还可以使用加热载体，如通过电子携热器或 Bunsen 火焰加热，将冷加压的材料逐步移至根管深处、软化材料尖端前面的部分，使冷加压器可以进行垂直加压。

使用与最终成形器械匹配的主尖进行热熔垂直加压是常规的加压方法。这可以通过单次加热或连续波热加压来完成。从根管中取少量的热软化材料，再用冷加压器压实——重复这个循环，直到距离工作长度 5~7mm。这种方法要求封闭剂在有热量的情况下有足够的工作时间。与冷侧牙充填相比，人们认为热熔加压超充的风险更大，通常建议少量使用封闭剂。

在牙髓摘除术中，内吸收需要特殊的处理。在这种情况下，根管的膨胀区域不适合使用冷侧压或单锥技术充填，而热塑方法则更可行（图10.21）。

再次强调，几乎没有令人信服的证据表明，在牙髓摘除术中任何特定的方法都会优于其他充

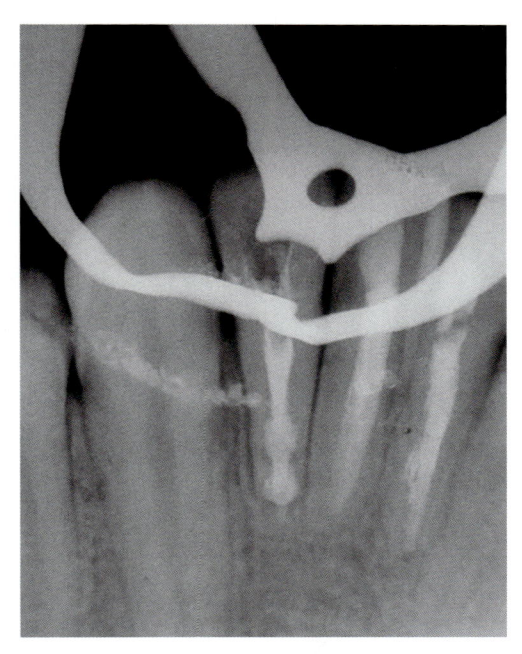

图 10.21　牙髓摘除术热充填后发生内吸收（感谢纽卡斯尔的 Geoff Seccombe 医生供图）

填方法。现有的证据指出，严密压实的根管充填物在X线片中显示延伸至根尖2mm以内，并且没有明显的超充，此时根管充填效果最好[54,76]。

所有技术可能执行得很好，也可能执行得不太好，医生应该在其有限的工作环境下，以可预测的质量来完成充填。操作中更重要的应该是有预期的完善一种技术，而不是纠结于哪种技术"最好"。

10.7.5 保护根管充填物和牙齿

经过牙髓治疗的牙齿可以使用很多年甚至几十年，术后长期预防感染是至关重要的。最好在根管口以下2~3mm处切断根管充填材料，并使用适应性良好的封闭剂封闭根管口[113]（图10.22）。同样，也可以在根管深处切断根内桩后，将根管塞置于根管口。应避免使用硬度和颜色都接近牙本质的材料，如流动复合材料，这可能会使后续再进入根管变得非常复杂。

所有类似步骤，如牙冠预备，无论是在根管充填后立即进行，还是在初次治疗多年之后再进行，都应该使用橡皮障来达到良好的封闭、避免污染。在临时或永久修复体周围可能存在渗漏，因此更应该放置这种内部屏障，以保护根管充填物不受口内液体和微生物的影响。然后，应尽一切努力来提高所有临时和永久冠修复的密封性，可以通过细致的清理洞壁、根据牙本质情况仔细地调整材料，以及优化粘接材料。在后牙边缘嵴缺失的情况下，强烈建议进行覆盖牙尖的修复，这可以防止严重的冠折，是可以延长患牙寿命的一种方法[74]。

10.8 结语

牙髓摘除术似乎是一种简单且可预测的治疗方法，用于保存受损或处于危险的牙髓。研究数据表明，无论对于根尖周健康还是牙齿保存率，医生都应该对治疗这样的牙齿有信心。在整个过程中严格遵守无菌操作的重要性不容忽视，硬软组织都应该小心处理。在这种复杂的干预中，医生无法从临床试验中确定哪些治疗元素对结果的影响最大。同样，医生也几乎不可能分辨出材料和技术的哪些微妙之处最有助于疗效。归根结底，可能是一系列的步骤中对细节和对无菌操作的关注促成了治疗的成功。重要的是要认识到，医生的行为在很大程度上受到他们工作环境的影响，这可能对治疗质量产生积极和消极的影响。教育工作者有很大的责任来传授最佳操作方法，本章概述的原则概括了活髓但患不可复性牙髓炎的患牙的最佳治疗方法。

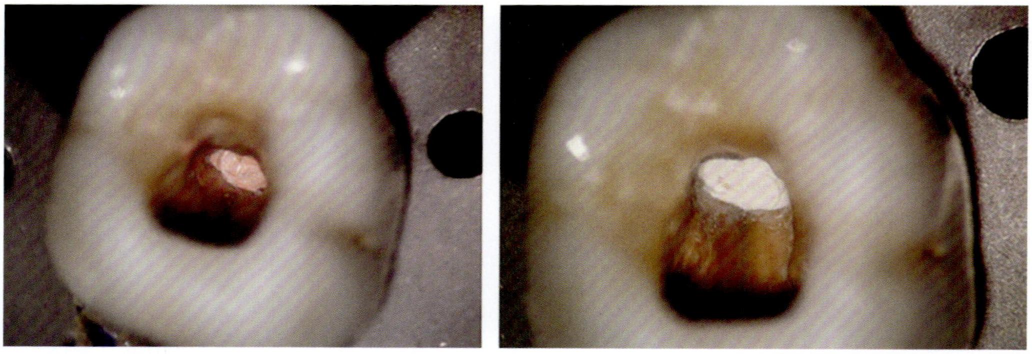

图10.22 根管口封闭，保护根管充填材料不受口腔环境影响的第二层防护。a. 将根管充填材料切至髓室底部以下2~3 mm处。b. 用IRM水门汀封闭根管口

参考文献

[1] Abbott P V. Assessing restored teeth with pulp and periapical diseases for the presence of cracks, caries and marginal breakdown. Aust Dent J, 2004, 49: 33–39; quiz 45.

[2] Abou-Rass M, Piccinino MV. The effectiveness of four clinical irrigation methods on the removal of root canal debris. Oral Surg Oral Med Oral Pathol, 1982, 54: 323–328.

[3] Akinosi J O. A new approach to the mandibular nerve block. Br J Oral Surg, 1977, 15: 83–87.

[4] Amato M, et al. Curved versus straight root canals: the benefit

[5] Anabtawi M F, et al. Rubber dam use during root canal treatment: findings from The Dental Practice-Based Research Network. J Am Dent Assoc, 2013, 144: 179–186.

[6] Bailey G C, et al. Root canal obturation by ultrasonic condensation of gutta-percha. Part II: an in vitro investigation of the quality of obturation. Int Endod J, 2004, 37: 694–698.

[7] Bao P, et al. In vitro efficacy of XP-endo finisher with 2 different protocols on biofilm removal from apical root canals. J Endod, 2017, 43: 321–325.

[8] Benatti O, et al. A histological study of the effect of diameter enlargement of the apical portion of the root canal. J Endod, 1985, 11: 428–434.

[9] Bergenholtz G. Evidence for bacterial causation of adverse pulpal responses in resin-based dental restorations. Crit Rev Oral Biol Med, 2000, 11: 467–480.

[10] Bergenholtz G, et al. Treatment of pulps in teeth affected by deep caries-A systematic review of the literature. Singapore Dent J, 2013, 34: 1–12.

[11] Bernardi A, Teixeira C S. The properties of chlorhexidine and undesired effects of its use in endodontics. Quintessence Int, 2015, 46: 575–582.

[12] Berutti E, et al. Energy consumption of ProTaper Next X1 after glide path with PathFiles and ProGlider. J Endod, 2014, 40: 2015–2018.

[13] Berutti E, et al. Use of nickeltitanium rotary PathFile to create the glide path: comparison with manual preflaring in simulated root canals. J Endod, 2009, 35: 408–412.

[14] Bogen G, Kim J S, Bakland L K. Direct pulp capping with mineral trioxide aggregate: an observational study. J Am Dent Assoc, 2008, 139: 305–315; quiz 305–15.

[15] Boutsioukis C, et al. The effect of needle-insertion depth on the irrigant flow in the root canal: evaluation using an unsteady computational fluid dynamics model. J Endod, 2010, 36: 1664–1668.

[16] Boutsioukis C, et al. Measurement and visualization of file-to-wall contact during ultrasonically activated irrigation in simulated canals. Int Endod J, 2013, 46: 1046–1055.

[17] Buchanan L S. The standardizedtaper root canal preparation-Part 1. Concepts for variably tapered shaping instruments. Int Endod J, 2000, 33: 516–529.

[18] Buehler C J C, Cross W B. 55-Nitinol unique wire alloy with a memory. Wire Journal, 1969, 2: 41–49.

[19] Charles T J, Charles J E. The "balanced force" concept for instrumentation of curved canals revisited. Int Endod J, 1998, 31: 166–172.

[20] Cochran M A, Miller C H, Sheldrake M A. The efficacy of the rubber dam as a barrier to the spread of microorganisms during dental treatment. J Am Dent Assoc, 1989, 119: 141–144.

[21] Cvek M. A clinical report on partial pulpotomy and capping with calcium hydroxide in permanent incisors with complicated crown fracture. J Endod, 1978, 4: 232–237.

[22] Cvek M, Granath L, Lundberg M. Failures and healing in endodontically treated non-vital anterior teeth with posttraumatically reduced pulpal lumen. Acta Odontol Scand, 1982, 40: 223–228.

[23] Davis W C. Partial Pulpectomy. Dental Items of Interest, 1922, 44: 801–809.

[24] De-Deus G. New directions in old leakage methods. Int Endod J, 2008, 41: 720–721; discussion 721–723.

[25] Didato A, et al. Time-based lateral hygroscopic expansion of a waterexpandable endodontic obturation point. J Dent, 2013, 41: 796–801.

[26] Editorial Board of the Journal of Endodontics. Wanted: a base of evidence. J Endod, 2007, 33: 1401–1402.

[27] Endodontists A A O AAE Position Statement. Dental Dam [Online]. American Association of Endodontists. [2010]. https://www.aae.org/ uploadedfiles/publications_ and_research/ guidelines_and_position_statements/ dentaldamstatement.pdf [Accessed 21.02.17 2017].

[28] Endodontology E S O. Quality guidelines for endodontic treatment: consensus report of the European Society of Endodontology. Int Endod J, 2006, 39: 921–930.

[29] Engelhardt J P, Grun L, Dahl H J. Factors affecting sterilization in glass bead sterilizers. J Endod, 1984, 10: 465–470.

[30] Engström B, Spångberg L. Wound healing after partial pulpectomy. A histologic study performed on contralateral tooth pairs. Odontol Tidskr, 1967, 75: 5–18.

[31] Fernandez R, et al. Impact of three radiographic methods in the outcome of nonsurgical endodontic treatment: a fiveyear follow-up. J Endod, 2013, 39: 1097–1103.

[32] Gesi A, et al. Incidence of periapical lesions and clinical symptoms after pulpectomy-a clinical and radiographic evaluation of 1-versus 2-session treatment. Oral Surg Oral Med Oral Pathol Oral Radiol Endod, 2006, 101: 379–388.

[33] Glossen C R, et al. A comparison of root canal preparations using Ni-Ti hand, Ni-Ti engine-driven, and K-Flex endodontic instruments. J Endod, 1995, 21: 146–151.

[34] Gluskin A H, Peters C I, Peters O A. Minimally invasive endodontics: challenging prevailing paradigms. Br Dent J, 2014, 216: 347–353.

[35] Gow-Gates G A. Mandibular conduction anesthesia: a new technique using extraoral landmarks. Oral Surg Oral Med Oral Pathol, 1973, 36: 321–328.

[36] Guivarc'h M, et al. Sodium Hypochlorite Accident: A Systematic Review. J Endod, 2017, 43: 16–24.

[37] Haapasalo M S, Shen Y A. Evolution of nickel-titanium instruments: from past to future. Endodontic Topics, 2013, 29: 3–17.

[38] Harty F J, Stock C J. The Giromatic system compared with hand instrumentation in endodontics. Br Dent J, 1974, 137: 239–244.

[39] Hauman C H, Chandler N P, Tong D C. Endodontic implications of the maxillary sinus: a review. Int Endod J, 2002, 35: 127–141.

[40] Hørsted P, Nygaard-Östby B. Tissue formation in the root canal after total pulpectomy and partial root filling. Oral Surg Oral Med Oral Pathol, 1978, 46: 275–282.

[41] Jacobsen I, Kerekes K. Longterm prognosis of traumatized permanent anterior teeth showing calcifying processes in the pulp cavity. Scand J Dent Res, 1977, 85: 588–598.

[42] Jiang L M, et al. Comparison of the cleaning efficacy of different final irrigation techniques. J Endod, 2012, 38: 838–841.

[43] Johnson E, et al. Comparison between a novel nickel-titanium alloy and 508 nitinol on the cyclic fatigue life of ProFile 25/.04 rotary instruments. J Endod, 2008, 34: 1406–1409.

[44] Kakehashi S, Stanley H R, Fitzgerald R J. The effects of surgical exposures of dental pulps in germ-free and conventional laboratory rats. Oral Surg Oral Med Oral Pathol, 1965, 20: 340–349.

[45] Kamel W H, Kataia E M. Comparison of the efficacy of Smear Clear with and without a canal brush in smear layer and debris removal from instrumented root canal using WaveOne versus ProTaper: a scanning electron microscopic study. J Endod, 2014, 40: 446–450.

[46] Kazemi R B, Stenman E, Spångberg L S. The endodontic file is a disposable instrument. J Endod, 1995, 21: 451–455.

[47] Kerekes K, Tronstad L. Morphometric observations on the root canals of human molars. J Endod, 1977, 3:114–118.

[48] Kerekes K, Tronstad L. Long-term results of endodontic treatment performed with a standardized technique. J Endod, 1979, 5: 83–90.

[49] Kersten H W, Fransman R, Thoden van Velzen S K. Thermomechanical compaction of gutta-percha. I. A comparison of several compaction procedures. Int Endod J, 1986, 19: 125–133.

[50] Keskin C, Sariyilmaz E, Sariyilmaz O. Efficacy of XP-endo Finisher File in Removing Calcium Hydroxide from Simulated Internal Resorption Cavity. J Endod, 2017, 43: 126–130.

[51] Ketterl W. Kriterien fur den Erfolg der Vitalextirpation. Deutsch Zahnarztliche Zeitschrift, 1965, 20: 407–416.

[52] Kirkevang L-L, Hørsted-Bindslev P. Technical aspects of treatment in relation to treatment outcome. Endodontic Topics, 2002, 2: 89–102.

[53] Koch J D, et al. Irrigant flow during photon-induced photoacoustic streaming (Pips, using Particle Image Velocimetry (PIV). Clin Oral Investig, 2016, 20: 381–386.

[54] Kojima K, et al. Success rate of endodontic treatment of teeth with vital and nonvital pulps. A meta-analysis. Oral Surg Oral Med Oral Pathol Oral Radiol Endod, 2004, 97: 95–99.

[55] Konstantinidi E, et al. Apical negative pressure irrigation versus syringe irrigation: a systematic review of cleaning and disinfection of the root canal system. Int Endod J, 2016.

[56] Kung J, Mcdonagh M, Sedgley C M. Does Articaine Provide an Advantage over Lidocaine in Patients with Symptomatic Irreversible Pulpitis? A Systematic Review and Meta-analysis. J Endod, 2015, 41: 1784–1794.

[57] Levine J M. Dakin's solution: past, present, and future. Adv Skin Wound Care, 2013, 26: 410–414.

[58] Lin P Y, et al. The effect of rubber dam usage on the survival rate of teeth receiving initial root canal treatment: a nationwide population-based study. J Endod, 2014, 40: 1733–1737.

[59] Linsuwanont P, et al. Treatment Outcomes of Mineral Trioxide Aggregate Pulpotomy in Vital Permanent Teeth with Carious Pulp Exposure: The Retrospective Study. J Endod, 2017, 43: 225–230.

[60] Liolios E, et al. The effectiveness of three irrigating solutions on root canal cleaning after hand mechanical preparation. Int Endod J, 1997, 30: 51–57.

[61] Lloyd A, et al. Shaping ability of the M4 handpiece and Safety Hedstrom files in simulated root canals. Int Endod J, 1997, 30: 16–24.

[62] Macedo R, et al. Cavitation measurement during sonic and ultrasonic activated irrigation. J Endod, 2014, 40: 580–583.

[63] Mancini M, et al. Smear layer removal and canal cleanliness using different Irrigation systems (EndoActivator, EndoVac, and passive ultrasonic irrigation): field emission scanning electron microscopic evaluation in an in vitro study. J Endod, 2013, 39: 1456–1460.

[64] Manfredi M, et al. Single versus multiple visits for endodontic treatment of permanent teeth. Cochrane Database Syst Rev, 2016, 12, Cd00(5296)

[65] Marending M, Attin T, Zehnder M. Treatment options for permanent teeth with deep caries. Swiss Dent J, 2016, 126: 1007–1027

[66] Martin H. Ultrasonic disinfection of the root canal. Oral Surg Oral Med Oral Pathol, 1976, 42: 92–99.

[67] Mejare B, Nyborg H, Palmkvist E. Amputation instruments for partial pulp extirpation. 3. A comparison between the efficiency of the Hedstrom file with cut tip and an experimental instrument. Odontol Revy, 1970, 21: 63–69.

[68] Mitchell R P, Baumgartner J C, Sedgley C M. Apical extrusion of sodium hypochlorite using different root canal irrigation systems. J Endod, 2011, 37: 1677–1681.

[69] Molina B, et al. Evaluation of Root Canal Debridement of Human Molars Using the GentleWave System. J Endod, 2015, 41: 1701–1705.

[70] Möller A J, et al. Influence on periapical tissues of indigenous oral bacteria and necrotic pulp tissue in monkeys. Scand J Dent Res, 1981, 89: 475–484.

[71] Möller A J R. Microbiological examination of root canals and periapical tissues of human teeth, methodological studies. Masters thesis, University of Lund, 1966.

[72] Nekoofar M H, et al. The fundamental operating principles of electronic root canal length measurement devices. Int Endod J, 2006, 39: 595–609.

[73] Neukermans M, et al. Endodontic performance by Flemish dentists: have they evolved? Int Endod J, 2015, 48: 1112–1121.

[74] Ng Y L, Mann V, Gulabivala K. Tooth survival following nonsurgical root canal treatment: a systematic review of the literature. Int Endod J, 2010, 43: 171–189.

[75] Ng Y L, Mann V, Gulabivala K. A prospective study of the factors affecting outcomes of nonsurgical root canal treatment: part 1: periapical health. Int Endod J, 2011, 44: 583–609.

[76] Ng Y L, et al. Outcome of primary root canal treatment: systematic review of the literature-Part 2. Influence of clinical factors. Int Endod J, 2008, 41: 6–31.

[77] Ng Y L, et al. Evaluation of protocols for field decontamination before bacterial sampling of root canals for contemporary microbiology techniques. J Endod, 2003, 29: 317–320.

[78] Niazi S A, Vincer L, Mannocci F. Glove Contamination during Endodontic Treatment Is One of the Sources of Nosocomial Endodontic Propionibacterium acnes Infections. J Endod, 2016, 42: 1202–1211.

[79] Nixdorf D, Moana-Filho E. Persistent dento-alveolar pain disorder (PDAP): Working towards a better understanding. Rev Pain, 2011, 5: 18–27.

[80] Nixdorf D R, et al. Frequency, impact, and predictors of persistent pain after root canal treatment: a national dental PBRN study. Pain, 2016, 157: 159–165.

[81] Nusstein J M, Reader A, Drum M. Local anesthesia strategies for the patient with a "hot" tooth. Dent Clin North Am, 2010, 54: 237–247.

[82] Nyborg H, Halling A. Amputation instruments for partial pulp extirpation. II. A comparison between the efficiency of the Anteos root canal reamer and the Hedstrom file with cut tip. Odontologisk Tidskrift, 1963, 71: 277–283.

[83] Nygaard-Östby B, Hjortdal O. Tissue formation in the root canal following pulp removal. Scand J Dent Res, 1971, 79: 333–349.

[84] Oliver C M, Abbott P V. Correlation between clinical success and apical dye penetration. Int Endod J, 2001, 34: 637–644.

[85] Ørstavik D, Horsted-Bindslev P. A comparison of endodontic treatment results at two dental schools. Int Endod J, 1993, 26: 348–354.

[86] Paqué F, Rechenberg D K, Zehnder M. Reduction of hard-tissue debris accumulation during rotary root canal instrumentation by etidronic acid in a sodium hypochlorite irrigant. J Endod, 2012, 38: 692–695.

[87] Patel S, et al. The detection of periapical pathosis using digital periapical radiography and cone beam computed tomography-part 2: a 1-year posttreatment follow-up. Int Endod J, 2012, 45: 711–723.

[88] Pedulla E, et al. Influence of continuous rotation or reciprocation of Optimum Torque Reverse motion on cyclic fatigue resistance of nickel-titanium rotary instruments. Int Endod J, 2017.

[89] Pedulla E, et al. Effects of 6 Single-File Systems on Dentinal Crack Formation. J Endod, 2017, 43: 456–461.

[90] Peng L, et al. Outcome of root canal obturation by warm gutta-percha versus cold lateral condensation: a meta-analysis. J Endod, 2007, 33: 106–109.

[91] Peters O A, et al. ProTaper rotary root canal preparation: effects of canal anatomy on final shape analysed by micro CT. Int Endod J, 2003, 36: 86–92.

[92] Pogrel M A. Damage to the inferior alveolar nerve as the result of root canal therapy. J Am Dent Assoc, 2007, 138: 65–69.

[93] Portenier I, Lutz F, Barbakow F. Preparation of the apical part of the root canal by the Lightspeed and step-back techniques. Int Endod J, 1998, 31: 103–111.

[94] Qudeimat M A, Alyahya A, Hasan A A. Mineral trioxide aggregate pulpotomy for permanent molars with clinical signs indicative of irreversible pulpitis: a preliminary study. Int Endod J, 2017, 50: 126–134.

[95] Ricucci D, Loghin S, Siqueira J F Jr. Correlation between clinical and histologic pulp diagnoses. J Endod, 2014, 40: 1932–1939.

[96] Ricucci D, et al. A prospective cohort study of endodontic treatments of 1, 369 root canals: results after 5 years. Oral Surg Oral Med Oral Pathol Oral Radiol Endod, 2011, 112: 825–842.

[97] Ricucci D, Siqueira J F Jr. Fate of the tissue in lateral canals and apical ramifications in response to pathologic conditions and treatment procedures. J Endod, 2010, 36: 1–15.

[98] Roane J B, Sabala C L, Duncanson M G Jr. The "balanced force" concept for instrumentation of curved canals. J Endod, 1985, 11: 203–211.

[99] Robertson A, et al. Incidence of pulp necrosis subsequent to

pulp canal obliteration from trauma of permanent incisors. J Endod, 1996, 22: 557–560.

[100] Rodig T, et al. Comparison of the Vibringe system with syringe and passive ultrasonic irrigation in removing debris from simulated root canal irregularities. J Endod, 2010, 36: 1410–1413.

[101] Saleh I M, et al. Survival of Enterococcus faecalis in infected dentinal tubules after root canal filling with different root canal sealers in vitro. Int Endod J, 2004, 37: 193–198.

[102] Sattar M M, Patel M, Alani A. Clinical applications of polytetrafluoroethylene (PTFE)tape in restorative dentistry. Br Dent J, 2017, 222: 151–158.

[103] Shahi S, et al. Effect of premedication with ibuprofen and dexamethasone on success rate of inferior alveolar nerve block for teeth with asymptomatic irreversible pulpitis: a randomized clinical trial. J Endod, 2013, 39: 160–162.

[104] Shen Y, et al. Three-dimensional numeric simulation of root canal irrigant flow with different irrigation needles. J Endod, 2010, 36: 884–889.

[105] Sigurdsson A, et al. 12-month Healing Rates after Endodontic Therapy Using the Novel GentleWave System: A Prospective Multicenter Clinical Study. J Endod, 2016, 42: 1040–1048.

[106] Simon S, et al. Should pulp chamber pulpotomy be seen as a permanent treatment? Some preliminary thoughts. Int Endod J, 2013, 46: 79–87.

[107] Sirtes G, et al. The effects of temperature on sodium hypochlorite short-term stability, pulp dissolution capacity, and antimicrobial efficacy. J Endod, 2005, 31: 669–671.

[108] Siu C, Baumgartner J C. Comparison of the debridement efficacy of the EndoVac irrigation system and conventional needle root canal irrigation in vivo. J Endod, 2010, 36: 1782–1785.

[109] Sjögren U, et al. Influence of infection at the time of root filling on the outcome of endodontic treatment of teeth with apical periodontitis. Int Endod J, 1997, 30: 297–306.

[110] Sjögren U, et al. Factors affecting the long-term results of endodontic treatment. J Endod, 1990, 16: 498–504.

[111] Sjögren U, et al. Factors affecting the long-term results of endodontic treatment. J Endod, 1990, 16: 498–504.

[112] Smart E R, Barnes I E. Tissue necrosis after using an arsenical endodontic preparation: a case report. Int Endod J, 1991, 24: 263–269.

[113] Stassen I G, et al. The relation between apical periodontitis and rootfilled teeth in patients with periodontal treatment need. Int Endod J, 2006, 39: 299–308.

[114] Stojicic S, et al. Antibacterial and smear layer removal ability of a novel irrigant, QMiX. Int Endod J, 2012, 45: 363–371.

[115] Subha N, et al. Efficacy of peracetic acid in rapid disinfection of Resilon and gutta-percha cones compared with sodium hypochlorite, chlorhexidine, and povidone-iodine. J Endod, 2013, 39: 1261–1264.

[116] Sundqvist G, et al. Microbiologic analysis of teeth with failed endodontic treatment and the outcome of conservative re-treatment. Oral Surg Oral Med Oral Pathol Oral Radiol Endod, 1998, 85: 86–93.

[117] Susini G, et al. Lack of correlation between ex vivo apical dye penetration and presence of apical radiolucencies. Oral Surg Oral Med Oral Pathol Oral Radiol Endod, 2006, 102, e19–23.

[118] Susini G, Pommel L, Camps J. Accidental ingestion and aspiration of root canal instruments and other dental foreign bodies in a French population. Int Endod J, 2007, 40: 585–589.

[119] Taha N A, Ahmad M B, Ghanim A. Assessment of Mineral Trioxide Aggregate pulpotomy in mature permanent teeth with carious exposures. Int Endod J, 2017, 50: 117–125.

[120] Tartari T, et al. Tissue dissolution and modifications in dentin composition by different sodium hypochlorite concentrations. J Appl Oral Sci, 2016, 24: 291–298.

[121] Tawakoli P N, et al. Effect of endodontic irrigants on biofilm matrix polysaccharides. Int Endod J, 2017, 50: 153–160.

[122] Tay F R, Pashley D H. Monoblocks in root canals: a hypothetical or a tangible goal. J Endod, 2007, 33: 391–398.

[123] Tay F R, et al. Susceptibility of a polycaprolactone-based root canal filling material to degradation. Evidence of biodegradation from a simulated field test. Am J Dent, 2007, 20: 365–369.

[124] Tay F R, et al. Susceptibility of a polycaprolactone-based root canal filling material to degradation. I. Alkaline hydrolysis. J Endod, 2005, 31: 593–598.

[125] Thompson S A. An overview of nickel-titanium alloys used in dentistry. Int Endod J, 2000, 33: 297–310.

[126] Topcuoglu H S, et al. Apically extruded debris during root canal preparation using Vortex Blue, K3XF, ProTaper Next and Reciproc instruments. Int Endod J, 2016, 49: 1183–1187.

[127] Van der Sluis L W, et al. Passive ultrasonic irrigation of the root canal: a review of the literature. Int Endod J, 2007, 40: 415–426.

[128] Van Nieuwenhuysen J P, Aouar M d'Hoore W. Retreatment or radiographic monitoring in endodontics. Int Endod J, 1994, 27: 75–81.

[129] Violich D R, Chandler N P. The smear layer in endodontics-a review. Int Endod J, 2010, 43: 2–15.

[130] Walia H M, Brantley W A, Gerstein H. An initial investigation of the bending and torsional properties of Nitinol root canal files. J Endod, 1988, 14: 346–351.

[131] Walker J T, et al. Cleanability of dental instruments-implications of residual protein and risks from Creutzfeldt-

Jakob disease. Br Dent J, 2007, 203: 395–401.

[132] Whitworth J M, et al. Use of rubber dam and irrigant selection in UK general dental practice. Int Endod J, 2000, 33: 435–441.

[133] Wu M K, Van der Sluis, L W, Wesselink P R. The capability of two hand instrumentation techniques to remove the inner layer of dentine in oval canals. Int Endod J, 2003, 36: 218–224.

[134] Yared G. Canal preparation using only one Ni-Ti rotary instrument: preliminary observations. Int Endod J, 2008, 41: 339–344.

[135] Yoshikawa T, et al. Effects of dentin depth and cavity configuration on bond strength. J Dent Res, 1999, 78: 898–905.

[136] Zehnder M, et al. Tissuedissolution capacity and dentin-disinfecting potential of calcium hydroxide mixed with irrigating solutions. Oral Surg Oral Med Oral Pathol Oral Radiol Endod, 2003, 96: 608–613.

[137] Zehnder M S, et al. Guided endodontics: accuracy of a novel method for guided access cavity preparation and root canal location. Int Endod J, 2016, 49: 966–972.

[138] Zhang K, et al. Effects of different exposure times and concentrations of sodium hypochlorite/ ethylenediaminetetraacetic acid on the structural integrity of mineralized dentin. J Endod, 2010, 36: 105–109.

[139] Zhou H, Bin P, Zheng,Y-F. An overview of the mechanical properties of nickel-titanium endodontic instruments. Endodontic Topics, 2013, 29: 42–54.

第 11 章　根尖周炎的根管治疗

Dag Ørstavik

11.1　概述

11.1.1　治疗的原因

通常，患牙诊断为根尖周炎时，不论何种类型都需要治疗。急性/有症状或慢性/无症状根尖周炎、伴或不伴有窦道的根尖周脓肿，以及根尖周囊肿都来自感染的根管系统，这是各种治疗措施的共同目标。

主诉疼痛或不适表明需要进行干预，如果疼痛是由根尖周炎所引起的，治疗方案显然是对疾病进行治疗。无症状的慢性根尖周炎本身也需要治疗。患者在没有疼痛或不适的情况下，认为不需要进行昂贵且复杂的治疗。以下是慢性无症状根尖周炎需要治疗的三个理由。

11.1.1.1　疼痛的控制

细菌引起的慢性炎症存在进一步恶化的可能。慢性根尖周炎可能在没有任何症状的情况下隐匿发展，形成大的囊肿，也可能保持稳定且大小不变。这种病损可能转变为急性炎症，伴有牙痛、肿胀和脓肿形成，这是人们倡导进行治疗的主要原因。然而，必须认识到，预测这种恶化的发生率及严重程度是困难的[7, 97, 198, 207]，并且受到许多可能超出患者和医生控制的因素的影响。

11.1.1.2　感染的局部扩散

治疗的第二个原因是感染有可能扩散到邻近区域和附近的组织和器官。颌骨的髓质可能被感染导致骨髓炎，这在许多情况下不易治疗。上颌窦也经常受累，许多鼻窦炎病例都是由根尖周炎所诱发或导致的[249-250]。据报道，超过30%的脑脓肿病例来源于牙齿感染，但牙齿感染的类型尚不明确[109]。急性感染沿着组织间隙或筋膜传播，可能到达纵隔腔，引发危及生命的并发症，免疫功能低下的个体更是如此[100, 156]。

11.1.1.3　与全身疾病的相关性

最后一个值得关注的问题是局部牙齿感染或炎症与心血管系统疾病的关系（参见第4章）。虽然牙齿感染导致全身疾病的风险很低，但毋庸置疑它是存在的[20, 112]。存在心脏瓣膜问题的患者在根管治疗后可能容易感染菌血症。因此，消除根尖周的炎症是必需的[42]。

11.1.2　治疗的目标和挑战

疾病本身和并发症的病因是微生物感染，这就决定了治疗的目标：清除感染的根管系统及感染根尖周组织中的微生物。治疗过程中所做的其他操作都是为了辅助这一主要目标，其他技术和临床手段（如疼痛控制、抗生素的应用或看似良好的根管充填）都不能弥补感染控制失败。

根尖周炎有多种治疗方案。本章的目的在于阐明治疗要素的原理和生物学基础，而不是详细阐述治疗的操作步骤。

11.1.2.1　消除感染微生物

根管系统的复杂性使治疗变得困难：物理和化学方法难以清理到峡部和根管分支表面的生物膜；牙体组织中的抗菌药物难以达到产生临床效果的浓度。除牙髓摘除术后根管充填的治疗原则

（第 10 章）外，感染牙齿还需要通过机械预备和化学消毒来确保最大的抗菌效果。

Sundqvist 及其同事在 20 世纪 70 年代到 90 年代期间的经典著作仍然是我们减少和消除牙髓感染概念和原则的基石。他们和其他研究者证实，在没有根管感染的情况下，人类不会发生根尖周炎 [18, 225]。他们接着记录了通过预备 [26]、冲洗 [27-28]、封药 [24, 212] 等系统性方法使根管内无菌，随后进行根管充填，治疗成功率与活髓摘除术相似 [25, 213]。

11.1.2.2 根管治疗的结果

临床细菌学研究表明：可以建立一种可预测的根尖周炎治愈率的治疗方案。此外，细菌学研究支持定性消毒方法的概念：即清除感染，重建健康无菌的根尖周组织是可行的。但随后的临床试验发现实际并不能达到同等的消毒水平，即使是在相同原则下进行治疗的后续研究并不总能产生同样良好的临床和影像学结果。人们还认识到，根管中样本的培养可能会产生假阳性和假阴性结果，尤其是在使用次优技术进行取样时 [195]。对于根尖周炎的治疗而言，要获得与牙髓摘除术后根管充填相同的高成功率仍然是一个挑战。

11.2 微生物的解剖定位

11.2.1 根管系统、牙本质和牙骨质的感染

感染微生物的解剖学位置（图 11.1）是导致根管系统和根尖周组织消毒困难的主要原因。大部分微生物存在于根管系统内，即使在长期和治疗后的根尖周炎中，根管系统内的细菌也是导致炎症反应的主要原因。这些牙髓腔中的细菌应该很容易受到机械和化学预备的影响，但是根管解剖的复杂性限制了器械和药物的作用范围。此外，微生物还以生物膜的形式有规律地定植在根管内最难以到达的区域 [259]。

如果根管内感染持续存在，微生物也会侵入侧支根管并侵入根管分叉中，这会使消毒工作变得更加复杂。

感染也会累及牙本质小管。当牙根表面的牙骨质完整且充满活力时，细菌仅会穿透牙本质小管到达有限的深度。如果感染长期存在，牙周膜发生破坏时，可能导致牙骨质坏死，进而发生牙本质小管的"彻底"感染。在这种情况下，根尖孔附近的近牙周膜侧的牙本质表面通常会发生不规则的吸收，这是由于多核细胞试图去接触感染牙本质小管和根管的微生物所造成的。幸运的是，

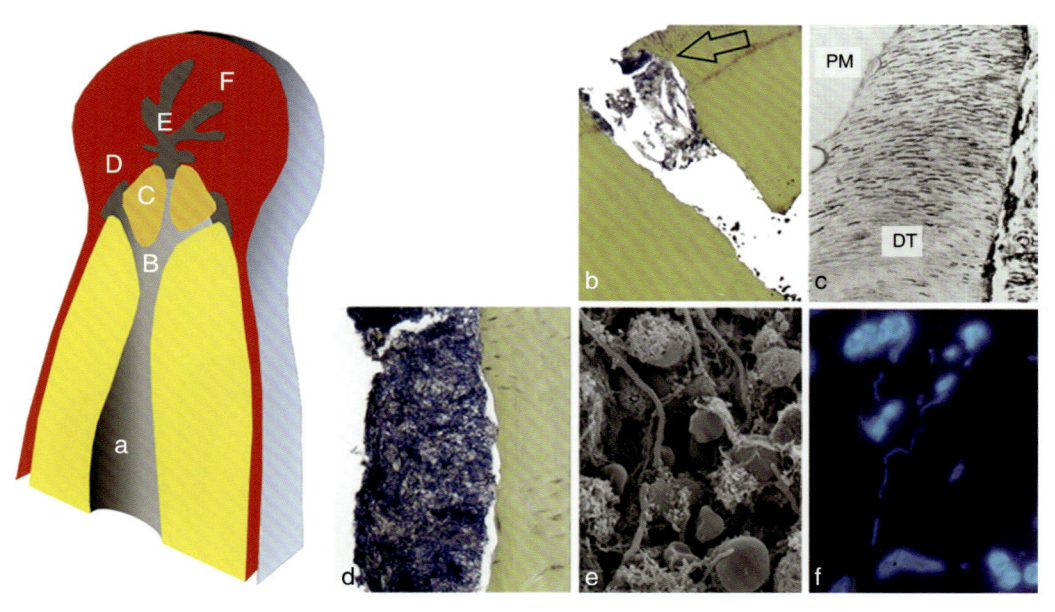

图 11.1 根尖周炎感染微生物的解剖位置。a. 大部分细菌位于髓腔内。b. 根管分支中的微生物（经许可引用 [176]）。c. 感染的牙本质小管（DT）中的细菌到达牙周膜（PM）（经许可引用 [244]）。d. 根外表面生物膜（经许可引用 [174]）。e. 肉芽肿中心的丝状菌和球菌以及红细胞（由 Pia T.Sunde 博士提供）。f. 牙髓病变结缔组织中根管外细菌的特异性荧光染色（经许可引用 [223]）

即使在广泛的根尖吸收后，成功消除感染仍然可使牙周组织得以重建[179]。

11.2.2 根外感染

现代细菌感染的概念强调细菌附着或繁殖的立足点或表面的重要性[63, 105]。皮肤、黏膜表面、血管和淋巴管内部都可以成为细菌附着的表面。在根尖处，致病性和毒性有限的细菌在周围组织中附着和增长的机会有限。在急性期，细菌毒力强于组织抵抗力，细菌与组织和免疫细胞间的相互作用导致液化和脓肿的形成。当窦道形成时，随着微生物通过窦道不断引流，感染也受到控制，但窦道的内表面可能会被细菌定植。

在慢性根尖周炎中，细菌生物膜可能会覆盖牙骨质表面[118, 134, 175]。这种生物膜类似于有钙化倾向的菌斑[165]。有理由推测，这种菌斑一旦形成，采取保守治疗消除感染不太可能成功。

脓肿、窦道和囊肿内的根管外细菌不容易受到机体的免疫防御的影响。此外，特殊类型的微生物能够在没有外部固体表面的情况下，在根尖周肉芽肿的软组织中存活[180]，如放线菌和丙酸杆菌菌落。这些细菌聚集并从内部生长，当聚集到足够多时，即使巨噬细胞对外部进行大规模攻击，也很难限制其中心区域的生长。此外，其他细胞也可能在软组织内联合起来形成集群，帮助细菌在宿主的防御中存活下来[50, 68, 180, 222–223, 238–240]。

全身性使用抗生素虽然可能会限制感染的增长和扩散，但是长期的成功率值得怀疑，因此，根尖切除手术是首选的治疗方式[177]。然而，应该注意的是，在活检证实之前，对根管外感染的临床诊断始终是一种推测。

11.2.3 根管治疗后牙齿的感染

已行根管充填的牙齿再次发生感染时，菌群可能与初次感染的菌群不同（见第4章）。第一次治疗时，根尖微环境受到干扰，根尖孔处或根尖孔外的根管充填材料提供了与原来不同的生态环境和物理表面。因此细菌能在根管充填材料、核材料和封闭剂表面生存[87]。

这可能更有利于兼性菌群的生存，其中链球菌，特别是粪肠球菌的相对数量增加[130, 278]。酵母菌也与持续性根尖周炎有关[256]，但其在治疗后疾病中占主导地位的初步发现尚未得到证实。如果治疗后炎症与根管欠填相关，残留的空间提供了一个类似于治疗前状态的环境，则定植的菌群很可能与初次感染的菌群相似。

细菌组成的差异可能是根尖周炎患牙再治疗成功率普遍低于初次治疗的原因之一[130, 226]，人们仍然尝试阐明这些感染持续存在的机制[89, 231]。然而，对不同牙髓感染的微生物菌群进行的分子生物学研究并没有显示任何明显差异[182]，总体而言，治疗后根管感染的微生物特征[274-275]与初次感染相似[191]。虽然微生物种类的相对比例也有可能存在系统性差异，但这种差异尚未有效地转化成疗效明确的差异化治疗策略。

11.3 治疗期间的细菌状态

鉴于根尖周炎的微生物病原学特点，从开髓到根管充填的整个治疗期间，监测感染的存在和程度具有重要意义。感染的过程如图 11.2 所示。"无细菌，无病变"这一已经证实的理念，因此，根管内无菌可以确保治疗成功，在根管填充时采

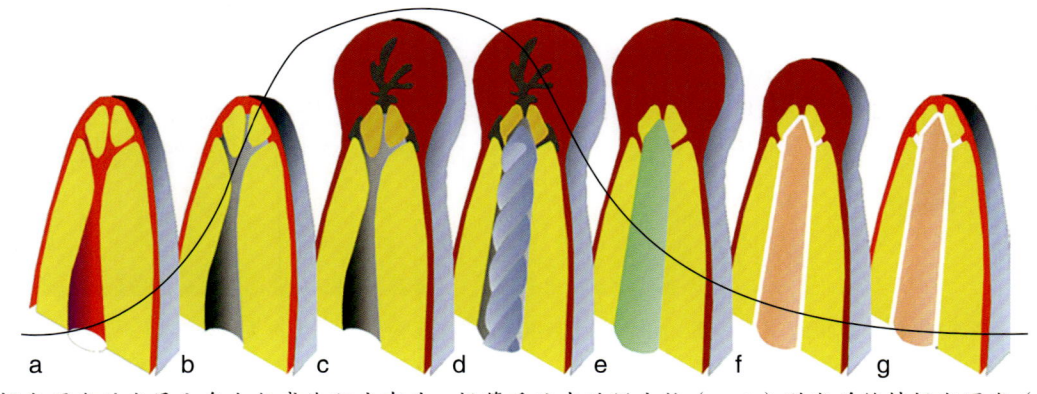

图 11.2 根尖周炎的发展和愈合与感染程度有关。根管系统中的微生物（a、b）引发并维持根尖周炎（c）。d. 机械预备。e. 冲洗和封药。f. 根管充填可充分降低感染水平，以使根尖周组织修复和再生（g）[148]

集的细菌样本不应显示任何生长迹象。

11.3.1 根管内微生物的历史与现状

细菌学样本可被视为治疗成功的替代指标，并被提倡作为根管适合充填前的常规程序[69]。然而由于多种原因，该程序在日常操作中已不再应用。原因是其操作麻烦、现有技术易于出错、且在充填阶段评估结果并不能提供准确的细菌学报告。然而，细菌取样仍然是对治疗的效果进行实验和对比研究的重要工具，根管内细菌的生长是与治疗结果直接相关的唯一病因学参数。目前，评估细菌状态的椅旁实时技术已经被研发出来，并且一些技术具有在临床实践中应用的潜力[74]。

人们有理由去评估不同技术和材料对牙本质壁的附着能力、清除坏死或活组织的能力、穿透牙本质小管的能力、限制碎屑排出的能力等，但是这些因素对根尖周炎愈合或发展的影响都次于微生物感染的效果。因此，近几十年，一种治疗期间标准化的检查感染的方法应运而生。该方法用于评估根管治疗的效果[26, 51, 153, 181, 225]。第一次进入根管时采集初始样本，这是为了确定根管确实受到感染，并且为后续样本提供参考。在治疗结束时采集第二个样本，细菌的减少或消除是衡量所用机械和（或）化学/生化方法有效性的标准。如果安排了第二次治疗，在再次就诊时采集另一份样本，以反映封药的效果；在根管充填前采集最终样本，这些样本通常标记为S1、S2、S3和S4。

样本的采集方法因患牙的临床状态而异，但基本原则是尽可能多的采集感染菌群。通常使用多个纸尖收集初始样本和根管预备后样本。在对根管充填牙齿和根管锉上牙本质碎屑取样时可以做出调整。可以取出无菌锉凹槽中的根充材料或牙本质碎屑，将其收集在培养基中生长[153, 275]。取样过程中严格遵守无菌操作可以避免假阳性样本，但是假阴性仍然是实验和临床应用中的一个重大问题：许多微生物无法用现有技术培养，生物膜可能位于远离取样点的位置。

采样技术最初记录了微生物的生长或不生长。随着生长条件的改善，灵敏度也随之提高，特别是厌氧菌。出于研究目的，取样还包括通过培养和生化方法鉴定菌属和菌种的表征。用于检测微生物遗传物质的分子生物学方法进一步提高了灵敏度。治疗结果与细菌状态之间的关联目前仍取决于培养检测到的细菌，即活的微生物。这种关联是定性的。虽然根管内微生物的数量与治疗预后可能存在某种关系，但已确定的是根管充填时可培养的细菌与预后显著相关[55, 131, 214, 246, 254]。死亡细菌或不可培养的微生物的遗传物质是否在原发性和治疗后根尖周炎的发病中发挥作用以及作用程度尚未确定，但人们普遍认为，为了维持疾病，必须具备足够数量和组织结构的活细菌[209]。

根管感染作为治疗效果替代指标的概念已应用于体外模型研究：将拔除的牙齿或牙根片段接种微生物（通常为粪肠球菌），并在实施各种机械和化学消毒程序后监测存活微生物。从此类体外研究到临床疗效验证还有很长的路要走，但该方法可能有助于发现不同产品和技术之间的效果差异，从而为利用这些变量进行临床研究提供理论依据。

11.4 治疗期间的感染控制

第10章中所概述的针对活髓、未感染牙齿的无菌基本原则和措施，也完全适用于患根尖周炎的感染牙齿，根管预备和充填的原则也相同。对感染根管进行根管治疗的另一个目的是最大限度地对根管系统进行彻底消毒，使根管在牙齿的整个生命周期内保持无菌状态。

11.4.1 局部隔离和消毒

专业技能和认知有限的从业者反复质疑使用橡皮障隔离患牙的必要性。鉴于牙髓炎和根尖周炎的感染特性，任何减少微生物感染的方法，包括使用橡皮障，都是有益的。忽略这个步骤的研究方案在伦理上是不合适的，在对使用和不使用橡皮障的治疗进行比较时，使用橡皮障的病例显示出更好的预后[116]。此外，在不使用橡皮障的治疗过程中，患者误吸或误吞尖锐器械和有害化学物质的风险更高[2]。必须准确地（通常是广泛地）去除可能藏匿细菌的修复体以及残留的龋坏牙本质，这可能需要进行复杂的牙体结构重建，以利于放置橡皮障（图11.3）。

通常采用氯己定或碘溶液消毒隔离患牙及其

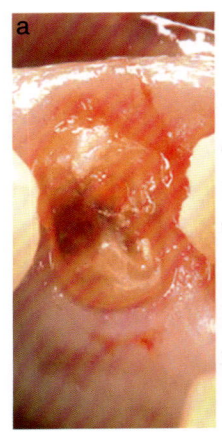

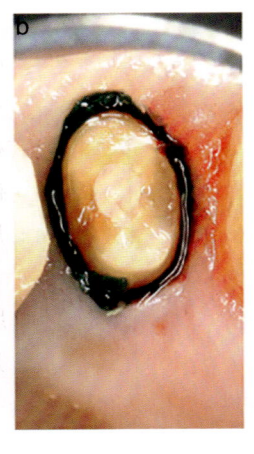

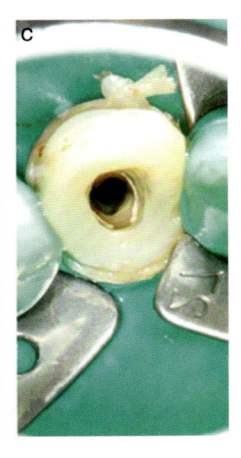

牙髓病学基础：根尖周炎的预防和治疗

图 11.3 根管治疗前重建。a. 入院时。b. 完全去除龋齿后，保护暴露的牙髓并控制出血。c. 原位粘接修复，橡胶障用夹子固定在邻牙上，以减少临时修复体上的应力（由 Nikola Petronijevic 供图）

周围环境。Möller 的研究表明，5% 碘酊与过氧化氢交替使用是有效的[133]；也有文献表明，用 3% 的过氧化氢和 2.5% 的次氯酸钠擦拭也能取得满意的消毒效果[275]。

11.4.2 机械预备

从数量上看，任何方式的机械预备，无论手用或者机用，无论不锈钢或镍钛器械，都能清除感染根管中的绝大多数微生物[26, 51, 153]。根管感染的初始负荷越大，越要付出更多努力才能最大限度地减少或彻底消除微生物[26, 275]。此外，即使细菌数量明显减少，但是残留细菌通常在所有或几乎所有仅使用机械预备的牙齿中检测到[26]。因此，需要采取补充性的抗菌措施进行有效消毒。

11.4.3 抗菌冲洗

在根管预备的过程中，冲洗液有多种用途，如溶解软组织或坏死组织，去除玷污层，润滑或润湿，开放牙本质小管等。这些功能对于治疗非常重要。牢记治疗目标，所有功能都是为了最大限度地减少根管内的微生物。

冲洗液包括了从无菌盐水到强效消毒剂。浓度为 0.5%~5.25% 的次氯酸钠溶液仍然是根管消毒的标准，它具有广谱杀菌作用，能溶解坏死组织，破坏并清除生物膜，有助于根管系统的清理[72]。浓度为 0.5%~2% 的氯己定溶液也有很强的抗菌活性，它对硬组织具有亲和性，使其在牙体组织中具有更长久的活性，但是对生物膜的效果较差[67, 72]。乙二胺四乙酸（EDTA）的抗菌活性较低，但是它能溶解和消除根管预备后的玷污层和牙本质碎屑。学者们经常提出不同的构想，并测试其在牙髓病学中的适用性。甲醛与戊二醛的抗菌效果与次氯酸钠相近，但由于其具有毒性和致癌性，已被放弃使用。经测试，其他化合物抗菌性能不如次氯酸钠，充其量只是根管消毒的辅助手段。

11.4.4 化学消毒的原理和作用机制

消毒是杀死病原微生物或使其失去活性的过程。最常见的方法是通过加热或化学方式来实现。消毒过程的一般原则，同样也适用于根管消毒。首先，消毒剂必须对病原微生物有作用效果。根尖周炎是一种非特异性疾病，所以消毒剂必须针对广谱的潜在病原体。

其次，消毒剂必须穿透相关组织并与微生物接触。这种溶液或悬浮液必须具有特殊的表面和化学特性，使其能够渗透活组织、坏死组织、生物膜和牙本质结构。

第三，消毒需要时间。消毒剂需要时间到达目标微生物，分解保护它们的细胞外基质，并破坏单个细胞。对消毒剂苯酚的经典研究表明，即使在悬浮液中，全效苯酚也需要 30min 才能杀灭大肠杆菌[82]。杀菌时间问题可能与单次就诊争议有关（见下文）。

第四，消毒剂的浓度越高，其抗微生物活性越强。然而，消毒剂的组织毒性会限制其安全使用浓度。醛类是最有效的消毒剂，但其组织毒性相对较高，因此不适合用于根管治疗[216]。由于消毒剂的活性成分可能被组织和碎片吸附，或通过化学反应而被消耗，因此，在使用过程中补充消毒剂可以维持足够的浓度，其效果类似于使用初始浓度较高但有潜在毒性的消毒剂。

第五，消毒剂可以通过物理或加热的方式活化。超声波活化通常被认为可以增强根管冲洗液的抗菌效果[139]，特别是所谓的被动超声冲洗（PUI）。用于根管冲洗的超声设备和方法已经被开发并广泛研究，但其效果可能甚微，且临床意义有限，而且对于根尖段的作用有限[252]。

11.4.5　生物力学预备原则

牙髓病学中，生物力学预备是指在充分考虑根管系统生物学和解剖学特征的基础上对根管进行机械预备。机械预备有三个目的：成形根管以利于根管充填；清除根管内残留的牙髓组织、碎屑以及微生物；促进冲洗液的抗菌作用。后两个目的直接与消除病原微生物的最终治疗目标相联系。

器械标准化　牙髓病学中，将根管预备器械和根管充填材料相协调有着悠久的历史。20世纪50年代[81]，Ingle提倡标准化，并在国际标准中确立了2%的基础锥度，20世纪70年代，在临床数据的支持下，Kerekes与Tronstad[91-94]重新提出了这一概念。对于大部分根管（但不是所有），都可以在根尖3~5mm的区域进行圆形预备以达到标准的根尖尺寸，并清除牙髓组织和感染的牙本质碎屑。标准化技术也显示出与传统的逐步后退技术同样良好的临床效果，甚至得到更好的效果[90, 94]。2%的锥度适合手用器械，可避免器械在冠方与根管壁广泛接触，从而防止了器械卡顿和折裂的风险，同时能对根尖部牙本质壁进行有效清除。

大锥度已被广泛用于机用器械，标准化手用器械的一个明显缺点是可能过度扩大根尖部分，有造成台阶和穿孔的风险。逐步后退技术[257]降低了这一风险，但是会产生与预制充填材料不相符的非标准化根尖预备。理论上，具有较大或者变化锥度的、旋转和往复运动器械所预备出的根管，能够使用相应尺寸的充填材料完全充填，从而将两种经典手用器械预备技术的理论优势结合起来。

机械效率　器械的切削能力取决于它的尺寸和与根管壁接触的能力，通常是通过扫描电镜进行测试[29, 77, 135, 159, 168, 190, 200, 248]，近来也通过微型计算机断层扫描[17, 22, 35, 49, 157-158, 162-164, 247, 279]来检测。虽然结果各不相同，一些器械系统的性能可能优于其他的系统，但结果普遍显示，预备器械没有接触到根管表面的大部分区域（30%~50%）。因此，在根尖周炎的治疗过程中，单靠机械预备并不能确保消毒的效果。在细菌对照临床研究中，不使用消毒剂时，大多数牙齿在机械预备后仍然处于感染状态[26, 153]。

促进消毒　机械预备通过促进消毒剂与生物膜的接触来增强消毒活性，声波和超声波设备则能够活化消毒剂。目前，将超声波直接作用于牙本质并不是首选的方法，超声波活化消毒剂主要是通过被动超声波激活来完成的，在这种情况下，仪器不应该接触牙本质壁。任何手用和机用的预备技术，都会使冲洗液向牙本质壁和根尖方向流动。随着更多的碎屑和感染物质的被机械预备所清除，消毒剂与残留微生物之间的距离变短，残留的细菌数量也随之减少。这些因素促成了根尖预备的基本原则：在不损害根尖完整性的情况下，应该尽可能将根尖预备到较大尺寸。这将更有可能消灭根尖三角区的大部分细菌，并促进冲洗液扩散到器械不易到达的区域[153]，从而提高愈合率和愈合速度[127]。相反的观点是，过度预备会削弱牙根，使其更易于产生微裂，从而导致根折，同时也具有很高的穿孔风险。

11.4.6　根管封药

为了治疗根尖周炎，根管内被放置了各种各样的物质，其中包括木榴油、甲醛、戊二醛、碘仿、氯胺、甲酚、甚至是放射性物质[137]。考虑到毒性、致癌性以及缺乏可证明的有效性，大多数药物已被排除。

20世纪60年代到70年代初期，根尖周炎的感染性得到证实[85, 225, 235-236]，但是封药能够辅助提高宿主愈合能力的观念一直存在。Cvek的开创性研究[43-48]表明，氢氧化钙糊剂有两方面作用：减少或消除牙齿中的细菌生长；未成熟牙齿在经过长期封药后（数月至一年以上），可形成硬组织屏障（根尖诱导成形术），从而达到愈合。

甲醛和樟脑氯苯酚化合物曾经被常规用作封药，部分原因是其良好的抗菌性和组织毒性比[216]。碘化钾比氯苯酚更有效，但其作用时间短，仅能在 2~4d 内短期使用。当对比试验表明氢氧化钙作为封药优于樟脑氯苯酚[24]和碘化钾时[189]，氢氧化钙成为诊间封药的首选药物。

氢氧化钙一开始就被认为是一种能够促进愈合的有效消毒剂。应用氢氧化钙封药数月，观察窦道愈合情况，疼痛不适的消除情况以及病变缩小的影像学表现。由于 3 个月内病变的愈合很难评估[95]，因此将 3 个月作为这种治疗方式的标准持续时间。但这样把重点转移到了强调抗菌效果上。通过微生物学监测，氢氧化钙实现抗菌效果的时间从数月[47]缩短到 4 周[24]，最终缩短到 7d[212]。在初次治疗结束时使用氢氧化钙 10min，没有观察到比冲洗更好的效果[212]。

11.4.7 单次和多次就诊的感染控制

封药周期的基本原理首先是将基于根管感染的替代测量作为预测成功的指标；其次是充填时根管内无细菌可以提高愈合率。随后的几项研究[1, 31, 37, 51, 84, 123-124, 126, 140, 155]采用了类似的方法优化消毒过程[161, 173, 181, 184-185, 201, 206, 254, 258, 264, 270]（图 11.4），但是事实证明，很难建立一个可预测的根管内细菌清除的方案。相反，氢氧化钙封药增加抗菌效果的重要性遭到质疑[107, 161]。如果封药不能将感染控制改善到具有临床意义的水平，那么在此期间使用临时填充物可能会带来新的感染风险，且这种风险可能超过封药的益处[275]。

单次就诊治疗根尖周炎可以节约时间和成本，大量精心设计的临床随机对照试验已经完成，这些试验比较了单次或两次法治疗后的短期和长期临床结果，其中包括有症状和无症状的根尖周炎病例。正如所预期的那样，各个临床实验结果存在差异，有的试验支持两次法治疗[186, 241]，有的试验支持单次法治疗[61]，还有许多试验发现没有显著性差异[21, 64, 262, 266, 268]。似乎可以得到这样的结论：就治疗后的主观（疼痛和镇痛药的使用）以及客观（影像学）愈合迹象而言，这两种治疗方法几乎没有差异。几乎所有关于有症状和无症状根尖周炎的系统评价中都反复证明了这一结论[59, 193-194, 197, 221, 267]。

虽然临床和传统影像学标准是判定成功的实用标准，但是组织病理学表现和 CBCT 在检测差异时更为敏感。来自动物[76-88]和人[245]的实验数据表明：氢氧化钙封药后，检测到的细菌更少，愈合效果更好，一项使用 CBCT 进行评估的随机研究表明，经过两次法治疗的患牙病变范围减小程度更大[52]。

控制成功治疗患牙所需的时间和精力是符合各方的利益的。无论如何，为了最大限度地减少根管内细菌，延长封药时间是无可争议的。但要实现完全无菌可能需要多次复诊或更长的间隔期[24]，且确定无菌的方案很复杂[138]。鉴于系统回顾和 meta 分析的结果，为了达到传统的临床和影像学成功的标准，将两次或多次就诊作为标准治疗方案变得越来越困难。当存在时间限制或特殊临床考虑时，氢氧化钙封药仍然是有效的措施。

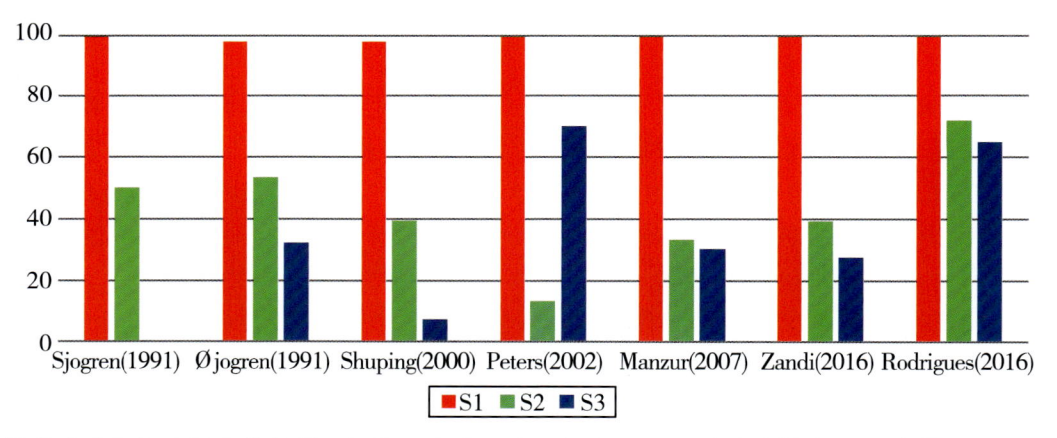

图 11.4 根管治疗期间的微生物控制。细菌阳性病例的百分比。S1. 开髓时的样本。S2. 在第一阶段的预备和冲洗之后的样本。S3. 用氢氧化钙进行诊间封药后的样本（数据引自文献 123、153、161、201、212、275。Zandi 和 Rodriguez 的数据来自分子技术和再治疗病例）

11.4.8 特殊技术

人们正在寻求和开发使用硬质锉进行机械预备的替代方法（见第10章）。学者们研发了一种"非器械"的根管清洁方法：开髓后在牙齿上建立一个密封环境，通过负压或可调节压力激活冲洗液来清洁根管[119-120]。这一概念的最新进展已在慢性根尖周炎病例中进行了体外和临床试验，在减少细菌和临床放射学方面均取得了良好的效果[32, 73, 132, 202-203, 261, 265]，但目前仍缺乏与其他技术的随机对照临床研究。

11.5 根管充填

11.5.1 根管充填的目的和作用

根管充填的主要目的是预防根管系统的再感染。实现这个目标有两种方式：一种是阻止微生物进入；另一种是在微生物穿透材料屏障时将其消灭。第一种方法取决于材料的完整性和它与牙本质的密合程度。第二种要求材料具备某种生物活性，这又取决于材料的溶解性。材料的抗菌特性也可能有助于通过生物力学方法对根管系统进行消毒[149]。

对于根尖孔闭合的成熟牙齿，充填材料与软组织的接触面积非常小，生物相容性显得不那么重要。然而，在牙髓暴露、穿孔、手术等情况下，材料和软组织的接触面积增大。此时，材料必须具有支持或促进相关组织愈合或再生的特性[60]，同时具有抑菌性。

满足临床要求的根管材料必须具备的三个特性：封闭性、抗菌性和生物相容性。此外，还必须具备优良的可操作性和耐久性[70]。

根管充填物的特性主要取决于封闭剂。大量文献描述了各种类型封闭剂的理化特性。一些临床对照研究比较了封闭剂的长期性能，差异并不显著[56, 78, 150, 152, 255]。然而，一些新产品的长期效果出现失败[14, 263]，这提醒医生在接受和推广新方法和新材料的过程中需要保持警惕。

核心材料应该被设计成具有惰性和稳定性，但必须具有一定的可塑性以适应预备后的根管。它们相当于封闭剂的活塞，决定了根管充填的功能特性。表11.1列举了一些用于根管充填的封闭剂材料。

11.5.2 抗菌性能

抗菌性能常常伴随着一定程度的组织毒性[217-218]，因此，研发具有强抗菌特性的封闭剂材料的需求有限。然而，大多数产品在凝固前具有抗菌作用，很多产品在凝固后或进入牙本质小管后仍有抗菌活性[39, 86, 167, 169]；在封闭剂中添加抗菌成分很常见[11, 16, 38, 187]。生物陶瓷封闭剂可在局部产生强碱性环境，可作为微生物生长的长效抑制剂[4, 260]。

表 11.1 糊剂类型、样品和临床试验

材料	亚类	样品	根尖周炎病例临床试验
氧化锌丁香油类		ProcoSol, Roth 811	Eriksen 等人 (1988)[56] Trope 等人 (1999)[241]
树脂类	环氧树脂	AH26, AH plus	Conner 等人 (2007)[14]
	甲基丙烯酸树脂	EndoRez, RealSeal	Barborka 等人 (2017)[14]
氢氧化钙类		Apexit, Sealapex	Waltimo 等人 (2001)[255]
硅酮类		RoekoSeal, GuttaFlow	Huumonen 等人 (2003)[78]
陶瓷类	钙-硅	BioRoot	
	钙-硅-磷	Endosequence	
牙胶尖	β 相	generic	
	α 相	GuttaFusion, GuttaCore, Herofill	
树脂核	全树脂	Resilon	Barborka 等人 (2017)[14]
	树脂衣	EndoRez, Endosequence	

11.5.3 生物学特性

根管封闭剂需要被组织所耐受,即使它们在凝固前可能具有很强的细胞毒性,但大多数在凝固后都很温和[117, 146-147, 280]。生物陶瓷封闭剂有刺激组织修复的作用[34, 269],这在与牙周组织接触面积较大的情况下很有意义,如根管倒充填、穿孔修补时[149]。

11.5.4 根管充填基本临床指南

根尖止点 虽然根管充填物的根尖止点位置对牙髓摘除术病例的预后影响不大[213],但是从后续的研究中可以清楚地发现,它对于根尖周炎的治疗至关重要[142, 145, 213](图11.5)。从影像学上讲,这意味着在感染病例中,根管充填物的末端应该在距离影像学根尖孔0~2mm处,这可能反映了大部分感染位于根尖狭窄的冠方。

根尖预备宽度 一些治疗理念主张将根尖预备至较大尺寸,以尽可能多地去除感染牙本质[31, 94];其他学者认为,根据测量的实际根尖宽度来选择终末锉的号数很重要[143, 257],同时可以避免出现台阶和穿孔的风险(图11.6)。关于根尖预备宽度的临床重要性的数据很少。大样本病例研究显示,充分预备的方法可以获得成功的结果[94, 152],其他人则报道使用逐步后退这种保守的根尖预备

技术可以取得良好甚至更好的效果[143]。无论选择何种方法,临床医生都应意识到,有病变的感染牙齿的根尖孔直径通常都比活髓牙齿大[62]。

通畅性 通畅性的观念是存在争议的[79]。用小号锉反复疏通根管至根尖孔以保持根尖通畅,似乎有利于冲洗液进入根尖的大部分区域。同时,可以防止感染碎屑堆积,有利于形成良好的根尖封闭。有数据表明,通畅性可能对预后产生积极影响[108, 128, 142, 230]。该操作有将感染物质运送到根尖周区域的风险,有可能会对病情发展及长期预后产生负面影响[80, 121, 128]。似乎可以得出这样的结论:如果在特定情况下需要保持根管通畅,则应使用较小号的锉(8#或10#的ISO标准器械),且适用于根尖孔足够大,能够允许根管锉畅通无阻通过的病例[79]。

充填密实性 通过根尖片的均匀程度评估根管充填质量,充填密实性似乎会影响根尖周炎患牙根管充填后的预后[94],但是不同研究的结果各不相同,可能对再治疗有特殊意义[142, 213]。

冠方封闭 治疗的长期疗效还取决于冠方修复的质量[101, 103-104, 171, 215, 237]。延伸至边缘骨水平下的严密冠方封闭与根尖周炎发生率较低相关[219];同时可以防止牙周袋内的细菌从侧根管和暴露的牙本质小管进入充填后的根管。

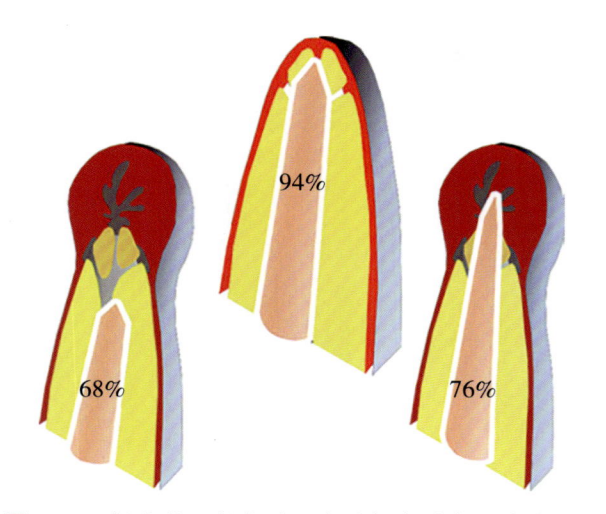

图11.5 根充物至根尖的距离对根尖周炎治疗结果的关键影响。根充物在距影像学根尖2mm范围内,结果类似于活髓牙根管充填。根充欠填或超填会大大降低成功率(改编更改自文献213)

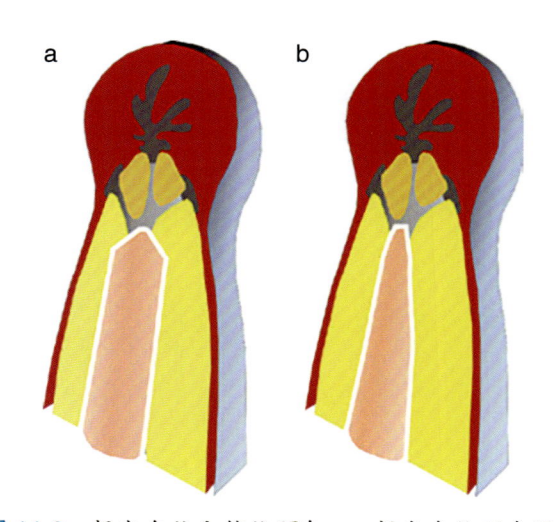

图11.6 根尖盒状和锥状预备。a. 根尖盒状理念强调大锥度预备,以最大限度地去除感染的牙本质,易于消毒剂进入。b. 锥形预备是为了更好地顺应原始根管形态

11.6 原发性根尖周炎诊断和治疗中的临床问题

成功消毒和有效填充可以使感染根管达到与活髓摘除术一样的成功率[94, 152, 213]。然而，在某些情况下，消毒变得相当困难或不可能，并且感染会引起一些在活髓切断术中不会遇到的特殊问题。

11.6.1 牙折

如果存在累及牙髓并且延伸到牙龈边缘的折裂或隐裂，则无法预测根管治疗的效果。根管消毒和充填可能会暂时掩盖症状，但微生物最终会沿着裂缝侵入并重新引发感染和炎症。

11.6.2 边缘性牙周炎

牙周牙髓联合病变（图 11.7）已经被广泛讨论和回顾[3, 196, 277]。牙髓状态决定了根管治疗方案：牙髓比较敏感表明不能诊断为根尖周炎。然而，如果牙周袋与根尖区域或根充物相交通，牙菌斑中的细菌就会持续侵入造成持续性根尖炎症。虽然有来源于牙周袋的牙髓感染的病例报告[276]，但这种情况很少见，通常不会影响根尖周炎根管治疗的成功。然而，在某些病例中，深牙周袋的继发感染可能会导致治疗后根尖周炎的发生[188]。

11.6.3 恶化

患者的主观症状通常在预备消毒后会迅速消退，但是该操作有引起感染急性加重的风险。根管内环境的改变可能有利于毒性更强的微生物的生长，超出根尖孔的器械可能会将微生物传播到根管外区域，导致短暂的疼痛，甚至剧痛的临床症状。治疗程序遵循急性口腔感染的一般处理原则，活髓摘除术一般不会发生明显的诊间疼痛[9]，这也证明了感染是所谓的急性发作的唯一原因，而不是过度预备所带来的物理效应或者冲洗液所带来的化学刺激[208, 210]。

11.6.4 解剖变异

同一牙根内根管间的峡部是感染物质持续存在的来源[98]，因此需要尽可能清洁和消毒这些区域[5, 54, 205]。简单类型的牙内陷很容易通过传统方法治疗（图 11.8），而更复杂的牙内陷则需要手术和其他辅助治疗的联合。

11.6.5 系统性疾病的影响

患有慢性疾病患者的愈合模式可能与健康个体不同。他们的病情也更容易恶化。比较典型的是糖尿病。根尖周炎似乎在糖尿病患者中发生率更高，治疗后的愈合也更慢[75, 113, 192, 199, 228]。

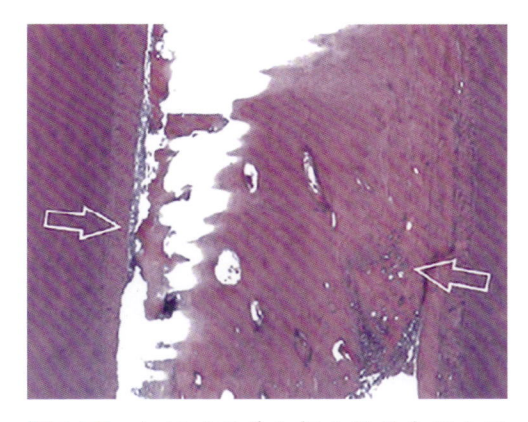

图 11.7 组织病理学分析人类牙齿再生治疗后，根管内产生的组织。图为根管中三分之一。根管被新形成的钙化组织部分占据（箭头之间；原图放大 950 倍）[115]（经许可引用）

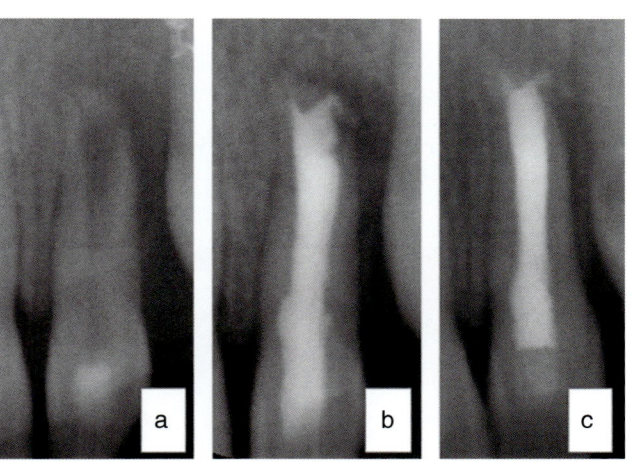

图 11.8 尽管根尖解剖高度不规则，但内陷牙的根尖周炎仍可以成功治疗。a. 入院时。b. 术后即刻。c. 5 个月的随访（由 Line Hardersen 博士提供）

11.7 持续性或复发性根尖周炎的治疗

再治疗病例中的所有治疗程序与原发性根尖周炎相同，但根管充填物的存在使问题变得复杂。根充物本身、封闭剂或核心材料可能是生物膜形成的基质，生物膜通常出现在充填材料和牙本质壁之间的界面上[178]。与残留根充材料相关的残留细菌很难被接触和消除，因此，清除所有根充材料至关重要。

11.7.1 根充材料的去除和根管预备

多种类型的旋转或手用器械可用于清除根材料。H锉是常用的手动方法[30, 83, 96, 125, 204, 272]，许多机用锉系统（包括旋转和往复运动器械）也用于根充材料的去除。

化学溶剂有助于去除牙胶。氯仿效果很好，但有毒且有潜在致癌性[229]。二甲苯也非常有效，但是也有毒。柠檬烯和橙油是从柑橘类水果中提取的物质，可以在市场上买到[170, 242, 243]，其效果虽然不如二甲苯和氯仿，但它的挥发性和毒性也更小。

鉴于封闭剂中含有各种化合物和化学成分，这些材料没有通用的溶剂。本质上，必须依靠机械程序才能最大限度地去除封闭剂，但是按照目前的方法，完全去除封闭剂几乎不可能[10]。

11.7.2 复发性根尖周炎的生物膜

与根充材料有关的细菌和物理清除残留物的困难解释了再治疗预后不佳的原因[19,141,144-145]。这也有助于解释对充填质量较差的根管行再治疗具有更好的预后[53]，因为材料更容易去除，且感染微生物主要存留在之前未充填的根管区域。

有人提出，持续性病变中的微生物组成不同于原发性根尖周炎（见第4章）。虽然可能存在更多兼性细菌，特别是链球菌和肠球菌，但是到目前为止，针对这些微生物来加强再治疗消毒过程的尝试[8, 129, 211, 227]还没有产生被验证的临床方案。

在根尖外感染中，细菌可在根尖孔以外的组织中定植[68, 165, 174, 175, 180, 183, 224, 238, 240]，并超出药物的作用范围。使用抗生素治疗此类病例的尝试并没有显示出可靠的愈合效果[15]，因此，通常采取根尖手术治疗[180]。

11.8 未成熟恒牙根尖周炎的治疗

采用传统方法能够成功治疗根尖孔开放的未成熟牙齿的根尖周炎，氢氧化钙封药可诱导硬组织形成[48]。然而，治疗后的牙齿根管壁薄，容易发生折裂。有口腔外伤史的儿童发生新外伤的风险会增加[166]。在使用抗生素糊剂治疗患有根尖周炎的未成熟牙齿中发现硬组织形成（图11.9），这有助于提升此类牙齿的抗折性[13]，并促进了对再生牙髓病学的广泛研究（见第8章）。

11.8.1 术语

与牙科中其他再生或组织工程方法一样，治疗程序尚未达到可以预测结果的标准化程序。此外，治疗涉及的许多生物学过程尚不清楚[99]，治疗的临床目标往往模糊不清。所涉及的细胞及激活机制已在第8章中详细阐述。在未成熟牙齿根尖周炎病例中，主要目标是刺激根尖发育[66]，以增加牙根长度和强度。其他方法也能

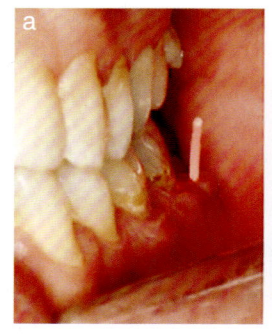

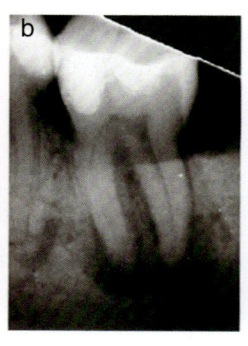

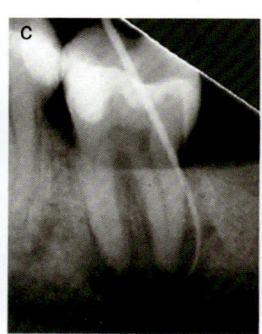

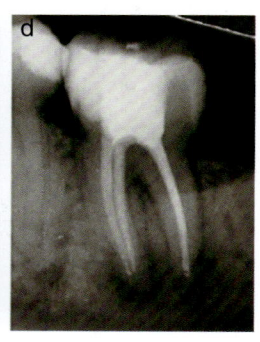

图11.9 a.将牙胶尖插入左下第二磨牙的颊部牙周袋。b.可见弥散透射影。c.示踪至远中根的根尖。d.根管治疗后12个月，病变已愈合（Dyveke Knudsen博士供图）

达到这个目的，氢氧化钙封药是标准步骤，如今，单次就诊时应用生物陶瓷材料也能得到类似的效果[41]。

牙髓血运重建是应用于无髓牙齿的最简单和生物学要求最低的治疗方法。首次尝试于1961年[154]，其目的是使血管化组织长入根管内，支持和促进根尖成形和发育[6]。牙髓血运重建是修复或再生的第一步。

当根管内形成了具有功能性成牙本质细胞的活髓组织时，可以说发生了真正意义上的再生。这充其量仍处于实验阶段，临床实践的实际目标是通过诱导根管内某种硬组织的形成而达到生物性修复。如果与前期牙本质结合，牙根可能通过类骨质组织加强，但是目前尚未实现与前期牙本质结合的新牙本质（图11.10）。

11.8.2 病例选择

第一例有明显硬组织形成的病例发生在无外伤史、有畸形中央尖的前磨牙[13]。龋坏会影响咬合面牙釉质的卷曲，由此引发的根尖周炎对再生治疗的反应可能优于创伤牙[114]，因为创伤牙通常伴随其他牙体组织损害。如果根尖诱导成形术（图11.11）或牙根成形术是治疗的主要临床目的，那么应用氢氧化钙和生物陶瓷材料，并结合常规充填冠部髓腔的经典治疗方案能够获得良好的预后[41]。

11.9 愈合监测和预后

第6章概述了根管治疗患牙的预后及其影响因素。许多随访研究并没有将初始根尖健康和有病变患牙的结果分开。虽然人们可能认为大多数因素对所有诊断都是共通的，但众所周知，有些因素只与术前病变有关，如根充物的根尖止点[213]。

根尖周炎的愈合主要体现在三个方面：疼痛缓解、临床症状（肿胀和窦道）消除以及骨组织替代病变软组织的影像学评估。此外，牙齿的存活率通常被用来记录治疗的临床成功率。

11.9.1 症状和体征

如果一开始就有症状和体征，大多数治疗方案通常能够使其减轻或消除，但在高达10%的病例中仍可能持续存在或发展[143]。由于炎症和（或）切断牙髓神经导致神经系统发生了一些变化，从而导致牙神经灵敏度改变，但有些轻微或有症状的牙齿可能隐藏着导致炎症的残留感染。

11.9.2 影像学监测

大多数关于根尖周炎患牙治疗结果的研究都特别关注影像学愈合。经典的成功/失败分析是利用术前根尖X线片和对照组X线片进行比较，但是强调硬骨板和正常牙周结构重建的重要性[143]。这些所谓的Strindberg标准[220]经过修改后，已被广泛使用。X线片的解读很容易受到

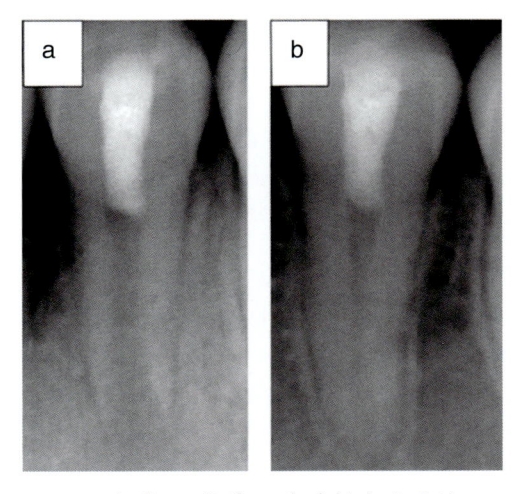

图 11.10 a.患牙35术前X线片根尖孔开放。b.术后12个月X线片。与术前图像相比，根管长度增加和管壁增厚[110]（经许可引用）

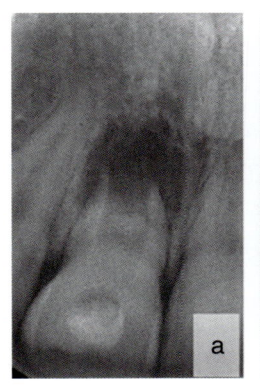

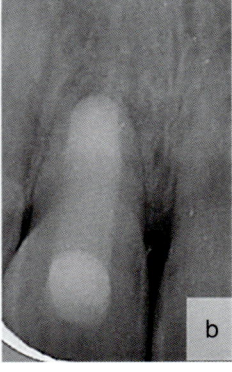

图 11.11 根尖诱导成形术。a.感染根管经过预备和大量冲洗，然后用氢氧化钙封药。b.在根尖部填充4mm的MTA，冠部树脂充填进行修复。15年的随访X线片显示牙齿硬组织形成，并形成完整的牙周膜[172]（经许可引用）

个人偏见的影响，对成功/失败的评判也不例外[65]。根尖周指数（PAI）[151]是一种通过将实验、影像和组织学证据[23]联系起来减少偏倚的方法，近年来被广泛使用。

不论采用何种评分系统，观察员都必须接受培训和校准，以便结果在时间和地域上具有可比性。此类校准应该标准化，并与公认的健康或疾病状态的影像相关联。很少有研究进行全球化校准，因此，在将一项研究结果与其他研究进行比较时必须谨慎。

11.9.3　CBCT

CBCT对根尖周疾病的检测更为敏感和准确（见第5章）。PAI分数与病损体积的比较显示出明显且显著的相关性，但同一项研究强调了二维根尖片与三维的CBCT影像相比的局限性[122]。此外，用于记录根尖病损的CBCT指数已被提出[57, 233]，这对比较不同研究结果有重要意义。

治疗的随访数据表明，在使用CBCT评估时，很多传统根尖片认为已经被治愈的患牙可能存在残留病变，其他因素可能与预后相关[111]。传统根尖片观察到的预后相关因素仍然存在，但是它们不能被自动转移到CBCT的类似研究中。此外，至少在手术病例中，CBCT检测到的一些病变可能是纤维化组织，而不是感染或炎症组织[106]。

11.9.4　患牙保存率

保存率是对根管治疗后患牙进行随访时的一种粗略的衡量方法。它经常用于比较根管治疗和其他治疗方法的研究，如种植[33, 234]。然而，根管治疗后牙齿保存率并不仅仅反映根管治疗本身，它在很大程度上取决于牙周状况和冠部牙体组织的丧失程度[12]。评估患牙的保存率对制定治疗计划至关重要，尤其是复杂的临床病例，但根尖周炎的治疗通常是非常成功的，因为该指标很少成为决策的决定性因素。

11.10　小结

11.10.1　病例选择和治疗决策的原则

预防胜于治疗。对于牙髓病学和其他疾病都是如此。尽管很多病变较大的患牙治疗[143]获得成功，但这并没有改变这样一个事实：即在所有前瞻性研究中，活髓摘除后进行根管充填的患牙预后明显更好[36]。根尖周病变越大，患牙预后越差[58, 102]。传统的、观望式的根管治疗方式在最终开始治疗时，存在预后降低的巨大风险。此外，CBCT检测出的病变数量大约是根尖片的两倍[111]，这放大了术前根尖周炎和非根尖周炎患牙间的预后差异。

此外，再治疗的预后普遍较差[213, 232]，这表明需要对牙髓炎和原发性根尖周炎进行高质量的根管治疗。在使用传统根尖片评价无根尖病损的患牙时，牙科学生[94, 152]和专家[143]通常会获得90%以上的成功率，因此，早期干预结合严格的灭菌、彻底的消毒和严密的充填技术是全面提升根尖周病变预后的关键。

参考文献

[1] Adl A, et al. Clinical investigation of the effect of calcium hydroxide intracanal dressing on bacterial lipopolysaccharide reduction from infected root canals. Aust Endod J, 2015, 41: 12–16.

[2] Ahmad I A. Rubber dam usage for endodontic treatment: a review. Int Endod J, 2009, 42: 963–972.

[3] Al-Fouzan K S. A new classification of endodontic-periodontal lesions. Int J Dent, 2014: 919173.

[4] Al-Haddad A, Che Ab Aziz Z A. Bioceramic-based root canal sealers: a review. Int J Biomater, 2016: 9753210.

[5] Alves F R, et al. Adjunctive steps for disinfection of the mandibular molar root canal system: a correlative bacteriologic, micro-computed tomography, and cryopulverization approach. J Endod, 2016, 42: 1667–1672.

[6] Araújo P R S, et al. Pulp revascularization: a literature review. The Open Dentistry Journal, 2017, 10: 48–56.

[7] Areai D M, et al. Self-reported oral health, dental self-care and dental service use among New Zealand secondary school students: findings from the Youth 07 study. N Z Dent J, 2011, 107: 121–126.

[8] Athanassiadis B, Abbott P V, Walsh L J. The use of calcium hydroxide, antibiotics and biocides as antimicrobial medicaments in endodontics. Aust Dent J, 2007, 52: S64–82.

[9] Azim A A, Azim K A, Abbott P V. Prevalence of inter-appointment endodontic flare-ups and host-related factors. Clin Oral Investig, 2017, 21: 889–894.

[10] Bago I, et al. Comparison of the effectiveness of various rotary and reciprocating systems with different surface treatments to remove gutta-percha and an epoxy resin-based

sealer from straight root canals. Int Endod J, 2018.
[11] Bailon-Sanchez M E, et al. Antibacterial and anti-biofilm activity of AH plus with chlorhexidine and cetrimide. J Endod, 2014, 40: 977–981.
[12] Balto K. Tooth survival after root canal treatment. Evid Based Dent, 2011, 12: 10–11.
[13] Banchs F, Trope M. Revascularization of immature permanent teeth with apical periodontitis: new treatment protocol? J Endod, 2004, 30: 196–200.
[14] Barborka B J, et al. Long-term clinical outcome of teeth obturated with resilon. J Endod, 2017, 43: 556–560.
[15] Barnett F, et al. Ciprofloxacin treatment of periapical Pseudomonas aeruginosa infection. Endod Dent Traumatol, 1988, 4: 132–137.
[16] Barros J, et al. Antibiofilm effects of endodontic sealers containing quaternary ammonium polyethylenimine nanoparticles. J Endod, 2014, 40: 1167–1171.
[17] Belladonna F G, et al. Microcomputed tomography shaping abilityassessment of the new blue thermal treated reciproc instrument. J Endod, 2018, 44: 1146–1150.
[18] Bergenholtz G. Micro-organisms from necrotic pulp of traumatized teeth. Odontol Revy, 1974, 25: 347–358.
[19] Bergenholtz G, et al. Retreatment of endodontic fillings. Scand J Dent Res, 1979, 87: 217–224.
[20] Berlin-Broner Y, Febbraio M, Levin L. Association between apical periodontitis and cardiovascular diseases: a systematic review of the literature. Int Endod J, 2017, 50: 847–859.
[21] Bharuka S B, Mandroli P S. Single-versus two-visit pulpectomy treatment in primary teeth with apical periodontitis: A double-blind, parallel group, randomized controlled trial. J Indian Soc Pedod Prev Dent, 2016, 34: 383–390.
[22] Brasil S C, et al. Canal transportation, unprepared areas, and dentin removal after preparation with BTRaCe and ProTaper next systems. J Endod, 2017, 43: 1683–1687.
[23] Brynolf I. A histological and roentgenological study of the periapical region of human upper incisors. Odontologisk revy, Supplement, 1967, 11: 176s.
[24] Byström A, Claesson R, Sundqvist G. The antibacterial effect of camphorated paramonochlorophenol, camphorated phenol and calcium hydroxide in the treatment of infected root canals. Endod Dent Traumatol, 1985, 1: 170–175.
[25] Byström A, et al. Healing of periapical lesions of pulpless teeth after endodontic treatment with controlled asepsis. Endod Dent Traumatol, 1987, 3: 58–63.
[26] Byström A, Sundqvist G. Bacteriologic evaluation of the efficacy of mechanical root canal instrumentation in endodontic therapy. Scand J Dent Res, 1981, 89: 321–328.
[27] Byström A, Sundqvist G. Bacteriologic evaluation of the effect of 0.5 percent sodium hypochlorite in endodontic therapy. Oral Surgery, Oral Medicine, Oral Pathology, Oral Radiology, 1983, 55: 307–312.
[28] Byström A, Sundqvist G. The antibacterial action of sodium hypochlorite and EDTA in 60 cases of endodontic therapy. International Endodontic Journal, 1985, 18: 35–40.
[29] Cameron J A. Factors affecting the clinical efficiency of ultrasonic endodontics: a scanning electron microscopy study. Int Endod J, 1995, 28: 47–53.
[30] Canali L C F, et al. Comparison of efficiency of the retreatment procedure between Wave One Gold and Wave One systems by Micro-CT and confocal microscopy: an in vitro study. Clin Oral Investig, 2018 .
[31] Card S J, et al. The effectiveness of increased apical enlargement in reducing intracanal bacteria. J Endod, 2002. 28: 779–783.
[32] Charara K, et al. Assessment of apical extrusion during root canal irrigation with the novel gentlewave system in a simulated apical environment. J Endod, 2016, 42: 135–139.
[33] Chatzopoulos G S, et al. Implant and root canal treatment: Survival rates and factors associated with treatment outcome. J Dent, 2018, 71: 61–66.
[34] Chen I, et al. Healing after root-end microsurgery by using mineral trioxide aggregate and a new calcium silicate-based bioceramic material as root-end filling materials in dogs. J Endod, 2015, 41: 389–399.
[35] Cheung L H, Cheung G S. Evaluation of a rotary instrumentation method for C-shaped canals with microcomputed tomography. J Endod, 2008, 34: 1233–1238.
[36] Chugal N, et al. Endodontic treatment outcomes. Dent Clin North Am, 2017, 61: 59–80.
[37] Cohenca N, et al. Microbiological evaluation of different irrigation protocols on root canal disinfection in teeth with apical periodontitis: an in vivo study. Braz Dent J, 2013, 24: 467–473.
[38] Collares F M, et al. Methacrylatebased root canal sealer containing chlorexidine and alpha-tricalcium phosphate. J Biomed Mater Res B Appl Biomater, 2018, 106: 1439–1443.
[39] Colombo M, et al. Biological and physico-chemical properties of new root canal sealers. J Clin Exp Dent, 2018, 10: e120–126.
[40] Conner D A, et al. Clinical outcome of teeth treated endodontically with a nonstandardized protocol and root filled with resilon. J Endod, 2007, 33: 1290–1292.
[41] Corbella S, et al. Apexification, apexogenesis and regenerative endodontic procedures: a review of the literature. Minerva Stomatol, 2014, 63: 375–389.
[42] Cotti E, et al. The perioperative dental screening and management of patients undergoing cardiothoracic, vascular surgery and other cardiovascular invasive procedures: A systematic review. Eur J Prev Cardiol, 2017, 24: 409–425.

[43] Cvek M. Treatment of non-vital permanent incisors with calcium hydroxide. I. Follow-up of periapical repair and apical closure of immature roots. Odontol Revy, 1972, 23: 27–44.

[44] Cvek M. Treatment of non-vital permanent incisors with calcium hydroxide. II. Effect on external root resorption in luxated teeth compared with effect of root filling with guttapercha. A follow-up. Odontol Revy, 1973, 24: 343–354.

[45] Cvek M. Treatment of non-vital permanent incisors with calcium hydroxide. IV. Periodontal healing and closure of the root canal in the coronal fragment of teeth with intra-alveolar fracture and vital apical fragment. A follow-up. Odontol Revy, 1974, 25: 239–246.

[46] Cvek M, Granath L E, Hollender L. Treatment of non-vital permanent incisors with calcium hydroxide. 3. Variation of occurrence of ankylosis of reimplanted teeth with duration of extraalveolar period and storage environment. Odontol Revy, 1974, 25: 43–56.

[47] Cvek M, Hollender L, Nord C E. Treatment of non-vital permanent incisors with calcium hydroxide. VI. A clinical, microbiological and radiological evaluation of treatment in one sitting of teeth with mature or immature root. Odontol Revy, 1976, 27: 93–108.

[48] Cvek M, Sundstrom B. Treatment of non-vital permanent incisors with calcium hydroxide. V. Histologic appearance of roentgenographically demonstrable apical closure of immature roots. Odontol Revy, 1974, 25: 379–391.

[49] da Silva Limoeiro A G, et al. Micro-computed tomographic evaluation of 2 nickel-titanium instrument systems in shaping root canals. J Endod, 2016, 42: 496–499.

[50] Dahle U R, Tronstad L, Olsen I. Spirochaetes in oral infections. Endod Dent Traumatol, 1993, 9: 87–94.

[51] Dalton B C, et al. Bacterial reduction with nickel-titanium rotary instrumentation. J Endod, 1998, 24: 763–767.

[52] de Castro Rizzi-Maia C, et al. Single vs two-session root canal treatment: a preliminary randomized clinical study using cone beam computed tomography. J Contemp Dent Pract, 2016, 17: 515–521.

[53] de Chevigny C, et al. Treatment outcome in endodontics: the Toronto study-phases 3 and 4: orthograde retreatment. J Endod, 2008, 34: 131–137.

[54] Endal U, et al. A high-resolution computed tomographic study of changes in root canal isthmus area by instrumentation and root filling. J Endod, 2011, 37: 223–227.

[55] Engström B, Lundberg M. The correlation between positive culture and the prognosis of root canal therapy after pulpectomy. Odontol Revy, 1965, 16: 193–203.

[56] Eriksen H M, Ørstavik D, Kerekes K. Healing of apical periodontitis after endodontic treatment using three different root canal sealers. Endod Dent Traumatol, 1988, 4: 114–117.

[57] Estrela C, et al. A new periapical index based on cone beam computed tomography. J Endod, 2008, 34: 1325–1331.

[58] Eyuboglu T F, Olcay K, Ozcan M. A clinical study on single-visit root canal retreatments on consecutive 173 patients: frequency of periapical complications and clinical success rate. Clin Oral Investig, 2017, 21: 1761–1768.

[59] Figini L, et al. Single versus multiple visits for endodontic treatment of permanent teeth: a Cochrane systematic review. J Endod, 2008, 34: 1041–1047.

[60] Floratos S, Kim S. Modern endodontic microsurgery concepts: a clinical update. Dental Clinics of North America, 2017, 61: 81–91.

[61] Fonzar F, et al. Single versus two visits with 1-week intracanal calcium hydroxide medication for endodontic treatment: One-year post-treatment results from a multicentre randomised controlled trial. Eur J Oral Implantol, 2017, 10: 29–41.

[62] Gesi A, et al. Apical dimension of root canal clinically assessed with and without periapical lesions. Int J Dent, 2014: 374971.

[63] Gibbons R J, Houte J V. Bacterial adherence in oral microbial ecology. Annu Rev Microbiol, 1975, 29: 19–44.

[64] Gill G S, et al. Single versus multi-visit endodontic treatment of teeth with apical periodontitis: an in vivo study with 1-year evaluation. Ann Med Health Sci Res, 2016, 6: 19–26.

[65] Goldman M, Pearson A H, Darzenta N. Endodontic success — who's reading the radiograph? Oral Surgery, Oral Medicine, Oral Pathology, Oral Radiology, 1972, 33: 432–437.

[66] Goldstein S, et al. Apexification and apexogenesis. N Y State Dent J, 1999, 65: 23–25.

[67] Gomes B P, et al. Chlorhexidine in endodontics. Braz Dent J, 2013, 24: 89–102.

[68] Grgurevic J, et al. Frequency of bacterial content finding in persistent periapical lesions. Acta Stomatol Croat, 2017, 51: 217–226.

[69] Grossman L I. Endodontic Practice. 9 ed. Philadelphia, Pennsylvania: Lea & Febiger, 1978.

[70] Grossman L I. Grossman's Endodontic Practice. [S. l.]: Lippincott Williams & Wilkin, 2013, s 544.

[71] Haapasalo M, et al. Irrigation in endodontics. Dent Clin North Am, 2010, 54: 291–312.

[72] Haapasalo M, et al. Irrigation in endodontics. Br Dent J, 2014, 216: 299–303.

[73] Haapasalo M, et al. Apical pressure created during irrigation with the GentleWave system compared to conventional syringe irrigation. Clin Oral Investig, 2016, 20: 1525–1534.

[74] Herzog D B, et al. Rapid bacterial detection during endodontic treatment. J Dent Res, 2017, 96: 626–632.

[75] Holland R, et al. Factors affecting the periapical healing process of endodontically treated teeth. J Appl Oral Sci,

2017, 25: 465–476.

[76] Holland R, et al. A comparison of one versus two appointment endodontic therapy in dogs' teeth with apical periodontitis. J Endod, 2003, 29: 121–124.

[77] Hülsmann M, Gressmann G, Schafers F. A comparative study of root canal preparation using FlexMaster and HERO 642 rotary Ni-Ti instruments. Int Endod J, 2003, 36: 358–366.

[78] Huumonen S, et al. Healing of apical periodontitis after endodontic treatment: a comparison between a silicone-based and a zinc oxide-eugenolbased sealer. International Endodontic Journal, 2003, 36: 296–301.

[79] Hülsmann M, Schäfer E. Apical patency: fact and fiction—a myth or a must? ENDO, 2009, 3: 171–184.

[80] Hülsmann M, Schäfer E. Apical patency: fact and fiction – a myth or a must? A contribution to the discussion. ENDO – Endodontic Practice Today, 2009, 3: 285–2307

[81] Ingle J I. The need for endodontic instrument standardization. Oral Surg Oral Med Oral Pathol, 1955, 8: 1211–1213.

[82] Jordan R C, Jacobs S E. Studies in the dynamics of disinfection; the reaction between phenol and Bact. coli; the true shape of the probit-log survival-time curve. Ann Appl Biol, 1945, 32: 221–229.

[83] Joseph M, et al. In vitro evaluation of efficacy of different rotary instrument systems for gutta-percha removal during root canal retreatment. J Clin Exp Dent, 2016, 8: e355–3660.

[84] Juric I B, et al. The antimicrobial effectiveness of photodynamic therapy used as an addition to the conventional endodontic re-treatment: a clinical study. Photodiagnosis Photodyn Ther, 2014, 11: 549–555.

[85] Kakehashi S, Stanley H R, Fitzgerald R J. The effect of surgical exposures of dental pulps in germ-free and conventional laboratory rats. Oral Surg Oral Med Oral Pathol, 1965, 20: 340–349.

[86] Kapralos V, et al. Antibacterial activity of endodontic sealers against planktonic bacteria and bacteria in biofilms. J Endod, 2018, 44: 149–154.

[87] Karygianni L, et al. Supplementary sampling of obturation materials enhances microbial analysis of endodontic treatment failures: a proof of principle study. Clin Oral Investig, 2015, 19: 319–327.

[88] Katebzadeh N, Hupp J, Trope M. Histological periapical repair after obturation of infected root canals in dogs. J Endod, 1999, 25: 364–368.

[89] Kayaoglu G, Erten H, Ørstavik D. Possible role of the adhesin ace and collagen adherence in conveying resistance to disinfectants on Enterococcus faecalis. Oral Microbiol Immunol, 2008, 23: 449–454.

[90] Kerekes K. Radiographic assessment of an endodontic treatment method. J Endod, 1978, 4: 210–213.

[91] Kerekes K, Tronstad L. Morphometric observations on root canals of human anterior teeth. J Endod, 1977, 3: 24–29.

[92] Kerekes K, Tronstad L. Morphometric observations on root canals of human premolars. J Endod, 1977, 3: 74–79.

[93] Kerekes K, Tronstad L. Morphometric observations on the root canals of human molars. J Endod, 1977, 3: 114–118.

[94] Kerekes K, Tronstad L. Long-term results of endodontic treatment performed with a standardized technique. J Endod, 1979, 5: 83–90.

[95] Kerosuo E, Ørstavik D. Application of computerised image analysis to monitoring endodontic therapy: reproducibility and comparison with visual assessment. Dentomaxillofac Radiol, 1997, 26: 79–84.

[96] Keskin C, Sariyilmaz E, Sariyilmaz O. Effect of solvents on apically extruded debris and irrigant during root canal retreatment using reciprocating instruments. Int Endod J, 2017, 50: 1084–1088.

[97] Kim S. Prevalence of apical periodontitis of root canal-treated teeth and retrospective evaluation of symptomrelated prognostic factors in an urban South Korean population. Oral Surg Oral Med Oral Pathol Oral Radiol Endod, 2010, 110:795–799.

[98] Kim S, et al. The influence of an isthmus on the outcomes of surgically treated molars: a retrospective study. J Endod, 2016, 42: 1029–1034.

[99] Kim S G, et al. Regenerative endodontics: a comprehensive review. Int Endod J, 2018.

[100] Kinzer S, et al. Severe deep neck space infections and mediastinitis of odontogenic origin: clinical relevance and implications for diagnosis and treatment. Acta Otolaryngol, 2009, 129: 62–70.

[101] Kirkevang L-L, et al. Periapical status and quality of root fillings and coronal restorations in a Danish population. Int Endod J, 2000, 33: 509–515.

[102] Kirkevang L-L, et al. Prognostic value of the full-scale Periapical Index. Int Endod J, 2014.

[103] Kirkevang L-L, et al. Risk factors for developing apical periodontitis in a general population. Int Endod J, 2007, 40: 290–299.

[104] Kirkevang L-L, Wenzel A. Risk indicators for apical periodontitis. Community Dent Oral Epidemiol, 2003, 31: 59–67.

[105] Krachler A M, Orth K. Targeting the bacteria-host interface: strategies in anti-adhesion therapy. Virulence, 2013, 4: 284–294.

[106] Kruse C, et al. Diagnostic validity of periapical radiography and CBCT for assessing periapical lesions that persist after endodontic surgery. Dentomaxillofac Radiol, 2017, 46: 20170210.

[107] Kvist T, et al. Microbiological evaluation of one- and two-visitendodontic treatment of teeth with apical periodontitis:

[108] Lambrianidis T, Tosounidou E, Tzoanopoulou M. The effect of maintaining apical patency on periapical extrusion. J Endod, 2001, 27: 696–698.
[109] Laulajainen-Hongisto A, et al. Intracranial abscesses over the last four decades; changes in aetiology, diagnostics, treatment and outcome. Infect Dis (Lond), 2016, 48: 310–316.
[110] Li L, et al. Clinical and radiographic outcomes in immature permanent necrotic evaginated teeth treated with regenerative endodontic procedures. J Endod, 2017, 43: 246–251.
[111] Liang Y H, et al. Endodontic outcome predictors identified with periapical radiographs and cone-beam computed tomography scans. J Endod, 2011, 37: 326–331.
[112] Liljestrand J M, et al. Association of endodontic lesions with coronary artery disease. J Dent Res, 2016, 95: 1358–1365.
[113] Lima S M, et al. Diabetes mellitus and inflammatory pulpal and periapical disease: a review. Int Endod J, 2013, 46: 700–709.
[114] Lin J, et al. Regenerative endodontics versus apexification in immature permanent teeth with apical periodontitis: a prospective randomized controlled study. J Endod, 2017, 43: 1821–1827.
[115] Lin L M, Ricucci D, Huang G T. Regeneration of the dentine-pulp complex with revitalization/ revascularization therapy: challenges and hopes. Int Endod J, 2014, 47: 713–724.
[116] Lin P Y, et al. The effect of rubber dam usage on the survival rate of teeth receiving initial root canal treatment: a nationwide population-based study. J Endod, 2014, 40: 1733–1737.
[117] Lodiene G, et al. Detection of leachables and cytotoxicity after exposure to methacrylate- and epoxy-based root canal sealers in vitro. Eur J Oral Sci, 2013, 121:488–496.
[118] Lomcali G, Sen B H, Cankaya H. Scanning electron microscopic observations of apical root surfaces of teeth with apical periodontitis. Endod Dent Traumatol, 1996, 12: 70–76.
[119] Lussi A, et al. A new noninstrumental technique for cleaning and filling root canals. Int Endod J, 1995, 28: 1–6.
[120] Lussi A, Nussbacher U, Grosrey J. A novel noninstrumented technique for cleansing the root canal system. J Endod, 1993, 19: 549–553.
[121] Machado R, et al. The impact of apical patency in the success of endodontic treatment of necrotic teeth with apical periodontitis: a brief review. Iran Endod J, 2016, 11: 63–66.
[122] Maia Filho E M, et al. Correlation between the periapical index and lesion volume in cone-beam computed tomography images. Iran Endod J, 2018, 13: 155–158.
[123] Manzur A, et al. Bacterial quantification in teeth with apical periodontitis related to instrumentation and different intracanal medications: a randomized clinical trial. J Endod, 2007, 33:114–118.
[124] Martinho F C, et al. Endodontic retreatment: clinical comparison of reciprocating systems versus rotary system in disinfecting root canals. Clin Oral Investig, 2015, 19: 1411–1417.
[125] Martins M P, et al. Effectiveness of the protaper next and reciproc systems in removing root canal filling material with sonic or ultrasonic irrigation: a microcomputed tomographic study. J Endod, 2017, 43: 467–471.
[126] McGurkin-Smith R, et al. Reduction of intracanal bacteria using GT rotary instrumentation, 5.25% NaOCl, EDTA, and $Ca(OH)_2$. J Endod , 2005, 31: 359–363.
[127] Mittal P, et al. Effect of apical clearing technique on the treatment outcome of teeth with asymptomatic apical periodontitis: A randomized clinical trial. J Conserv Dent , 2016, 19: 396–401.
[128] Mohammadi Z, et al. Establishing apical patency: To be or not to be? J Contemp Dent Pract, 2017, 18: 326–329.
[129] Molander A, Reit C, Dahlén G. The antimicrobial effect of calcium hydroxide in root canals pretreated with 5% iodine potassium iodide. Endod Dent Traumatol, 1999, 15: 205–209.
[130] Molander A, et al. Microbiological status of root-filled teeth with apical periodontitis. Int Endod J, 1998, 31: 1–7.
[131] Molander A, et al. Clinical and radiographic evaluation of one- and twovisit endodontic treatment of asymptomatic necrotic teeth with apical periodontitis: a randomized clinical trial. J Endod 3, 2007, 3: 1145–1148.
[132] Molina B, et al. Evaluation of root canal debridement of human molars using the gentlewave system. J Endod , 2015, 41: 1701–1705.
[133] Möller Å J R. Microbiological examination of root canals and periapical tissues of human teeth, methodological studies. University of Lund: Sweden, 1966.
[134] Molven O, Olsen I, Kerekes K. Scanning electron microscopy of bacteria in the apical part of root canals in permanent teeth with periapical lesions. Endod Dent Traumatol, 1991, 7: 226–229.
[135] Moodnik R M, et al. Efficacy of biomechanical instrumentation: a scanning electron microscopic study. J Endod, 1976, 2: 261–266.
[136] Mozo S, Llena C, Forner L. Review of ultrasonic irrigation in endodontics: increasing action of irrigating solutions. Med Oral Patol Oral Cir Bucal, 2012, 17: e512–516.
[137] Münch J. Pulpa-und Wurzelbehandlung. 3 ed. Leipzig: Arbeitsgemeinschaft Medizinischer Verlage Gmbh, 1952.

[138] Möller Å J R. Microbiological examination of root canals and periapical tissues of human teeth. Methodological studies. Odontologisk Tidskrift, 1966, 74 (5): 1–380.

[139] Nagendrababu V, et al. Effectiveness of ultrasonically activated irrigation on root canal disinfection: a systematic review of in vitro studies. Clin Oral Investig, 2018, 22: 655–670.

[140] Neves M A, Rôças I N, Siqueira J F Jr. Clinical antibacterial effectiveness of the self-adjusting file system. Int Endod J, 2014, 47: 356–365.

[141] Ng Y L, Mann V, Gulabivala K. Outcome of secondary root canal treatment: a systematic review of the literature. Int Endod J, 2008, 41: 1026–1046.

[142] Ng Y L, Mann V, Gulabivala K. A prospective study of the factors affecting outcomes of nonsurgical root canal treatment: part 1: periapical health. Int Endod J, 2011, 44: 583–609.

[143] Ng Y L, Mann V, Gulabivala K. A prospective study of the factors affecting outcomes of nonsurgical root canal treatment: part 1: periapical health. International Endodontic Journal, 2011, 44: 583–609.

[144] Ng Y L, et al. Outcome of primary root canal treatment: systematic review of the literature – part 1. Effects of study characteristics on probability of success. Int Endod J, 2007, 40: 921–939.

[145] Ng Y L, et al. Outcome of primary root canal treatment: systematic review of the literature – Part 2. Influence of clinical factors. Int Endod J, 2008, 41: 6–31.

[146] Ørstavik D. Antibacterial properties of root canal sealers, cements and pastes. International Endodontic Journal, 1981: 14: 125–133.

[147] Ørstavik D. Antibacterial properties of endodontic materials. International Endodontic Journal, 1988, 21: 161–169.

[148] Ørstavik D. Intracanal medication//Pitt Ford T R.Harty's Endodontics in Clinical Practice. Oxford: Wright, 1977: 106–122.

[149] Ørstavik D. Endodontic filling materials. Endodontic Topics, 2014, 31: 53–67.

[150] Ørstavik D, Horsted-Bindslev P. A comparison of endodontic treatment results at two dental schools. International Endodontic Journal, 1993, 26: 348–354.

[151] Ørstavik D, Kerekes K, Eriksen H M. The periapical index: a scoring system for radiographic assessment of apical periodontitis. Endod Dent Traumatol, 1986, 2: 20–34.

[152] Ørstavik D, Kerekes K, Eriksen H M. Clinical performance of three endodontic sealers. Endod Dent Traumatol, 1987, 3: 178–186.

[153] Ørstavik D, Kerekes K, Molven O. Effects of extensive apical reaming and calcium hydroxide dressing on bacterial infection during treatment of apical periodontitis: a pilot study. International Endodontic Journal, 1991, 24: 1–7.

[154] Ostby B N. The role of the blood clot in endodontic therapy. An experimental histologic study. Acta Odontol Scand, 1961, 19: 324–353.

[155] Paiva S S, et al. Molecular microbiological evaluation of passive ultrasonic activation as a supplementary disinfecting step: a clinical study. J Endod, 2013, 39: 190–194.

[156] Palma D M, et al. Clinical features and outcome of patients with descending necrotizing mediastinitis: prospective analysis of 34 cases. Infection, 2016, 44: 77–84.

[157] Paqué F, Peters O A. Microcomputed tomography evaluation of the preparation of long oval root canals in mandibular molars with the self-adjusting file. J Endod, 2011, 37: 517–521.

[158] Paqué F, Zehnder M, De-Deus G. Microtomography-based comparison of reciprocating single-file F2 ProTaper technique versus rotary full sequence. J Endod, 2011, 37: 1394–1397.

[159] Paranjpe A, et al. Efficacy of the self-adjusting file system on cleaning and shaping oval canals: a microbiological and microscopic evaluation. J Endod, 2012, 38: 226–231.

[160] Persoon I F, Crielaard W, Ozok A R. Prevalence and nature of fungi in root canal infections: a systematic review and meta-analysis. Int Endod J, 2017, 50:1055–1066.

[161] Peters L B, et al. Effects of instrumentation, irrigation and dressing with calcium hydroxide on infection in pulpless teeth with periapical bone lesions. Int Endod J, 2002, 35: 13–21.

[162] Peters O A, Arias A, Paqué F. A micro-computed tomographic assessment of root canal preparation with a novel instrument, TRUShape, in mesial roots of mandibular molars. J Endod, 2015, 41:1545–1550.

[163] Peters O A, Boessler C, Paqué F. Root canal preparation with a novel nickel-titanium instrument evaluated with micro-computed tomography: canal surface preparation over time. J Endod, 2010, 36: 1068–1072.

[164] Peters O A, Schonenberger K, Laib A. Effects of four Ni-Ti preparation techniques on root canal geometry assessed by micro computed tomography. Int Endod J, 2001, 34: 221–230.

[165] Petitjean E, et al. Multimodular assessment of a calcified extraradicular deposit on the root surfaces of a mandibular molar. Int Endod J, 2018, 51:375–385.

[166 Pissiotis A, Vanderas A P, Papagiannoulis L. Longitudinal study on types of injury, complications and treatment in permanent traumatized teeth with single and multiple dental trauma episodes. Dent Traumatol, 2007, 23: 222–225.

[167] Poggio C, et al. Antibacterial activity of different root canal sealers against Enterococcus faecalis. J Clin Exp Dent, 2017, 9: e743–748.

[168] Pradeepkumar M, et al. Efficacy of F file compared to ultrasonic techniques using scanning electron microscopy. N Y State Dent J, 2012, 78: 54–57.

[169] Prestegaard H, et al. Antibacterial activity of various root canal sealers and root-end filling materials in dentin blocks infected ex vivo with Enterococcus faecalis. Acta Odontologica Scandinavica in press, 2014.

[170] Ramos T I, Camara A C, Aguiar C M. Evaluation of capacity of essential oils in dissolving protaperuniversal gutta-percha points. Acta Stomatol Croat, 2016, 50: 128–133.

[171] Ray H A, Trope M. Periapical status of endodontically treated teeth in relation to the technical quality of the root filling and the coronal restoration. Int Endod J, 1995, 28: 12–18.

[172] Ree M H, Schwartz R S. Long-term success of nonvital, immature permanent incisors treated with a mineral trioxide aggregate plug and adhesive restorations: a case series from a private endodontic practice. J Endod, 2017, 43: 1370–1377.

[173] Rico-Romano C, et al. An analysis in vivo of intracanal bacterial load before and after chemo-mechanical preparation: A comparative analysis of two irrigants and two activation techniques. J Clin Exp Dent, 2016, 8: e9–13.

[174] Ricucci D, et al. Complex apical intraradicular infection and extraradicular mineralized biofilms as the cause of wet canals and treatment failure: report of 2 cases. J Endod, 2016, 42: 509–515.

[175] Ricucci D, et al. Histobacteriologic conditions of the apical root canal system and periapical tissues in teeth associated with sinus tracts. J Endod, 2018, 44: 405–413.

[176] Ricucci D, Loghin S, Siqueira J F Jr. Exuberant Biofilm infection in a lateral canal as the cause of short-term endodontic treatment failure: report of a case. J Endod, 2013, 39: 712–718.

[177] Ricucci D, et al. Large bacterial floc causing an independent extraradicular infection and posttreatment apical periodontitis: a case report. J Endod, 2018, 44: 1308–1316.

[178] Ricucci D, et al. Histologic investigation of root canal-treated teeth with apical periodontitis: a retrospective study from twenty-four patients. J Endod, 2009, 35: 493–502.

[179] Ricucci D, et al. Repair of extensive apical root resorption associated with apical periodontitis: radiographic and histologic observations after 25 years. J Endod, 2014, 40: 1268–1274.

[180] Ricucci D, et al. Extraradicular infection as the cause of persistent symptoms: a case series. J Endod, 2015, 41: 265–273.

[181] Rôças I N, Lima K C, Siqueira J F Jr. Reduction in bacterial counts in infected root canals after rotary or hand nickel-titanium instrumentation – a clinical study. Int Endod J, 2013, 46: 681–687.

[182] Rôças I N, Siqueira J F Jr. Frequency and levels of candidate endodontic pathogens in acute apical abscesses as compared to asymptomatic apical periodontitis. PLoS One, 2018, 13: e0190469.

[183] Rocha C T, et al. Biofilm on the apical region of roots in primary teeth with vital and necrotic pulps with or without radiographically evident apical pathosis. Int Endod J, 2008, 41: 664–669.

[184] Rodrigues R C, et al. Infection control in retreatment cases: in vivo antibacterial effects of 2 instrumentation systems. J Endod, 2015, 41: 1600–1605.

[185] Rodrigues R C V, et al. Influence of the apical preparation size and the irrigant type on bacterial reduction in root canal-treated teeth with apical periodontitis. J Endod, 2017, 43: 1058–1063.

[186] Rudranaik S, Nayak M, Babshet M. Periapical healing outcome following single visit endodontic treatment in patients with type 2 diabetes mellitus. J Clin Exp Dent, 2016, 8: e498–504.

[187] Ruiz-Linares M, et al. Physical properties of AH Plus with chlorhexidine and cetrimide. J Endod, 2013, 39: 1611–1614.

[188] Ruiz X F, et al. Development of periapical lesions in endodontically treated teeth with and without periodontal involvement: a retrospective cohort study. J Endod, 2017, 43: 1246–1249.

[189] Safavi K E, et al. A comparison of antimicrobial effects of calcium hydroxide and iodine-potassium iodide. J Endod, 1985, 11:454–456.

[190] Sant'Anna Junior A, et al. The effect of larger apical preparations in the danger zone of lower molars preparedusing the Mtwo and Reciproc systems. J Endod, 2014, 40: 1855–1859.

[191] Santos A L, et al. Comparing the bacterial diversity of acute and chronic dental root canal infections. PLoS One, 2011, 6:e28088.

[192] Sasaki H, et al. Interrelationship between periapical lesion and systemic metabolic disorders. Curr Pharm Des, 2016, 22:2204–2215.

[193] Sathorn C, Parashos P, Messer H. The prevalence of postoperative pain and flare-up in single- and multiplevisit endodontic treatment: a systematic review. Int Endod J, 2008, 41: 91–99.

[194] Sathorn C, Parashos P, Messer H H. Effectiveness of single- versus multiple-visit endodontic treatment of teeth with apical periodontitis: a systematic review and meta-analysis. Int Endod J, 2005, 38: 347–355.

[195] Sathorn C, Parashos P, Messer H H. How useful is root canal culturing in predicting treatment outcome? J Endod,

2007, 33: 220–225.
[196] Schmidt J C, et al. Treatment of periodontal-endodontic lesions – a systematic review. J Clin Periodontol, 2014, 41: 779–790.
[197] Schwendicke F, Gostemeyer G. Single-visit or multiple-visit root canal treatment: systematic review, meta-analysis and trial sequential analysis. BMJ Open, 2017, 7: e013115.
[198] Sebring D, et al. Characteristics of teeth referred to a public dental specialist clinic in endodontics. Int Endod J, 2017, 50:629–635.
[199] Segura-Egea J J, et al. Association between diabetes and the prevalence of radiolucent periapical lesions in rootfilled teeth: systematic review and metaanalysis. Clin Oral Investig, 2016, 20:1133–1141.
[200] Seixas F H, et al. Determination of root canal cleanliness by different irrigation methods and morphometric analysis of apical third. J Contemp Dent Pract, 2015, 16: 442–450.
[201] Shuping G B, et al. Reduction of intracanal bacteria using nickel-titanium rotary instrumentation and various medications. J Endod, 2000, 26: 751–755.
[202] Sigurdsson A, et al. Healing of periapical lesions after endodontic treatment with the gentlewave procedure: a prospective multicenter clinical study. J Endod, 2018, 44: 510–517.
[203] Sigurdsson A, et al. 12-month healing rates after endodontic therapy using the novel gentlewave system: a prospective multicenter clinical study. J Endod, 2016, 42: 1040–1048.
[204] Silva E, et al. Micro-computed tomographic evaluation of canal retreatments performed by undergraduate students using different techniques.Restor Dent Endod, 2018, 43: e5.
[205] Silva E, et al. Micro-CT evaluation of different final irrigation protocols on the removal of hard-tissue debris from isthmus-containing mesial root of mandibular molars. Clin Oral Investig, 2018.
[206] Silva L A, et al. Antibacterial effect of calcium hydroxide with or without chlorhexidine as intracanal dressing in primary teeth with apical periodontitis. Pediatr Dent, 2017, 39: 28–33.
[207] Sindet-Pedersen S, Petersen J K, Gotzsche P C. Incidence of pain conditions in dental practice in a Danish county. Community Dent Oral Epidemiol, 1985, 13: 244–246.
[208] Siqueira J F Jr. Microbial causes of endodontic flare-ups. Int Endod J, 2003, 36: 453–463.
[209] Siqueira J F Jr, Rôças I N. Clinical implications and microbiology of bacterial persistence after treatment procedures. J Endod, 2008, 34: 1291–301.e3.
[210] Siqueira J F Jr, et al. Incidence of postoperative pain after intracanal procedures based on an antimicrobial strategy. J Endod, 2002, 28: 457–460.
[211] Siren E K, et al. In vitro antibacterial effect of calcium hydroxide combined with chlorhexidine or iodinepotassium iodide on Enterococcus faecalis. Eur J Oral Sci, 2004, 112: 326–331.
[212] Sjögren U, et al. The antimicrobial effect of calcium hydroxide as a shortterm intracanal dressing. Int Endod J, 1991, 24:119–125.
[213] Sjögren U, et al. Factors affecting the long-term results of endodontic treatment. J Endod, 1990, 16: 498–504.
[214] Sjögren U, et al. Influence of infection at the time of root filling on the outcome of endodontic treatment of teeth with apical periodontitis. International Endodontic Journal, 1997, 30: 297–306.
[215] Song M, et al. Periapical status related to the quality of coronal restorations and root fillings in a Korean population. J Endod, 2014, 40: 182–186.
[216] Spångberg L, Engström B, Langeland K. Biologic effects of dental materials. 3. Toxicity and antimicrobial effect of endodontic antiseptics in vitro. Oral Surg Oral Med Oral Pathol, 1973, 36: 856–871.
[217] Spångberg L. Biological effects of root canal filling materials. 5. Toxic effect in vitro of root canal filling materials on HeLa cells and human skin fibroblasts. Odontol Revy, 1969, 20: 427–436.
[218] Spångberg L, Engström B, Langeland K. Biologic effects of dental materials. 3. Toxicity and antimicrobial effect of endodontic antiseptics in vitro. Oral Surgery, Oral Medicine, Oral Pathology, Oral Radiology, 1973, 36: 856–871.
[219] Stassen I G, et al. The relation between apical periodontitis and rootfilled teeth in patients with periodontal treatment need. Int Endod J, 2006, 39: 299–308.
[220] Strindberg L. The dependence of the results of pulp therapy on certain factors. Acta Odontol Scand, 1956, 14 (Suppl 21,: 1–175.
[221] Su Y, Wang C, Ye L. Healing rate and post-obturation pain of singleversus multiple-visit endodontic treatment for infected root canals: a systematic review. J Endod, 2011, 37: 125–132.
[222] Sunde P T, et al. Microbiota of periapical lesions refractory to endodontic therapy. J Endod, 2002, 28: 304–310.
[223] Sunde P T, et al. Fluorescence in situ hybridization (FISH, for direct visualization of bacteria in periapical lesions of asymptomatic root-filled teeth. Microbiology, 2003, 149: 1095–1102.
[224] Sunde P T, et al. Assessment of periradicular microbiota by DNA-DNA hybridization. Endod Dent Traumatol, 2000, 16: 191–196.
[225] Sundqvist G. Bacteriological Studies of Necrotic Dental Pulps. Umeå Univ Odontological Dissertations, 7. Umeå Department of Oral Microbiology, University of Umeå,

1976,

[226] Sundqvist G, et al. Microbiologic analysis of teeth with failed endodontic treatment and the outcome of conservative re-treatment. Oral Surg Oral Med Oral Pathol Oral Radiol Endod, 1998, 85: 86–93.

[227] Tello-Barbaran J, et al. The antimicrobial effect of iodine-potassium iodide after cleaning and shaping procedures in mesial root canals of mandibular molars. Acta Odontol Latinoam, 2010, 23: 244–247.

[228] Tiburcio-Machado C D, et al. Influence of diabetes in the development of apical periodontitis: a critical literature review of human studies. J Endod, 2017, 43:370–376.

[229] Tilley S K, Fry R C. Priority environmental contaminants: Understanding their sources of exposure, biological mechanisms, and impacts on health// Fry R C. Systems Biology in Toxicology and Environmental Health . Boston MA: Academic Press, 2015: 117–169.

[230] Tinaz A C, et al. The effect of disruption of apical constriction on periapical extrusion. J Endod, 2005, 31: 533–535.

[231] Tong Z, et al. Relevance of the clustered regularly interspaced short palindromic repeats of Enterococcus faecalis strains isolated from retreatment root canals on periapical lesions,resistance to irrigants and biofilms. Exp Ther Med, 2017, 14: 5491–5496.

[232] Torabinejad M, et al. Outcomes of nonsurgical retreatment and endodontic surgery: a systematic review. J Endod, 2009, 35: 930–937.

[233] Torabinejad M, et al. Prevalence and size of periapical radiolucencies using cone-beam computed tomography in teeth without apparent intraoral radiographic lesions: a new periapical index with a clinical recommendation. J Endod, 2018, 44: 389–394.

[234] Torabinejad M, White S N. Endodontic treatment options after unsuccessful initial root canal treatment: alternatives to single-tooth implants. J Am Dent Assoc, 2016, 147: 214–220.

[235] Torneck C D. Reaction of rat connective tissue to polyethylene tube implants. I. Oral Surg Oral Med Oral Pathol, 1966, 21: 379–387.

[236] Torneck C D. Reaction of rat connective tissue to polyethylene tube implants. II. Oral Surg Oral Med Oral Pathol, 1967, 24: 674–683.

[237] Tronstad L, et al. Influence of coronal restorations on the periapical health of endodontically treated teeth. Endod Dent Traumatol, 2000, 16: 218–221.

[238] Tronstad L, Barnett F, Cervone F. Periapical bacterial plaque in teeth refractory to endodontic treatment. Endod Dent Traumatol, 1990, 6:73–77.

[239] Tronstad L, et al. Extraradicular endodontic infections. Endod Dent Traumatol, 1987, 3: 86–90.

[240] Tronstad L, Kreshtool D, Barnett F. Microbiological monitoring and results of treatment of extraradicular endodontic infection. Endod Dent Traumatol, 1990, 6: 129–136.

[241] Trope M, Delano E O, Ørstavik D. Endodontic treatment of teeth with apical periodontitis: single vs. multivisit treatment. Journal of Endodontics, 1999, 25: 345–350.

[242] Uemura M, et al. Effectiveness of eucalyptol and d-limonene as guttapercha solvents. J Endod, 1997, 23: 739–741.

[243] Vajrabhaya L O, et al. Cytotoxicity evaluation of gutta-percha solvents: chloroform and GP-solvent (limonene). Oral Surg Oral Med Oral Pathol Oral Radiol Endod, 2004, 98: 756–759.

[244] Valderhaug J. A histologic study of experimentally induced periapical inflammation in primary teeth in monkeys. Int J Oral Surg, 1974, 3: 111–123.

[245] Vera J, et al. One- versus two-visit endodontic treatment of teeth with apical periodontitis: a histobacteriologic study. J Endod, 2012, 38: 1040–1052.

[246] Verma P, et al. Effect of residual bacteria on the outcome of pulp regeneration in vivo. J Dent Res, 2017, 96:100–106.

[247] Versiani M A, et al. Micro-computed tomography study of oval-shaped canals prepared with the self-adjusting file, Reciproc, WaveOne, and ProTaper universal systems. J Endod, 2013, 39: 1060–1066.

[248] Versumer J, Hülsmann M, Schafers F. A comparative study of root canal preparation using Profile.04 and Lightspeed rotary Ni-Ti instruments. Int Endod J, 2002, 35: 37–46.

[249] Vestin Fredriksson M, et al. When maxillary sinusitis does not heal: findings on CBCT scans of the sinuses with a particular focus on the occurrence of odontogenic causes of maxillary sinusitis. Laryngoscope Investig Otolaryngol, 2017, 2:442–446.

[250] Vidal F, et al. Odontogenic sinusitis: a comprehensive review. Acta Odontol Scand, 2017, 75: 623–633.

[251] Violich D R, Chandler, N.P. The smear layer in endodontics–a review. Int Endod J, 2010, 43: 2–15.

[252] Virdee S S, et al. Efficacy of irrigant activation techniques in removing intracanal smear layer and debris from mature permanent teeth: a systematic review and meta-analysis. Int Endod J, 2018, 51:605–621.

[253] Walsh L J, George R. Activation of alkaline irrigation fluids in endodontics. Materials (Basel), 2017, 10.

[254] Waltimo T, et al. Clinical efficacy of treatment procedures in endodontic infection control and one year follow-up of periapical healing. Journal of Endodontics, 2005, 31: 863–866.

[255] Waltimo T M, et al. Clinical performance of 3 endodontic

[255] sealers. Oral Surg Oral Med Oral Pathol Oral Radiol Endod, 2001, 92: 89–92.
[256] Waltimo T M, et al. Fungi in therapy-resistant apical periodontitis. Int Endod J, 1997, 30: 96–101.
[257] Walton R E. Current concepts of canal preparation. Dent Clin North Am, 1992, 36: 309–326.
[258] Wang C S, et al. Clinical efficiency of 2% chlorhexidine gel in reducing intracanal bacteria. J Endod, 2007, 33:1283–1289.
[259] Wang J, et al. Imaging of extraradicular biofilm using combined scanning electron microscopy and stereomicroscopy. Microsc Res Tech, 2013, 76: 979–983.
[260] Wang Z, Shen Y, Haapasalo M. Dental materials with antibiofilm properties. Dent Mater, 2014, 30: e1–16.
[261] Wang Z, Shen Y, Haapasalo M. Root canal wall dentin structure in uninstrumented but cleaned human premolars: a scanning electron microscopic study. J Endod, 2018, 44: 842–848.
[262] Weiger R, Rosendahl R, Lost C. Influence of calcium hydroxide intracanal dressings on the prognosis of teeth with endodontically induced periapical lesions. Int Endod J, 2000, 33:219–226.
[263] Whatley J D, et al. Susceptibility of methacrylate-based root canal filling to degradation by bacteria found in endodontic infections. Quintessence Int, 2014, 45: 647–652.
[264] Williams J M, et al. Detection and quantitation of E. faecalis by real-time PCR (qPCR), reverse transcription-PCR (RTPCR, and cultivation during endodontic treatment. J Endod, 2006, 32: 715–721.
[265] Wohlgemuth P, et al. Effectiveness of the gentlewave system in removing separated instruments. J Endod, 2015, 41:1895–1898.
[266] Wong A W, et al. Treatment outcomes of single-visit versus multiplevisit non-surgical endodontic therapy: a randomised clinical trial. BMC Oral Health, 2015, 15: 162.
[267] Wong A W, Zhang C, Chu C H. A systematic review of nonsurgical single-visit versus multiple-visit endodontic treatment. Clin Cosmet Investig Dent, 2014, 6: 45–56.
[268] Wong A W, et al. Incidence of post-obturation pain after single-visit versus multiple-visit non-surgical endodontic treatments. BMC Oral Health, 2015, 15: 96.
[269] Wongwatanasanti N, et al. Effect of bioceramic materials on proliferation and odontoblast differentiation of human stem cells from the apical papilla. J Endod, 2018.
[270] Yared G M, Dagher F E. Influence of apical enlargement on bacterial infection during treatment of apical periodontitis. J Endod, 1994, 20: 535–537.
[271] Yaylali I E, Kececi A D, Ureyen Kaya B. Ultrasonically activated irrigation to remove calcium hydroxide from apical third of human root canal system: a systematic review of in vitro studies. J Endod, 2015, 41: 1589–1599.
[272] Yilmaz F, et al. Evaluation of 3 different retreatment techniques in maxillary molar teeth by using microcomputed tomography. J Endod, 2018, 44: 480–484.
[273] Yuanyuan C, et al. Cleaning effect of ultrasonic activation as an adjunct to syringe irrigation of root canals: a systematic review. Hua Xi Kou Qiang Yi Xue Za Zhi, 2015, 33: 145–152.
[274] Zandi H, et al. Microbial analysis of endodontic infections in root-filled teeth with apical periodontitis before and after irrigation using pyrosequencing. J Endod, 2018, 44: 372–378.
[275] Zandi H, et al. Antibacterial effectiveness of 2 root canal irrigants in root-filled teeth with infection: a randomized clinical trial. J Endod, 2016, 42:1307–1313.
[276] Zehnder M. Endodontic infection caused by localized aggressive periodontitis: a case report and bacteriologic evaluation. Oral Surg Oral Med Oral Pathol Oral Radiol Endod, 2001, 92: 440–445.
[277] Zehnder M, Gold S I, Hasselgren G. Pathologic interactions in pulpal and periodontal tissues. J Clin Periodontol, 2002, 29: 663–671.
[278] Zhang C, Du J, Peng Z. Correlation between enterococcus faecalis and persistent intraradicular infection compared with primary intraradicular infection: a systematic review. J Endod, 2015, 41: 1207–1213.
[279] Zhao D, et al. Root canal preparation of mandibular molars with 3 nickel-titanium rotary instruments: a micro-computed tomographic study. J Endod, 2014, 40: 1860–1864.
[280] Zhou H M, et al. In vitro cytotoxicity of calcium silicate-containing endodontic sealers. J Endod, 2015, 41: 56–61.

第 12 章 根管外科

Frank C. Setzer, Bekir Karabucak

12.1 概述

根尖周炎的手术治疗已有几个世纪的历史。19 世纪 80 年代，为了去除根尖的坏死部分，医生引入了根尖切除的方法 [17, 34, 70]；为了去除病变的根尖周组织，医生又采用了根尖刮治的方法。然而，这两种手术方法均未去除来自根管系统内的感染源 [199]。19 世纪 90 年代，Partsch 发表了多例关于根尖切除术的报告 [181-183]，促进这一术式在欧洲被广泛接受 [71]。

为了使手术更安全、操作更简单、更可预测，多种手术技术被提出并投入使用 [79]。多年来形成的标准的手术方法包括：使用手术车针建立术区入路并行根尖切除，使用银汞合金作为根尖充填材料 [43, 64, 103, 176]。

随着初次根管治疗和非手术再治疗的化学和机械清理能力的提高，一些临床研究结果显示牙髓外科的疗效极低，因此其有效性受到了质疑 [7, 76]。

牙髓外科治疗的失败是由于导致根尖周炎的生物学问题未能解决。大多数情况下，非手术和手术治疗失败的主要原因是牙根内和（或）根外感染的持续存在。这两种治疗方法的成功取决于消除感染，或至少将微生物菌群的数量降低到机体能自愈的阈值以下，并将它们严密封闭在根管内。

如果使用的方法和材料不能提供有效的密封作用，持续的根管内感染将是手术失败的一个原因。如果根尖切除术后遗留大量的牙本质小管及管间分支，微生物可通过这些通道侵入并引起根尖周炎 [51]，进而加重病情。使用手术显微镜来识别这些解剖细节并联合新的根管倒充填材料可提供更好的治疗和更佳的预后结果 [79]。

根管治疗外科已发展成为显微根管外科 [125]。外科手术显微镜具有高放大倍数和直接照明功能。这一方法减小了根切斜面的角度，减少了牙本质小管暴露的数量 [51]。将超声器械用于根管倒预备可以减少损伤，实现更好的根管清理 [239]。生物相容性好、性能稳定的倒填充材料比传统水门汀类材料更有利于术后愈合 [203]。本章通过一个循证综述，以外科再治疗为重点，对比其与传统、历史治疗技术和其他外科根管治疗技术之间的差异。

12.2 牙髓外科的治疗程序

公认的牙髓外科包括根尖刮治术、根尖周手术、冠根切除术以及牙齿再植术。过去，根尖周手术包括根尖切除术（单纯根尖切除而不逆行填充），而现在，探查性手术和手术穿孔修补，以及结合根尖切除和根尖填充的经典根尖手术均包含在内。冠根切除包括截根、完全根切、半切或三切和分牙术。再植包括移植和意向再植，意向再植属于牙髓治疗的范畴。

12.3 适应证

12.3.1 牙齿相关因素

在非手术再治疗不可行或失败的情况下，手

术干预是一个有效的替代方案。非手术或手术再治疗干预的一般指征是根尖周炎的存在。在选择牙髓外科手术作为治疗方案之前，必须仔细评估任何持续性病理表现的病因[120]，包括对已存在的无症状病变进行适当随访。如果最初的根管治疗质量不佳，例如有遗漏根管的迹象或需要重新行永久修复，应该首选非手术再治疗。大多数牙源性根尖周病变，包括肉芽肿[22,228,236]、囊肿[195]和脓肿，通过适当的非手术再治疗均可获得积极的疗效。但以下情况可能会阻止非手术再治疗后的根尖周愈合，或在初次根管治疗失败后建议行手术治疗。

复杂的根管解剖结构

牙根重度弯曲（>30°）S形根管、根中或根尖三分之一分叉、牙根较长（>25mm）或根尖敞开（>直径1.5mm）的牙齿可能会给非手术再治疗带来困难甚至无法进行再治疗。此外，钙化根管、牙根内吸收和外吸收更适合行手术治疗。原始根管解剖结构的医源性改变，如堵塞、管间交通、台阶或穿孔，导致微生物遗留在根管系统的峡区[274]或根尖孔处[227]，可能使生物力学消毒不彻底[87]。

根尖周病的病理生理学

绝大多数根尖周病变是炎症性的[18]。Nair等人[195]将拔除牙的病损分为三类，其中35%为根尖周脓肿，50%为肉芽肿，15%为囊肿。根尖周囊肿可以是与感染根管系统直接相连的袋状囊肿，也可以是与根管分离的根尖真性囊肿[164, 195]。在所有根尖周病变中，9%被描述为根尖真性囊肿，6%被描述为根尖袋状囊肿[195]。真性囊肿不能通过根管治疗或非手术再治疗来解决[195]，需要手术干预。残留银汞合金、牙胶、其他根管充填和封闭材料、纸尖或伴有囊性病变相关的胆固醇结晶均可引起根尖周异物反应[163-165]。根管外感染可能以附着在牙根外表面的生物膜的形式发生[257]，也可能以软组织损伤本身内放线菌和丙酸杆菌菌落的形式发生[194, 200, 229, 240]。如果根尖周缺损的初始直径超过5mm，非手术治疗的愈合可能会受到影响[168-169]。当上述这些情况都不能通过非手术再治疗来解决时，即考虑行牙髓外科手术治疗。

改变的根管解剖结构阻碍非手术器械

许多再治疗病例中显示的微生物谱可能更难以根除（见第5章）。此外，由于初次治疗后原始根管的解剖结构可能会发生改变，这些改变可能会阻碍器械和冲洗液进入根管系统的所有区域。这些改变包括管间交通、台阶、穿孔和分离器械。虽然其中一些障碍可能只有在开始进行常规的根管再治疗时才很明显，但有些障碍在制定治疗计划时就已经很明显了。根尖周炎合并根管解剖结构发生改变而不能重新找到原根管通路的病例，行非手术再治疗的成功率仅为40%左右[87]。因此，根据残留的牙齿结构和现有的冠方修复体的情况，可以在先行非手术再治疗之再行手术治疗，抑或在直接进行手术治疗之间做出选择。非感染的分离器械可能不需要取出，当存在根尖病变的情况下，应考虑取出。一般来说，对于不锈钢或镍钛分离器械应首先尝试进行非手术治疗取出，但治疗时必须考虑牙齿结构的损失是否合理[219]。当分离器械在根管弯曲处或弯曲以下时，传统镍钛器械的超弹性可能会将其楔入根管弯曲外侧，从而使一些分离器械的取出变得非常困难或不可能实现[179]，有时直接手术的创伤可能较小[120]。

硬质根管充填材料

各种各样的根管充填材料，包括硬质糊剂和银尖，可能会阻碍非手术再治疗的进行。间苯二酚甲醛膏剂（俄罗斯红）[6]以前常用于东欧国家，通常不能从根管系统中去除，需要行根管外科手术治疗。众所周知，新型的硅酸钙基密封材料固化后也非常坚硬，但目前尚无相关再治疗的临床研究。

桩和核重建

当患牙存在长桩、预制金属桩、分体式铸造桩核冠行再治疗时，需要拆除原修复体，这可能会带来根折、牙齿组织过度丧失或穿孔的风险，此时更倾向于行外科手术治疗。

吸收、穿孔和根折

内外部吸收以及穿孔的修复取决于其在根管或根内的位置[219, 226]。吸收的位置越靠近冠方，非手术再治疗成功的可能性越大[155, 170, 193, 219]；越靠近根尖，越有利于手术治疗。根尖吸收通常在非手术再治疗后停止，但是，如果再吸收仍旧继续，还需要手术治疗。牙根纵裂的临床确诊需要手术探查。在多根牙中，根据缺损的大小和位置，手术切除受损伤的牙根可以挽救剩余的根和牙冠。活髓牙的牙根横折不需要进行手术干预，因为即使冠方牙髓坏死，根尖段牙髓仍可保存活力[111]。但是，如果牙齿在外伤前就已经感染，手术可能是必要的[72]。

12.3.2　患者对治疗方案的抉择

告知患者治疗替代方案的相关预后和风险。对于根管外科手术，应该向患者说明这是一个真正的手术过程，具有潜在的风险，如对邻近解剖结构的损伤、术后肿胀、不适和伤口愈合。患者将根据对治疗方案利弊的权衡、自身对患牙的重视程度、对长时间牙科手术的承受程度和治疗费用的承担意愿，做出最终决定[138]。

12.3.3　医生在决策中的作用

临床医生的决策必须包括详细的病史、牙科治疗史以及临床检查。冠方修复的类型、根管桩存在与否，以及医生的技能水平都可能影响治疗计划的制定[39, 238]。众所周知，牙髓病专家和普通医生之间是存在差异的[230]。医生可能会致力于在学术上成功治愈根尖周病变，而患者则更关心牙齿的留存和功能。对于有症状的患牙，推荐治疗方案比较容易，但对于无症状的根尖周炎则比较复杂。尤其是，如果推荐手术治疗，临床医生应该具备完成手术所需要的充足的知识、技能、经验和设备。尽管病例选择适当即可获得一个较好的预后，但外科手术必须经过充分的培训才能进行。

12.4　禁忌证

在某些情况下，根管外科手术可能受到限制或无法实施。包括手术部位邻近的解剖结构可能遭受严重或永久性损伤，如颏神经和下牙槽神经、鼻腔或窦腔、腭部神经血管束。冠根比不佳、松动度增加或牙周病晚期的牙齿预后较差。系统性疾病，如心血管疾病行局部麻醉时禁止使用血管收缩剂；先天性血液病，有静脉注射二磷酸盐治疗史，患者处于双磷酸盐相关颌骨骨坏死高风险中，这些情况下禁止手术。其他情况，如糖尿病、免疫缺陷或抗凝治疗均会增加患者术后并发症或伤口愈合受损的风险。在这些情况下，牙科医生必须与患者的内科医生合作[219]。

12.5　手术准备

12.5.1　CBCT 评估

在牙髓病学中，CBCT 已经成为一种被广泛接受的评估工具[213, 218]（见第 6 章），但使用中受较高辐射照射的限制。在手术治疗计划设计中，CBCT 有助于评估根尖周炎的范围和位置，病变缺损区的骨质厚度，与相邻解剖结构（如下牙槽神经和颏神经、鼻腔和窦腔、邻牙的牙根结构）的位置关系[74, 218]。由于根充材料的分辨率和光束硬化效应的限制，CBCT 无法准确检测到牙根纵裂，但狭窄的垂直骨缺损[44, 156]可以指示根裂的存在。CBCT 软件还可以提供让临床医生准确测量出颊侧骨面到根尖的距离和根的长度等功能[28]。引导显微外科技术已经发展起来，它使用术前 CBCT 和传统或数字印模导板，使手术车针直接切除目标根尖。这对于极其接近重要解剖结构的根尖切除术尤其有用[4, 83]（图 12.1）。

12.5.2　设备

现代根管外科是一种需要专业器械的显微外科技术[125]。标准的显微外科器械包含标准外科器械的微缩版本，这些器械是专门为在牙科显微镜下工作而设计的。必要的器械包括以下内容。

- 牙科口镜
- 牙周探针
- 根管探针和显微探针
- 手术刀片、刀柄、翻瓣器
- 牙周刮匙、外科刮匙、用于去除病变组织的微型刮匙
- 显微口镜和手柄
- 倒充填输送器和加压器

除了这些手持仪器外，还需要下文中列举器械，这些器械在本章的手术部分进行了详细描述。

- 骨开窗和根尖切除的手机和车针

根管外科 | 第 12 章

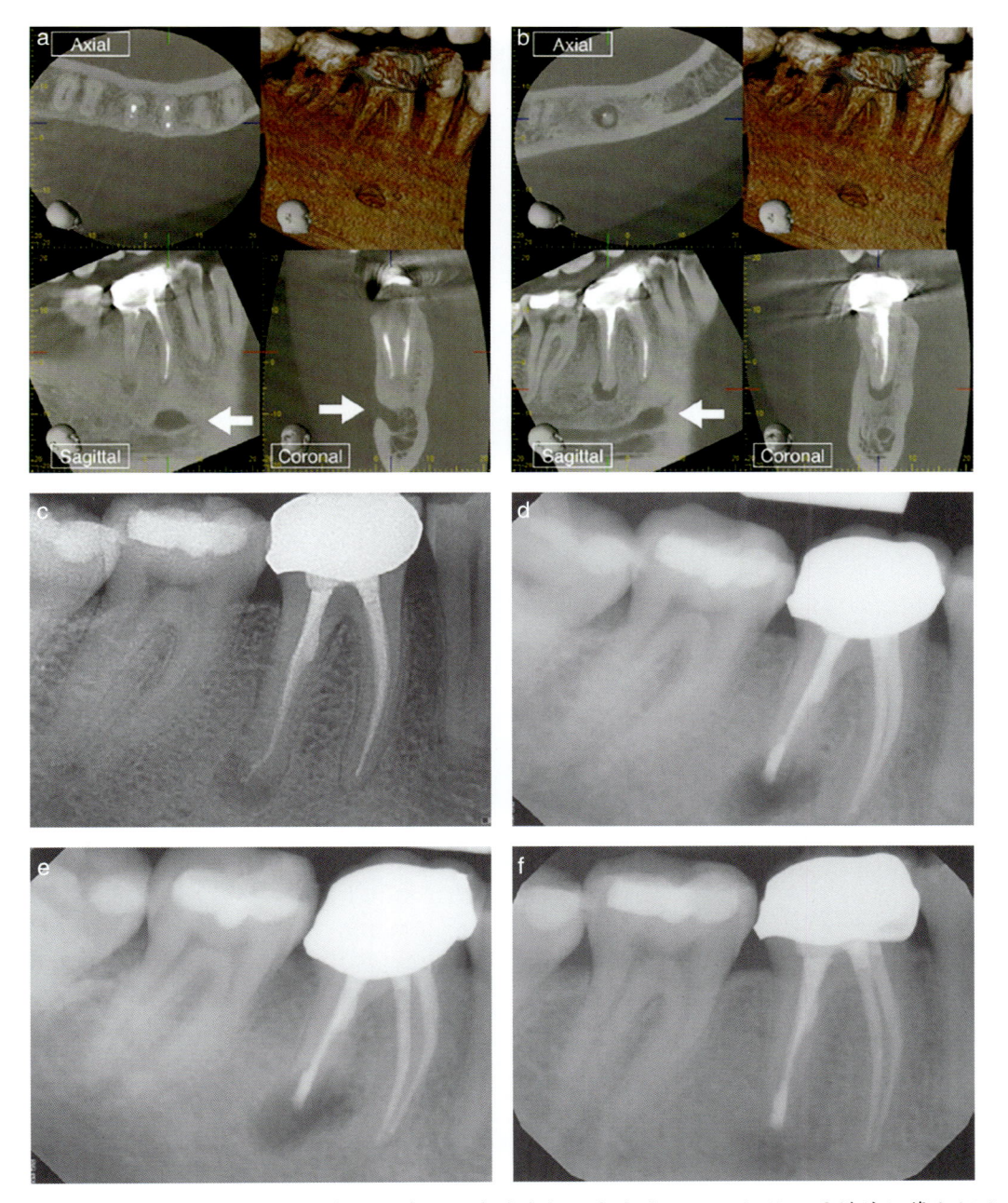

图 12.1 使用 CBCT 对右下第一磨牙远中根根管制定外科手术治疗计划。a、b. 评估下牙槽神经管和颏孔（箭头）的位置，在矢状面和冠状面上测量距离。c. 术前 X 线片。d、e. 术后 X 线片，原位倒充填。f. 术后 12 个月随访，影像学显示根尖已愈合，无临床症状（美国费城 Frank Setzer 医生提供）

- 拉钩
- 用于根尖倒预备的超声工作仪和工作尖
- 显微的镊子、持针器和剪刀
- 其他器械，如麻醉注射器、镊子、三用枪头和微型冲洗器。

一次性物品包括以下内容。

- 局麻药物
- 纱布和棉球
- 止血剂、染色剂、生理盐水
- 根管倒充填和穿孔修补材料
- 骨粉骨膜材料
- 缝线

特定截骨技术也可使用超声骨刀。

12.5.3 患者体位

根管外科手术适用于除需要行根管倒预备和倒充填的上下颌第二、第三磨牙外的大多数患牙。患者、医生和助手的正确位置是手术的关键[119,134]。患者的舒适度和医生充分执行手术的能力均要兼顾。对于显微根管外科手术，牙科显微镜可提供高倍放大、共轴照明、符合临床医生人体工程学的座椅，直视截根面无须斜切[125,220]。在整个软组织翻瓣、去骨开窗和牙根切除过程中，患者应保持患牙的牙齿长轴处于水平位置。根切和探查完成后，超声倒预备工作尖开始工作，必须直视截根面以避免超声工作尖错位，并将截骨范围控制在合适的大小。治疗上颌牙时调直椅位，治疗下颌牙时倾斜椅位能实现直视根面。根管倒充填完成后恢复至初始的体位。

12.6 麻醉

在根管外科手术中，局部麻醉用于深度镇痛和止血[127]。根切表面的探查需要在高倍率显微镜下进行。局麻药物的止血作用是通常通过添加1∶50 000的肾上腺素血管收缩剂来实现的，也可用1∶80 000替代[35,93,126]。如果将高浓度的血管收缩剂注射到黏膜下层可减少出血[93,113,280]。

高浓度的肾上腺素是否对体循环有影响已引起关注[258,280]。含1∶50 000肾上腺素的局麻药应注射于患牙近远中各1~2颗邻牙的颊黏膜（或腭侧黏膜）下层。由于较高浓度的肾上腺素浓度并不促进术区止血，因此它不适用于下牙槽神经阻滞麻醉[35,93,126]。如果药物能避免直接注射进血管，对大多数患者的心血管影响就较微小，且作用时间短、患者耐受良好。对于患有严重心血管疾病或做过心血管手术的患者，较高的肾上腺素浓度是禁忌的，术前需咨询患者的内科医生以建立不同的麻醉方案[23,128,283]。

12.7 手术解剖

12.7.1 软组织解剖

除上颌磨牙的腭根外，一般外科手术均可从颊侧入路。颊侧有三种软组织：牙槽黏膜、附着龈和边缘龈。牙槽黏膜是覆盖在上下颌骨的牙槽突上的一层薄薄的无角化的黏膜，其松弛地附着在下方骨面上，可随着脸颊或嘴唇的运动而被牵拉。附着龈是指牙龈从游离龈沟延伸至牙槽黏膜交界处的部分，它与下面的骨和牙骨质紧密相连，不可移动。边缘牙龈是游离牙龈的嵴，呈颈圈状包绕牙颈部，形成龈沟的软组织部分。在根管外科手术中，必须非常小心，尽量减少手术过程中潜在的损伤。

12.7.2 瓣膜设计

适当的皮瓣设计和翻瓣的主要目的是允许对基底骨、牙根结构和病变组织提供充分的手术入路，并提供简单且无瘢痕的软组织愈合[147,160]。

多年来，人们提出了各种瓣膜设计[189,263-264,271]。现在半月瓣已被淘汰，这种设计的弧形切口完全在黏膜上[332,96]。这种皮瓣的缺点包括：对于较大的根尖周围病变的手术入路有限，复位困难；经常由肉芽组织继发性愈合，术后产生更多的肿胀和疼痛，皮瓣收缩；由于切口跨越血管和纤维束，造成皮瓣的血供减少，更易留下瘢痕[132]。还有一种瓣膜设计是在牙根上方做单个垂直切口，并向外剥离组织以暴露根尖上的骨[36,277]。虽然该方法有利于手术入路较长的牙根，且不穿过血管，但由于其切口通常位于术后骨腔内充盈的血凝块之上，难以进入较大病变，而且增加了术后感染的风险。

目前应用最广的两种切口是沟内皮瓣和边缘下皮瓣。

沟内切口

沟内切口可追溯到20世纪30年代[105]。这是一种全厚皮瓣设计，有利于初期愈合，并保持血液供应完整[96]（图12.2）。使用一个或两个垂直切口，可设计为三角瓣或矩形瓣。三角瓣对于常规手术位点的暴露已足够，但若根尖周病损范围较大或多颗患牙手术，需设计为矩形瓣。沟内瓣可以很好地实现皮瓣的重新附着，且由于阻隔了骨开窗部位血凝块的感染，使得术后疼痛和肿胀反应极小[96]。沟内瓣的缺点包括轻微的牙龈退缩，特别是在上颌前牙区，当涉及全冠修复体边缘时可能影响美学问题[132]。也有报道说这种皮瓣会造成牙龈乳头受损[91,262]，特别是当组织角化

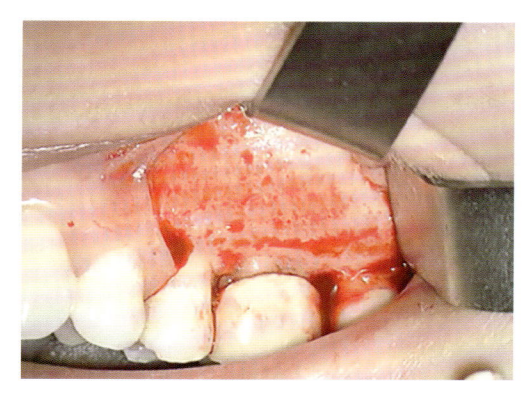

图12.2 后牙手术的三角沟内瓣，用于左上第一磨牙的颊根（感谢美国费城 Frank Setzer 医生供图）

不良、乳头很薄或软组织处理不仔细时。如果垂直切口与龈乳头外侧的水平切口成90°时，这种皮瓣设计可以保证龈乳头足够的血液供给。要特别关注微笑线高或薄-扇形牙周生物型的患者。为了避免这些问题的出现，有学者提出了一种改良的龈乳头基底部切口，原龈沟内切口改为颊侧颈部切口，切口通过龈乳头的基部以保持乳头完整，翻瓣时不将乳头分离[261]。采用这种切口可能会明显减少龈乳头的退缩[262]。

龈缘下切口

龈缘下切口于20世纪20年代被引入[167]，由 Ochsenbein-Luebke 进一步提出[148]。与沟内切口不同的是，这种皮瓣无须损伤牙齿周围的游离龈，其水平切口沿牙冠边缘形态设置在附着龈中间（图12.3）。与上述适应证相同，也可设计为三角瓣或矩形瓣。这种皮瓣设计更适用于附着龈

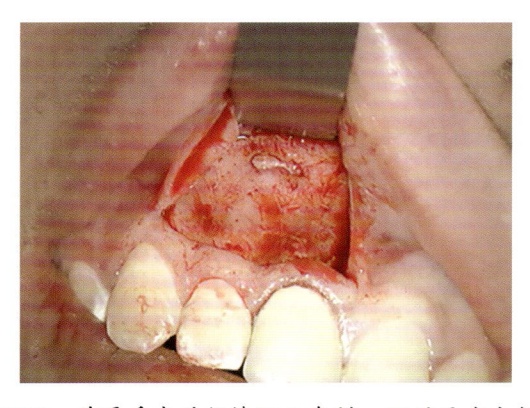

图12.3 前牙手术的龈缘下三角瓣，可用于右上侧切牙相关的根尖周病变。注意颊板缺损（美国费城 Frank Setzer 医生供图）

较宽的区域，特别是上颌前牙区或存在修复体边缘的区域，或其他有利于保持牙龈组织不受损伤的较高美学要求的病例[91]。这种皮瓣设计不适用于手术入路受限或存在较大的根尖周病变（尤其是冠状-根尖方向上）时。虽然皮瓣设计通常具有良好的预适应和伤口愈合能力，但在软组织容易撕裂的区域也会产生术后瘢痕[132]。

12.7.3 常规颌骨解剖结构

在某些情况下，由于根尖周病变已经导致皮质骨板缺损，行简单的软组织刮除术即可定位根尖。如果根尖没有暴露，临床医生根据术前临床检查和根尖周 X 线片或 CBCT 的测量，也可有效的定位根尖。行根尖手术时，应考虑患牙根尖与邻牙根尖、颏孔、下牙槽神经或上颌窦的相邻关系[112, 136, 174]。一般来说，在保证去除炎症组织，充分实施根切术、探查根切表面、根管逆行预备和根管逆行充填的基础上，去骨开窗的范围应尽可能小。

另类去骨开窗技术已经出现。在骨板无开窗或预期皮质骨板较厚的情况下，可以采用骨窗技术[123]。这种开窗技术可以使用手术锯或超声骨刀进行。开一个矩形的骨窗，露出根尖，将取出的骨质储存在合适的盐溶液中，并在手术结束时放回其原始位置。近年来，随着 CBCT 扫描与成像技术及3D-打印导板引导手术技术的应用使得邻近重要解剖结构的术区手术路径更易获得[4, 83]。

12.7.4 特殊解剖结构

上颌窦

如果根尖周病变到达或穿破上颌窦，去除炎症组织后可在口腔内形成上颌窦漏口[104]。当穿孔发生或可能发生时，应采取预防措施，不要将任何残留组织或异物进入窦腔。对于是否可以切除根尖存在争议，因此必须密切注意不要使牙本质碎屑进入窦腔内[142]，或者采取更好的技术在固定根尖的同时仔细切除整个根尖[92]。可通过放置缝线固定的无菌纱布垫作为临时屏障，来防止任何碎屑或异物进入窦腔内[125]（图12.4）。牙髓手术的结果不会因窦口本身而受到影响[276]，因为瓣膜重新复位后将在手术后提供保护，对于较

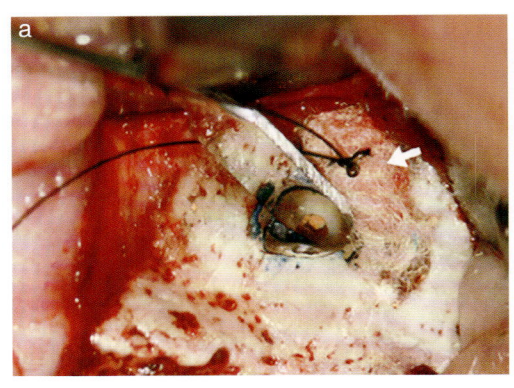

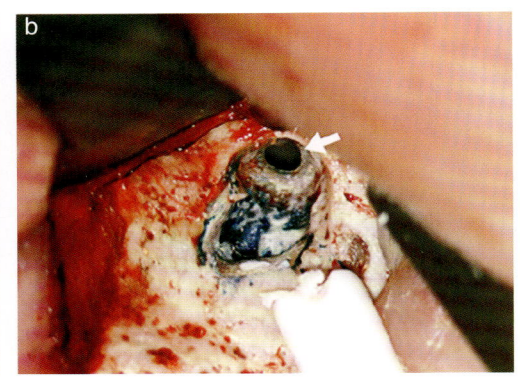

图 12.4　左上第二前磨牙根尖周病变切除后上颌窦开口的术中保护。a. 根管预备的显微探查。由手术缝线固定的棉球阻塞穿孔区。b. 根管逆行填充和取出棉球后的情况。注意箭头所示上颌窦穿孔（该病例由美国得克萨斯州奥斯汀市的 Karla Sermeño de Castillo 医生提供）

大的漏口建议使用骨移植材料，如骨胶原或骨膜覆盖颊侧缺损区。健康的患者不必服用抗生素，但建议使用减充血剂以防止窦腔内的压力问题干扰伤口愈合。

腭部神经血管束

腭部手术大多局限于第一磨牙。上颌前磨牙通常可以从颊侧行手术入路。由于解剖风险，第二磨牙手术几乎在所有情况下都无法从腭侧入路。腭大孔位于硬腭后缘前 3~4mm 处，神经和血管约在腭中线和牙龈边缘中间的黏膜下层向前方走行。第一磨牙腭根手术的软组织翻瓣可能包括皮瓣内的神经血管束，但任何试图对第二磨牙进行手术后部入路的去骨开窗都可能损伤此血管束，并大大增加严重出血或神经损伤的风险。为预防这些风险，可在尖牙和第一前磨牙之间设计一个腭瓣的松弛切口[95-96]。经上颌窦到达腭根的手术已有报道[8, 275]，但实际上仅限于远颊根和腭根融合的病例，因为从颊侧入路到腭尖的距离较大，根尖逆行预备和根尖逆行填充会变得非常困难，并且可能存在在窦腔中残留牙本质碎屑和异物材料的风险。

下牙槽神经血管束

影像学评估和（或）CBCT 影像资料以及周密的治疗计划是下颌前磨牙和磨牙区根管外科手术的先决条件[108-109, 162, 223, 267]。颏孔多位于下颌第二前磨牙的根尖附近，偶见于第一磨牙或第一前磨牙的根尖附近。颏孔与最近的牙根间距离是 0.3~9.8 mm[10]。少数报道显示，颏孔可与邻牙根尖处于同一水平或位于其冠方，甚至存在副颏孔[1, 174]。下颌管位于下颌磨牙根尖的下方偏舌侧。在大多数情况下，下颌管与下颌第一磨牙的根尖保持安全距离。但其邻近第二磨牙的根尖，加之第二磨牙的位置靠后，下颌骨升支部骨板较厚，使其成为手术禁忌牙位。

为保护下颌后牙手术中颏孔不受损伤，应选择沟内切口来获得更好的手术视野，行第二前磨牙和第一磨牙的手术时，垂直切口应设计在第一前磨牙的近中。为保护颏神经免受损伤，建议使用手术车针或超声骨刀在骨面上制作一个凹槽来固定手术拉钩，以防止意外滑动造成的组织损伤[1]（图 12.5）。

12.8　根尖手术的临床操作步骤

12.8.1　根尖刮治术

根尖刮治术包括去除根尖周围的软组织病变，不行根尖切除或根管逆行充填[144]。虽然炎症组织的去除是根尖手术的一个必要组成部分，但传统的根尖刮除术单独作为一种手术术式的适应证较局限。无须根尖切除或根管逆行填充的病例仅适用于探查性手术，如确定牙根纵裂或牙齿不可修复的其他原因。根管治疗失败的病例，特别是非手术再治疗后失败的病例，计划行外科手术治疗，来解决导致失败的潜在的根内和根外感染的原因。因此，除了牙冠或牙根切除术外，根管外科手术必须要包括根尖切除和根管逆行充填术，以最大限度地提高预后。根管治疗失败的病

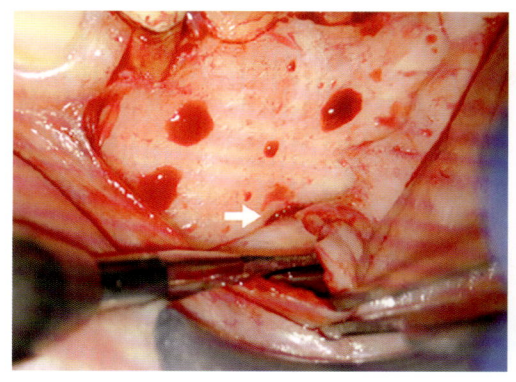

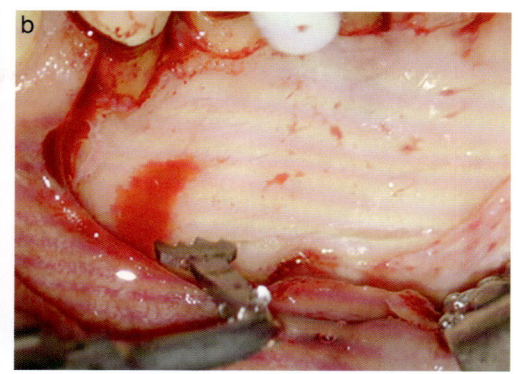

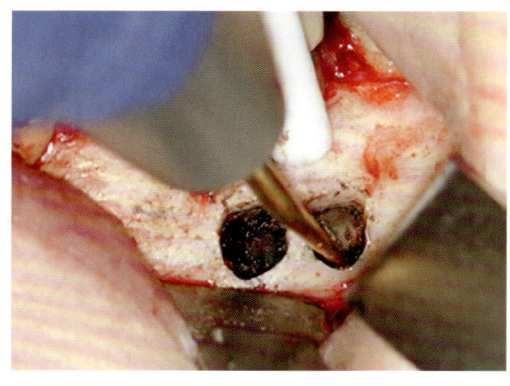

图 12.5 颏神经血管束的术中保护。a. 临床可见颏孔和神经血管束插入颊侧软组织内。b. 使用超声骨刀制备用于固定手术拉钩的凹槽。c. 在左下第一磨牙手术过程中将拉钩牢固固定在凹槽中来保护颏神经。在超声逆行预备远中根时，注意使用含有肾上腺素的棉球进行近中骨腔的止血（该病例由美国宾夕法尼亚州费城 Frank Setzer 医生提供）

因去除后不管是根尖周肉芽肿或脓肿都可以愈合，但在手术过程中无法确定是否存在根外感染。因此，作为外科手术的一部分，应尽可能去除整个根周病灶[32, 144, 171, 206-207]，包括任何可能引起囊性病变增殖或根外感染的上皮残留物。

12.8.2 根尖切除

去除根周炎症组织后，根尖清晰可辨。根尖切除术将切除以下病变：①可能存在根管内感染的复杂解剖结构，如根尖分歧、副根管或重度根尖弯曲；②非手术再治疗过程中阻碍清理根管系统的医源性因素，包括穿孔、台阶、管间交通或异物材料；③根尖断裂或微裂；④或在常规根管治疗中影响严密封闭效果的根尖吸收。根尖切除术还有助于去除组织中的致病因素，如异物和根管外感染。使用裂钻或 Lindemann 骨切削钻进行根尖切除，可获得光滑的根切表面，进而探查牙根内部解剖结构，从而确定先前治疗失败的可能原因。到底应该切除多少根尖结构，在文献中尚未达成共识。没有必要切除到病变底部[37, 95-96]。应尽可能多地暴露颊侧骨质。根尖孔、副根管以及根管侧支是根内感染传播到根周组织的主要途径。细菌可以穿过牙本质小管，但可能无法穿过完整的牙骨质层到达牙周组织。牙本质小管中的微生物通过根尖切除暴露于根周组织中，被认为是根管外科手术后周围组织中的潜在感染源。然而，尚无证据表明牙本质小管中微生物的存在与根周炎症程度之间的相关性[206]。最小的斜切角度有助于将根切后开放的牙本质小管数量保持在最低限度。此外，由于根尖三分之一处的多数细菌已被证实紧邻根管系统，因此根管逆行预备也将大大减少牙本质小管中的细菌数量[117, 225]。

解剖学研究显示，根尖切除 3mm 可消除 98% 的根尖分歧和 93% 的根管侧支[125]，此研究可作为临床指南。但根切长度因具体情况不同需做调整，例如，根尖可能邻近颏神经等解剖结构，或需要磨除折裂线，又或根管桩过长导致根尖可用长度有限。根切角度应为 0°~10°，而不是传统的 45°[42, 125, 206]，这样可以保留根尖结构，减少舌侧根管和副根管的遗漏概率；保证牙根切除完整；暴露较少的可能有助于传播根管内感染的牙本质小管[51, 85, 97, 245]；并使得超声工作尖可以更容易地沿牙体长轴行根管逆行预备。

骨腔内彻底止血后行根切面探查。生理盐水

冲洗骨腔后,使用浸有肾上腺素或止血剂(如硫酸铁或氯化铝)的棉球止血。手术结束后必须彻底去净止血剂,以清除任何可能对愈合产生潜在不利影响的有毒成分[98, 110, 114, 141],并使血液充盈骨腔内。使用微型冲洗器(例如 Stropko 装置[237])仔细吹干后,用亚甲蓝或其他染料对根切表面进行染色[125]。染色后不仅能显示出牙周韧带的轮廓以确保根切完全,而且有助于识别遗漏的根管,微裂,峡部(主根管之间的狭窄连接,通常包含组织残留和感染物质),其他解剖细节,变异或医源性损伤(图 12.6a)。应在高倍率(16~24 倍)下对切除的牙根表面进行探查[272]。在原始牙尖切除 3mm 的水平,90% 的上颌第一磨牙近颊根、30% 的上下颌前磨牙、超过 80% 的下颌第一磨牙近中根存在峡部[107, 279](图 12.7)。

12.8.3 根管倒预备

根管倒预备旨在清理根管系统中术前常规根管治疗未能触及的部分,包含先前遗漏的根管和根管充填质量不佳,或者由于根充糊剂不足以封闭根充材料和根管壁之间的所有间隙或管间吻合区。在根管倒预备时,管间峡部也应得到预备[153](图 12.6b)。

使用超声工作尖进行根管倒预备。在管腔预备之前,操作者应在低倍率(4~8 倍)下将超声工作尖端对准牙根长轴方向(图 12.5b)。颌骨不同部位对应有不同角度的特定工作尖。尽管有人担心超声倒预备根管后牙根会出现微裂纹[75, 140],但其似乎与临床结果无关[19, 122]。根据根管的原始形状和大小,选用不同大小的工作尖。在进行根管倒充填之前,应干燥管腔,并使用显微口镜在高倍镜下检查管腔中是否残留填充材料,特别是在管壁的颊侧,因为这部分区域在超声预备时无法直视[237]。

12.8.4 根管倒充填的需求

理想的根管倒充填材料需要满足多种特性。生物相容性和密封能力是首要性能;要有杀菌或抑菌能力来协助达到总体治疗目的。此外,还需这些基本功能:对根管表面的黏附能力;尺寸稳定性;无腐蚀性;抗溶解性;操作方便,有足够的可操作时间;牙齿或组织不染色;成骨和成牙骨质特性;阻射性。

目前已有多种根管倒充填材料[50, 118, 253]被研

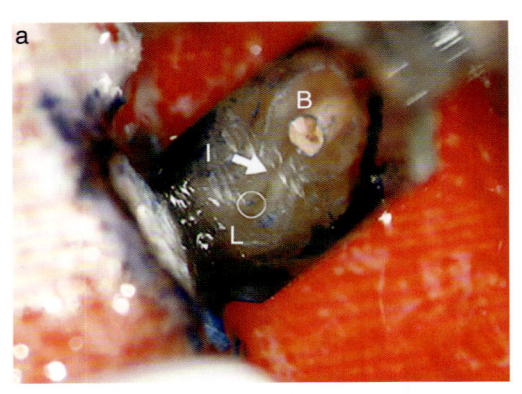

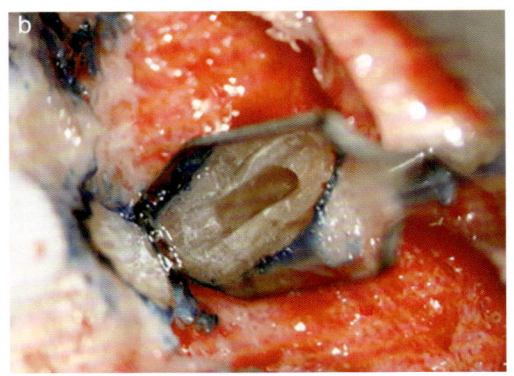

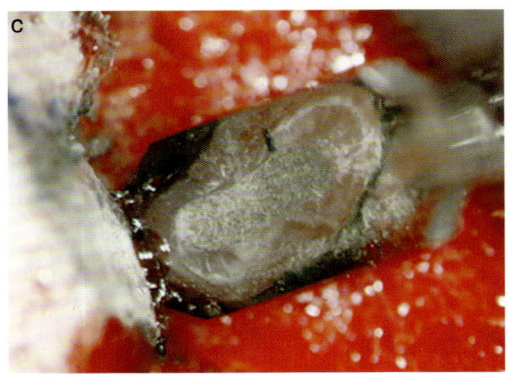

图 12.6 左下第一前磨牙根切后探查、根管倒预备和根管倒充填的临床步骤。a.亚甲蓝染色后显微口镜观察根切表面。注意已行根管填充的颊侧根管(B)、遗漏的舌侧根管(L)(圆圈)和连接颊舌根管的峡部(I)(箭头)。b.倒预备的洞形,包括峡部预备。c.根管倒填充(MTA)(该病例由美国宾夕法尼亚州费城 Frank Setzer 医生提供)

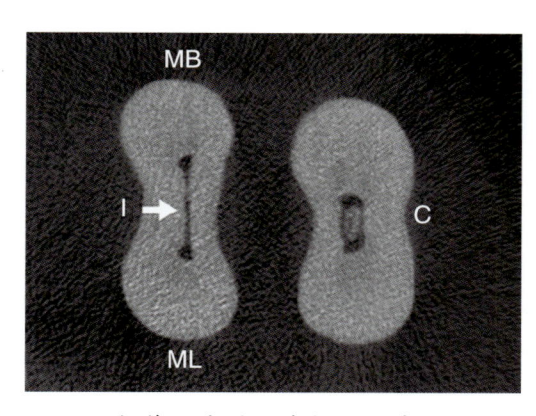

图 12.7 下颌第一磨牙近中根和远中根的显微 CT（μ-CT）轴向视图。峡部（I）（箭头）连接近颊根管（MB）和近舌根管（ML）。注意远中根管内的钙化（C）（该病例由美国宾夕法尼亚州费城 Vanessa Cabrera Saez 医生提供）

究和使用。已广泛用于临床研究的材料包括银汞合金、牙胶尖[173, 186]、氧化锌/硫酸钙水门汀（Cavit）[73, 172, 187]、聚乙烯树脂（Diaket）[244]、玻璃离子水门汀[116]、复合树脂（Geristore、Retroplast）[9]、氧化锌/丁香酚水门汀（IRM、SuperEBA）[101]、硅酸钙基水门汀[三氧化矿物凝聚体（MTA）]、生物牙本质、生物陶瓷牙根修复材料（BC, RRM）。除了银汞合金由于其历史原因包含在内，并且至今仍被一些从业者使用[33]之外，本部分仅详细讨论最现代的根管逆行填充材料。

12.8.5 根管倒充填材料

银汞合金

多年来，银汞合金是最受欢迎和使用最广泛的根管倒填充材料[26, 77, 273]。银汞合金因其缺乏生物相容性、有腐蚀性、可能在根尖形成裂纹、银盐扩散导致软硬组织着色[100]，以及预后不佳而受到批评[7, 63, 73, 116, 178, 221]（图 12.8）。染色渗透实验[77, 177]或流体过滤模型[234, 282]已证实银汞合金在体外条件下存在渗漏。尽管有人批评这些研究并不是体内条件[188, 201]，但银汞合金也显示出细菌渗漏[53, 255]，与其他的研究材料相比，不管实验方法如何，它始终显示出更明显的渗漏[53]。因此，银汞合金作为根管倒充填材料很可能会导致渗漏[13, 53, 96]。银汞合金缺乏生物相容性是由于其汞含量具有环境危害性，其作为修复填充材料使用有严格的限制[66]。在组织学上，银汞合金或其腐蚀产物被认为是炎症组织反应的原因[16, 51, 188, 252, 256]，从根端仍可检测到银汞合金痕迹[188]。在所有材料的对比中，银汞合金的根尖周组织炎症反应最严重也最广泛[51, 188, 192, 252, 254]。

复合树脂

体外研究表明复合树脂在倒预备的管腔中具有良好的密封性能[3, 150-151]，并且双固化亲水改良复合树脂 Geristore 已被用作传统的根管倒充填材料，也被用于龈下或骨下缺损修复，以及作为引导组织再生（GTR）的屏障材料。

Rud 等人率先引入了一种通过复合树脂材料封闭切除根尖的技术。1991 年[209]，最近 von Arx 等人也使用这种技术[268]。在使用显微镜或内窥镜高倍放大时，与其他传统或现代手术方法不同，该技术并不做传统的根管倒预备和充填。取而代之的是，该技术使用球钻在根切表面制作一个凹形窝洞，然后用 EDTA 进行蚀刻，并以圆顶状方式放置粘接树脂材料。该技术使用的材料是 Retroplast，这是一种牙本质粘接的双固化复合树脂[209, 268]。虽然与传统的根尖手术技术相比，该技术显示出良好的愈合效果[115, 209-210, 211]，但与现代技术相比疗效尚有差距[130]，并且仅限于无法使用超声进行根管倒预备的患牙。该技术的主要缺点在于它依赖于精确的湿度控制，否则材料将无法与根切面粘接[210-211]。

氧化锌/丁香油酚

几十年来，氧化锌/丁香酚（ZOE）水门汀被推荐为根尖手术的充填材料[81, 171]。有两种最常用的中间修复材料（IRM），一种通过向粉剂中添加聚甲基丙烯酸酯而增强的 ZOE 水门汀；另一种为超级乙氧基苯甲酸（SuperEBA），通过丁香酚液体部分取代原乙氧基苯甲酸，并添加熔融石英或氧化铝（氧化铝）粉末。两种材料均表现出明显优于银汞合金的治疗效果[63, 204-205]，组织学已证实，尽管牙根表面仍存在一些炎症细胞，但其比未改良的 ZOE 具有更高的生物相容性[188, 191-192]。IRM 和 SuperEBA 均表现出低溶解度[48]、良好的抗菌作用[49, 251]，并且在染料渗透测试中几乎没有渗漏[47, 175]。与银汞合金相比，SuperEBA 充填微渗漏显著减少，与根管壁也有更好的结合。使

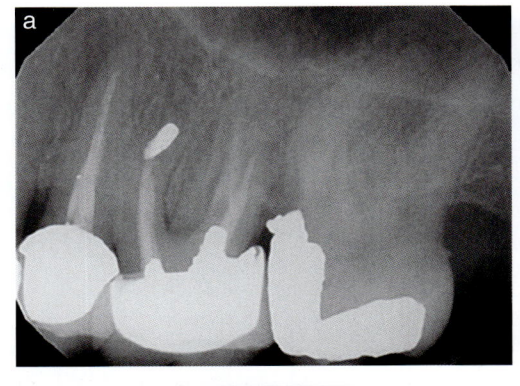

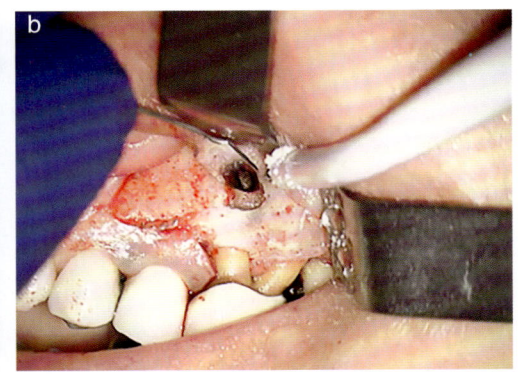

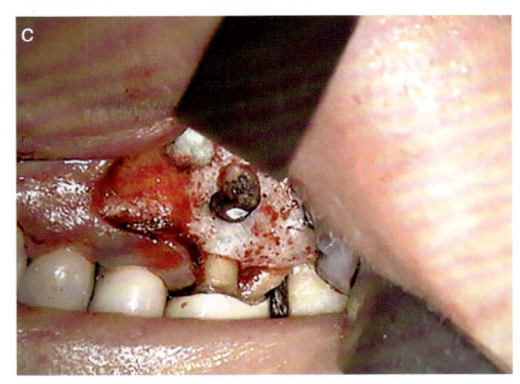

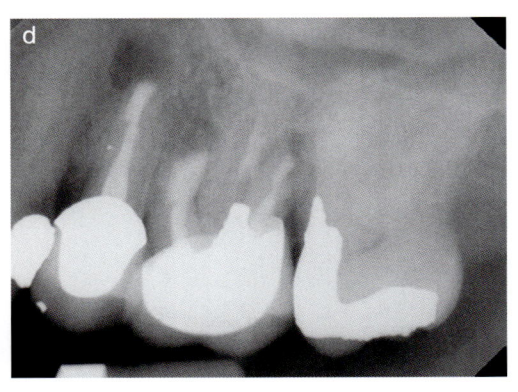

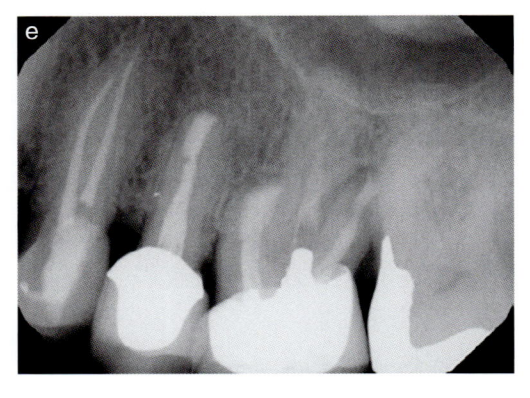

图 12.8 左上颌区手术治疗。第二前磨牙和第一磨牙的颊根上的根尖周炎（通过 CBCT 证实）。传统的根尖手术治疗史，用银汞合金充填第一磨牙近颊根。第二磨牙银汞合金悬突引起颊侧肿胀。a. 术前 X 线片。b. 临床可见银汞合金逆行充填材料。c. 新的根管逆行充填（RRM）。d. 前磨牙和磨牙逆行根管充填的术后 X 线片。对第二磨牙上现有的银汞合金填充物重新修整后的情况。e. 12 个月随访 X 线片。影像学显示愈合，无临床症状。注意第一前磨牙的牙髓治疗和新的冠修复体（该病例由美国宾夕法尼亚州费城的 Frank Setzer 医生提供）

用 IRM 或 SuperEBA 作为根管倒充填材料，使用超声工作仪进行根管倒预备，使用高放大倍数的研究通常才有资格纳入评估显微根管外科手术疗效的 meta 分析[130, 220-221]。

硅酸钙基水门汀

该材料最初源自硅酸盐水门汀，一种二氧化硅、氧化铝和钙复合建筑材料，现已开发出多种牙科充填和修复材料，包括三氧化矿物凝聚体（MTA）、BioDentine 或生物陶瓷牙根修复材料（BC、RRM）。所有材料都是亲水性的，凝固时间和准备方法上有所不同。硅酸钙基水门汀比氧化锌/丁香酚水门汀具有显著的改进，优点包括降低了细胞毒性[29, 55]，增加了生物相容性[84, 158]，增加了细胞附着[55]，诱导牙骨质和骨组织形成[46, 84]，还提高了 pH[88]。

MTA 是第一个被引入的材料[252]，已被全面研究。对动物根管倒充填材料的几项组织学研究[16, 197, 252, 254]表明：MTA 比银汞合金显示出明显更少的炎症，并且在切除的牙根表面和充填材料上形成新的牙骨质（图 12.9，图 12.10）[252, 254]。近期研究表明，在材料凝固期间，与组织液接触的 MTA 表面上会形成羟基磷灰石（HA）层，称为"生物矿化"[25]。该层在 MTA 和牙本质界面之间形成生物密封，从而增强 MTA 的长期密

根管外科 | 第12章

至 2h。RRM 和 MTA 在抗菌功效[146]、生物相容性[5]和封闭能力[166]方面没有显著差异。在一项比较 RRM 和 MTA 作为根管倒充填材料的体内研究中[45]，愈合后手术部位没有明显的炎症或炎症范围较小，与 MTA 类似，在 RRM 附近也观察到牙骨质样组织（图 12.11）。两项研究显微根管外科手术的随机对照试验证实 RRM 疗效显著[224, 285]。

12.8.6 伤口的闭合及术后护理

手术完成后，伤口的闭合和术后护理将很大程度上决定的生物学和美学愈合过程。在骨窗部位应检查和清除多余的材料和止血剂，避免异物反应，并清除硫酸铁等材料中的任何有毒副产物。血液充盈骨窗部位，以形成血凝块并引导后期的骨愈合。任何移植材料或膜都应该在手术的这一阶段放置。在皮瓣复位之前，用含有生理盐水的湿纱布湿润软组织，因为软组织可能在手术过程中已经脱水，软组织再次湿润将有助于恢复组织的自然弹性。软组织管理可能对美学效果有很大的影响。为了将黏膜瓣恢复到原来的位置，缝合是必须的。通过使用显微镜或放大镜来提高缝合的准确性，特别是对于较小直径的缝线。常用 5-0 或 6-0 的缝线，在美学要求的区域，如上颌骨前部；如果选择乳头基底皮瓣，可能建议使用 7-0 缝合线复位乳头。任何皮瓣设计都需要与

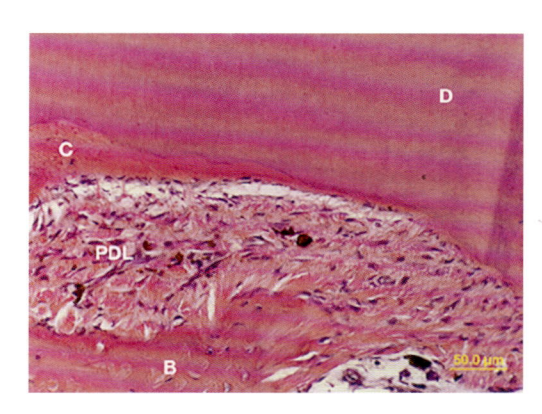

图 12.9 在截面的牙本质 [D] 上沉积新的牙骨质 [C] 层。观察到周围骨质 [B] 和牙周韧带结构 [PDL] 无炎症（引自文献 45）

封能力。不管是灰色还是白色配方的 MTA，它们的共同缺点包括操作性能差和可能引起牙齿变色[131]。调拌好的 MTA 具有湿润的颗粒糊状物的稠度，难以将其放置在管腔中。当存在出血或出血过多，或其他体液影响的情况下，MTA 容易产生冲洗效应，影响封闭效果。

硅酸钙基水门汀、BioDentine（一种可在研磨机中混合的胶囊材料）和预混的 RRM 材料解决了MTA 使用中遇到的一些问题。两种材料的牙齿变色效果都比 MTA 小[131]，RRM 作为根管逆行充填材料比 BioDentine 更受关注，BioDentine 更常用于穿孔修补。RRM 尺寸稳定，pH 高，凝固时间短

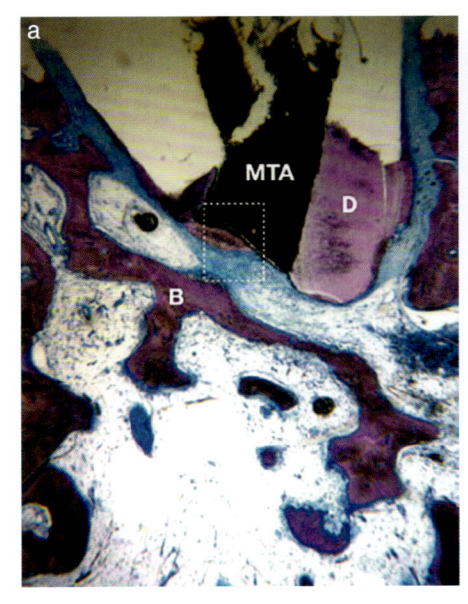

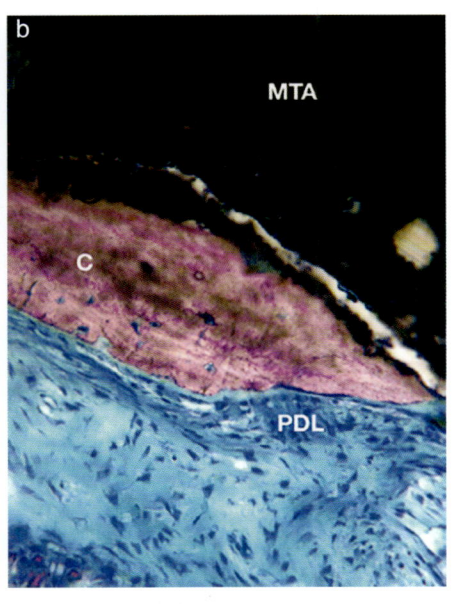

图 12.10 充填 MTA 后牙根和根尖周区域的组织学表现。a. 充填材料（MTA）的根部截面。b. 图 a 中标记区域的特写。新沉积的矿化细胞牙骨质（C）在 MTA 上生长（由 Baek 等人提供[16]）

261

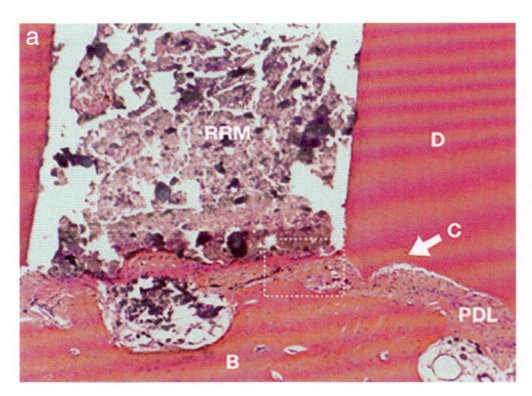

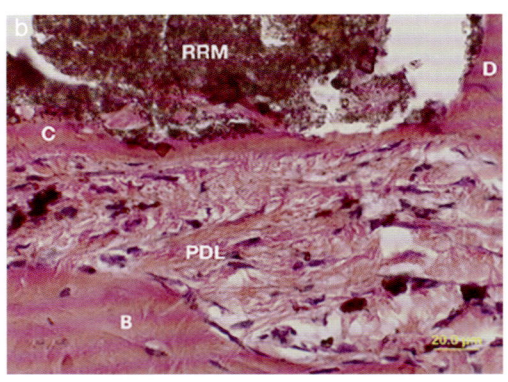

图 12.11 根管倒充填 RRM 后牙根和根尖周区域的组织学表现。a. 充填材料（RRM）的根截面。b. 图 a 中标记区域的特写，RRM 表面形成矿化组织。注意牙周韧带结构（PDL）和周围骨质（引自文献 45）

底层骨组织密切接触，以最小化骨膜下血块的厚度，并根据主要意图愈合。尼龙、聚丙烯或聚四氟乙烯（PTFE）单丝缝合线或有涂层的单丝缝合线是首选材料[265]，因为传统的丝线可能会促进细菌定植，阻碍伤口愈合。可吸收缝线（如肠线）减少了就诊的次数，但其吸收为伤口愈合过程增加了炎症成分。是否拆除缝线需要临床医生在手术干预后 48h[96] 至 4d[95, 263] 检查评估，并密切控制愈合过程。据报道，如果缝线留下的时间过长，感染可能会损害一些皮瓣边缘[91,96]。缝合针的形状、大小和曲率对于特定的手术过程很重要，但它的选择可能会随着牙周的生物类型、手术入路和术者的偏好而变化[265]。间断缝合通常比连续缝合更可取，因为它有更可控的重新适应性。悬吊缝合可用于后牙区域的邻接区的缝合。应指导患者在术后前 1~2d 避免运动和掀起嘴唇，因为这可能会导致出血或撕裂皮瓣边缘，引起疼痛、肿胀和血肿，同时增加血肿感染的风险和延迟愈合。患者应尽可能长时间地避免吸烟，同时近期应进食容易通过常规口腔清洁方法从术区清理的食物。间隔冰敷能预防过度肿胀[94,96]。除了肿胀和疼痛外，还应告知少数患者软组织可能会出现暂时的变色和瘀伤。如果患者能耐受非甾体类消炎药，首选此类镇痛药，因为它具有抗炎和镇痛药的双重作用。不建议常规使用抗生素[94]，但可以根据患者的医疗或牙科史给予相应的用药指导。术后第二天开始使用氯己定溶液仔细漱口，有利于伤口愈合，因其可减少口腔内的细菌含量，从而减少术后手术部位感染的风险。给予患者紧急联系方式。最后，应告知患者，如果在初始愈合阶段后出现任何复发症状，应及时复诊。患者应在术后 4 周后复诊，以确保软组织的成功愈合、无任何临床症状。术后 1 年、2 年和 4 年后进行影像学检查检测愈合过程，确保长期的手术成功。

12.9 穿孔的修复

穿孔是指牙髓与牙根周围组织之间的异常连通[198]。穿孔通常发生在医源性穿孔、器械选择不当、桩道预备不当或激进的根管扩大。正确治疗导致的与吸收性缺损或龋损相通而产生的穿孔较少见。穿孔的位置可能从龈沟到牙槽嵴顶下、根中或根尖区。能否成功修复穿孔主要取决于穿孔部位是否存在感染、穿孔的大小，能否选择合适入路和可视化操作。即刻穿孔修复比有微生物进入穿孔区并伴有炎症和严重出血损伤恢复后再行穿孔修复的预后更好[170, 216]。龈沟内的穿孔可以通过常规的修复方式完成，或通过一个小翻瓣良好地控制修复的边缘。根据水分控制，粘接复合树脂或改性复合树脂都是可选择的穿孔修复材料。牙槽嵴顶下方穿孔的修复可从根管内进行非手术修复[198]；如果无法应用注射器或微型插入器、或因根管弯曲无法可视化、或因根周组织出血无法控制的穿孔，可选择手术修复。牙槽嵴顶下穿孔修复材料的理想性能与根尖倒充填材料基本相同。因 MTA[193, 254] 或 RRM[45] 等材料上可形成牙骨质或骨水泥样组织，硅酸钙基水门汀成为合适的材料[198, 248]。大多数穿孔不需要手术修复[20, 24, 137]。如果需要手术修复，手术方案通常将遵循根尖手术流程，根尖切除范围需要包括穿孔区域。在冠根比可能受到损害的情况下，选择不接近垂直的切除角度是可取的，这样可以保留更多的牙根结构以提供牙周支持。

12.10 意向再植

意向再植是指有目的拔牙，在根尖预备和根尖倒充填后立即再植[90]。意向再植不是再治疗的首选方案[278]，但对于因修复或根管的原因不能进行非手术再治疗，非手术治疗方案失败，或者由于解剖限制不能进行常规的手术再治疗，可以选择意向再植以避免拔牙[2, 68, 89, 133]。最新的综述和荟萃分析（纳入1966至2014年的研究）显示：意向再植后牙齿的生存率为88%，而治疗后牙根吸收的发生率为11%[247]。治疗方案包括：缓慢而小心地拔牙，以避免根折、冠方修复体的脱落以及牙槽骨、牙槽窝内牙周韧带和牙骨质层的损伤（图12.12）。应避免搔刮牙槽窝，以便牙周韧带的重建。拔牙后，必须非常小心，不要接触牙根表面，以防止牙周组织损伤和牙根吸收[12, 121]。

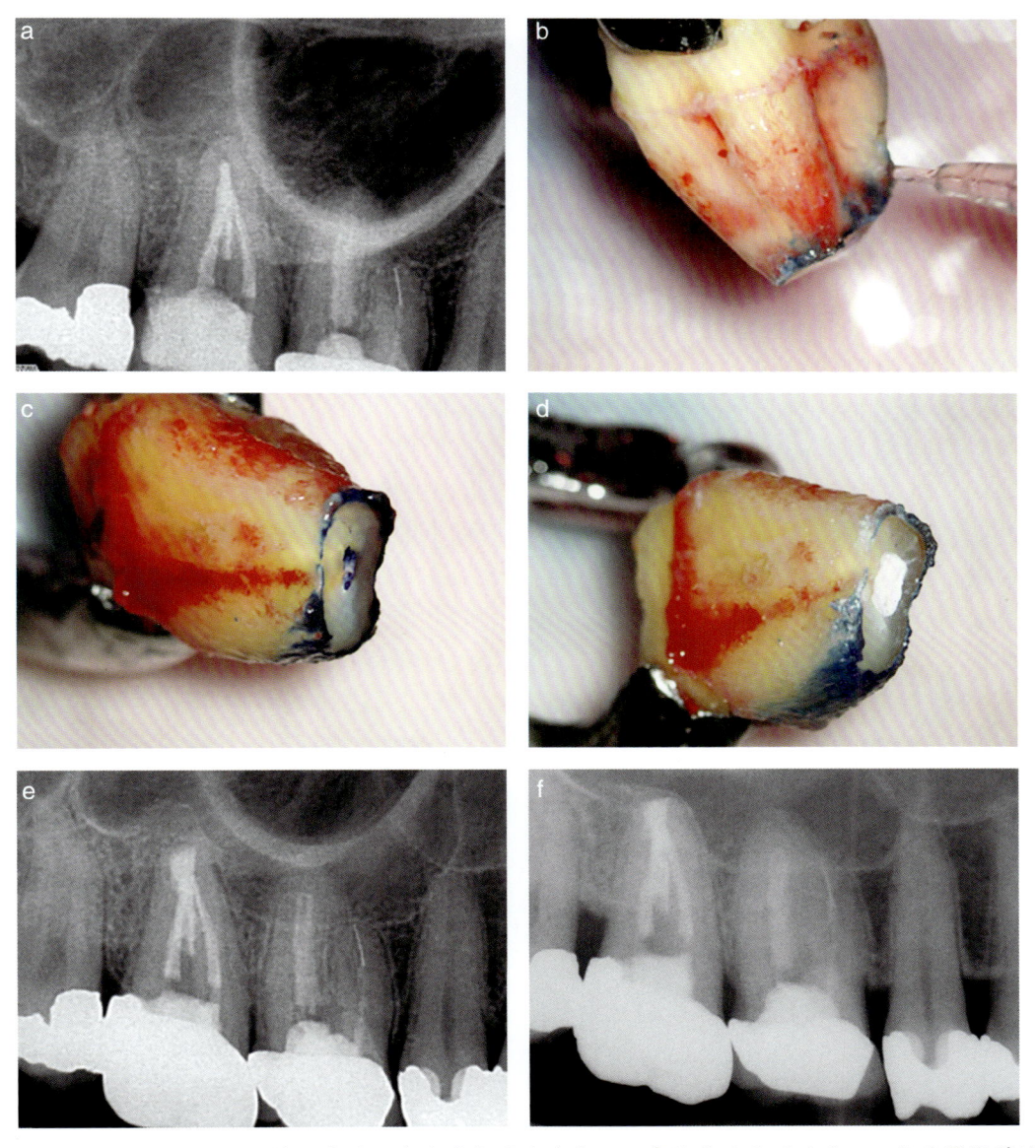

图12.12 意向再植术完成右上颌第二磨牙。有非手术再治疗失败且有临床症状的病史。a. 术前影像学检查。b. 用生理盐水冲洗拔出的牙齿。c. 亚甲基蓝染色后的牙根表面。注意长椭圆形根管横截面和未填充的根管部分。d. 用RRM进行根管倒充填。e. 术后X线片。f. 随访18个月，观察到影像学愈合，无临床症状（该病例由美国宾夕法尼亚州费城的Bekir karabucak医生提供）

出于同样的原因，洁治和根面平整也是禁忌的。再植后2~4周会发生短暂的牙根表面吸收，大约2个月后减少。在供牙体外阶段，应仔细检查牙齿是否有根折或其他医源性损伤，并确定之前根管治疗失败的可能原因。与根尖外科手术不同，因为没有空间限制需要使用超声工作尖来预备根尖区，所以可选择裂钻来进行根尖区预备。口腔外操作时间不应超过15min[129]，以避免牙根表面的牙周韧带结构变性。使用生理盐水持续冲洗牙齿，以便牙根保持湿润[86]。再植后，必须小心地将牙齿放置在正确的方向，最好是轻咬合，因为牙齿根尖区已经被切除。如果牙齿在愈合阶段有轻微的脱离咬合，随着咬合力被最小化，PDL可能会更好的重新附着。意向再植牙齿的移动性应保持在最低限度；只有在动度增加的情况下才需要夹板固定。建议患者术后至少两周避免患侧咀嚼，并按照根尖外科手术的方案进行定期随访。

12.11 牙根截除、半切

截根术最早在19世纪80年代被提出用于治疗多根牙[71]。截根术被认为是一种"根切除"技术，因为它只切除齐平或位于釉牙骨质界下方的牙根结构，而不去除部分牙冠组织[222]。相比之下，"冠切除"包括半切、三切和前磨牙化（premolarization）（分牙术），即它们在术中都要穿过多根牙的牙冠和根分叉，以便切除冠和根的相关部分（半切、三切）或所有根/冠部分被保留（预磨化、双化）[222]。冠切除术和根切除术的适应证和禁忌证如下文所述[159,222,235]。

（1）适应证
· 严重的骨丧失，影响一个牙根，不适合接受其他形式的治疗。
· 中度至重度多根牙的根分叉病变。
· 与邻牙牙根距离较近。
· 根折、穿孔、根面龋、涉及一个根或根分叉区域的牙根外吸收。
· 特殊牙根无法完成根管治疗，且根尖手术是禁忌的。
· 去除一个特定牙根后能被保留的桥体基牙。
· 当解剖因素妨碍种植体植入时。

（2）禁忌证

· 剩余牙根周围或根分叉区域的骨组织支撑力不足。
· 根分叉太靠近根尖，牙根没有充分分开，或牙根融合。
· 剩余牙根无法完成根管治疗，剩余牙根的解剖结构不良。
· 根分叉区域有广泛的龋坏或牙根吸收。
· 剩余牙根无保留价值。

术前应进行完善的根管治疗[159]。如果切除时需要切割金属修复体或涉及切除大量的牙冠结构，这些操作应在切开翻瓣之前进行，以防止牙齿颗粒和金属碎屑残留在软组织中。手术入路应通过颊侧和舌侧全厚黏膜皮瓣，以便有足够的手术通路和良好的视野完成切除和伤口闭合。炎症组织必须被切除，使用长细的裂钻或者Lindeman骨切割钻，完全切除牙根。通过使用牙周探针仔细探查根分叉区域和检查每个牙根的动度来检查牙根是否被完全分离。一旦牙根被完全的分开，小心地移除它，避免损害剩余的牙齿结构。剩余牙冠结构保持原有轮廓，以确保没有凸出的牙齿结构，因为这些地方可能堆积菌斑。清洁牙根表面，清除所有肉芽组织，并对剩余骨组织进行骨成形术，以消除任何不规则的外形轮廓，同时为愈合后的齿龈复合体提供生物学宽度。然后，皮瓣重新复位、缝合。随访遵循根尖手术指南。永久修复应便于患者进行口腔清洁。目前有许多临床研究[21,38,40-41,61,69-80,99,106,139,180,241,284]、系统性综述和meta分析对牙根切除术的预后进行了分析，将在下面详细讨论[222]。

12.12 引导组织再生

引导组织再生（GTR）或骨移植材料和（或）屏障膜已广泛被用于牙周病学和牙科种植学，但在牙髓病学中应用较少[259]。20世纪50年代引入了将骨愈合和结缔组织愈合分开的屏障膜，到20世纪60年代该技术应用到牙槽外科[30]。对于根管外科手术，屏障膜在动物实验[58,59,149]和患者[67,185]中均已开展研究。任何移植材料或屏障膜的放置都应发生在手术结束时，伤口闭合之前。常见的膜材料包括聚四氟乙烯（聚四氟乙烯、Goretex）、胶原蛋白膜或聚乳酸膜；常见的移植材料包括冻干同种异体骨移植、脱矿冻干同种异体骨移植、羟基磷灰石、磷酸三钙、生物玻璃或硫酸钙。与不使用屏障材料[14,82,266]的对照组病变相比，GTR有效地组织了上皮细胞长入病变，允许骨再生。

已有综述回顾了GTR在根管外科手术中的应用[143,259]。在根管外科手术中，骨缺损可以分为简单缺损、复杂缺损和累及牙周缺损。

简单缺损是没有任何牙周组织受累的牙髓病变，例如牙周探针深度，或牙周与牙髓缺损之间的关系。在术后1年的随访中可见，术中是放置屏障膜[83,149]还是膜联合移植材料，愈合率未见差异[243]。同样，在术后6个月的随访中，CT扫描显示根尖周骨愈合和骨密度也没有差异[212]。

复杂缺损不涉及牙周组织的牙髓病变，但缺损直径超过10mm，表现为颊舌"贯通"缺损、和（或）鼻腔穿通的、或大的上颌窦穿通。这些病变可能受益于GTR技术。与对照组不放屏障膜没有愈合相比，颊舌侧放置屏障膜的大鼠颅骨缺损的贯通伤显示出完全愈合[66]。在类似的缺损中，在根管外科手术后使用屏障膜的病例显示完全愈合，而对照组[57-58]仅显示纤维结缔组织愈合。在人类中，GTR技术治疗的贯通型病变的愈合率为88%，而不使用的为57%[242]。这些发现表明，贯通型病变应有颊舌屏障以促进有效愈合[27]。相较于对照组，从临床、影像学和组织学结果的多方面来看[185,196,246]，使用GTR技术时，缺损直径超过10 mm的病变显示出更快的愈合和更好的结果[184-185]。

累及牙周的缺损表现为根分叉区骨丢失、根尖破损或牙周牙髓联合缺损，或由于根裂或牙根完全外露导致的颊侧骨板丧失。与单纯的牙髓病变相比[124,233]，牙周病受累性缺损的牙髓病变手术的总体成功率显著降低。在根管外科手术的总体成功率中，与单纯的牙髓病变相比，累及牙周的缺损的成功率显著降低[124,233]。GTR对改善牙齿牙周状态的有效性已被组织学和临床研究结果证实。在颊侧骨板缺失的犬类中放置屏障膜能显著提高牙槽骨再生量[65]，放置膜的同时增加移植材料可以显著增加牙骨质沉积[31,60]。

总之，使用GTR技术对于复杂缺损和累及牙周组织的缺损有益。

12.13 手术失败病例的再治疗

初次手术失败最常见的原因是没有放置或不正确地放置倒充填材料[133]。在对短期随访成功的病例进行长期随访中发现，长期随访中失败主要与术者的错误有关[232]。如果失败的原因是不完善的根管充填，发生冠方微渗漏，可进行根管再治疗，此时，非手术再治疗应是首选治疗方案[231]。Mente等人评估了手术失败后的非手术再治疗[157]。在这个前瞻性病例系列中，25例患者进行了再治疗和根尖MTA填充，总成功率为87%。然而，前牙的成功率为100%，而后牙的成功率为80%，说明多根牙手术的困难和挑战性[157]。如果非手术再治疗不是首选或可预测的选择，应考虑再次手术或拔除患牙[207]。如果是某一个特殊牙根治疗失败，牙冠或牙根切除就可能是保存牙齿的选择[222]。一些研究报道，再次手术预后很差，通常是禁忌证[215,270]，对再次手术的系统回顾报告显示，包括传统的二次手术在内，加权合并成功率仅为36%[190]。如果采用显微外科技术和生物相容性的根尖填充材料如使用MTA和Super-EBA，再次手术的成功率可更高一些，接近首次手术[231]。

12.14 愈合方式

根尖周组织的愈合需要从骨髓、骨内膜、骨膜和牙周韧带中招募干细胞/祖细胞来分化为成骨细胞、牙周韧带（PDL）细胞和成牙骨质细胞。术后切除性伤口区域的愈合比非手术治疗后肉芽肿或囊肿的消退更快，因在非手术治疗中，炎症组织必须首先被吞噬细胞分解[143]。根尖手术后，骨缺损区域充满血液，并通过重新定位的皮瓣来保护血凝块免受口腔感染。上皮细胞增殖以闭合手术切口处的伤口。建议患者在术后第一周使用口内消毒剂，以减少手术部位感染的风险。软组织下，骨的愈合和牙槽愈合是两个独立的过程。

12.14.1 骨愈合

通过血管收缩和血小板聚集的止血机制，达

到手术干预后的骨愈合[143]。伤口愈合有三个基本阶段，在两个阶段之间有相当大的重叠：炎症、增殖和重塑[54, 60, 135, 152, 281]。在这三个阶段中，发生了一系列复杂而协调的事件。炎症期包括趋化和吞噬作用[135, 152]。在增殖阶段，新胶原形成、上皮化和血管生成导致来自 PDL 和骨内膜的肉芽组织的形成[52, 102, 135, 152]。最后，在重塑阶段，活跃的胶原重塑和组织成熟发生，导致修复或再生的发生[135]。对于骨性伤口，这将转化为初始血凝块血运重建和矿化基质的形成，从编织骨最终成熟为松质骨。新骨形成开始于内部区域，并向前皮质板的水平发展。当新的编织骨到达固有层时，覆盖的膜成为功能性牙周组织，这是骨愈合过程的一部分。此过程与牙槽愈合是不同的，因为它是对手术切除的反应。

12.14.2 牙槽愈合

在根尖周炎的发展过程中，牙周韧带、牙骨质和牙本质在根尖被吸收。来自邻近牙根表面的牙周韧带细胞在牙槽愈合过程中增殖，并覆盖切除后的牙根表面[143, 145]。从这些组织中，PDL 干细胞将分化成牙骨质样细胞，使牙骨质再生[143, 145]。同时涉及牙骨质和牙本质的牙根吸收只能通过类牙骨质组织来修复，因为 PDL 干细胞不能分化为产生牙本质的成骨细胞[217]。在没有感染或严重炎症反应的情况下，牙骨质已被证明可以恢复为覆盖切除的牙本质表面[11, 13, 102, 202]。牙骨质可以直接附着在 MTA 和 RRM 的材料表面[45, 252, 254]。此外，MTA 可能支持重建与其厚度相当的 PDL 宽度，而骨到材料的距离是 SuperEBA 的两倍，是汞合金的4倍[15]。

12.15 牙髓外科学的结果

与非手术牙髓学一样，牙髓学手术的目的是消除根尖周炎和预防其复发。最广泛使用的评估手术的分类是基于 Rud 和 Molven 的标准[161, 208]。成功的定义在放射学上表现为完全愈合或不完全愈合（瘢痕组织形成），在临床上表现为没有疼痛、肿胀、叩痛或窦道（图 12.13）。失败包括影像学的愈合不确定（病变范围减小）或愈合不理想（病变范围保持不变或增加），以及临床上存在上述任何症状。根据 Molven 等人的研究[161]：术后愈合相关的变化多发生在手术干预后的第 1 年内。完全或不完全愈合的无症状病例被认为是成功的，而愈合不确定的病例应重新评估至第 4 年，然后确定为成功或失败。牙齿留存已被证实是切除治疗积极结果的衡量指标[222]。牙髓外科学手术后根尖周围愈合的三维评估标准最近被引入[45,214]并得到验证[269]（图 12.14）。然而，大多数评估外科手术结果的研究都依赖于临床评价及二维影像学表现。

一项关于手术结果的系统回顾发现：因操作者和手术过程中使用的具体技术而异，包括所有传统技术，成功率为 37%~91%[78]。然而，由于不同研究之间的治疗方案和方法存在许多变量，包括研究设计、样本量、纳入和排除标准、随访期、缺乏标准化的临床和影像学愈合参数、术前牙周状况、既往根管治疗质量的变化、冠方修复以及手术材料和技术本身，结果评估必须谨慎进行。此外，许多报道根尖手术成功和失败的研究都是系列病例或其他证据水平较低的研究[154]。然而，已经证明对于相同的研究主题，与随机对照试验相比，设计良好的观察性研究的结果、队列或病例对照设计没有高估治疗的影响[56]，系统回顾和 meta 分析被认为是有效的评估证据。

很少有牙科技术经历了像根尖手术这样的实质性的发展。许多系统的综述和 meta 分析证明了根尖手术中使用的技术对手术结果的影响。传统的，如今已经过时的（使用直角手机、牙根斜向切除、汞合金逆行填充）技术，显示加权合并成功率为 59.0%[221]。使用放大镜、超声器械预备、更好的生物相容性材料将根尖周愈合的成功率提高至 86%[220]。牙髓显微外科使用相同技术，但用牙科显微镜替代放大镜，能够提供高倍放大的视野，根管病损的成功率从 91.4%~94.4%[130, 221, 250, 260]。此外，最近的一项系统综述和 meta 分析评估了基于树脂处理的牙髓外科手术的结果，该手术使用高放大倍数制备根尖浅凹状充填区，并使用粘接树脂材料填充，如倒充填技术，有 82.2% 的病例成功，失败的原因可能是由于潮湿的根周环境导致粘

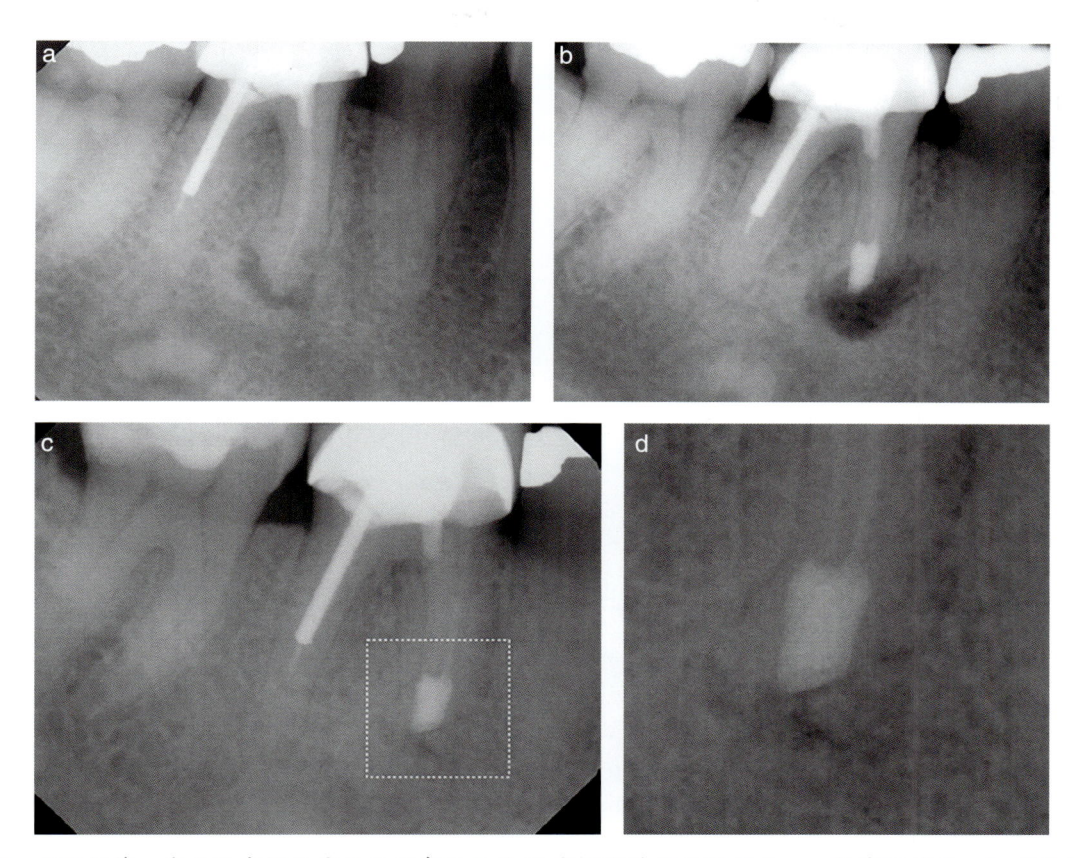

图 12.13 右下颌第一磨牙近中根治疗后使用常规二维 X 线摄影进行结果评估。a. 术前 X 线片。b. 术后 X 线片。注意峡部的预备和填充（RRM）。c. 随访 12 个月，观察到影像学愈合，无临床症状。d. 图 c 中标记区域的愈合。注意牙周膜轮廓的影像学重建和根尖区的骨愈合（由美国费城 Frank Setzer 医生提供）

接失败[130]。生物陶瓷牙根修复材料已成功地用作三氧化矿物聚合物材料的替代品，成功率为 92.0%~94.4%[224, 285]。

根尖周手术后愈合的逆转经常存在争议。2007 年，DelFabbro 等人比较了非手术再治疗和手术再治疗，发现一年后手术治疗比非手术再治疗愈合更快，但在 4 年随访期间发现，手术成功病例数下降[62]。Friedman[79] 也提出了类似的观点。然而，大多数愈合逆转的出现与过时的技术有关，例如：牙胶或汞合金倒充。现在有大量的数据证实，使用现代技术和选择适当的病例的外科手术不会有过高的失败率，这是因为在随访中成功的病例人数流失率最小。根据 Song 等人的研究：在 2012 年使用显微手术技术进行过手术的牙齿研究中，6 年以上的成功率为 93.3%。在再次手术中对不成功组的病例进行了分析，发现失败主要与根折和操作者错误有关，包括初始手术中没有进行根尖充填、根尖预备错误、根管遗漏或未处理、峡部微渗漏[232]。

然而，对牙周状况不佳的牙实施根尖周手术和切除术治疗的预期成功率较低。将牙周健康的牙齿与出现中到重度骨缺失的牙齿进行比较，健康牙齿的手术成功率为 95.2%，牙周受损牙齿的手术成功率为 77.5%，具有统计学意义[124]。基于这项研究，探针达根尖区、或颊侧皮质骨完全缺失的病例成功率最低，这表明在这些情况下需要谨慎的治疗计划。最近的一项评估冠切除和根切除结果的系统综述和 meta 分析显示：患牙累积生存率为 85.6%，冠切除和根切除技术之间无统计学差异[222]。

总之，虽然牙髓外科手术适用于非手术再治疗失败的或由于技术原因不能进行非手术再治疗的牙齿[249]，但利用现代技术的研究结果证明：选择适当的病例进行牙髓外科手术是合理的。

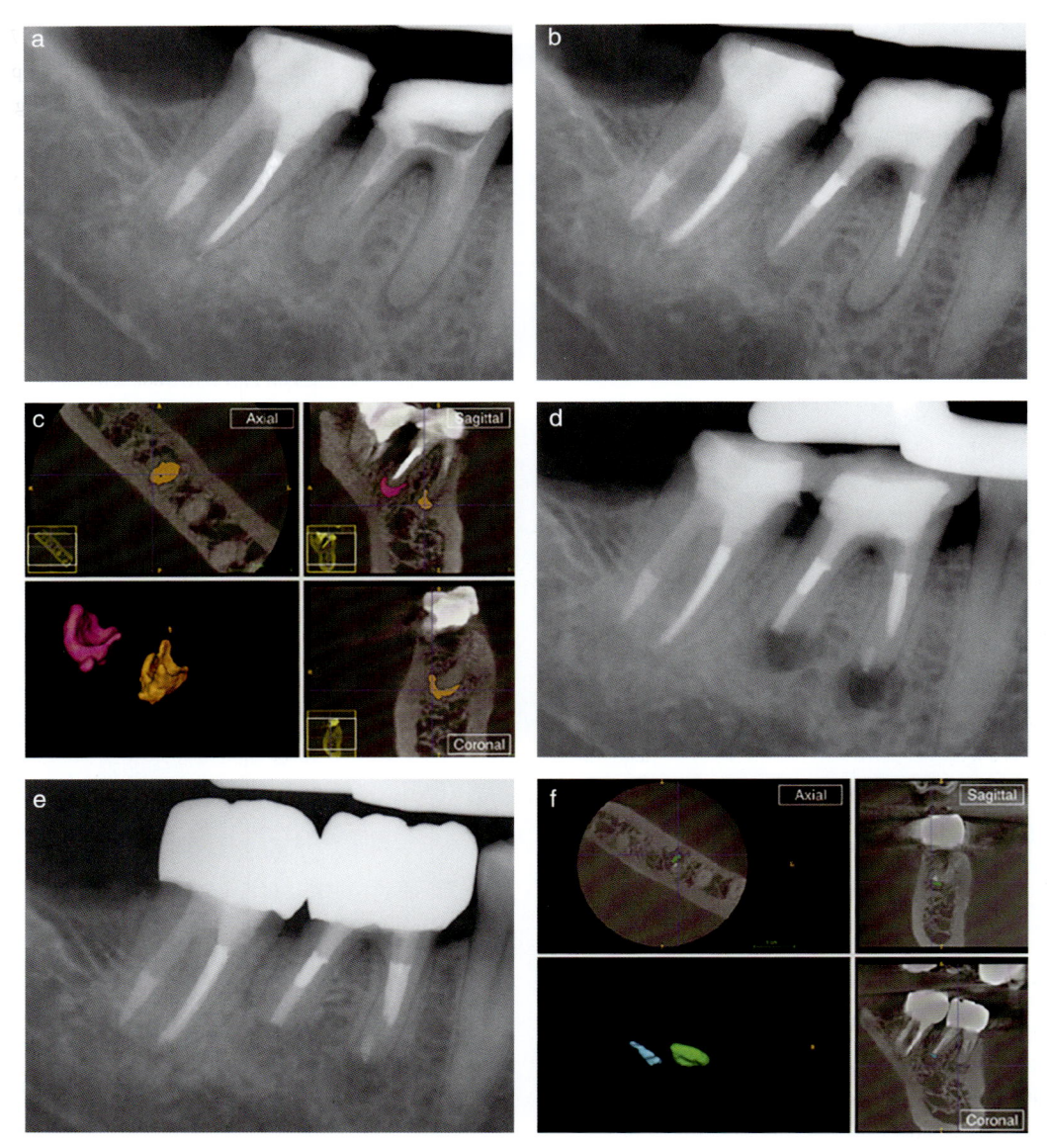

牙髓病学基础：根尖周炎的预防和治疗

图 12.14　比较右下颌第一磨牙近中根术后，常规二维影像与三维 CBCT 影像的评估。a. 非手术再治疗前的术前 X 线片。b. 再治疗后的术后 X 线片。请注意，近中根根管无法疏通。仍然存在临床症状。c. 术前根尖周围病变的三维分析。d. 术后近中根根尖填充（MTA）的 X 线片。e. 随访 18 个月的 X 线片。影像学愈合，无临床症状。f. 对 CBCT 图像中识别的剩余低密度区域进行三维分析，允许进行体积比较和对根尖周围区域进行更精确的评估（经机构审查委员会批准的后续 CBCT 成像）（由德国纽伦堡的 Tom Schloss 医生提供）

参考文献

[1] Abella F, et al. Applications of piezoelectric surgery in endodontic surgery: a literature review. Journal of Endodontics, 2014, 40: 325–332.

[2] Abid W K. Post-surgical outcomes and prognosis of intentionally replanted lower posterior teeth. Al-Rafidain Dental Journal, 2010, 10: 332–340.

[3] Adamo H L, et al. A comparison of MTA, Super-EBA, composite and amalgam as root-end filling materials using a bacterial microleakage model. International Endodontic Journal, 1999, 32: 197–203.

[4] Ahn S Y, et al. Computer-aided design/computer-aided manufacturingguided endodontic surgery: guided osteotomy and apex localization in a mandibular molar with a thick buccal bone plate. Journal of Endodontics, 2018, 44: 665–670.

[5] Alanezi A Z, et al. Cytotoxicity evaluation of endosequence root repair material. Oral Surgery, Oral Medicine, Oral Pathology, Oral Radiology and Endodontology, 2010, 109, e122–5.

[6] Albrecht J. Verfärbung durch Resorzin-Formalin-Alkali-

Wurzelfüllung. Deutsche Zahnärztliche Wochenschrift, 1915, 18:577–82.

[7] Allen R K, Newton C W, Brown C E Jr. A statistical analysis of surgical and nonsurgical endodontic retreatment cases. Journal of Endodontics, 1989, 15: 261–266.

[8] Altonen M. Transantral, subperiosteal resection of the palatal root of maxillary molars. International Journal of Oral Surgery, 1975, 4: 277–283.

[9] Al-Sabek F, Shostad S, Kirkwood K L. Preferential attachment of human gingival fibroblasts to the resin ionomer Geristore. Journal of Endodontics, 2005, 31: 205–208.

[10] Aminoshariae A, Su A, Kulild J C. Determination of the location of the mental foramen: a critical review. Journal of Endodontics, 2014, 40: 471–475.

[11] Andreasen J O. Cementum repair after apicoectomy in humans. Acta Odontologia Scandinavia, 1973, 31: 211–221.

[12] Andreasen J O. Relationship between cell damage in the periodontal ligament after replantation and subsequent development of root resorption: A time related study in monkeys. Acta Odontologia Scandinavia, 1981, 39: 15–25.

[13] Andreasen J O, Rud J. Modes of healing histologically after endodontic surgery in 70 cases. International Journal of Oral Surgery, 1972, 1: 148–160.

[14] Baek S-H, Kim S. Bone repair of experimentally induced through-andthrough defects by Gore-Tex, Guidor, and Vicryl in ferrets: A pilot study. Oral Surgery, Oral Medicine, Oral Patholology, Oral Radiology and Endodontology, 2001, 91: 710–714

[15] Baek S-H, et al. Periapical bone regeneration after endodontic microsurgery with three different root-end filling materials: amalgam, SuperEBA, and mineral trioxide aggregate. Journal of Endodontics, 2010, 36: 1323–1325.

[16] Baek S-H, et al. Periapical tissue responses and cementum regeneration with amalgam, SuperEBA, and MTA as root-end filling materials. Journal of Endodontics, 2005, 31: 444–449.

[17] Beal M. De la resection de l'apex. Revue de Stomatologie, 1908, 15: 439–446.

[18] Beccosall-Ryan K, Tong D, Love R M. Radiolucent inflammatory jaw lesions: a twenty-year analysis. International Endodontic Journal, 2010, 43: 859–865.

[19] Beling K L, et al. Evaluation for cracks associated with ultrasonic root-end preparation of gutta-percha filled canals. Journal of Endodontics, 1997, 23: 323–326.

[20] Benenati F W, et al. Recall evaluation of iatrogenic root perforations repaired with amalgam and gutta-percha. Journal of Endodontics, 1986, 12: 161–166.

[21] Bergenholtz A. Radectomy of multirooted teeth. Journal of the American Dental Association, 1972, 85: 870–875.

[22] Bergenholtz G, et al. Retreatment of endodontic fillings. Scandinavian Journal of Dental Research, 1979, 87: 217–224.

[23] Besner E. Systemic effects of racemic epinephrine when applied to the bone cavity during periapical surgery. Virginia Dental Journal, 1972, 49: 9–12.

[24] Biggs J T, Benenati F W, Sabala C L. Treatment of iatrogenic root perforations with associated osseous lesions. Journal of Endodontics, 1988, 14: 620–624.

[25] Bird D C, et al. In vitro evaluation of dentinal tubule penetration and biomineralization ability of a new root-end filling material. Journal of Endodontics, 2012, 38: 1093–1096.

[26] Block R M, Bushell A. Retrograde amalgam procedures for mandibular posterior teeth. Journal of Endodontics, 1982, 8: 107–112.

[27] Bohning B P, Davenport W D, Jeansonne B G. The effect of guided tissue regeneration on the healing of osseous defects in rat calvaria. Journal of Endodontics, 1999, 25: 81–84.

[28] Bornstein M M, et al. Comparison of periapical radiography and limited conebeam computed tomography in mandibular molars for analysis of anatomical landmarks before apical surgery. Journal of Endodontics, 2011, 37: 151–157.

[29] Bortoluzzi E A, et al. Cytotoxicity and osteogenic potential of silicate calcium cements as potential protective materials for pulpal revascularization. Dental Materials, 2015, 31: 1510–1522.

[30] Boyne P J. Restoration of osseous defects in maxillofacial casualities. Journal of the American Dental Association, 1969, 78: 767–776.

[31] Britain S K, et al. The use of guided tissue regeneration principles in endodontic surgery for induced chronic periodontic-endodontic lesions: a clinical, radiographic, and histologic evaluation. Journal of Periodontology, 2005, 76: 450–460.

[32] Brock D O. Minor oral surgery in general practice. VII-Apicoectomy. British Dental Journal, 1961, 110: 216–218.

[33] Bronkhorst M A, et al. Use of root-end filling materials in a surgical apical endodontic treatment in the Netherlands. Nederlands Tijdschrift voor Tandheelkunde, 2008, 115:423–427.

[34] Brophy T W. Caries of the superior maxilla. Chicago Medical Journal and Examiner, 1880, 41: 582–586.

[35] Buckley J A, Ciancio S G, McMullen J A. Efficacy of epinephrine concentration on local anesthesia during periodontal surgery. Journal of Periodontology, 1984, 55: 653–657.

[36] Buckley J P. The rational treatment of chronic dentoalveolar abscess, with root and bone complications. Dental Review, 1911, 25: 755–776.

[37] Buckley J P. Root amputation. Dental Summary, 1914, 34: 964–965.

[38] Bühler H. Evaluation of rootresected teeth. Results after 10 years. Journal of Periodontology, 1988, 59: 805–810.

[39] Burns L, et al. Long-term evaluation of treatment planning decisions for non-healing endodontic cases by different groups of practitioners. Journal of Endodontics, 2018, 44: 226–232.

[40] Carnevale G, et al. A retrospective analysis of the periodontal-prosthetic treatment of molars with interradicular lesions. International Journal of Periodontics and Restorative Dentistry, 1991, 11: 189–205.

[41] Carnevale G, Pontoriero R, di Febo G. Long-term effects of root-resective therapy in furcationinvolved molars. A 10-year longitudinal study. Journal of Clinical Periodontology, 1998, 25: 209–214.

[42] Carr G B. Surgical endodontics// Cohen, Burns R C. Pathways of the Pulp. 6ed. S St Louis MO: Mosby, 1994:531–67.

[43] Castenfelt T. Om retrograd rotfyllningvid radikaloperation av kronisk apikal parentit. Svensk Tandlakare Tidskrift, 1939, 32: 227–260.

[44] Chang E, et al. Cone-beam computed tomography for detecting vertical root fractures in endodontically treated teeth: a systematic review. Journal of Endodontics, 2016, 42: 177–185.

[45] Chen I, et al. Healing after root-end microsurgery by using mineral trioxide aggregate and a new calcium silicate-based bioceramic material as root-end filling materials in dogs. Journal of Endodontics, 2015, 41: 389–399.

[46] Chen I, et al. A new calcium silicate-based bioceramic material promotes human osteo-and odontogenic stem cell proliferation and survival via the extracellular signal-regulated kinase signaling pathway. Journal of Endodontics, 2016, 42: 480–486.

[47] Chong B S, et al. Sealing ability of potential retrograde root filling materials. Dental Traumatology, 1995, 11: 264–269.

[48] Chong B S, et al. Cytotoxicity of potential retrograde root-filling materials. Dental Traumatology, 1994, 10: 129–133.

[49] Chong B S, et al. Antibacterial activity of potential retrograde root filling materials. Endodontics and Dental Traumatology, 1994, 10: 66–70.

[50] Chong B S, Pitt Ford T R. Root end filling materials: rationale and tissue response. Endodontic Topics, 2005, 11: 114–130.

[51] Chong B S, Pitt Ford T R, Kariyawasam S P. Tissue response to potential root-end filling materials in infected root canals. International Endodontic Journal, 1997, 30: 102–114.

[52] Chong B S, Pitt Ford T R, Kariyawasam S P. Short-term tissue response to potential root-end filling materials in infected root canals. International Endodontic Journal, 1997, 30: 240–249.

[53] Chong B S, et al. Sealing ability of potential retrograde root filling materials. Endodontics and Dental Traumatology, 1995, 11: 264–269.

[54] Clark R A F. The molecular and cellular biology of wound repair. 2nd ed. New York: Plenum Press, 1996.

[55] Collado-González M, et al. Cytotoxicity and bioactivity of various pulpotomy materials on stem cells from human exfoliated primary teeth. International Endodontic Journal, 2017, 50(Suppl 2): 19–e30.

[56] Concato J, Shah N, Horwitz R I. Randomized, controlled trials, observational studies, and the hierarchy of research designs. New England Journal of Medicine, 2000, 342: 1887–1992.

[57] Cotran R S, Kumar V, Collins T. Robbin's pathologic basis of disease. 6th ed. Philadelphia: WB Saunders, 1999.

[58] Dahlin C, et al. Healing of maxillary and mandibular bone defects using a membrane technique. An experimental study in monkeys. Scandinavian Journal of Plastic and Reconstructive Surgery and Hand Surgery, 1990, 24: 13–19.

[59] Dahlin C, et al. Healing of bone defects by guided tissue regeneration. Plastic and Reconstructive Surgery, 1988, 81: 672–676.

[60] Da Silva Pereira S L, et al. Comparison of bioabsorbable and non-resorbable membranes in the treatment of dehiscence-type defects. A Histomorphometric study in dogs. Journal of Periodontology, 2000, 71: 1306–1314.

[61] De Beule F, et al. Periodontal treatment and maintenance of molars affected with severe periodontitis (DPSI = 4): An up to 27-year retrospective study in a private practice. Quintessence International, 2017, 48: 391–405.

[62] Del Fabbro M, et al. Surgical versus non-surgical endodontic re-treatment for periradicular lesions. Cochrane Database of Systematic Reviews, 2007, 18, CD005511.

[63] Dorn S O, Gartner A H. Retrograde filling materials: a retrospective success-failure study of amalgam, EBA, and IRM. Journal of Endodontics, 1990, 16: 391–393.

[64] Dorn S O, Gartner A H. Surgical endodontic and retrograde procedures. Current Opinions in Dentistry, 1991, 1: 750–753.

[65] Douthitt J C, Gutmann J L, Witherspoon D E. Histologic assessment of healing after the use of a bioresorbable membrane in the management of buccal bone loss concomitant with periradicular surgery. Journal of Endodontics, 2001, 27: 404–410.

[66] Eley B M, Cox S W. The release, absorption and possible health effects of mercury from dental amalgam: a review of recent findings. British Dental Journal, 1993, 175: 355–362.

[67] El-Fayomy S, et al. Healing of bone defects by guided bone regeneration (GBR,: an experimental study. Egyptian Journal of Plastic and Reconstructive Surgery, 2003, 27: 159–166.

[68] Emmertsen E, Andreasen J O. Replantation of extracted molars. A radiographic and histological study. Acta Odontologia Scandinavia, 1966, 24: 327–346.

[69] Erpenstein H. A 3-year study of hemisectioned molars. Journal of Clinical Periodontology, 1983, 10: 1–10.

[70] Farrar J M. Radical and heroic treatment of alveolar abscess by amputation of roots of teeth. Dental Cosmos, 1884, 26: 79–81.

[71] Faulhaber B, Neumann R. Die chirurgische Behandlung der Wurzelerkrankungen, 19. Berlin: Hermann Meusser, 1912.

[72] Floratos S G, Kratchman S I. Surgical management of vertical root fractures for posterior teeth: report of four cases. Journal of Endodontics, 2012, 38: 550–555.

[73] Finne K, et al. Retrograde root filling with amalgam and Cavit. Oral Surgery, Oral Medicine, Oral Pathology, 1977, 43:621–26.

[74] Forni A, Sánchez-Garcés M A, Gay-Escoda C. Identification of the mental neurovascular bundle: a comparative study of panoramic radiography and computer tomography. Implant Dentistry, 2012, 21: 516–521.

[75] Frank R J, Antrim D D, Bakland L K. Effect of retrograde cavity preparations on root apexes. Endodontics and Dental Traumatology, 1996, 12: 100–103.

[76] Frank A L, et al. Long-term evaluation of surgically placed amalgam fillings. Journal of Endodontics, 1992, 18: 391–398.

[77] Friedman S. Retrograde approaches in endodontic therapy. Endodontics and Dental Traumatology, 1991, 7: 97–107.

[78] Friedman S. The prognosis and expected outcome of apical surgery. Endodontic Topics, 2005, 11: 219–262.

[79] Friedman S. Outcome of endodontic surgery: a meta-analysis of the literature-part 1: comparison of traditional root-end surgery and endodontic microsurgery. Journal of Endodontics, 2011, 37: 577–578.

[80] Fugazzotto P A. A comparison of the success of root resected molars and molar position implants in function in aprivate practice: results of up to 15-plus years. Journal of Periodontology, 2001, 72: 1113–1123.

[81] Garcia G F. Apicoectomia experimental. Revista Odontológica, 1937, 25: 145–160.

[82] Garrett K, et al. The effect of a bioresorbable matrix barrier in endodontic surgery on the rate of periapical healing: an in vivo study. Journal of Endodontics, 2002, 28: 503–506.

[83] Giacomino C M, Ray J J, Wealleans J A. Targeted endodontic microsurgery: a novel approach to anatomically challenging scenarios using 3-dimensional-printed guides and trephine burs-a report of 3 cases. Journal of Endodontics, 2018, 44: 671–677.

[84] Giacomino C M, et al. Comparative biocompatibility and osteogenic potential of two bioceramic sealers. Journal of Endodontics, 2019, 45: 51–56.

[85] Gilheany P A, Figdor D, Tyas M J. Apical dentin permeability and microleakage associated with root end resection and retrograde filling. Journal of Endodontics, 1994, 20: 22–26.

[86] Gomez S M, Lallier T. Pedialyte promotes periodontal ligament cell survival and motility. Journal of Endodontics, 2013, 39: 202–207.

[87] Gorni F G, Gagliani M M. The outcome of endodontic retreatment: a 2-yr follow-up. Journal of Endodontics, 2004, 30: 1–4.

[88] Grech L, Mallia B, Camilleri J. Characterization of set intermediate restorative material, biodentine, bioaggregate and a prototype calcium silicate cement for use as root-end filling materials. International Endodontic Journal, 2013, 46: 632–641.

[89] Grossman L I. Replantation of teeth: A clinical evaluation. Journal of the American Dental Association, 1966, 104: 633–636.

[90] Grossman L I, Chacker F M. Clinical evaluation and histologic study of intentionally replanted teeth. Transactions of the Fourth International Conference on Endodontics.Philadelphia, PA: University of Pennsylvania., 1968: 127–144.

[91] Grung B. Healing of gingival mucoperiosteal flaps after marginal incision in apicoectomy procedures. International Journal of Oral Surgery, 1973, 2: 20–25.

[92] Guess G, Kratchman S. Maxillary posterior surgery, the sinus, and managing palatal access// Kim S, et al Microsurgery in Endodontics.Hoboken NJ: John Wiley & Sons Ltd, 2017:151–162.

[93] Gutmann J L. Parameters of achieving quality anesthesia and hemostasis in surgical endodontics. Anesthesia and Pain Control in Dentistry, 1993, 2: 223–226.

[94] Gutmann J L. Surgical endodontics: post-surgical care. Endodontic Topics, 2005, 11: 196–205.

[95] Gutmann J L, Harrison J W. Posterior endodontic surgery: anatomical considerations and clinical techniques. International Endodontic Journal, 1985, 18: 8–34.

[96] Gutmann J L, Harrison J W. Surgical Endodontics. Cambridge MA: Blackwell, 1991.

[97] Gutmann J L, et al. Ultrasonic root-end preparation. Part 1. SEM analysis. International Endodontic Journal, 1994, 27: 318–324.

[98] Haasch G C, Gerstein H, Austin B P. Effect of two hemostatic agents on osseous healing. Journal of Endodontics, 1989, 15: 310–314.

[99] Hamp S E, Nyman S, Lindhe J. Periodontal treatment of multirooted teeth. Results after 5 years. Journal of Clinical Periodontology, 1989, 2: 126–135.

[100] Harrison J D, Rowley P S, Peters P D. Amalgam tattoos: light and electron microscopy and electron-probe micro-analysis. Journal of Pathology, 1977, 121: 83–92.

[101] Harrison J W, Johnson S A. Excisional wound healing following the use of IRM as a root-end filling material. Journal of Endodontics, 1997, 23: 19–27.

[102] Harrison J W, Jurosky K A. Wound healing in the tissues of the periodontium following periradicular surgery. III. The

osseous excisional wound. Journal of Endodontics, 1992, 18: 76–81.

[103] Harty F J, Parkins B J, Wengraf A M. The success rate of apicectomy: a retrospective study of 1, 016 cases. British Dental Journal, 1970, 129: 407–413.

[104] Hauman C H, Chandler N P, Tong D C. Endodontic implications of the maxillary sinus: a review. International Endodontic Journal, 2002, 35: 127–141.

[105] Hofer O. Wurzelspitzenresektion und Zystenoperationen. Zeitschrift für Stomatologie, 1935, 32: 513–533.

[106] Hou G L, Tsai C C, Weisgold A S. Treatment of molar furcation involvement using root separation and a crown and sleeve - coping telescopic denture. A longitudinal study. Journal of Periodontology, 1999, 70: 1098–1109.

[107] Hsu Y Y, Kim S. The resected root surface. The issue of canal isthmuses. Dental Clinics of North America, 1997, 41: 529–540.

[108] Hu K S, et al. Branching patterns and intraosseous course of the mental nerve. Journal of Oral and Maxillofacial Surgery, 2007, 65: 2288–2294.

[109] Imada T S, et al. Accessory mental foramina: prevalence, position and diameter assessed by cone-beam computed tomography and digital panoramic radiographs. Clinical Oral Implants Research, 2014, 25: e94–99.

[110] Ibarrola J L, et al. Osseous reaction to three hemostatic agents. Journal of Endodontics, 1985, 11: 75–83.

[111] Jacobsen I, Kerekes K. Diagnosis and treatment of pulp necrosis in permanent anterior teeth with root fracture. Scandinavian Journal of Dental Research, 1980, 88: 370–376.

[112] Jang J K, et al. Anatomical relationship of maxillary posterior teeth with the sinus floor and buccal cortex. Journal of Oral Rehabilitation, 2017, 44: 617–625.

[113] Jastak J T, Yagiela J A. Vasoconstrictors and local anesthesia: a review and rationale for use. Journal of the American Dental Association, 1983, 107: 623–630.

[114] Jeansonne B G, Boggs W S, Lemon R R. Ferric sulfate hemostasis: Effect on osseous wound healing. II. With curettage and irrigation. Journal of Endodontics, 1993, 19: 174–176.

[115] Jensen S S, et al. A prospective, randomized, comparative clinical study of resin composite and glass ionomer cement for retrograde root filling. Clinical Oral Investigations, 2002, 6: 236–243.

[116] Jesslén P, Zetterqvist L, Heimdahl A. Long-term results of amalgam versus glass ionomer cement as apical sealant after apicectomy. Oral Surgery, Oral Medicine, Oral Pathololgy, Oral Radiology and Endodontology, 1995, 79: 101–103.

[117] Jolly M, Sullivan H R. A basic approach to endodontic practice. Australian Dental Journal, 1956, 1: 151–160.

[118] Johnson B R. Considerations in the selection of a root-end filling material. Oral Surgery, Oral Medicine, Oral Pathololgy, Oral Radiology and Endodontology, 1999, 87: 398–404.

[119] Jouanny G, Safi C. Ergonomie et organization du cabinet en endodontie. Realities Cliniques, 2014, 25: 279–289.

[120] Karabucak B, Setzer F. Criteria for the ideal treatment option for failed endodontics: surgical or nonsurgical? Compendium for Continuing Education in Dentistry, 2007, 28: 391–397.

[121] Kawanami M, Sugaya T, Gama H. Periodontal healing after replantation of intentionally rotated teeth with healthy and denuded root surfaces. Dental Trauma, 2001, 17: 127–133.

[122] Khabbaz M G, et al. Evaluation of different methods for the root-end cavity preparation. Oral Surgery, Oral Medicine, Oral Pathololgy, Oral Radiology and Endodontology, 2004, 98: 237–242.

[123] Khoury F, Hensher R. The bony lid approach for the apical root resection of lower molars. International Journal of Oral and Maxillofacial Surgery, 1987, 16: 166–170.

[124] Kim E, et al. Prospective clinical study evaluating endodontic microsurgery outcomes for cases with lesions of endodontic origin compared with cases with lesions of combined periodontal-endodontic origin. Journal of Endodontics, 2008, 34: 546–551.

[125] Kim S, Kratchman S. Modern endodontic surgery concepts and practice: a review. Journal of Endodontics, 2006, 32: 601–623.

[126] Kim S, Pecora G, Rubinstein R. Comparison of traditional and microsurgery in endodontics// Kim S, Pecora G, Rubinstein R. Color Atlas of Microsurgery in Endodontics. Philadelphia PA: W B Saunders, 2001:5–11.

[127] Kim S, Rethnam S. Hemostasis in endodontic microsurgery. Dental Clinics of North America, 1997, 41: 499–511.

[128] Knoll-Kohler E, et al. Changes in plasma epinephrine concentration after dental infiltration anesthesia with different doses of epinephrine. Journal of Dental Research, 1989, 68: 1097–1101.

[129] Koenig K H, Nguyen N T, Barkhordar R A. Intentional replantation: a report of 192 cases. General Dentistry, 1988, 36: 327–331.

[130] Kohli M R, et al. Outcome of endodontic surgery: a meta-analysis of the literature-part 3: comparison of endodontic microsurgical techniques with two different root-end filling materials. Journal of Endodontics, 2018, 44: 923–931.

[131] Kohli M R, et al. Spectrophotometric analysis of coronal tooth discoloration induced by various bioceramic cements and other endodontic materials. Journal of Endodontics, 2015, 41: 1862–1866.

[132] Kramper B J, et al. A comparative study of the wound healing of three types of flap design used in periapical

surgery. Journal of Endodontics, 1984, 10: 17–25.
[133] Kratchman S. Intentional replantation. Dental Clinics of North America, 1997, 41: 603–617.
[134] Kratchman S, Kim S. Positioning// Kim S, et al. Microsurgery in Endodontics. Hoboken NJ: John Wiley & Sons Ltd, 2017: 221–226.
[135] Kumar V, et al. Robbins and Cotran Pathologic Basis of Disease. 8th edn. Philadelphia PA: Saunders, 2009.
[136] Kuzmanovic D V, et al. Anterior loop of the mental nerve: a morphological and radiographic study. Clinical Oral Implants Research, 2003, 14: 464–471.
[137] Kvinnsland I, et al. A clinical and roentgenological study of 55 cases of root perforation. International Endodontic Journal, 1989, 22: 75–84.
[138] Kvist T. Endodontic retreatment. Aspects of decision making and clinical outcome. Swedish Dental Journal, 2001, 144: 1–57.
[139] Langer B, Stein S D, Wagenberg B. An evaluation of root resections. A ten-year study. Journal of Periodontology, 1981, 52: 719–722.
[140] Layton C A, et al. Evaluation of cracks associated with ultrasonic rootend preparation. Journal of Endodontics, 1996, 22: 157–160.
[141] Lemon R R, Steele P J, Jeansonne B G. Ferric sulfate hemostasis: Effect on osseous wound healing. I. Left in situ for maximum exposure. Journal of Endodontics, 1993, 19: 170–173.
[142] Lin L, et al. Oroantral communication in periapical surgery of maxillary posterior teeth. Journal of Endodontics, 1985, 11: 40–44.
[143] Lin L, et al. Guided tissue regeneration in periapical surgery. Journal of Endodontics, 2010, 36: 618–625.
[144] Lin L M, Gaengler P, Langeland K. Periradicular curettage. International Endodontic Journal, 1996, 29: 220–227.
[145] Lin L M, Rosenberg P A. Repair and regeneration in endodontics. International Endodontic Journal, 2011, 44: 889–906.
[146] Lovato K F, Sedgley C M. Antibacterial activity of endosequence root repair material and proroot MTA against clinical isolates of Enterococcus faecalis. Journal of Endodontics, 2011, 37: 1542–1546.
[147] Lubow R M, Wayman B E, Cooley R L. Endodontic flap design: analysis and recommendations for current usage. Oral Surgery, Oral Medicine, Oral Pathology, 1984, 58: 207–212.
[148] Luebke R G. Surgical endodontics. Dental Clinics of North America, 1974, 18: 379–391.
[149] Maguire H, et al. Effects of resorbable membrane placement and human osteogenic protein-1 on hard tissue healing after periradicular surgery in cats. Journal of Endodontics, 1998, 24: 720–725.
[150] McDonald N J, Dumsha T C. A comparative retrofill leakage study utilizing a dentin bonding material. Journal of Endodontics, 1987, 13: 224–227.
[151] McDonald N J, Dumsha T C. Evaluation of the retrograde apical seal using dentine bonding materials. International Endodontic Journal, 1990, 23: 156–162.
[152] Majno G, Joris I. Cell, Tissue, and Disease. 2nd ed. Oxford: Oxford University Press, 2004 .
[153] Mannocci F, et al. The isthmuses of the mesial root of mandibular molars: a micro-computed tomographic study. International Endodontic Journal, 2005, 38: 558–563.
[154] Mead C, et al. Levels of evidence for the outcome of endodontic surgery. Journal of Endodontics, 2005, 31: 19–24.
[155] Meister F Jr, et al. Endodontic perforations which resulted in alveolar bone loss. Report of five cases. Oral Surgery, Oral Medicine, Oral Pathology, 1979, 47: 463–470.
[156] Menezes R F, et al. Detection of vertical root fractures in endodontically treated teeth in the absence and in the presence of metal post by cone-beam computed tomography. BMC Oral Health, 2016, 14: 16–18.
[157] Mente J, et al. Outcome of orthograde retreatment after failed apicoectomy: use of a mineral trioxide aggregate apical plug. Journal of Endodontics, 2015, 41: 613–620.
[158] Mestieri L B, et al. Biocompatibility and bioactivity of calcium silicate-based endodontic sealers in human dental pulp cells. Journal of Applied Oral Sciences, 2015, 23: 467–471.
[159] Minsk L, Polson A M. The role of root resection in the age of dental implants. Compendium of Continuing Education in Dentistry, 2006, 27: 384–388.
[160] Mitsis F J. Flap operation techniques for the treatment of certain endodontic and periodontic problems. Journal of the British Endodontic Society, 1970, 4: 6–9.
[161] Molven O, Halse A, Grung B. Observer strategy and the radiographic classification of healing after endodontic surgery. International Journal of Oral and Maxillofacial Surgery, 1987, 16: 432–439.
[162] Moiseiwitsch J R D. Avoiding the mental foramen during periapical surgery. Journal of Endodontics, 1995, 21: 340–342.
[163] Nair P N. New perspectives on radicular cysts: do they heal? International Endodontic Journal, 1998, 3: 155–160.
[164] Nair P N. On the causes of persistent apical periodontitis: a review. International Endodontic Journal, 2006, 39: 249–281.
[165] Nair P N, et al. Radicular cyst affecting a root-filled human tooth: a long-term post-treatment follow-up. International Endodontic Journal, 1993, 26: 225–233.
[166] Nair U, et al. A comparative evaluation of the sealing ability of 2 root-end filling materials: an in vitro leakage study

using Enterococcus faecalis. Oral Surgery, Oral Medicine, Oral Patholology, Oral Radiology and Endodontology, 2011, 112, e74–7.

[167] Neumann R. Atlas der radikalchirurgischen Behandlungen der Paradentosen. Berlin: Hermann Meusser, 1926:14

[168] Ng Y L, Mann V, Gulabivala K. Outcome of secondary root canal treatment: a systematic review of the literature. International Endodontic Journal, 2008, 41: 1026–1046.

[169] Ng Y L, et al. Outcome of primary root canal treatment: systematic review of the literature-Part 2. Influence of clinical factors. International Endodontic Journal, 2008, 41: 6–31.

[170] Nicholls E. Treatment of traumatic perforations of the pulp cavity. Oral Surgery, Oral Medicine, Oral Pathology, 1962, 15: 603–612.

[171] Nichols E. The role of surgery in endodontics. British Dental Journal, 1965, 19, Suppl, 118:59–71.

[172] Nord P G. Retrograde rootfilling with Cavit: a clinical and roentgenological study. Svensk Tandlakare Tidskrift, 1970, 63: 261–273.

[173] Nygaard-Östby B. Introduction to Endodontics. Oslo: Universitetsverlaget, 1971: 73–75.

[174] Oberli K, Bornstein M, von Arx T. Periapical surgery and the maxillary sinus: radiographic parameters for clinical outcome. Oral Surgery, Oral Medicine, Oral Patholology, Oral Radiology and Endodontology, 2007, 103: 848–853.

[175] O'Connor R P, Hutter J W, Roahen J O. Leakage of amalgam and Super-EBA root-end fillings using two preparation techniques and surgical microscopy. Journal of Endodontics, 1995, 21: 74–78.

[176] Oginni A O, Olusile A O. Follow-up study of apicectomised anterior teeth. South African Dental Journal, 2002, 57: 136–140.

[177] Olson A K, et al. An in vitro evaluation of injectable thermoplasticized gutta-percha, glass ionomer, and amalgam when used as retrofilling materials. Journal of Endodontics, 1990, 16: 361–364.

[178] Pantschev A, et al. Retrograde root filling with EBA cement or amalgam: a comparative clinical study. Oral Surgery, Oral Medicine, Oral Pathology, 1994, 78: 101–104.

[179] Parashos P, Messer H H. Rotary NiTi instrument fracture and its consequences. Journal of Endodontics, 2006, 32: 1031–1043.

[180] Park S Y, et al. Factors influencing the outcome of root-resection therapy in molars: a 10-year retrospective study. Journal of Periodontology, 2009, 80: 32–40.

[181] Partsch C. Dritter Bericht der Poliklinik für Zahn-und Mundkrankheiten des zahnärztlichen Instituts der Königl. Universität Breslau. Deutsche Monatsschrift für Zahnheilkunde, 1896, 14: 486–499.

[182] Partsch C. Über Wurzelspitzenresection. Deutsche Monatszeitschrift für Zahnheilkunde, 1898, 16: 80–86.

[183] Partsch C. Über Wurzelspitzenresection. Deutsche Monatszeitschrift für Zahnheilkunde, 1899, 17: 348–367.

[184] Pecora G, et al. The use of calcium sulphate in the surgical treatment of a "through and through" periradicular lesion. International Endodontic Journal, 2001, 34: 189–197.

[185] Pecora G, et al. The guided tissue regeneration principle in endodontic surgery: one‐year postoperative results of large periapical lesions. International Endodontic Journal, 1995, 28: 41–46.

[186] Persson G. Efterundersökning av rot-amputerade tänder. Odontologiska Foereningens Tidskrift, 1964, 28: 323–357.

[187] Persson G, Lennartson B, Lundström I. Results of retrograde root-filling with special reference to amalgam and Cavit as root-filling materials. Svensk Tandlakare Tidskrift, 1974, 67: 123–313.

[188] Peters L B, Harrison J W. A comparison of leakage of filling materials in demineralized and non-demineralized resected root ends under vacuum and non-vacuum conditions. International Endodontic Journal, 1992, 25: 273–278.

[189] Peters L B, Wesselink P R. Soft tissue management in endodontic surgery. Dental Clinics of North America, 1997, 41: 513–518.

[190] Peterson J, Gutmann J L. The outcome of endodontic resurgery: a systematic review. International Endodontic Journal, 2001, 34: 169–175.

[191] Pitt Ford T R, et al. Effect of super-EBA as a root end filling on healing after replantation. Journal of Endodontics, 1995, 21: 13–15.

[192] Pitt Ford T R, et al. Effect of various zinc oxide materials as root-end fillings on healing after replantation. International Endodontic Journal, 1995, 28: 273–278.

[193] Pitt Ford T R, et al. Use of mineral trioxide aggregate for repair of furcal perforations. Oral Surgery, Oral Medicine, Oral Pathology, Oral Radiology, and Endodontology, 1995, 79: 756–763.

[194] Ramachandran Nair P N. Light and electron microscopic studies of root canal flora and periapical lesions. Journal of Endodontics, 1987, 13: 29–39.

[195] Ramachandran Nair P N, Pajarola G, Schroeder H E. Types and incidence of human periapical lesions obtained with extracted teeth. Oral Surgery, Oral Medicine, Oral Patholology Oral Radiology and Endodontology, 1996, 81: 93–102.

[196] Rankow H J, Krasner P R. Endodontic applications of guided tissue regeneration in endodontic surgery. Journal of Endodontics, 1996, 22: 34–43.

[197] Regan J D, Gutmann J L, Witherspoon D E. Comparison of Diaket and MTA when used as root-end filling materials

to support regeneration of the periradicular tissues. International Endodontic Journal, 2002, 35: 840–847.

[198] Regan J D, Witherspoon D E, Foyle D. Surgical repair of root and tooth perforations. Endodontic Topics, 2005, 11: 152–178.

[199] Rhein M L. Cure of acute and chronic alveolar abscess. Dental Items of Interest, 1897, 19: 688–702.

[200] Ricucci D, Siqueira J F Jr. Apical actinomycosis as a continuum of intraradicular and extraradicular infection: case report and critical review on its involvement with treatment failure. Journal of Endodontics, 2008, 34: 1124–1129.

[201] Roda R S, Gutmann J L. Reliability of reduced air pressure methods used to assess the apical seal. International Endodontic Journal, 1995, 28: 154–162.

[202] Rowe A H R. Postextraction histology of root resections. Dental Practitioner and Dental Record, 1967, 17: 343–349.

[203] Rubinstein R. Magnification and illumination in apical surgery. Endodontic Topics, 2005, 11: 56–77.

[204] Rubinstein R A, Kim S. Short-term observation of the results of endodontic surgery with the use of a surgical operation microscope and super-EBA as root-end filling material. Journal of Endodontics, 1999, 25: 43–48.

[205] Rubinstein R A, Kim S. Long-term follow-up of cases considered healed one year after apical microsurgery. Journal of Endodontics, 2002, 28: 378–383.

[206] Rud J, Andreasen J O. Operative procedures in periapical surgery with contemporaneous root filling. International Journal of Oral Surgery, 1972, 1: 297–310.

[207] Rud J, Andreasen J O, Möller Jensen J E. A follow-up study of 1 000 cases treated by endodontic surgery. International Journal of Oral Surgery, 1972, 1: 215–228.

[208] Rud J, Andreasen J O, Jensen J E. Radiographic criteria for theassessment of healing after endodontic surgery. International Journal of Oral Surgery, 1972, 1: 195–214.

[209] Rud J, et al. Retrograde root filling with composite and a dentin-bonding agent. Dental Traumatology, 1991, 7: 118–125.

[210] Rud J, Rud V, Munksgaard E C. Long-term evaluation of retrograde root filling with dentin-bonded resin composite. Journal of Endodontics, 1996, 22: 90–93.

[211] Rud J, Rud V, Munksgaard E C. Retrograde root filling with dentin-bonded modified resin composite. Journal of Endodontics, 1996, 22: 477–480.

[212] Santamaria J, et al. Bone regeneration after radicular cyst removal with and without guided bone regeneration. International Journal of Oral and Maxillofacial Surgery, 1998, 1998: 118–120.

[213] Scarfe W C, et al. Use of cone beam computed tomography in endodontics. International Journal of Dentistry, 2009, 1: 1–20.

[214] Schloss T, et al. A comparison of 2-and 3-dimensional healing assessment after endodontic surgery using cone-beam computed tomographic volumes or periapical radiographs. Journal of Endodontics, 2017, 43: 1072–1079.

[215] Schwatz-Arad D, et al. A retrospective radiographic study of root-end surgery with amalgam and intermediate restorative material. Oral Surgery, Oral Medicine, Oral Pathololoy, Oral Radiology and Endodontology, 2003, 96: 472–477.

[216] Seltzer S, Sinai I, August D. Periodontal effects of root perforations before and during endodontic procedures. Journal of Dental Research, 1970, 49: 332–339.

[217] Seo B M, et al. Investigation of multipotent postnatal stem cells from human periodontal ligament. Lancet, 2004, 364: 149–155.

[218] Setzer F C, et al. A survey of CBCT use amongst endodontic practitioners in the United States. Journal of Endodontics, 2017, 43: 699–704.

[219] Setzer F C, Karabucak B. Endodontic retreatment-the decision making process// Bjørndal L, Kirkevang L-L, Whitworth J. Textbook of Endodontology. 3ed. Chichester: John Wiley & Sons Ltd, 2018: 327–341.

[220] Setzer F C, et al. Outcome of endodontic surgery: a meta-analysis of the literature-Part 2: Comparison of endodontic microsurgical techniques with and without the use of higher magnification. Journal of Endodontics, 2012, 38: 1–10.

[221] Setzer F C, et al. Outcome of endodontic surgery: a meta-analysis of the literature-part 1: comparison of traditional root-end surgery and endodontic microsurgery. Journal of Endodontics, 2010, 36: 1757–1765.

[222] Setzer F C, et al. Outcome of crown and root resection: a systematic review and meta-analysis of the literature. Journal of Endodontics, 2019, 45: 6–19.

[223] Shibli J A, et al. Detection of the mandibular canal and the mental foramen in panoramic radiographs: intraexaminer agreement. Journal of Oral Implantology, 2010, 38: 27–31.

[224] Shinbori N, et al. Clinical outcome of endodontic microsurgery that uses EndoSequence BC root repair material as the root-end filling material. Journal of Endodontics, 2015, 41: 607–612.

[225] Shovelton D S. The presence and distribution of microorganisms within non-vital teeth. British Dental Journal, 1964, 117: 101–107.

[226] Sinai I H. Endodontic perforations: their prognosis and treatment. Journal of the American Dental Association, 1977, 95: 90–95.

[227] Siqueira J F Jr, Lopes H P. Bacteria on the apical root surfaces of untreated teeth with periradicular lesions: a scanning electron microscopy study. International Endodontic Journal, 2001, 34: 216–220.

[228] Sjögren U, et al. Factors affecting the long-term results of endodontic treatment. Journal of Endodontics, 1990, 16:

498–504.

[229] Sjögren U, et al. Survival of Arachnia propionica in periapical tissue. International Endodontic Journal, 1988, 21: 277–282.

[230] Smith J, Crisp J, Torney D. A survey: controversies in endodontic treatment and retreatment. Journal of Endodontics 1981,7: 477–483.

[231] Song J S, Shin S J, Kim E. Outcomes of endodontic microresurgery: a prospective clinical study. Journal of Endodontics, 2011, 37: 316–320.

[232] Song M, et al. Long-term outcome of the cases classified as successes based on short-term follow-up in endodontic microsurgery. Journal of Endodontics, 2012, 38: 1192–1196.

[233] Song M, et al. Prognostic factors for clinical outcomes in endodontic microsurgery: a retrospective study. Journal of Endodontics, 2011, 37: 927–933.

[234] Spångberg L S, et al. Influence of entrapped air on the accuracy of leakage studies using dye penetration methods. Journal of Endodontics, 1989, 15: 548–551.

[235] Staffileno H Jr. Surgical management of the furca invasion. Dental Clinics of North America, 1969, 13: 103–119.

[236] Strindberg L L. The dependence of the results of pulp therapy on certain factors. Acta Odontologia Scandinavia, 1956, 14, Suppl 21:1–175.

[237] Stropko J J, Doyon G E, Gutmann J L. Root-end management: resection, cavity preparation, and material placement. Endodontic. Topics, 2005, 11: 131–151.

[238] Su H, et al. Factors affecting treatment planning decisions for compromised anterior teeth. International Journal of Periodontology and Restorative Dentistry, 2014, 34: 389–398.

[239] Sultan M, Pitt Ford T R. Ultrasonic preparation and obturation of root-end cavities. International Endodontic Journal, 1995, 28: 231–238.

[240] Sunde P T, et al. Fluorescence in situ hybridization (FISH) for direct visualization of bacteria in periapical lesions of asymptomatic root-filled teeth. Microbiology, 2003, 149: 1095–1102.

[241] Svärdström G, Wennström J L. Periodontal treatment decisions for molars: an analysis of influencing factors and long-term outcome. Journal of Periodontology, 2000, 71: 579–585.

[242] Taschieri S, et al. Efficacy of guided tissue regeneration in the management of through-and-through lesions following surgical endodontics: a preliminary study. International Journal of Periodontics and Restorative Dentistry, 2008, 028: 265–271.

[243] Taschieri S, et al. Efficacy of xenogeneic bone grafting with guided tissue regeneration in the management of bone defects after surgical endodontics. Journal of Oral and Maxillofacial Surgery, 2007, 65: 1121–1127.

[244] Tetsch P. Wurzelspitzenresektionen. Munich Wien: Hanser, 1986.

[245] Tidmarsh B G, Arrowsmith M G. Dentinal tubules at the root ends of apicected teeth: a scanning electron microscopic study. International Endodontic Journal, 1989, 22: 184–189.

[246] Tobon S I, et al. Comparison between a conventional technique and two bone regeneration techniques in periradicular surgery. International Endodontic Journal, 2002, 35: 635–641.

[247] Torebinejad M. Survival of intentionally replanted teeth and implantsupported single crowns: A systematic review. Journal of Endodontics, 2015, 41: 992–998.

[248] Torabinejad M, Chivian N. Clinical applications of mineral trioxide aggregate. Journal of Endodontics, 1999, 25: 197–205.

[249] Torabinejad M, et al. Outcomes of nonsurgical retreatment and endodontic surgery: a systematic review. Journal of Endodontics, 2009, 35: 930–937.

[250] Torabinejad M, et al. Survival of intentionally replanted teeth and implant-supported single crowns: a systemic review. Journal of Endodontics, 2015, 41:992–98.

[251] Torabinejad M, et al. Antibacterial effects of some root end filling materials. Journal of Endodontics, 1995, 21: 403–406.

[252] Torabinejad M, et al. Physical and chemical properties of a new root-end filling material. Journal of Endodontics, 1995, 21: 349–353.

[253] Torabinejad M, Pitt Ford T R. Root end filling materials: a review. Dental Traumatology, 1996, 12: 161–178.

[254] Torabinejad M, et al. Histologic assessment of mineral trioxide aggregate as a root-end filling in monkeys. Journalof Endodontics, 1997, 23: 225–228.

[255] Torabinejad M, et al. Bacterial leakage of mineral trioxide aggregate as a root-end filling material. Journal of Endodontics, 1995, 21: 109–112.

[256] Torabinejad M, et al. Sealing ability of a mineral trioxide aggregate when used as a root end filling material. Journal of Endodontics, 1993, 19: 591–595.

[257] Tronstad L, Barnett F, Cervone F. Periapical bacterial plaque in teeth refractory to endodontic treatment. Endodontics and Dental Traumatology, 1990, 6: 73–77.

[258] Troullos E S, et al. Plasma epinephrine levels and cardiovascular response to high administered doses of epinephrine contained in local anesthesia. Anesthesia Progress, 1987, 34: 10–13.

[259] Tsesis I, et al. Effect of guided tissue regeneration on the outcome of surgical endodontic treatment: a systematic review and meta-analysis. Journal of Endodontics, 2011, 37: 1039–1045.

[260] Tsesis I, et al. Outcomes of surgical endodontic treatment performed by a modern technique: an updated meta, analysis of the literature. Journal of Endodontics, 2013, 39: 332–339.

[261] Velvart P. Papilla base incision: a new approach to recession-free healing of the interdental papilla after endodontic surgery. International Endodontic Journal, 2002, 35: 453–460.

[262] Velvart P, Ebner-Zimmermann U, Ebner J P. Comparison of long-term papilla healing following sulcular full thickness flap and papilla base flap in endodontic surgery. International Endodontic Journal, 2004, 37: 687–693.

[263] Velvart P, Peters C I. Soft tissue management in endodontic surgery. Journal of Endodontics, 2005, 31: 4–16.

[264] Velvart P, Peters C I, Peters O A. Soft tissue management: flap design, incision, tissue elevation, and tissue retraction. Endodontic Topics, 2005, 11: 78–97.

[265] Velvart P, Peters C I, Peters O A. Soft tissue management: suturing and wound closure. Endodontic Topics, 2005, 11: 179–195.

[266] Villar C, Cochran D. Regeneration of periodontal tissues: guided tissue regeneration. Dental Clinics of North America, 2010, 54: 73–92.

[267] Von Arx T, et al. Location and dimensions of the mental foramen: a radiographic analysis by using cone-beam computed tomography. Journal of Endodontics, 2013, 39: 1522–1528.

[268] Von Arx T, Hanni S, Jensen S S. Clinical results with two different methods of root-end preparation and filling in apical surgery: mineral trioxide aggregate and adhesive resin composite. Journal of Endodontics, 2010, 36: 1122–1129.

[269] Von Arx T, et al. Evaluation of new cone-beam computed tomographic criteria for radiographic healing evaluation after apical surgery: assessment of repeatability and reproducibility. Journal of Endodontics, 2016, 42: 236–242.

[270] Von Arx T, Penarrocha M, Jensen S. Prognostic factors in apical surgery with root-end filling: a meta-analysis. Journal of Endodontics, 2010, 36: 957–973.

[271] Von Arx T, Salvi G E. Incision techniques and flap designs for apical surgery in the anterior maxilla. European Journal of Esthetic Dentistry, 2008, 3: 110–126.

[272] Von Arx T, Steiner G R, Tay F R. Apical surgery: endoscopic findings at the resection level of 168 consecutively treated roots. International Endodontic Journal, 2011, 44: 290–302.

[273] Von Hippel R. Zur Technik der Granulomoperation. Deutsche Monatsschrift für Zahnheilkunde, 1914, 32: 255–265.

[274] Walton R E, Ardjmand K. Histological evaluation of the presence of bacteria in induced periapical lesions in monkeys. Journal of Endodontics, 1992, 18: 216–227.

[275] Walton R E, Wallace J A. Transantral endodontic surgery. Oral Surgery, Oral Medicine, Oral Pathology, Oral Radiology and Endodontology, 1996, 82: 80–83.

[276] Watzek G, Bernhart T, Ulm C. Complications of sinus perforations and their management in endodontics. Dental Clinics of North America, 1997, 41: 563–583.

[277] Weaver S M. Root canal treatment with visual evidence of histologic repair. Journal of the American Dental Association, 1949, 35: 483–497.

[278] Weine F S. The case against intentional replantation. Journal of the American Dental Association, 1980, 100: 664–668.

[279] Weller R N, Niemczyk S P, Kim S. Incidence and position of the canal isthmus: part 1. Mesiobuccal root of the maxillary first molar. Journal of Endodontics, 1995, 21: 380–383.

[280] Witherspoon D E, Gutmann J L. Haemostasis in periradicular surgery. International Endodontic Journal, 1996, 29: 135–149.

[281] Witte M B, Barbul A. General principle of wound healing. Surgical Clinics of North America, 1997, 77: 509–528.

[282] Wu M K, Kean S D, Kersten H W. Quantitative microleakage study on a new retrograde filling technique. International Endodontic Journal, 1990, 23: 245–249.

[283] Yagiela J A. Vasoconstrictor agents for local anesthesia. Anesthesia Progress, 1995, 42: 116–120.

[284] Zafiropoulos G G, et al. Mandibular molar root resection versus implant therapy: a retrospective nonrandomized study. Journal of Oral Implantology, 2009, 35: 52–62.

[285] Zhou W, et al. Comparison of mineral trioxide aggregate and iRoot BP plus root repair material as root-end filling materials in endodontic microsurgery: a prospective randomized controlled study. Journal of Endodontics, 2017, 43: 1–6.